Tumors of
the Esophagus
and Stomach

AFIP Atlas
of
Tumor Pathology

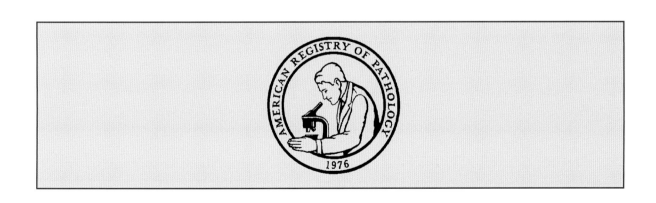

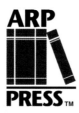

ARP PRESS

Arlington, VA

Senior Editorial Director: Mirlinda Q. Caton
Production Editor: Dian S. Thomas
Technical Editor and Subscription Manager: Magdalena C. Silva
Copyeditor: Audrey Kahn
Editorial Assistant: Elizabeth Tomlinson

Available from the American Registry of Pathology
Arlington, VA 22209
www.arppress.org
ISBN 1-933477-40-7
978-1-933477-40-4

Printed in South Korea

AFIP ATLAS OF TUMOR PATHOLOGY

Fourth Series
Fascicle 28

TUMORS OF THE ESOPHAGUS AND STOMACH

by

Robert D. Odze, MD, FRCP
Professor of Pathology; Chief, GI Pathology
Brigham and Women's Hospital
Harvard Medical School
Boston, Massachusetts

Elizabeth A. Montgomery, MD
Director, Gastrointestinal and Liver Pathology
Professor of Pathology, Oncology, and Orthopedic Surgery
Johns Hopkins Medical Institutions
Baltimore, Maryland

Helen H. Wang, MD
Professor of Pathology
Medical Director, Cytology
Beth Israel Deaconess Medical Center
Boston, Massachusetts

Gregory Y. Lauwers, MD
Senior Pathologist, Department of Oncologic Sciences
Department of Pathology and Cell Biology
H. Lee Moffitt Cancer Center and Research Institute
University of South Florida, Tampa, Florida

Joel K. Greenson, MD
Professor, Gastrointestinal and Hepatobiliary Pathology
University of Michigan Medical School
Ann Arbor, Michigan

Fátima Carneiro, MD, PhD
Faculty of Medicine of the University of Porto, Centro Hospitalar de São João
Institute of Molecular Pathology and Immunology at the University of Porto
Institute for Research Innovation in Health
Porto, Portugal

Jason L. Hornick, MD, PhD
Director, Surgical Pathology and Immunohistochemistry Laboratory
Associate Professor of Pathology
Brigham and Women's Hospital and Harvard Medical School
Boston, Massachusetts

Published by the
American Registry of Pathology
Arlington, VA
2019

AFIP ATLAS OF TUMOR PATHOLOGY

EDITORS' NOTE

The Atlas of Tumor Pathology has a long and distinguished history. It was first conceived at a cancer research meeting held in St. Louis in September 1947, as an attempt to standardize the nomenclature of neoplastic diseases. The first series was sponsored by the National Academy of Sciences-National Research Council. The organization of this formidable effort was entrusted to the Subcommittee on Oncology of the Committee on Pathology, and Dr. Arthur Purdy Stout was the first editor-in-chief. Many of the illustrations were provided by the Medical Illustration Service of the Armed Forces Institute of Pathology (AFIP), the type was set by the Government Printing Office, and the final printing was done at the Armed Forces Institute of Pathology. The American Registry of Pathology (ARP) purchased the Fascicles from the Government Printing Office and sold them virtually at cost. Over a period of 20 years, approximately 15,000 copies each of nearly 40 Fascicles were produced. The worldwide impact of these publications over the years has largely surpassed the original goal. They quickly became among the most influential publications on tumor pathology, primarily because of their overall high quality, but also because their low cost made them easily accessible the world over to pathologists and other students of oncology.

Upon completion of the first series, the National Academy of Sciences-National Research Council handed further pursuit of the project over to the newly created Universities Associated for Research and Education in Pathology (UAREP). A second series was started, generously supported by grants from the AFIP, the National Cancer Institute, and the American Cancer Society. Dr. Harlan I. Firminger became the editor-in-chief and was succeeded by Dr. William H. Hartmann. The second series' Fascicles were produced as bound volumes instead of loose leaflets. They featured a more comprehensive coverage of the subjects, to the extent that the Fascicles could no longer be regarded as "atlases" but rather as monographs describing and illustrating in detail the tumors and tumor-like conditions of the various organs and systems.

Once the second series was completed, with a success that matched that of the first, ARP, UAREP, and AFIP decided to embark on a third series. Dr. Juan Rosai was appointed as editor-in-chief, and Dr. Leslie Sobin became associate editor. A distinguished Editorial Advisory Board was also convened, and these outstanding pathologists and educators played a major role in the success of this series, the first publication of which appeared in 1991 and the last (number 32) in 2003.

The same organizational framework applies to the current fourth series, but with UAREP and AFIP no longer functioning, ARP is now the responsible organization. New features include a hardbound cover and illustrations almost exclusively in color. There is also an increased emphasis on the cytopathologic (intraoperative, exfoliative, or fine needle aspiration) and molecular features that are important in diagnosis and prognosis. What does not change from the three previous series, however, is the goal of providing the practicing pathologist with thorough, concise, and up-to-date information on the nomenclature and classification; epidemiologic, clinical, and pathogenetic features; and, most importantly, guidance in the diagnosis of the tumors and tumorlike lesions of all major organ systems and body sites.

As in the third series, a continuous attempt is made to correlate, whenever possible, the nomenclature used in the Fascicles with that proposed by the World Health Organization's Classification of Tumors, as well as to ensure a consistency of style. Close cooperation between the various authors and their respective liaisons from the Editorial Board will continue to be emphasized in order to minimize unnecessary repetition and discrepancies in the text and illustrations.

Particular thanks are due to the members of the Editorial Advisory Board, the reviewers, the editorial and production staff, and the individual Fascicle authors for their ongoing efforts to ensure that this series is a worthy successor to the previous three.

Steven G. Silverberg, MD
Ronald A. DeLellis, MD
Leslie H. Sobin, MD

PREFACE

Since the publication of the third series of the Armed Forces Institute of Pathology (AFIP) Fascicle on Tumors of the Esophagus and Stomach, great advances in many areas of tumor biology have led to a better understanding of the pathogenesis, pathology, and molecular biology of epithelial and stromal malignancies of the upper gastrointestinal tract. Many of these advances have led to specific improvements in diagnosis, prognosis, treatment, and thus, survival in patients affected by these tumors. This edition of the Fascicle was written to highlight these advances, and more specifically, to help pathologists diagnose diseases more accurately and understand how pathology contributes to clinical treatment in the new age of personalized and targeted therapy.

Notable advances described in this publication include: 1) expansion of our understanding of the pathologic features and molecular pathogenesis of carcinomas of the esophagus and stomach, most of which develop through a chronic inflammation-metaplasia-dysplasia-carcinoma sequence. Important refinements in the classification of neoplastic precursor lesions have been made since the last AFIP series, including the morphologic and endoscopic subtypes, and this has led to improvements in surgical treatment with a strong trend toward minimization in the form of endoscopic mucosal and submucosal dissections; 2) discovery of new diseases, such as gastric adenocarcinoma and proximal polyposis syndrome (GAPPS), a special variant of familial adenomatous polyposis, and significant advances in our knowledge regarding the molecular characterization of genetic polyposis syndromes; 3) great expansion in the molecular-pathology correlation, morphologic diversity, classification, and therapeutic options of gastrointestinal stromal tumors (GISTs); 4) reclassification and refinement of prognostic factors related to neuroendocrine tumors; and 5) improvements in the role of cytology in the diagnosis of tumors of the upper gastrointestinal tract.

We wrote this book with the pathologist in mind first by using tables that illustrate salient pathologic, molecular, and differential diagnostic features of key entities that are often difficult to distinguish from each other. We also used many specific color photographs of classic tumors and morphologic variants often difficult to recognize.

This book represents the long and hard dedication of many investigators in tumor biology worldwide, but also serves to highlight the many areas that still need research, such as how Eastern and Western pathologists differ in their interpretation of morphologic diagnostic criteria. This book will be useful not only for pathologists, but for any health care individual who is dedicated to helping patients prevent and treat cancer.

The authors of this series are very grateful to Dr. Steven Silverberg for his patience, wisdom, and guidance and to Ms. Mirlinda Caton and her staff for their expert editorial assistance in the production of this book. We would also like to thank Dr. Ronald DeLellis for his editorial assistance and helpful reviews of the manuscript.

Finally, we would like to thank the vast number of colleagues worldwide, who in one way or another contributed to this book by their research, thoughtful insights, inspiration, and excellent photographs. We are the messengers of their work.

Robert D. Odze, MD, FRCP

Elizabeth A. Montgomery, MD

Helen H. Wang, MD

Gregory Y. Lauwers, MD

Joel K. Greenson, MD

Fátima Carneiro, MD, PhD

Jason L. Hornick, MD, PhD

ACKNOWLEDGMENTS

Dr. Odze would like to thank Drs. Donald Antonioli and the late Harvey Goldman for their lifelong inspiration, guidance, and support, and his late mother Natasha Odze, who remains his hero in life. Dr. Joel Greenson would like to thank his lifelong mentor Dr. Henry Appelman for his support. Dr. Helen Wang would like to thank Drs. German Pihan and Karen Chang for their careful review and valuable input to her manuscript.

Permission to use copyrighted illustrations has been granted by:

CONTENTS

1 EVALUATION OF ESOPHAGEAL AND GASTRIC CYTOLOGY AND TISSUE SPECIMENS

To obtain maximum information from a specimen, in addition to adequate and representative sampling of the lesion, optimal handling and proper evaluation are required. Handling of the specimen involves all of the steps that begin when a specimen is removed from the patient to the time a report is issued. Handling of a specimen depends on the type of specimen and the information pathologists/clinicians need from the specimen for proper management of the patient. Special handling may be required to perform special studies for specific purposes. Specific requirements relating to the handling of distinctive tumor types are included in the respective chapters of these tumors.

Esophageal and gastric specimens arrive in the pathology department as one of four main types: cytologic specimens, endoscopic mucosal biopsies and resections, and surgically resected specimens. This chapter covers handling and evaluating gastric and esophageal specimens for optimum diagnosis and prognosis.

CYTOLOGIC SPECIMENS

Fine-Needle Aspirations

Endoscopic fine-needle aspiration (FNA), with or without ultrasound guidance, is increasingly used to sample mucosal and intramural esophagogastric lesions as well as periluminal lesions. Endoscopic FNA is useful for sampling lesions underneath necrotic debris or involving lamina propria, such as lymphomas and endocrine tumors, and is complimentary to forceps biopsies and brushings to increase the diagnostic yield (1). Endoscopic ultrasound-guided FNA to sample periluminal lymph nodes helps preoperatively to stage malignancies, reduce unnecessary surgeries, and triage patients for treatment protocols (2).

The material in the needle can be expelled onto a clean slide to make direct smears that are then either air dried for a Romanowsky stain, or immediately fixed with 95 percent ethanol for a Papanicolaou stain. Alternatively, the material can be rinsed into a preservative (CytoLyt® or CytoRich®) for liquid-based preparations (through either a ThinPrep® processor or a SurePath PrepStain System®) and Papanicolaou stain.

Endoscopic Brushings

This is the most common exfoliative type of cytologic specimen. Endoscopic washings have fallen out of favor due to their poor quality and cumbersome processing. Brushing of the mucosal surface allows larger areas of esophageal epithelium to be sampled (3). In addition, dysplastic/malignant cells tend to break free more readily than normal cells, thus enriching the sample with cells of interest. Similar to FNA material, the material on the brush can be either rolled onto a clean slide to make direct smears or immersed into a preservative for liquid-based preparations (4).

Nonendoscopic Cytologic Specimens

Patients with an increased risk of esophageal squamous cell carcinoma and adenocarcinoma can be surveyed with nonendoscopic cytologic sampling, which samples the entire esophagus at a low cost. Three samplers have been designed for this purpose: esophageal balloon cytology, encapsulated sponge cytology (Biosearch® Medical Products, Inc.), and encapsulated sponge-mesh cytology (Cytosponge®) (5,6). In a microsimulation model based on the assumption of a higher response rate (6) to invitation to participate in screening by Cytosponge (45 percent) than by endoscopy (23 percent), screening 50-year-old men with symptoms of gastroesophageal reflux disease by Cytosponge is more cost effective than screening by endoscopy (7). The traditional esophageal balloon cytology sampler (CICAMS) consists of a disposable, single-lumen rubber tube attached to an expandable rubber balloon covered with a cotton mesh net. When inflated with 15 to 20 mL of air, it turns into a near-perfect sphere with a diameter of 35 mm.

A new mechanical balloon (Cytomesh Esophageal Cytology Device) is a mechanically expandable, plastic mesh-covered balloon attached to two semirigid plastic catheters (8). The outer catheter acts as a sleeve through which the inner catheter passes, and it terminates at the proximal end of the mesh. The inner catheter contains a lumen that connects to the balloon, and this catheter terminates at the distal end of the mesh. The other two samplers consist of a gelatin capsule attached to a flexible plastic stylet. The gelatin capsule contains a compressed polyurethane sponge in the sponge sampler, and a polyurethane sponge covered with cotton mesh in the sponge-mesh sampler. The material collected on these samplers can be processed in the same way as that from endoscopic brushings.

Immunohistochemical and Molecular Studies on Cytologic Specimens

Immunocytochemical and molecular studies of cytologic materials can be applied on direct smears, various liquid-based preparations, and sections cut from cell blocks (9). Advantages and disadvantages exist for each preparation (9,10). When the available material is extremely limited, cytospin slides can be made for a limited panel of antibodies. Since cell blocks retain most materials for multiple studies, and protocols of most immunohistochemical and molecular tests are established on formalin-fixed and paraffin-embedded tissues, if sufficient material is available, cell block preparations are preferable for a more complete panel and more predictable results (11).

Cell blocks can be prepared by a number of methods (9,12). Most are suitable, if not optimal, for immunohistochemical and molecular studies. The thromboplastin-plasma cell block technique seems to be the easiest to prepare with the highest yield of cellularity (13). It is also of high quality in terms of cell distribution and background. A commercially available automated cell block processor, the Cellient™ processor, prepares a cell block within 1 hour, with minimal labor time. The product from this processor has been shown to provide materials for immunohistochemical stains with reliable results that are concordant with the standard

formalin-fixed paraffin-embedded material for at least 80 percent of the commonly used antibodies (14–16).

Reporting

Cytologic specimens are examined primarily to detect malignant cells; results complement those of biopsy specimens (17). However, a definitive diagnosis is not always possible due to the limited amount of material and the lack of architecture. Cytopathologists should not feel compelled to issue a definitive diagnosis when in doubt.

The interpretation of cytologic specimens can be reported as one of four categories: benign (negative for malignant cells), atypical (indeterminate but favor benign), suspicious (indeterminate but favor malignant), and malignant (positive for malignant cells). A more detailed description of the cytologic findings follows the diagnostic categories to give more specific information, such as type of benign changes (nonspecific reaction or specific infection) and differentiation of the tumor.

ENDOSCOPIC MUCOSAL SPECIMENS

Endoscopic Biopsy Specimens

The size of the forceps determines the size and quality of the biopsy specimen. The standard biopsy forceps is 2.4 mm in diameter and is usually sufficient to obtain diagnostic material (18). The 3.4-mm jumbo forceps obtains larger specimens that are best for diagnostic purposes (18); this forceps requires the 3.6-mm channel therapeutic endoscope, which is less comfortable for patients (19).

Proper orientation of biopsy specimens is usually not necessary for the diagnosis of a grossly visible tumor. Optimal orientation becomes important, however, in order to distinguish dysplasia from a superficially invasive tumor in surveillance biopsies from patients with Barrett esophagus. It is preferable to orient the specimen immediately after it is removed from the patient and before fixation. The specimen can be placed submucosal side down on a piece of mounting material, such as a thin plastic card, Millipore filter®, Gelfoam®, or the inside of the lid of a standard plastic cassette used for histologic tissue processing (18,20).

Ideally, specimens taken from different sites should be put into separate appropriately labeled containers of fixative as soon as possible. Separate labels assure correct identification of the origin of the lesions. Immediate fixation avoids autolytic changes that may damage histologic features and impair pathologists' ability to render a definitive diagnosis.

The standard fixative for tissue specimens is 10 percent buffered formalin. It is inexpensive, preserves tissue for a sustained period of time, and is compatible with all of the stains commonly used for morphologic assessment (19). Although protein precipitant fixatives, such as Hollande solution, B5, and Bouin fixative, result in better preservation of nuclear morphology compared to formalin (18), their heavy metal content creates biohazard disposal problems. Furthermore, these fixatives interfere with the isolation of nucleic acids from tissue and thus render samples unsuitable for molecular studies.

Lesions suspected of representing a lymphoproliferative process may be processed for flow cytometry. A small piece of tissue can be placed in a sterile culture medium and delivered as soon as possible, no longer than several hours later, to the flow cytometry laboratory. When this is not possible, storage of specimens at 4°C overnight is an acceptable alternative.

The number and largest dimension of the samples submitted to the pathology department should be documented. With the exception of samples submitted for special studies, all tissue fragments should be put into cassettes and submitted for microscopic examination in their entirety. It is best not to put more than four or five tissue fragments in the same cassette/block as it is difficult to assure that they are all present on the step-serial sections.

The plastic cassettes containing the tissue samples are processed on automated tissue processors. Most of the standard processing schedules should provide satisfactory results. When embedding oriented specimens, the tissue fragments should be put into paraffin on edge so that subsequent microtome sectionings can be cut perpendicular to the mucosal surface. If two or more tissue samples are embedded in the same block, they should be placed close together at a similar level. Step-serial sectioning can

regain to some extent the information lost as a result of lack of orientation in most specimens.

Each individual laboratory determines the number of routine step-serial sections. Although, the probability of finding significant lesions increases with an increasing number of levels, the yield does reach a point of diminishing return. In one study, goblet cell (intestinal) metaplasia was identified in three levels in 95 percent of 261 endoscopic esophageal mucosal biopsies (21). At four levels, an additional 4.7 percent were identified. Deeper sections, however, uncovered goblet cell metaplasia in only 1 (0.8 percent) of 120 blocks that did not show goblet cell metaplasia in the initial four levels. In 32 blocks from patients with a history of documented Barrett esophagus, deeper sections revealed initially undetected goblet cell metaplasia in 4 (13 percent) of 32 blocks. Therefore, it may be worthwhile to routinely cut a few serial sections from at least two different levels, and additional sections can be cut as indicated in individual cases.

The hematoxylin and eosin (H&E) stain is the only routine stain used on tissue sections in most laboratories. Additional stains, such as alcian blue at pH of 2.5 (for acid mucin), saffron (for collagen) (18), periodic acid–Schiff with diastase (PAS-D for both acid and neutral mucin), and Genta stains (triple Steiner, H&E, and alcian blue stain) (22,23) have been proposed as routine stains for various purposes. It may be most cost-effective to examine H&E-stained sections first before using other stains as a diagnosis is rendered based on the H&E stain alone in most cases.

ENDOSCOPIC ABRASIVE TRANSEPITHELIAL BRUSH BIOPSY SPECIMENS

An abrasive, transepithelial brush biopsy (EndoCDx®) technology with computer-assisted analysis was recently introduced (24,25). This brush biopsy device consists of an abrasive sampling instrument, which obtains a sample of the entire thickness of the squamous or glandular epithelium down to the muscularis mucosae, enclosed in a 2.5-mm sheath that is passed through the operating channel of a standard endoscope. A neural network computer system is programmed to detect esophageal abnormalities. The device is then placed against the surface of the mucosa. Sampling of any visualized columnar mucosa is performed by maintaining pressure against the mucosa, and rotating the brush circumferentially along the epithelial surface. Pinkish red tissue or pinpoint bleeding at the biopsy site is evidence of proper technique. Up to 4 cm of the columnar-lined mucosa is sampled with a single brush.

The resultant specimen is a disaggregated combination of intact tissue fragments, cell clusters, and individual cells. The cellular material collected on the brush is transferred to a glass slide and immersed in fixative. A second brush is used to collect a new specimen, which is immersed into a fixative with the brush. Cellular material is harvested from the brush by mechanical abrasion to make cell blocks. The slide with cellular material and the cell blocks are processed for cytologic and histologic examination, respectively, as described above for cytologic and biopsy specimens.

Microscopic examination of this complex tissue sample is aided by a multiple focal plane, neural network-based computer-assisted scan of each slide, which highlights potentially abnormal cells for presentation on a video monitor to a pathologist, who also examines the specimen with a standard manual microscope. The addition of this brush biopsy technique to the standard forceps biopsy technique has been reported to increase the detection of Barrett esophagus by up to 70 percent and the detection of dysplasia by 87 percent in a screening population (24,25, 25a), but these figures may be high (26).

Endoscopic Mucosal Resection Specimens

Endoscopic resections are carried out for polyps, biopsy-proven dysplasias, and even superficial small carcinomas (27–29). Gross examination of the specimen can include the size of the specimen and the lesion, and a description of the configuration of any lesion (for example: flat but thickened, bosselated, villiform, or ulcerated). The base of the specimen or any stalk should be inked. Preferably and, in particular, for endoscopic mucosal resection specimens, the specimen can be gently stretched and pinned on a firm surface, such as a wax block, cork board, or styrofoam. If a photograph is desired, it is best to photograph the specimen in its fresh state after it has been pinned and before it is fixed. Then, the specimen is fixed overnight or for at least 2 hours.

The base and the lateral margins of the specimen can be inked before the specimen is

sliced at 2-mm intervals along the long axis. The slices are then serially and sequentially put into labeled cassettes to facilitate reconstruction, if necessary. For small endoscopic mucosal resection specimens, both ends need to be submitted en face.

Fragments from piecemeal endoscopic mucosal resection specimens may be too small to stretch and challenging to reconstruct. In this situation, direct communication with the gastroenterologist is important. Up to 26 percent of the endoscopic mucosal resection specimens may be fragmented (27).

Large polyps (over 1 cm in diameter) with clearly identifiable stalks may be bisected along their long axis instead of being pinned before fixing overnight. The sides of the polyp may be trimmed from the stalk on a vertical axis and submitted in separate labeled cassettes. The middle of the polyp with the base should be sectioned vertically and submitted in appropriately labeled cassettes. The remainder of the process, including embedding, sectioning, and staining, is the same as described above with the exception of step-serial sections. For large polyps and mucosal resection specimens, routine step-serial sections may not be necessary.

Reporting

A definitive diagnosis should be issued to the extent possible based on the material. A thorough evaluation of the prognostic factors, such as tumor grade and depth of invasion, usually is not possible on biopsy specimens. However, endoscopic mucosal resection specimens for superficial neoplasms, whether dysplasia or carcinoma, should be treated as surgical specimens. The report can include size of the specimen, size of the lesion, status of the margins (lateral and deep), grade of the lesion, degree of differentiation, depth of invasion, and presence or absence of lymphovascular invasion.

SURGICALLY RESECTED SPECIMENS

Gross Examination

Surgically resected esophageal and gastric specimens for curative purpose contain a variable amount of adjacent uninvolved segments of esophagus and stomach (margins) (figs. 1-1–1-3). It is important to orient the specimen

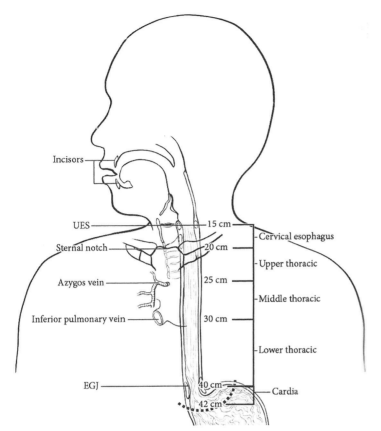

Figure 1 1

ESOPHAGUS: ANATOMIC SUBSITES

Anatomy of esophageal cancer primary site, including typical endoscopic measurements of each region measured from the incisors. Exact measurements depend on body size and height. (Fig. 16.1 from Amin M, Edge S, Greene F, Schilsky R, Gaspar L, Washington M, et al. AJCC Cancer Staging Manual, 8th ed. AG Switzerland: Springer International Publishing; 2017:188.)

and to locate the tumor by palpation before opening the specimen. It is useful to ink the margin(s) nearest to the tumor, if not the entire surgical margin. The ink should be blotted dry before any further manipulation of the specimen. Opening the specimen should avoid cutting through the tumor. Without violating this prerequisite, it is best to open gastric resections along the greater curvature for viewing and photographing the tumor and its surroundings. Samples for special studies, such as flow cytometric, cytogenetic, and electron microscopic studies, should be taken as soon as possible and preserved in appropriate medium before fixing the entire specimen in formalin. Measurements of the specimen size, lesion size, and distances to various margins as well as photography can be done in the fresh state as fixation results in shrinkage and muting of colors. It is also best to look for other significant findings, such as Barrett esophagus, in the fresh state.

For best fixation, the specimen can be stretched and pinned to a firm surface and fixed overnight as described above for endoscopic

mucosal resection specimens. Bulky, solid tumors may be sliced in the fresh state with a formalin-soaked paper towel inserted between slices to ensure thorough fixation. After the specimen has been fixed, it can be sliced further to examine the relationship between tumor and margins, and tumor and different layers of esophagus and stomach as well as involvement of adjacent organs, if any.

Opinions differ as to whether lymph nodes should be identified and dissected in the fresh or fixed state. Efforts should be made to identify all lymph nodes in the specimen. The number of lymph nodes and their size and location should be determined as described in figures 1-2 and 1-4. All grossly uninvolved lymph nodes should be entirely submitted and at least one H&E-stained section for each node should be obtained for microscopic examination.

Microscopic Examination

In addition to evaluating the lymph node status, microscopic examination of resected specimens achieves the following: a definitive

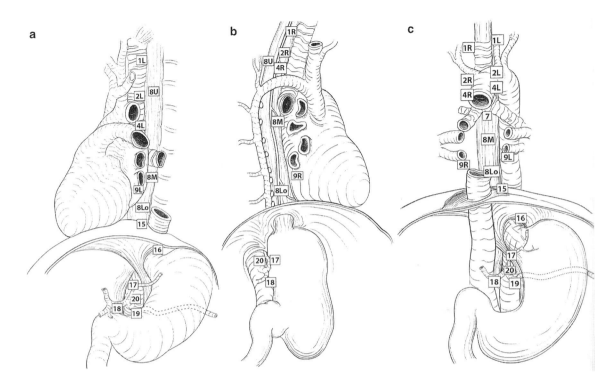

Figure 1-2

ESOPHAGUS: REGIONAL LYMPH NODES

A–C: Lymph node maps for esophageal cancer. Regional lymph node stations for staging esophageal cancer from left (A), right (B), and anterior (C). IR = right lower cervical paratracheal nodes, between the supraclavicular paratracheal space and apex of the lung. IL = left lower cervical paratracheal nodes, between the supraclavicular paratracheal space and apex of the lung. 2R = right upper paratracheal nodes, between the intersection of the caudal margin of the brachiocephalic artery with the trachea and the apex of the lung. 2L = left upper paratracheal nodes, between the top of the aortic arch and the apex of the lung. 4R = right lower paratracheal nodes, between the intersection of the caudal margin of the brachiocephalic artery with the trachea and cephalic border of the azygos vein. 4L = left lower paratracheal nodes, between the top of the aortic arch and the carina. 7 = subcarinal nodes, caudal to the carina of the trachea. 8U = upper thoracic paraesophageal lymph nodes, from the apex of the lung to the tracheal bifurcation. 8M = middle thoracic paraesophageal lymph nodes, from the tracheal bifurcation to the caudal margin of the inferior pulmonary vein. 8Lo = lower thoracic paraesophageal lymph nodes, from the caudal margin of the inferior pulmonary vein to the EGJ. 9R = pulmonary ligament nodes, within the right inferior pulmonary ligament. 15 = diaphragmatic nodes, lying on the dome of the diaphragm and adjacent to or behind its crura. 16 = paracardial nodes, immediately adjacent to the gastroesophageal junction. 17 = left gastric nodes, along the course of the left gastric artery. 18 = common hepatic nodes, immediately on the proximal common hepatic artery. 19 = splenic nodes, immediately on the proximal splenic artery. 20 = celiac nodes, at the base of the celiac artery. (Fig. 16.3 from Amin M, Edge S, Greene F, Schilsky R, Gaspar L, Washington M, et al. AJCC Cancer Staging Manual, 8th ed. AG Switzerland: Springer International Publishing; 2017:190.)

diagnosis (including histology type and grade), margin status, extent of tumor, and other significant findings (please see diagnostic checklist for details). If a tumor can be submitted in its entirety in less than five sections, it should be submitted entirely. Otherwise, four or five sections of large tumors are usually enough to ensure a diagnosis. These should include sections that demonstrate the maximal depth of invasion. The proximal, distal, and radial resection margins should be represented. If a margin is grossly less than 1 cm

from the tumor, a section should be submitted to include both the tumor and the inked margin for microscopic measurement of the distance between the margin and the tumor.

Synoptic Reporting

The College of American Pathologists (CAP) has issued protocols/recommendations for examination and reporting of specimens containing esophageal and gastric carcinomas (30,31). Standardized reporting maintains the

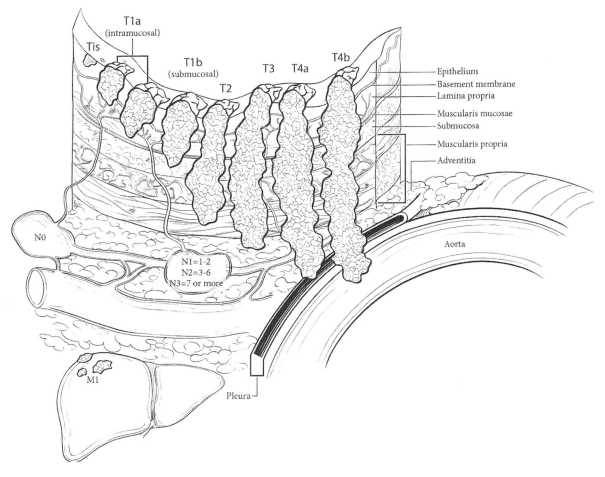

Figure 1-3

ESOPHAGUS: T, N, AND M CATEGORIES

Primary tumor (T) is classified by depth of tumor invasion. Regional lymph node categories are determined by metastatic burden. Distant metastatic sites are designated M1. (Fig. 16.5 from Amin M, Edge S, Greene F, Schilsky R, Gaspar L, Washington M, et al. AJCC Cancer Staging Manual, 8th ed. AG Switzerland: Springer International Publishing; 2017:192.)

consistency of content and quality of reports, and facilitates communication with clinicians. The diagnostic checklists recommended by the CAP are shown in Tables 1-1 and 1-2 for esophageal and gastric carcinomas, respectively (30,31). Standardized reporting for biomarkers (especially HER2) has also been endorsed by the CAP (32,33).

TNM CLASSIFICATION AND CARCINOMA STAGING

According to recommended checklists, synoptic pathologic reports provide detailed information on resected tumors. Nevertheless, a succinct summary to characterize the extent of the tumor for prognostic and treatment planning purposes as well as for facilitating exchange of information and comparison of treatment results is necessary.

The TNM (tumor, node, metastasis) classification system, proposed by International Union Against Cancer (UICC) and endorsed by the American Joint Committee on Cancer (AJCC), incorporates the most important prognostic factors, including the extent of the primary tumor, the absence or presence and extent of regional lymph node metastasis, and the absence or presence of distant metastasis (34,35). The prognostic significance of the TNM classification has been validated in outcome studies (34).

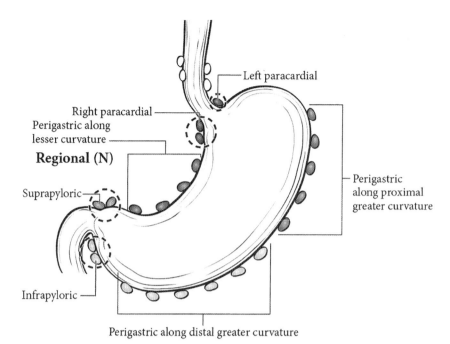

Figure 1-4

REGIONAL LYMPH NODES OF THE STOMACH

(Fig. 17.3 Amin M, Edge S, Greene F, Schilsky R, Gaspar L, Washington M, et al. AJCC Cancer Staging Manual, 8th ed. AG Switzerland: Springer International Publishing; 2017: 207.)

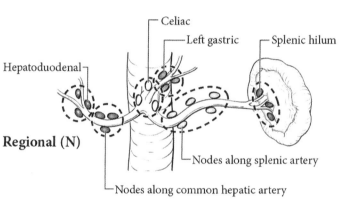

AJCC uses various prefixes and suffixes to indicate different situations. A prefix of "c" indicates that the TNM is based on clinical evidence acquired before primary treatment, such as physical examination, imaging, endoscopy, biopsy, and surgical exploration. A prefix of "p" indicates that the TNM is based on the evidence acquired before treatment and supplemented or modified by the additional evidence acquired during and from surgery, particularly from pathologic examination of the resected specimen. A prefix of "r" is assigned when a tumor recurs after a disease-free interval and is staged for further treatment. All the information available at the time of retreatment is used in determining the TNM of the recurrent tumor (rTNM). A prefix of "y" before the "c" or "p" prefix indicates the TNM classification during or following initial multimodality therapy. The ycTNM or ypTNM categorizes the extent of tumor actually present at the time of the examination after the multimodality therapy. A suffix of "m" in parentheses after T (T(m)) indicates the presence of multiple primary tumors in a single site. A prefix of "a" designates the extent determined at autopsy. The AJCC also groups tumors with similar prognosis into four stages (I, II, III, and IV) for easy comparison.

The TNM classification and AJCC staging of esophageal and gastric carcinomas are shown in Tables 1-1, 1-2.

Table 1-1

SUGGESTED DIAGNOSTIC CHECKLIST FOR RESECTED ESOPHAGEAL CARCINOMAS[a,b]

Surgical Pathology Cancer Case Study

Protocol posting date: June 2017

ESOPHAGUS:

Select a single response unless otherwise indicated.

Procedure
_____ Endoscopic resection
_____ Esophagectomy
_____ Esophagogastrectomy
_____ Other (specify): _____
_____ Not specified

Tumor Site (select all that apply)
_____ Cervical (proximal) esophagus
_____ Mid esophagus, upper thoracic esophagus
_____ Mid esophagus, middle thoracic esophagus
_____ Mid esophagus, not otherwise specified
_____ Distal esophagus (low thoracic esophagus)
_____ Esophagogastric junction (EGJ)
_____ Proximal stomach/cardia
_____ Other (specify): _____
_____ Esophagus, not otherwise specified

Relationship of Tumor to Esophagogastric Junction
_____ Tumor is entirely located within the tubular esophagus and does not involve the esophagogastric junction
_____ Tumor midpoint lies in the distal esophagus and tumor involves the esophagogastric junction
_____ Tumor midpoint is located at the esophagogastric junction
_____ Tumor midpoint is 2 cm or less into the proximal stomach or cardia and tumor involves the esophagogastric junction[c]
_____ Not specified
_____ Cannot be assessed

Distance of tumor center from esophagogastric junction (specify, if applicable) (centimeters): ____ cm

Tumor Size
Greatest dimension (centimeters): _____ cm
+[d]Additional dimensions (centimeters): _____ x _____ cm
____ Cannot be determined (explain): _____

Histologic Type
_____ Adenocarcinoma
_____ Adenoid cystic carcinoma
_____ Mucoepidermoid carcinoma
_____ Mixed adenoneuroendocrine carcinoma
_____ Undifferentiated carcinoma with glandular component
_____ Squamous cell carcinoma
_____ Basaloid squamous cell carcinoma
_____ Adenosquamous carcinoma
_____ Spindle cell (squamous) carcinoma
_____ Verrucous (squamous) carcinoma
_____ Undifferentiated carcinoma with squamous component
_____ Undifferentiated carcinoma
_____ Large cell neuroendocrine carcinoma

[a]Modified from the College of American Pathologists Protocol for the Examination of Specimens from Patients with Carcinoma of the Esophagus, June 2017.
[b]Includes pTNM requirements from the 8th edition, AJCC Staging Manual.
[c]Use the stomach cancer protocol if either 1) the tumor involves the EGJ, but the midpoint is more than 2 cm into the proximal stomach; or 2) the midpoint is less than 2 cm into the proximal stomach, but the tumor does not involve the EGJ.
[d]Data elements preceded by this symbol (+) are not required for accreditation purposes. These optional elements may be clinically important but are not yet validated or regularly used in patient management.

Table 1-1 continued

Histologic Type, continued
_____ Small cell neuroendocrine carcinoma
_____ Neuroendocrine carcinoma (poorly differentiated)[e]
_____ G1: Well-differentiated neuroendocrine tumor
_____ G2: Well-differentiated neuroendocrine tumor
_____ G3: Well-differentiated neuroendocrine tumor
_____ Other histologic type not listed (specify): _____
_____ Carcinoma, type cannot be determined

Histologic Grade (required only if applicable)[f]
_____ G1: Well differentiated
_____ G2: Moderately differentiated
_____ G3: Poorly differentiated, undifferentiated
_____ GX: Cannot be assessed

Tumor Extension
_____ No evidence of primary tumor
_____ High-grade dysplasia/carcinoma in situ, defined as malignant cells confined to the epithelium by the basement membrane
_____ Tumor invades the lamina propria
_____ Tumor invades the muscularis mucosae
_____ Tumor invades the submucosa
_____ Tumor invades the muscularis propria
_____ Tumor invades adventitia
_____ Tumor invades adjacent structures/organs[g] (specify): _____
_____ Cannot be assessed

Margins
Note: Use this section only if all margins are uninvolved and all margins can be assessed.
_____ All margins are uninvolved by the invasive carcinoma, dysplasia, and intestinal metaplasia
Margins examined: _____
(Note: margins may include proximal, distal, radial, mucosal, deep, and others.)
+[d]Distance of invasive carcinoma from closest margin (millimeters or centimeters: ___ mm or ___ cm)
+Specify closest margin: _____

Individual margin reporting required if any margins are involved or margin involvement cannot be assessed.
For esophagectomy and esophagogastrectomy specimens only.

Proximal Margin
_____ Cannot be assessed
_____ Involved by invasive carcinoma
_____ Uninvolved by invasive carcinoma
    _____ Uninvolved by dysplasia
    _____ Involved by low-grade squamous dysplasia
    _____ Involved by high-grade squamous dysplasia
    _____ Involved by low-grade glandular dysplasia
    _____ Involved by high-grade glandular dysplasia
    _____ Involved by intestinal metaplasia (Barrett's esophagus) without dysplasia

Distal Margin
_____ Cannot be assessed
_____ Uninvolved by invasive carcinoma
    _____ Uninvolved by dysplasia
    _____ Involved by low-grade squamous dysplasia
    _____ Involved by high-grade squamous dysplasia
    _____ Involved by low-grade glandular dysplasia
    _____ Involved by high-grade glandular dysplasia
    _____ Involved by intestinal metaplasia (Barrett's esophagus) without dysplasia

[e]Select this option only if large cell or small cell cannot be determined.
[f]Histologic grade is not applicable to adenoid cystic carcinoma, mucoepidermoid carcinoma, well-differentiated neuroendocrine tumor, and high-grade neuroendocrine carcinoma.
[g]The adjacent structures of the esophagus include the pleura, pericardium, azygos vein, diaphragm, peritoneum, aorta, vertebral body, and airway.

Table 1-1 continued

Radial Margin
____ Cannot be assessed
____ Uninvolved by invasive carcinoma
____ Involved by invasive carcinoma

Other Margin(s) (required only if applicable)
Specify margin(s): _____
____ Cannot be assessed
____ Uninvolved by invasive carcinoma
____ Involved by invasive carcinoma

For endoscopic resection specimens only.

Mucosal Margin
____ Cannot be assessed
____ Involved by invasive carcinoma
____ Uninvolved by invasive carcinoma
    ____ Uninvolved by dysplasia
    ____ Involved by low-grade squamous dysplasia
    ____ Involved by high-grade squamous dysplasia
    ____ Involved by low-grade glandular dysplasia
    ____ Involved by high-grade glandular dysplasia
    ____ Involved by intestinal metaplasia (Barrett's esophagus) without dysplasia

Deep Margin
____ Cannot be assessed
____ Uninvolved by invasive carcinoma
____ Involved by invasive carcinoma

Other Margin(s) (required only if applicable)
Specify margin(s): _____
____ Cannot be assessed
____ Uninvolved by invasive carcinoma
____ Involved by invasive carcinoma

Treatment Effect
____ No known presurgical therapy
____ Present
    +[d]____ No viable cancer cells (complete response, score 0)
    +____ Single cells or rare small groups of cancer cells (near complete response, score 1)
    +____ Residual cancer with evident tumor regression, but more than single cells or rare small groups of cancer cells (partial response, score 2)
____ Absent
    +____ Extensive residual cancer with no evident tumor regression (poor or no response, score 3)
____ Cannot be determined

Lymphovascular Invasion
____ Not identified
____ Present
____ Cannot be determined

+Perineural Invasion
+____ Not identified
+____ Present
+____ Cannot be determined

Regional Lymph Nodes
____ No nodes submitted or found

Lymph Node Examination (required only if lymph nodes present in specimen)

---

[d]Data elements preceded by this symbol (+) are not required for accreditation purposes. These optional elements may be clinically important but are not yet validated or regularly used in patient management.

Table 1-1, continued

Number of lymph nodes involved: _____
_____ Number cannot be determined (explain): _____

Number of lymph nodes examined: _____
_____ Number cannot be determined (explain): _____

Pathologic Stage Classification (pTNM, AJCC 8th Edition)

Note: Reporting of pT, pN, and (when applicable) pM categories is based on information available to the pathologist at the time the report is issued. Only the applicable T, N, or M category is required for reporting; their definitions need not be included in the report. The categories (with modifiers when applicable) can be listed on 1 line or more than 1 line.

Pathologic Stage Classification, continued

TNM Descriptors (required only if applicable) (select all that apply)
_____ m (multiple primary tumors)
_____ r (recurrent)
_____ y (posttreatment)

Primary Tumor (pT)
_____ pTX: Tumor cannot be assessed
_____ pT0: No evidence of primary tumor
_____ pTis: High-grade dysplasia, defined as malignant cells confined to the epithelium by basement membrane
_____ pT1: Tumor invades the lamina propria, muscularis mucosae, or submucosa
_____ pT1a: Tumor invades the lamina propria, or muscularis mucosae
_____ pT1b: Tumor invades the submocosa
_____ pT2: Tumor invades the muscularis propria
_____ pT3: Tumor invades the adventitia
_____ pT4: Tumor invades the adjacent structures
_____ pT4a: Tumor invades the pleura, pericardium, azygos vein, diaphragm, or peritoneum
_____ pT4b: Tumor invades other adjacent structures, such as aorta, vertebral body, or airway

Regional Lymph Nodes (pN)
_____ pNX: Regional lymph nodes cannot be assessed
_____ pN0: No regional lymph node metastasis
_____ pN1: Metastasis in one or two regional lymph nodes
_____ pN2: Metastasis in three to six regional lymph nodes
_____ pN3: Metastasis in seven or more regional lymph nodes

Distant Metastasis (pM) (required only if confirmed pathologically in this case)
_____ pM1: Distant metastasis
Specify site(s), if known: _____

+dAdditional Pathologic Findings (select all that apply)
+_____ None identified
+_____ Intestinal metaplasia (Barrett's esophagus)
+_____ Low-grade squamous dysplasia
+_____ High-grade squamous dysplasia
+_____ Low-grade glandular dysplasia
+_____ High-grade glandular dysplasia
+_____ Esophagitis (type): _____
+_____ Gastritis (type): _____
+_____ Other (specify): _____

+Ancillary Studies
Note: For HER2 reporting, the CAP Gastric HER2 template should be used. Pending biomarker studies should be listed in the Comments section of this report.

+Comment(s):

---

dData elements preceded by this symbol (+) are not required for accreditation purposes. These optional elements may be clinically important but are not yet validated or regularly used in patient management.

Table 1-2

SUGGESTED DIAGNOSTIC CHECKLIST FOR RESECTED GASTRIC CARCINOMAS[a,b]

Surgical Pathology Cancer Case Summary

Protocol posting date: June 2017

STOMACH:

Select a single response unless otherwise indicated.

Procedure

_____ Endoscopic resection
_____ Partial gastrectomy, proximal
_____ Partial gastrectomy, distal
_____ Partial gastrectomy, other (specify): _____
_____ Total gastrectomy
_____ Other (specify): _____
_____ Not specified

Tumor Site (select all that apply)

_____ Cardia
_____ Fundus
  +[c]_____ Anterior wall
  +_____ Posterior wall
_____ Body
  +_____ Anterior wall
  +_____ Posterior wall
  +_____ Lesser curvature
  +_____ Greater curvature
_____ Antrum
  +_____ Anterior wall
  +_____ Posterior wall
  +_____ Lesser curvature
  +_____ Greater curvature
_____ Pylorus
_____ Other (specify): _____
_____ Not specified

Note: Use the esophageal cancer protocol if the tumor involves the EGJ and the tumor midpoint is 2 cm or less into the proximal stomach.

Tumor Size

Greatest dimension (centimeters): ___ cm
+Additional dimensions (centimeters): ____ x ____ cm
_____ Cannot be determined (explain): _____

Histologic Type

_____ Adenocarcinoma
    Lauren classification of adenocarcinoma:
        _____ Type
        _____ Diffuse type (includes signet-ring carcinoma, classified as >50% signet-ring cells)
        _____ Mixed (approximately equal amounts of intestinal and diffuse)
    +Alternative optional classification (based on WHO classification):
        +____ Tubular (intestinal) adenocarcinoma
        +____ Poorly cohesive carcinoma (including signet-ring cell carcinoma and other variants)
        +____ Mucinous adenocarcinoma (>50% mucinous)
        +____ Papillary adenocarcinoma
        +____ Mixed carcinoma (mixture of discrete glandular [tubular/papillary] and signet-ring/poorly cohesive cellular histologic components)

[a]Modified from the College of American Pathologists Protocol for the Examination of Specimens from Patients with Carcinoma of the Stomach, June 2017.
[b]Includes pTNM requirements from the 8th edition, AJCC Staging Manual.
[c]Data elements preceded by this (+) symbol are not required. However, these elements may be clinically important but are not yet validated or regularly used in patient management.

Table 1-2, continued

Histologic Type, continued:
_____ Hepatoid adenocarcinoma
_____ Carcinoma with lymphoid stroma (medullary carcinoma)
_____ Large cell neuroendocrine carcinoma
_____ Small cell neuroendocrine carcinoma
_____ Neuroendocrine carcinoma (poorly differentiated)[d]
_____ Mixed adenoneuroendocrine carcinoma
_____ Squamous cell carcinoma
_____ Adenosquamous carcinoma
_____ Undifferentiated carcinoma
_____ Other (specify): _____

Histologic Grade
_____ G1: Well differentiated
_____ G2: Moderately differentiated
_____ G3: Poorly differentiated, undifferentiated
_____ Other (specify): _____
_____ GX: Cannot be assessed
_____ Not applicable

Tumor Extension
_____ No evidence of primary tumor
_____ Carcinoma in situ: intraepithelial tumor without invasion of the lamina propria, high-grade dysplasia
_____ Tumor invades the lamina propria
_____ Tumor invades the muscularis mucosae
_____ Tumor invades the submucosa
_____ Tumor invades muscularis propria
_____ Tumor penetrates the subserosal connective tissue without invasion of the visceral peritoneum or adjacent
        structures
_____ Tumor invades the serosa (visceral peritoneum)
_____ Tumor invades adjacent structures/organs[e] (specify): _____
_____ Cannot be assessed

Margins
Note: Use this section only if all margins are uninvolved and all margins can be assessed.
_____ All margins are uninvolved by invasive carcinoma and dysplasia
        Margins examined: _____
Note: Margins may include proximal, distal, omental (radial), mucosal, deep, and others.
        [c]+Distance of invasive carcinoma from closest margin (millimeters or centimeters): ___ mm or ___ cm
        +Specify closest margin: _____

Individual margin reporting required if any margins are involved or margin involvement cannot be assessed.

For gastrectomy specimens only:

Proximal Margin
_____ Cannot be assessed _____ involved by invasive carcinoma
_____ Uninvolved by invasive carcinoma
        _____ Uninvolved by dysplasia
        _____ Involved by carcinoma in situ (high-grade dysplasia)
        _____ Involved by low-grade dysplasia

Distal Margin
_____ Cannot be assessed _____ involved by invasive carcinoma
_____ Uninvolved by invasive carcinoma
        _____ Uninvolved by dysplasia
        _____ Involved by carcinoma in situ (high-grade) dysplasia
        _____ Involved by low-grade dysplasia

[c]Data elements preceded by this (+) symbol are not required. However, these elements may be clinically important but are not yet validated or regularly used in patient management.
[d]Note: select this option only if large cell or small cell cannot be determined.
[e]The adjacent structures of the stomach include the spleen, transverse colon, liver, diaphragm, pancreas, abdominal wall, adrenal gland, kidney, small intestine, and retroperitoneum. Intramural extension to the duodenum or esophagus is not considered invasion of an adjacent structure, but is classified using the depth of the greatest invasion in any of these sites.

Table 1-2, continued

Omental (Radial) Margins
_____ Cannot be assessed
_____ Uninvolved by invasive carcinoma
_____ Involved by invasive carcinoma
    +c___ Greater omental margin involved by invasive carcinoma
    +____ Lesser omental margin involved by invasive carcinoma

Other Margin(s) (required only if applicable)
Specify margin(s): _____
_____ Cannot be assessed
_____ Involved by invasive carcinoma
_____ Uninvolved by invasive carcinoma

For endoscopic resection specimens only
Mucosal Margin
_____ Cannot be assessed
_____ Uninvolved by invasive carcinoma
_____ Involved by invasive carcinoma
    _____ Uninvolved by dysplasia
    _____ Involved by carcinoma in situ (high-grade dysplasia)
    _____ Involved by low-grade dysplasia

Deep Margin
_____ Cannot be assessed
_____ Uninvolved by invasive carcinoma
_____ Involved by invasive carcinoma

Other Margin(s) (required only if applicable)
Specify margin(s): _____
_____ Cannot be assessed
_____ Involved by invasive carcinoma
_____ Uninvolved by invasive carcinoma

Treatment Effect
_____ No known presurgical therapy
_____ Present
    +_____ No viable cancer cells (complete response, score 0)
    +_____ Single cells or rare small groups of cancer cells (near complete response, score 1)
    +_____ Residual cancer with evident tumor regression, but more than single cells or rare small groups of cancer cells (partial response, score 2)
_____ Absent
    +_____ Extensive residual cancer with no evident tumor regression (poor or no response, score 3)
_____ Cannot be determined

Lymphovascular Invasion
_____ Not identified
_____ Present
_____ Cannot be determined

+Perineural Invasion
+_____ Not identified
+_____ Present
+_____ Cannot be determined

Regional Lymph Nodes
_____ No lymph nodes submitted or found

Lymph Node Examination (required only if lymph nodes present in specimen)

Number of lymph nodes involved: _____
_____ Number cannot be determined (explain): _____

Number of lymph nodes examined: _____
_____ Number cannot be determined (explain): _____

cData elements preceded by this (+) symbol are not required. However, these elements may be clinically important but are not yet validated or regularly used in patient management.

Table 1-2, continued

Pathologic Stage Classification (pTNM, AJCC 8th Edition)

Note: reporting of pT, pN, and (when applicable) pM categories is based on information available to the pathologist at the time the report is issued. Only the applicable T, N, or M category is required for reporting; their definitions need not be included in the report. The categories (with modifiers when applicable) can be listed on 1 line or more than 1 line.

TNM Descriptors (required only if applicable) (select all that apply)
____ m (multiple primary tumors)
____ r (recurrent)
____ y (post treatment)

Primary Tumor (pT)
____ pTX: Primary tumor cannot be assessed
____ PT0: No evidence of primary tumor
____ pTis: Carcinoma in situ: intraepithelial tumor without invasion of the lamina propria, high-grade dysplasia
____ pT1: Tumor invades the lamina propria, muscularis mucosae, or submucosa
____ pT1a: Tumor invades the lamina propria or muscularis mucosae
____ pT1b: Tumor invades the submucosa
____ pT2: Tumor invades the muscularis propria[f]
____ pT3: Tumor penetrates the submucosal connective tissue without invasion of the visceral peritoneum or adjacent structures[g,h]
____ pT4: Tumor invades the serosa (visceral peritoneum) or adjacent structures[g,h]
____ pT4a: Tumor invades the serosa (visceral peritoneum)
____ pT4b: Tumor invades adjacent structures/organs

Regional Lymph Nodes (pN)[i]
____ pNX: Regional lymph node(s) cannot be assessed
____ pN0: No regional lymph node metastasis
____ pN1: Metastasis in one or two regional lymph nodes
____ pN2: Metastasis in three to six regional lymph nodes
____ pN3: Metastasis in seven or more regional lymph nodes
____ pN3a: Metastasis in seven to 15 regional lymph nodes
____ pN3b: Metastasis in 16 or more regional lymph nodes

Distant Metastasis (pM) (required only if confirmed pathologically in this case)
____ pM1: Distant metastasis
        Specify site(s), if known: _____

+[c]*Additional Pathologic Findings (select all that apply)*
+____ None identified
+____ Intestinal metaplasia
+____ Low-grade dysplasia
+____ High-grade dysplasia
+____ *Helicobacter pylori* gastritis
+____ Autimmune atrophic chronic gastritis
+____ Polyp(s) (type[s]): _____
+____ Other (specify): _____

+Ancillary Studies
Note: For HER2 reporting, the CAP Gastric HER2 template should be used. Pending biomarker studies should be listed in the Comments section of this report.

*Comment(s):

---

[f]A tumor may penetrate the muscularis propria with extension into the gastrocolic or gastrohepatic ligaments, or into the greater or lesser omentum, without perforation of the visceral peritoneum covering these structures. In this case, the tumor is classified as T3. If there is perforation of the visceral peritoneum covering the gastric ligaments or the omentum, the tumor should be classified as T4

[g]The adjacent structures of the stomach include the spleen, transverse colon, liver, diaphragm, pancreas, abdominal wall, adrenal gland, kidney, small intestine, and retroperitoneum.

[h]Intramural extension to the duodenum or esophagus is not considered invasion of an adjacent structure, but is classified using the depth of the greatest invasion in any of these sites.

[i]Note: Metastatic tumor deposits in the subserosal fat adjacent to a gastric carcinoma, without evidence of residual lymph node tissue, are considered regional lymph node metastases for purposes of gastric cancer staging.

REFERENCES

1. Kochhar R, Rajwanshi A, Malik AK, Gupta SK, Mehta SK. Endoscopic fine needle aspiration biopsy of gastroesophageal malignancies. Gastrointest Endosc 1988;34:321-3.
2. Jhala N, Jhala D. Gastrointestinal tract cytology: advancing horizons. Adv Anat Pathol 2003;10:261-77.
3. Falk GW. Cytology in Barrett's esophagus. Gastrointest Endosc Clin N Am 2003;13:335-48.
4. Walavalkar V, Patwardhan R, Owens C, et al. Utility of liquid bases cytology examination of distal esophageal brushings in the management of barett's esophagus: a prospective study of 45 cases. J Am Soc Cytopathol 2015;4:113-21.
5. Sepehr A, Razavi P, Saidi F, Salehian P, Rahmani M, Shamshiri A. Esophageal exfoliative cytology samplers. A comparison of three types. Acta Cytol 2000;44:797-804.
6. Kadri SR, Lao-Sirieix P, O'Donovan M, et al. Acceptability and accuracy of a non-endoscopic screening test for Barrett's oesophagus in primary care: cohort study. BMJ 2010;341:c4372.
7. Pan QJ, Roth MJ, Guo HQ, et al. Cytologic detection of esophageal squamous cell carcinoma and its precursor lesions using balloon samplers and liquid-based cytology in asymptomatic adults in Llinxian, China. Acta Cytol 2008;52:14-23.
8. Benaglia T, Sharples LD, Fitzgerald RC, Lyratzopoulos G. Health benefits and cost effectiveness of endoscopic and nonendoscopic cytosponge screening for Barrett's esophagus. Gastroenterology 2013;144:62-73 e6.
9. Jain D, Mathur SR, Iyer VK. Cell blocks in cytopathology: a review of preparative methods, utility in diagnosis and role in ancillary studies. Cytopathology 2014;25:356-71.
10. Bellevicine C, Vita GD, Malapelle U, Troncone G. Applications and limitations of oncogene mutation testing in clinical cytopathology. Semin Diagn Pathol 2013;30:284-97.
11. Lindeman NI, Cagle PT, Beasley MB, et al. Molecular testing guideline for selection of lung cancer patients for EGFR and ALK tyrosine kinase inhibitors: guideline from the College of American Pathologists, International Association for the Study of Lung Cancer, and Association for Molecular Pathology. J Thorac Oncol 2013;8:823-59.
12. Nigro K, Tynski Z, Wasman J, Abdul-Karim F, Wang N. Comparison of cell block preparation methods for nongynecologic ThinPrep specimens. Diagn Cytopathol 2007;35:640-3.
13. Kulkarni MB, Desai SB, Ajit D, Chinoy RF. Utility of the thromboplastin-plasma cell-block technique for fine-needle aspiration and serous effusions. Diagn Cytopathol 2009;37:86-90.
14. Gorman BK, Kosarac O, Chakraborty S, Schwartz MR, Mody DR. Comparison of breast carcinoma prognostic/predictive biomarkers on cell blocks obtained by various methods: Cellient, formalin and thrombin. Acta Cytol 2012;56:289-96.
15. Montgomery E, Gao C, de Luca J, Bower J, Attwood K, Ylagan L. Validation of 31 of the most commonly used immunohistochemical antibodies in cytology prepared using the Cellient((R)) automated cell block system. Diagn Cytopathol 2014;42:1024-33.
16. van Hemel BM, Suurmeijer AJ. Effective application of the methanol-based PreservCyt® fixative and the Cellient® automated cell block processor to diagnostic cytopathology, immunocytochemistry, and molecular biology. Diagn Cytopathol 2013;41:734-41.
17. Geisinger KR. Endoscopic biopsies and cytologic brushings of the esophagus are diagnostically complementary. Am J Clin Pathol 1995;103:295-9.
18. Bronner MP, Haggitt RC, Rubin CE. Endoscopy and endoscopic biopsy. In: Ming SC, Goldman H, eds. Pathology of the gastrointestinal tract, 2nd ed. Baltimore: Williams & Wilkins, 1998:35-46.
19. Jacobson BC, Crawford JM, Farraye FA. Gastrointestinal tract endoscopic and tissue processing techniques. In: Odze RD, Goldblum JR, Crawford JM, eds. Surgical pathology of the GI tract, liver, biliary tract, and pancreas. Philadelphia: Saunders, 2004:3-18.
20. Lewin KJ, Appelman HD. Handling of esophageal and gastric biopsy and resection specimens. In: Tumors of the esophagus and stomach. AFIP Atlas of Tumor Pathology, 3rd Series, Fascicle 18. Washington, DC: American Registry of Pathology; 1996:3-16.
21. Chitkara YK, Eyre CL. Evaluation of initial and deeper sections of esophageal biopsy specimens for detection of intestinal metaplasia. Am J Clin Pathol 2005;123:886-8.
22. Genta RM, Robason GO, Graham DY. Simultaneous visualization of Helicobacter pylori and gastric morphology: a new stain. Hum Pathol 1994;25:221-6.
23. el-Zimaity HM, Wu J, Graham DY. Modified Genta triple stain for identifying Helicobacter pylori. J Clin Pathol 1999;52:693-4.

24. Anandasabapathy S, Sontag S, Graham DY, et al. Computer-assisted brush-biopsy analysis for the detection of dysplasia in a high-risk Barrett's esophagus surveillance population. Dig Dis Sci 2011;56:761-6.

25. Johanson JF, Frakes J, Eisen D, EndoCDx Collaborative Group. Computer-assisted analysis of abrasive transepithelial brush biopsies increases the effectiveness of esophageal screening: a multicenter prospective clinical trial by the EndoCDx Collaborative Group. Dig Dis Sci 2011;56:767-72.

25a. Vennalaganti PR, Kaul V, Wang KK, et al. Increased detection of Barrett's esophagus-associated neoplasia using wide-area trans-epithelial sampling: a multicenter, prospective, randomized trial. Gastrointest Endosc 2018;87:348-55.

26. Canto MI, Montgomery E. Wide-area transepithelial sampling with 3-dimensional cytology: Does it detect more dysplasia or yield more hype? Gastrointest Endosc 2018;87:356-9.

27. Lauwers GY, Forcione DG, Nishioka NS, et al. Novel endoscopic therapeutic modalities for superficial neoplasms arising in Barrett's esophagus: a primer for surgical pathologists. Mod Pathol 2009;22:489-98.

28. Hull MJ, Mino-Kenudson M, Nishioka NS, et al. Endoscopic mucosal resection: an improved diagnostic procedure for early gastroesophageal epithelial neoplasms. Am J Surg Pathol 2006;30:114-8.

29. Namasivayam V, Wang KK, Prasad GA. Endoscopic mucosal resection in the management of esophageal neoplasia: current status and future directions. Clin Gastroenterol Hepatol 2010;8:743-54; quiz e96.

30. http://www.cap.org/ShowProperty?nodePath=UCMCon/Contribution Folders/WebContent/pdf/cp-esophagus-17protocol-4000.pdf.

31. http://www.cap.org/ShowProperty?nodePath=UCMCon/Contribution Folders/WebContent/pdf/cp-stomach-17protocol-4000.pdf.

32. Simpson RW, Berman MA, Foulis PR, et al. Cancer biomarkers: the role of structured data reporting. Arch Pathol Lab Med 2015;139:587-93.

33. Bartley AN, Christ J, Fitzgibbons PL, et al. Template for reporting results of HER2 (ERBB2) biomarker testing of specimens from patients with adenocarcinoma of the stomach or esophagogastric junction. Arch Pathol Lab Med 2015;139:618-20.

34. Amin M, Edge S, Greene F, Schilsky R, Gaspar L, Washington M, et al. AJCC Cancer Staging Manual. 8th ed: AG Switzerland: Springer International Publishing; 2017.

35. Brierley J, Gospodarowicz MK, Wittekind C, eds. TNM classification of malignant tumours, 8th ed. Hoboken, NJ: John Wiley & Sons; 2017.

2 THE NORMAL ESOPHAGUS

The esophagus is a muscular tube that connects the oropharynx with the stomach. While this simple fact seems irrefutable, there is now considerable debate as to where exactly the esophagus ends and the stomach begins (1–3). Regardless of the exact endpoint, the function of the esophagus is simply to pass food from the mouth to the stomach in order to facilitate digestion. A brief review of the embryology, anatomy, and normal histology of the esophagus is provided below. A basic understanding of this is critical for developing expertise in diagnostic surgical pathology of this region.

EMBRYOLOGY

The esophagus develops from the endoderm of the foregut. The prevailing theory is that around the 20th day of gestation, septa from the lateral walls of the foregut fuse and separate the trachea from the esophagus (4,5). This process is thought to begin at the carina and spread cephalad over several weeks (6). At this early stage of development, the esophagus is lined by columnar epithelium that proliferates and occludes the lumen (7). Between 6 and 8 weeks' gestation, this columnar epithelium is thought to become vacuolated and replaced by ciliated epithelium, leading to reformation of the esophageal lumen.

Unfortunately, while this sequence of events is the one most often quoted in the literature, it is not supported by animal model studies of tracheoesophageal fistulae and atresias (8). While it appears as though the exact mechanisms by which the esophagus and trachea form and separate are still somewhat of a mystery, we know that the sonic hedgehog, bone morphogenetic protein, and Wnt signaling pathways are vital to this process (9). Studies in knockout mice have shown that *SOX2* is vital to esophageal development while *NKX2.1* and *BMP* are critical for airway development (9).

The esophageal mucosal glands (cardiac-type glands) form at 4 months' gestation via downward growth of the surface epithelium into the lamina propria. The ciliated epithelial cells persist until the 5th month of gestation at which time stratified squamous epithelial cells replace them (10,11). The submucosal glands develop after the formation of this squamous epithelium (7,10,11). The muscularis propria develops at about 6 weeks' gestation. The circular muscle appears first, followed by the outer longitudinal layer at about 9 weeks' gestation. The striated muscle normally present in the upper third of the esophagus is not fully formed until the 5th month (11).

ANATOMY

The esophagus begins in the pharynx and ends in the stomach. Its length ranges from 25 to 30 cm, depending on the height of the individual (shorter in children) (12,13). Endoscopically, the average gastroesophageal junction (GEJ) is 40 cm from the incisors, with the distance from the incisors to the beginning of the esophagus being approximately 15 cm (12). The diameter of the esophagus varies from 13 to 30 mm depending on the amount of distention (12).

The esophagus begins at the level of the 6th cervical vertebra and the cricoid cartilage where the cricopharyngeus muscle forms the upper esophageal sphincter (fig. 2-1) (5,14). The esophagus follows the vertebral column through the thorax and exits the posterior mediastinum via the diaphragmatic hiatus at the level of the 7th thoracic vertebra. The phrenoesophageal ligament attaches the diaphragm to the esophagus and is thought to keep a muscular seal between the two structures (15).

The GEJ has been defined anatomically as the junction of the tubular esophagus and the saccular stomach. Endoscopists typically refer to the squamocolumnar junction or Z-line as

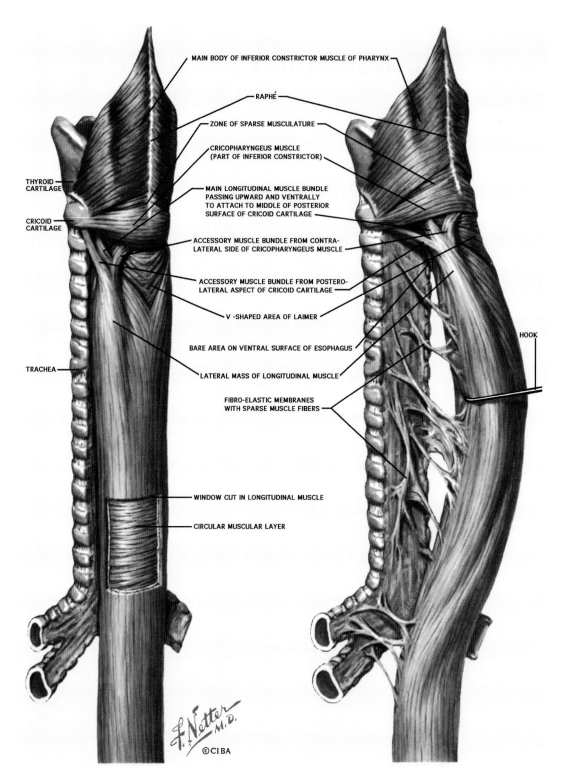

Figure 2-1

DIAGRAMMATIC ILLUSTRATION OF ESOPHAGEAL MUSCULATURE

(Plate 3 from Netter F. Ciba collection of medical illustrations, Digestive System: Part 1. West Caldwell, NJ: Ciba Geigy; 1959:36.) (Courtesy of Frank H. Netter.)

LYMPHATIC DRAINAGE

The esophagus has a rich network of mucosal and submucosal lymphatics that connect with branches in the muscular and adventitial layers. The lymphatics in the muscularis propria are oriented longitudinally, which helps explain the frequent finding of intramucosal and submucosal spread of tumors in this region. The lymphatics in the cervical esophagus tend to drain to paratracheal and internal jugular lymph nodes while the lymphatics in the thoracic esophagus drain into the superior, middle, and lower mediastinal lymph nodes and, ultimately, the thoracic duct or right lymph duct. The lymphatics of the abdominal portion of the esophagus drain into the superior gastric, celiac, common hepatic, and splenic artery lymph nodes. Because of the extensive interconnections between these lymphatic channels, the pattern of metastatic spread of tumors in this region may be unpredictable.

NERVES

The esophagus has both sympathetic and parasympathetic innervation as well as its own intrinsic innervation from the Auerbach (between layers of muscularis propria) and Meissner (submucosal) plexi (4). The vagus nerve provides both parasympathetic and sympathetic innervation to the esophagus. These vagal trunks give rise to the right and left recurrent laryngeal nerves which run between the esophagus and trachea, and innervate the cervical esophagus. In the thorax, the vagi break into a meshwork of nerves on the anterior and posterior surfaces of the esophagus. This meshwork reunites into several vagal nerve trunks on the anterior and posterior surfaces proximal to the GEJ.

Ganglion cells may be found in both Meissner and Auerbach plexi, although these tend to be less well developed than in the rest of the gut. Destruction of the myenteric plexus in achalasia leads to decreased peristalsis and a failure of the lower esophageal sphincter to relax (19).

HISTOLOGY

Mucosa

The esophageal mucosa consists of nonkeratinizing squamous epithelium, the lamina propria, and the muscularis mucosae (fig. 2-7). The squa-

mous epithelium is composed of three zones: the basal, the prickle, and the functional (fig. 2-8).

The basal layer is about three cell layers thick and comprises up to 15 percent of the thickness of the epithelium. Thickening of this layer typically occurs in the distal 3 cm of esophagus (normally) as well as more proximally in patients with reflux (20). Basal cells have hyperchromatic nuclei with scant cytoplasm, and mitotic activity is common. When marked basal cell hyperplasia occurs in response to mucosal injury, the appearance can mimic squamous dysplasia/carcinoma. Rare argyrophilic cells and melanocytes are found within the basal layer. These cells may give rise to rare cases of primary small cell carcinoma and melanoma of the esophagus (22–24). By definition, the basal layer gives way to the prickle layer when nuclei become separated by a distance of at least one nuclear diameter (21).

The prickle cell layer contains cells with flattened nuclei and glycogen-rich cytoplasm. As these cells move toward the luminal surface they become flatter and clearer. Once the cells lose their nuclei they become part of the functional layer.

T lymphocytes are frequently seen within the esophageal mucosa (25,26). These cells interdigitate between the squamous epithelial cells and may take on a squiggled appearance (fig. 2-9). Care must be taken not to mistake these cells for neutrophils on low-power microscopy. Langerhans cells are also found in the normal esophageal mucosa (26).

Patches of heterotopic gastric mucosa, known as inlet patches, may be found in the cervical esophagus. While these are composed of benign fundic or antral mucosae (fig. 2-10), rare complications, such as peptic ulceration or carcinoma, may occur. In neonates, small patches of ciliated mucosa may be found in the cervical esophagus at birth (5). These foci are replaced by squamous mucosa within a few days postpartum. Heterotopic sebaceous glands as well as heterotopic parathyroid and thyroid tissue have also been described. The latter are more typically found in the cervical esophagus (27,28).

The lamina propria of the esophagus consists of loose connective tissue containing a few lymphocytes, macrophages, and plasma cells, as well as rare lymphoid follicles. The overlying

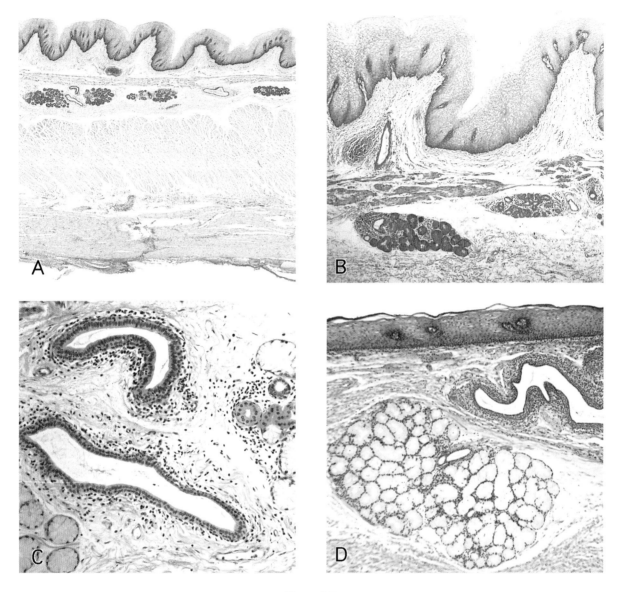

Figure 2-7

HISTOLOGIC FEATURES OF THE ESOPHAGUS

A: Scanning power of the full thickness of the esophagus. The mucosa is composed of squamous epithelium, lamina propria, and muscularis mucosae. The latter separates the mucosa from the submucosa. The muscularis propria consists of two layers, namely, the inner circular and outer longitudinal coats. The circular muscle layer is thicker than the longitudinal. Also visible are lymphoid follicles just above the muscularis mucosae.

B: Higher-power magnification shows the three layers of the mucosa and the submucosal glands stained by hematoxylin eosin (H&E) and alcian blue stains.

C: Higher-power magnification of the submucosal glands and their ducts stained with H&E.

D: Section of esophageal mucosa shows a duct originating from the submucosal glands beneath the overlying squamous epithelium.

epithelium has invaginations of lamina propria called dermal papillae. These papillae normally extend up to two thirds of the thickness of the epithelium. In reflux esophagitis and other in-flammatory conditions, these papillae typically become elongated, coursing closer to the luminal surface of the epithelium. In the proximal and distal esophagus, esophageal cardiac glands are

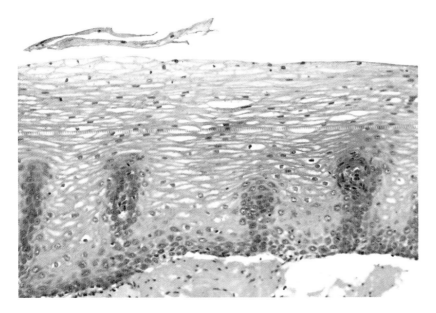

Figure 2-8

NORMAL ESOPHAGEAL SQUAMOUS EPITHELIUM

The epithelium is nonkeratinizing and has a thin basal zone, a prickle cell zone composed of glycogen-rich flattened cells that occupy most of the epithelium, and a few flattened cells on the surface that are devoid of nuclei. There is no granular cell layer.

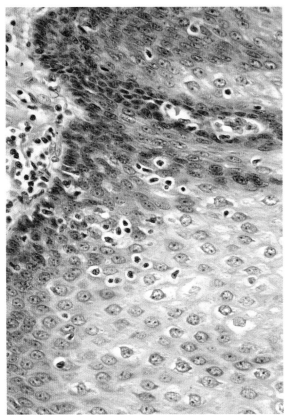

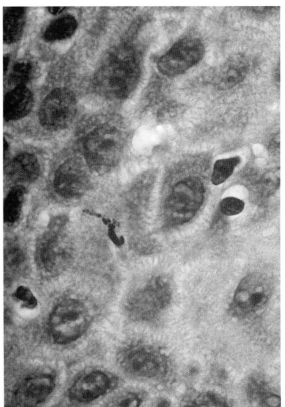

Figure 2-9

SQUAMOUS EPITHELIUM WITH INTRAEPITHELIAL LYMPHOCYTES

Intraepithelial lymphocytes can occur normally within the epithelium and do not necessarily indicate esophagitis.

Left: Low-power view of squamous epithelium containing scattered lymphocytes just above the basal layer.

Right: High-power magnification showing lymphocytes with round nuclei surrounded by a clear halo. A "squiggle cell" is in the center of the field.

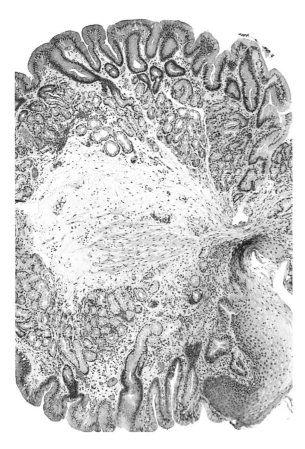

Figure 2-10

ESOPHAGEAL INLET PATCH

Mucosal biopsy showing antral-type mucosa and a small fragment of squamous epithelium.

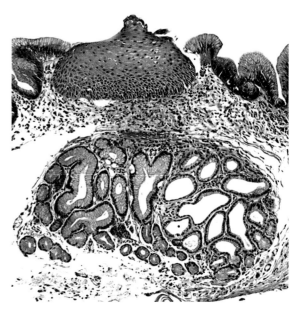

Figure 2-11

ESOPHAGEAL CARDIAC GLANDS

Low-power view of the gastroesophageal junction showing cardiac-type mucous glands beneath the squamous mucosa.

commonly found in the lamina propria (fig. 2-11). These glands secrete neutral mucins and should not be confused with Barrett metaplasia.

The muscularis mucosae (fig. 2-12) consists of a thin band of longitudinally oriented smooth muscle that separates the mucosa from the submucosa. It becomes progressively thicker in the distal esophagus and may be mistaken for muscularis propria in biopsy specimens. The muscularis mucosae often becomes duplicated in cases of Barrett esophagus.

Submucosa

The submucosa consists of loose connective tissue containing blood and lymphatic vessels, nerve fibers, scattered lymphocytes, and small lymphoid follicles. In addition, the submucosa contains submucosal glands and ducts (fig. 2-7). These glands are felt to be minor salivary glands and are more common at the proximal and distal ends of the esophagus.

Submucosal glands are largely lined by mucinous cells but may have a minor component of serous cells. The glands contain acidic mucins that stain with alcian blue pH 2.5 (fig. 2-7B). The deep ducts are lined by columnar epithelium that gives way to stratified squamous epithelium as they course through the lamina propria (2-7C,D).

Muscularis Propria

As discussed previously in this chapter, the muscularis propria is composed of a mixture of striated and smooth muscle, with striated muscle present proximally and smooth muscle present distally.

General and Clinical Features. The most common forms of heterotopia in the esophagus are gastric, sebaceous gland, and pancreatic; rarely, other forms, such as thyroid, parathyroid, or even tracheobronchial remnants, are found as well (15–21). Up to 10 percent of the general population may show esophageal heterotopia, particularly gastric, which occurs most commonly in the upper third of the esophagus.

In a study by Terada et al. (15) in 2011 of 1,008 cases of heterotopia involving the esophagus, a total of 158 cases of heterotopic gastric mucosa were identified. The male to female ratio was 112 to 36, and the mean age of the patients was 62 years. Microscopically, two types of heterotopia were identified. The first consisted of gastric glands and foveolar-type epithelium, and the second was composed only of foveolar-type epithelium. Goblet cell metaplasia occurred in 11 of the 158 cases.

The pathogenesis of most, if not all, heterotopias is presumed to be congenital. Some associations have been noted with other clinical and pathologic conditions, particularly in patients with gastric heterotopia (15,22–24). Most of the published literature focuses on gastric and sebaceous heterotopias, which are the two most common types.

Gastric heterotopia occurs in patients of all age groups, roughly equally in males and females, and may be located anywhere in the esophagus, but is particularly common in the upper third where the heterotopia is often referred to as an "inlet patch" at endoscopy (15,24). Gastric heterotopia is normally an asymptomatic lesion, although it may give rise to symptoms that result from complications of acid secretion in the heterotopic mucosa, such as heartburn, dysphagia, esophagitis, ulceration, bleeding, stricture formation, and rarely, perforation (25,26). In one retrospective analysis of 487,229 patients who had upper endoscopy, 870 (0.18 percent) were found to have an inlet patch (22). In this study, inlet patches were significantly associated with male gender, dysphagia, upper respiratory complaints, a globus sensation, Barrett esophagus (22,29), and Barrett esophagus-associated adenocarcinoma. In patients with Barrett esophagus, caution should be used to rule out the possibility that heterotopic gastric mucosa simply represents a proximal, possibly disconnected, island of metaplastic

mucosa. Gastric heterotopia may give rise to hyperplastic/inflammatory polyp formation (27). Rarely, adenocarcinoma may develop in heterotopia (28–30). Patients with *Helicobacter pylori* gastritis may show colonization of heterotopic gastric mucosa as well (23).

Heterotopic sebaceous glands are the second most common form of heterotopia in the esophagus. To date, more than 30 cases have been reported in the literature (31). Sebaceous heterotopia may occur at any level of the esophagus and is frequently multiple. It is also presumed to be congenital in origin, although one study suggested that it may represent a metaplastic process because of the frequent association with reflux esophagitis (32). Malignant transformation has not been reported in cases of esophageal sebaceous heterotopia.

Gross and Microscopic Findings. As mentioned above, gastric heterotopia occurs most commonly in the upper third of the esophagus, where it appears as a "patch" of erythematous, velvety gastric mucosa which may be flat, nodular, or rarely, polypoid in appearance (33). Microscopically, gastric heterotopia is usually composed of oxyntic-type glands, sometimes in combination with pyloric-type mucous glands, mucinous columnar epithelium, and lamina propria (fig. 3-3). Heterotopic epithelium may be present underneath squamous mucosa as well.

Ectopic sebaceous tissue usually appears as 1 to 2 mm lesions, often multiple, that are slightly elevated and yellowish in color. The sebaceous glands are composed of cells with microvesicular and vacuolated cytoplasm, often located around an excretory duct lined by squamous epithelium (fig. 3-4) (34). It also may be located in the lamina propria or even the submucosa. The sebaceous glands may, or may not, connect to the luminal surface, but in either case, active and particularly chronic inflammation is usually present.

Other forms of heterotopia, such as thyroid, parathyroid, pancreatic, and even tracheobronchial remnants, are rarely found in the esophagus. Most previously reported cases of thyroid or parathyroid heterotopia probably represent ectopic tissue within the mediastinum in close proximity to the outer layers of the esophageal wall. Ectopic thyroid or parathyroid tissue may be functional and, rarely, may lead to the development of endocrine tumors (18–20).

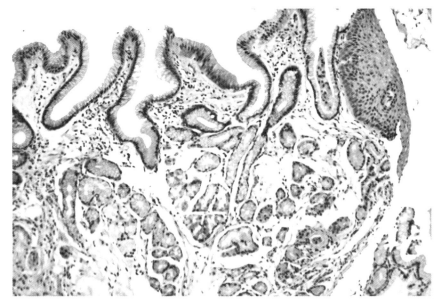

Figure 3-3

GASTRIC HETEROTOPIA IN UPPER THIRD OF ESOPHAGUS

Adjacent to the squamous epithelium is an area of columnar epithelium showing surface and foveolar epithelium and underlying glands with mixed mucinous and oxyntic differentiation. There is a mild degree of chronic inflammation in the lamina propria.

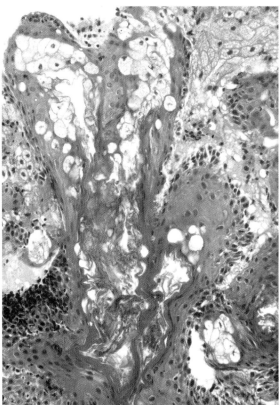

Figure 3-4

SEBACEOUS HETEROTOPIA IN PROXIMAL ESOPHAGUS

The sebaceous glands are composed of cells with microvesicular and vacuolated cytoplasm in combination with squamous cells that have a reactive appearance. The lumen of the heterotopic focus shows necrotic mucinous debris mixed with inflammatory cells.

Microscopically, this tissue appears identical to normal thyroid, parathyroid, or pancreatic tissue. One case of an intraductal papillary mucinous neoplasm was reported to arise from pancreatic heterotopia (35).

Tracheobronchial remnants are associated with congenital esophageal stenosis, and in this setting, are thought to develop as a result of esophageal sequestration of a tracheobronchial anlage prior to embryologic separation (21). These cases are frequently associated with esophageal atresia. The heterotopic tissue is usually present deep in the mucosa or in the wall of the esophagus.

Differential Diagnosis. The diagnosis of heterotopia in the esophagus is usually straightforward. Ultimately, it depends on the recognition of the specific tissue type in the esophagus. Heterotopia that shows intestinal-type columnar epithelium should be distinguished from Barrett esophagus, especially if the latter is of the long segment type. Gastric heterotopia is best distinguished from Barrett esophagus by the demonstration of normal squamous mucosa between the inlet patch and the GEJ or distal Barrett esophagus. Conversely, a diagnosis of Barrett esophagus may be erroneously established if a biopsy from the upper esophagus with gastric heterotopia is presumed to be due to metaplasia. Sebaceous heterotopia may be mistaken for a mixed adenosquamous or mucoepidermoid carcinoma.

SQUAMOUS PAPILLOMA

Definition. *Esophageal squamous papilloma* (ESP) is characterized by acanthotic squamous epithelium that is usually in a papillary configuration, a variable amount of acute and chronic inflammation, and often human papillomavirus (HPV)-like cellular changes.

General and Clinical Features. ESPs are benign epithelial tumors. The prevalence rate ranges from 0.01 to 0.43 percent, although this reaches 1 percent in autopsy studies (36–39). One recent paper suggests an increased prevalence rate in recent years, from 0.13 percent in 2000 to 0.57 percent in 2013, so the incidence may be on the rise (36,37).

Most occur in isolation, however, a small proportion may be multiple, and rarely, diffuse (40–43). They occur at all levels of the esophagus, but are more common in the distal and mid-esophagus rather than the proximal esophagus (41,44,45). In one recent study, 58 percent occurred in the distal esophagus, 28 percent in the mid-esophagus, and 13 percent in the proximal esophagus (44).

ESPs affect patients of all ages and both genders, but some studies show a slight male predominance (37–39). The mean age of patients is in the 5th and 6th decades of life. Patients generally have no symptoms, but symptoms may arise when either the lesion is large or multiple and diffuse, such as in the rare cases of esophageal papillomatosis (37,40,42,43,46,49). Some cases have been reported to cause dysphagia (42,43).

The pathogenesis of ESP is controversial. Chronic mucosal irritation, or more likely, infection, are the two leading theories of pathogenesis (45,47,48). Many studies have shown an association with HPV of both low- and high-risk oncogenic types (44,45,48,49). Two recent studies showed that more than 40 percent of ESPs are positive for HPV, and in one study, more than 50 percent contained high-risk HPV types (types 16, 18, 31, 81) in comparison to low risk types (types 6 or 11) (39,44,49). Some studies failed to show a strong association with HPV, but in those studies, it is presumed that differences in techniques used to evaluate HPV, or the possibility that previously unidentified novel subtypes of HPV caused the ESP, are potential reasons for the discrepant results (40,50). For instance, one study showed an association with

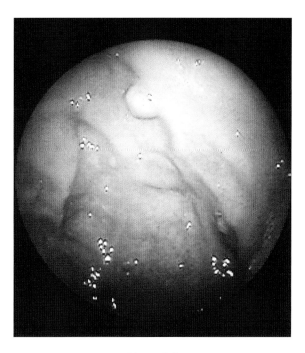

Figure 3-5

ESOPHAGEAL SQUAMOUS PAPILLOMA

A small, discrete and well-circumscribed dome-shaped lesion has a slightly gray to tan appearance endoscopically.

rare HPV types, such as DL284 and DL436, not previously identified in other studies (40). One recent study showed a lack of hypermethylation of the *CDKN2A* gene, which plays a role in the development of squamous cell carcinoma (48). Some studies showed a potential association with GERD or hiatus hernia but these are uncontrolled studies and may be prone to selection bias based on the fact that many of the patients were identified to have ESP based on endoscopy performed for reflux type symptoms (36,47).

Gross Findings. Endoscopically, ESPs are typically small, discrete, well-circumscribed, often dome-shaped, sessile lesions that have a gray or tan appearance (fig. 3-5). The surface may be variegated or verrucoid. They most commonly measure 3 to 5 mm, but larger lesions and even giant papillomas have been reported (46,51). Most are isolated lesions, but 20 percent of patients have multiple lesions (40,42,43). Rarely, children with HPV-related nasopharyngeal squamous papillomas also have numerous lesions in the esophageal wall (45,52); these lesions are associated with low-risk HPV types 6 or 11 (45).

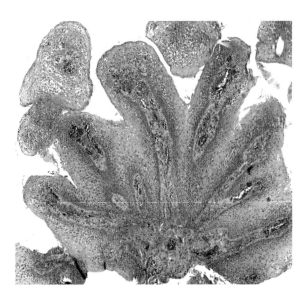

Figure 3-6

EXOPHYTIC (PAPILLARY) TYPE OF SQUAMOUS PAPILLOMA

A finger-like papillary frond of acanthotic and reactive-appearing squamous epithelium and an elongated fibrovascular core of lamina propria containing increased inflammation are present. The papilloma shows decreased maturation, with nucleated cells at the surface and slight parakeratosis. The epithelium shows areas of cellular degeneration and acantholysis. The basal and superbasal cells are reactive in appearance.

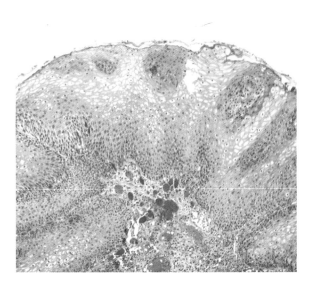

Figure 3-7

INVERTED SQUAMOUS PAPILLOMA

A smooth surface contour is combined with an inverted squamous papillomatous proliferation in which the basal epithelium extends deep into lamina propria.

Microscopic Findings. Three distinct histologic types of ESP have been described (45). The most common is the classic *exophytic*, or *papillary*, type, which is composed of finger-like papillary fronds of acanthotic reactive-appearing squamous epithelium overlying lamina propria, with a variable degree of acute and chronic inflammation (fig. 3-6). The *inverted*, or *endophytic*, type has a smooth contour, combined with an inverted squamous papillomatous proliferation that extends deep into the lamina propria (fig. 3-7). These lesions often show increased inflammation in the lamina propria and a robust granulation tissue response. Much less commonly, ESPs are *spiked* or *verrucoid* in appearance, showing acanthotic squamous epithelium containing a spiked surface contour with a prominent granular cell layer and marked hyperkeratosis (fig. 3-8). It is this type that is most commonly misdiagnosed as well-differentiated (verrucous) carcinoma because of the prominent degree of hyperkeratosis.

All ESPs show acanthotic squamous epithelium, basal cell hyperplasia, reactive epithelial changes, and a branching fibrovascular core of lamina propria with a variable degree of acute and chronic inflammation (fig. 3-9). The papillary fronds typically show a prominent basal and suprabasal layer, but with complete surface maturation. Variable features include hyperkeratosis, parakeratosis, dyskeratosis, and a prominent granular cell layer, as mentioned above. Up to 50 percent show histologic features of HPV infection, such as koilocytosis, binucleation, and multinucleation (fig. 3-10). The spiked type of papilloma occurs more commonly in children with HPV 6 and 11 infection (45,52). Rarely, papillomas are associated with dysplasia, which is most often low grade, or even with squamous cell carcinoma (see below) (37,40,53,54).

Differential Diagnosis. In most patients, ESPs are recognized easily both endoscopically and pathologically. Rare examples that are either large, multiple, or associated with dysplasia, may be difficult to differentiate from a verrucous carcinoma, particularly if the pathologist is unaware of the endoscopic findings and is only evaluating mucosal biopsies. Verrucous carcinomas lack cytologic atypia, but show an expansile growth pattern at the base of the lesion. Carcinomas often show stricture

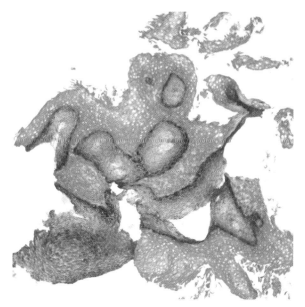

Figure 3-8

SPIKED TYPE OF PAPILLOMA

A spiked surface contour and epithelium with a prominent granular cell layer and marked hyperkeratosis are seen.

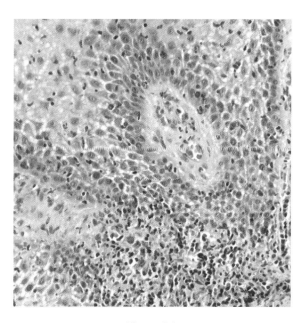

Figure 3-9

SQUAMOUS PAPILLOMA

Markedly reactive epithelial changes are seen in the basal and superbasal layers. An inflamed fibrovascular core of lamina propria with a variable degree of acute and chronic inflammation infiltrates the basal portion of the epithelium.

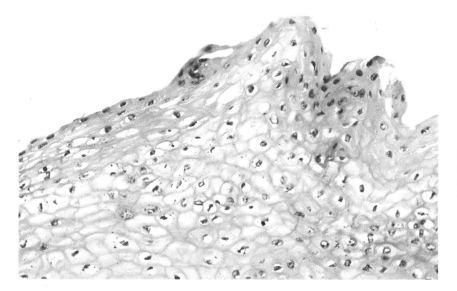

Figure 3-10

SQUAMOUS PAPILLOMA

Prominent human papillomavirus (HPV)-like changes, such as koilocytosis, binucleation, and perinuclear clearing, are seen at high-power magnification.

formation, unlike ESPs, which are well-circumscribed nodules. Verrucous carcinomas usually contain a central crater of keratin which is not a feature of ESPs. Correlation with the clinical and endoscopic findings is essential.

Treatment and Prognosis. The treatment of ESP is polypectomy, although rare examples have been removed by radiofrequency ablation,

particularly when the patient has multiple lesions such as papillomatosis (53). Most ESPs are benign, without malignant potential. Occasional cases have been shown to regress with time (55). Due to their benign nature there is no clinical necessity to ensure adequacy of excision.

The association with squamous cell carcinoma is controversial, but if present, is extremely

37

rare (37,53,54,56). In one study by d'Huart (37), two squamous cell cancers were detected in 78 patients with ESP over a 9-year period, but only one of those showed an association with a prior ESP. In two other studies, one of which followed 19 patients long term, no association was noted between squamous papilloma and squamous cell cancer upon follow-up (36,39). Rare cases with cancer have been associated with papillomatosis and with high-risk HPV types (54).

PSEUDOEPITHELIOMATOUS HYPERPLASIA

Definition. *Pseudoepitheliomatous hyperplasia* is reactive squamous epithelium characterized by the presence of parallel, elongated, and often evenly spaced and uniform columns (pegs) of reactive basilar squamous cells that extend deep into the lamina propria, most often adjacent to healing ulcers.

General and Clinical Features. Pseudoepitheliomatous hyperplasia is a common pathologic tissue reaction which always occurs secondary to injury or ulceration of the esophageal squamous mucosa (57,58), most commonly GERD, infection, or pill-induced esophagitis (2,57). The prevalence of pseudoepitheliomatous hyperplasia is unknown, but in one series by Terada et al. (2), it was noted in 1.9 percent of consecutive esophageal biopsies from 910 patients over a 15-year period. Because of its association with inflammation and ulceration, it occurs most commonly in middle-aged and older individuals; patients of both genders are affected.

Since the symptoms and signs are due to the underlying inflammatory disorder, pseudoepitheliomatous hyperplasia is most commonly noted incidentally at the time of evaluation of mucosal biopsy specimens by the pathologist. It is believed that as a response to surface ulceration, the basal cells of the preserved squamous epithelium proliferate laterally and downward into the lamina propria in an attempt to heal and re-epithelialize the ulcerated mucosa.

Gross Findings. Endoscopically, pseudoepitheliomatous hyperplasia may be visible as an area of heaped up or variegated mucosa at the edge of mucosal ulcers. When particularly prominent, it appears nodular or polypoid (termed hyperplastic or inflammatory polyp by some [59]) at which time it may be confused with a malignant lesion.

Microscopic Findings. Microscopically, pseudoepitheliomatous hyperplasia is characterized by the presence of multiple, typically parallel, elongated, and occasionally irregular columns of highly reactive basaloid squamous cells that extend for a variable distance into the lamina propria of the affected area of mucosa (fig. 3-11, left). The columns of reactive basal cells are usually smooth in contour and show blunt ends and a sharp demarcation from the surrounding lamina propria. The reactive squamous cells are usually cuboidal or pyramidal shaped, with enlarged round to oval-shaped hyperchromatic nuclei and hypereosinophilic dense cytoplasm with an increased nuclear/cytoplasmic (N/C) ratio (fig. 3-11, right). Mitoses may be numerous. A lack of surface maturation (nucleated cells at the surface) and parakeratosis may be present as well. Inflammation, both acute and chronic, is usually present and this assists in recognizing the reactive nature of the cell proliferation.

With maturation and healing of the mucosa, the reactive pegs of epithelium mature and become separated by collagen rather than by inflammatory cells and granulation tissue. At this point it may take on more of a "basaloid" appearance, showing cells that are smaller, contain round normochromatic nuclei without mitoses, and arrange themselves in a linear fashion in the basal layer of the squamous epithelium.

Differential Diagnosis. The main entities in the differential diagnosis of pseudoepitheliomatous hyperplasia are benign esophageal squamous papilloma, squamous dysplasia, and squamous cell carcinoma. Squamous papillomas, particularly the endophytic type, usually have a smooth surface and marked hyperkeratosis and parakeratosis, and are not typically associated with mucosal ulcers or an underlying inflammatory disorder. In contrast to dysplasia and carcinoma, pseudoepitheliomatous hyperplasia shows cells with nuclear enlargement, hyperchromasia, and increased mitoses, but without atypical mitoses. There is smooth and even expansion of the basal layer, in contrast to dysplasia or carcinoma. The reactive cells lack pleomorphism, overlapping or crowding of the nuclei, loss of polarity, and atypical mitoses. The mucosal architecture in hyperplasia retains its uniformity, showing squamous pegs that expand roughly to equal depths within the deep lamina propria. Unlike dysplasia,

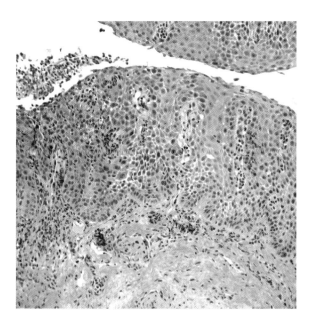 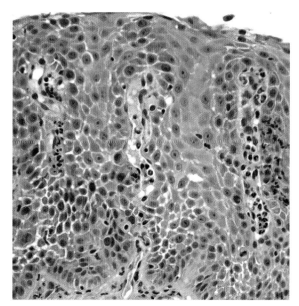

Figure 3-11

PSEUDOEPITHELIOMATOUS HYPERPLASIA

Left: Esophageal biopsy from a patient with severe gastroesophageal reflux disease (GERD) shows an area of surface erosion and marked pseudoepitheliomatous hyperplasia. There are marked basal and suprabasal reactive changes in the epithelium with lack of surface maturation. The pegs of hyperplastic basal cells extend into the lamina propria in a parallel and regular fashion. The columns of reactive basal cells are smooth in contour and have blunt ends and a sharp demarcation from the lamina propria. The squamous cells are enlarged and show an increased N/C ratio, but maintain their polarity with an absence of overlapping with adjacent cells and atypical mitoses. Prominent nucleoli are apparent.

Right: High-power view of the basal portion of pseudoepitheliomatous hyperplasia shows hyperreactive basal cells containing enlarged, round to oval hyperchromatic nuclei with prominent nucleoli, hyperdense eosinophilic cytoplasm, and increased mitoses.

the chromatin pattern in pseudoepitheliomatous hyperplasia is generally fine and homogeneous, and the nucleoli, when present, are typically isolated, small, and centrally located.

Dysplastic squamous epithelium typically displays irregular architectural distortion with sharply angulated or markedly irregular pegs of squamous epithelium in terms of their length and width. Compared to pseudoepitheliomatous hyperplasia, dysplastic squamous cells are typically more pleomorphic in size and shape, more hyperchromatic, more irregular in nuclear contour, and reveal nuclear overlapping and loss of polarity. Occasionally, the basal portion of reactive squamous epithelium may contain bizarre-shaped multinucleated epithelial giant cells that are most often situated immediately adjacent to areas of ulceration (60). Despite their multinucleated appearance, these cells have a low N/C ratio and have an open chromatin pattern with prominent nucleoli, in contrast to

neoplastic cells that have an irregular nuclear contour and hyperchromatic nuclei.

ADENOMAS

Definition. *Esophageal adenomas* are benign epithelial tumors located within the anatomic esophagus.

General and Clinical Features. Adenomas of the esophagus are rare benign neoplasms, although rare carcinomas have been reported to develop within these lesions (73). In the esophagus, there are several morphologic types, separated into two broad categories. The first are those associated with cystic dilatation or neoplastic alteration of the submucosal gland duct system; the second are adenoma-like polypoid dysplastic lesions that arise in Barrett esophagus. The latter lesions are not considered true adenomas of the esophagus since they develop as a result of neoplastic complications of underlying Barrett esophagus (61–65). These

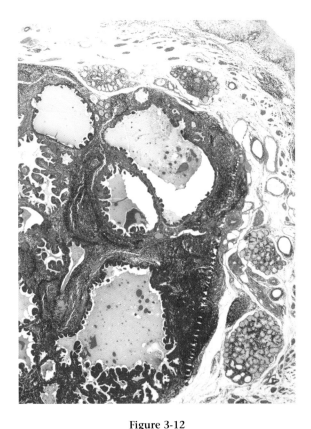

Figure 3-12

ESOPHAGEAL ADENOMA

This benign adenoma in the esophageal submucosa appears similar to a Warthin tumor of the salivary glands. The lesion is composed of micropapillary epithelium situated within microcystic spaces lined by abundant chronic inflammatory cells and reactive lymphoid tissue. The cells are hypereosinophilic and have an oncocytic appearance. The lesion is well circumscribed without infiltration into the surrounding tissues.

polyps are composed of tubular or tubulovillous proliferations of dysplastic intestinal or foveolar epithelium, and have a high association with adenocarcinoma both within the polyp and in the adjacent Barrett esophagus (61,64). Some may show a serrated phenotype and, thus, resemble traditional serrated adenomas, while others may appear similar to pyloric gland adenomas of the stomach (66,67). These lesions are discussed more completely in chapter 4.

True esophageal adenomas, those that develop from the submucosal gland duct system, are extremely rare. They are similar histologically to those that arise from the salivary glands (68–76). They have been variously termed (or

diagnosed as) submucosal gland duct adenoma, serous cystadenoma, canalicular adenoma, tubular adenoma, sialadenoma papilliferum, and Warthin tumor (fig. 3-12). Little is known of their pathogenesis. In one series of 19 cases identified from 786 endoscopic mucosal resection specimens over a 7-year period, the median age of the patients was 58 years and there was a male predominance. These lesions are usually asymptomatic. They usually come to clinical attention at the time of endoscopy performed for upper gastrointestinal symptoms.

Gross and Microscopic Findings. Grossly, esophageal adenomas are typically well-circumscribed submucosal nodules or bulges that generally measure between 1 and 5 cm. Microscopically, many appear similar to tumors that arise in the minor salivary glands, which is not surprising considering that the esophageal submucosal glands are considered by some authorities to represent a continuation of the minor salivary glands of the oropharynx.

Several histologic types of adenoma have been described. Lesions that resemble pleomorphic adenomas of the salivary gland are the most common (68). Others resemble sialadenoma papilliferum or canalicular adenoma of the salivary glands (figs. 3-13, 3-14) (69,72). Rarely, pancreatic or ovarian-like cystadenomas have been described. Other lesions lack a salivary gland appearance, but instead show features reminiscent of the normal submucosal gland duct system (66,67,69,75). These lesions often show a mixture of tubal, cystic, and papillary growth, and are composed of epithelium containing two cell layers, similar to the normal submucosal gland ducts. The superficial (luminal) layer is composed of small cuboidal-shaped cells with small centrally located nuclei and eosinophilic cytoplasm, without significant nuclear atypia. The underlying basal layer resembles myoepithelial cells, and shows the characteristic immunostaining pattern of that cell lineage. The surface epithelium usually shows little or no cytologic atypia, may be flattened or cuboidal in shape, and contains bland oval-shaped nuclei with an open chromatin pattern and slightly eosinophilic cytoplasm. Mitoses are uncommon. These lesions show a mild degree of chronic inflammation, both surrounding and within the body of the tumor.

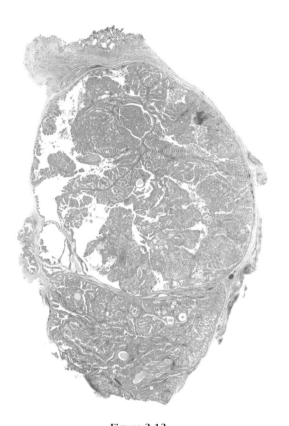

Figure 3-13

ESOPHAGEAL ADENOMA

There is a well-circumscribed and organized submucosal proliferation of epithelium within microcystic spaces and a papillary and micropapillary pattern of growth. Multiple glandular spaces containing eosinophilic luminal material are present.

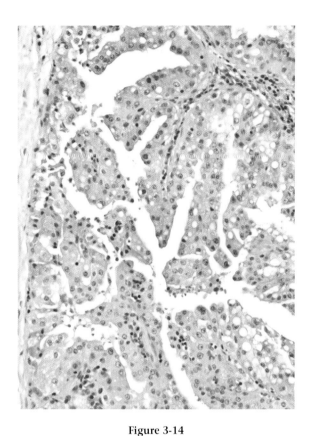

Figure 3-14

ESOPHAGEAL ADENOMA

High-power microscopy shows a micropapillary, cord-like and solid arrangement of cells with prominent round to oval nuclei, prominent nucleoli, and amphophilic cytoplasm. The nuclei are regular in size and shape, without significant pleomorphism. In some areas, the epithelium is arranged in trabeculae that are two or three cells thick.

The duct lining and basal cells of adenomas are typically positive for cytokeratins (CK) 5, 6, 7, 17, 18, 19, and P63, but are negative for CK20. They usually show strong staining with high molecular weight cytokeratins. The underlying basal layer stains similar to myoepithelial cells, showing positivity for smooth muscle actin and S-100 protein. Negative markers include P53, CDX2, MUC5AC, MUC6, MUC2, and MUC1. Non-neoplastic gland/duct cysts may be erroneously diagnosed as an "adenoma," but instead are believed to develop secondary to duct inspissation or obstruction (fig. 3-15).

Differential Diagnosis. The differential diagnosis of esophageal gland duct adenomas includes polypoid dysplasia associated with Barrett esophagus, well-differentiated ductal or tubular adenocarcinomas, and metastasis. In contrast to adenomas, adenocarcinomas show more cytologic atypia, nuclear pleomorphism, mitoses, and atypical mitoses and usually show an infiltrative pattern of growth characteristic of malignant tumors. Recognition of the characteristic two-cell layer typical of most gland duct adenomas, combined with a lack of atypia and histologic similarity to salivary gland tumors, is the key to establishing a correct diagnosis.

PSEUDODIVERTICULOSIS

Definition. *Pseudodiverticulosis* is a disorder characterized by squamous metaplasia, cystic dilatation, and inflammation of the esophageal submucosal glands and ducts. It mimics diverticulosis, or carcinoma, upon radiologic examination (such as barium swallow), due to the presence of stricture formation or diverticula.

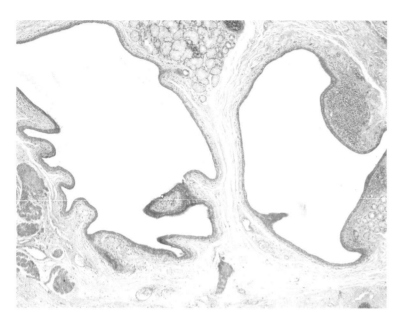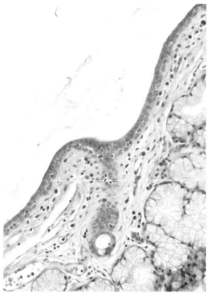

Figure 3-15

DILATED SUBMUCOSAL GLAND DUCTS

Left: Low-power view of non-neoplastic dilated submucosal gland ducts which may be erroneously diagnosed as an adenoma. This lesion appears to represent cystic dilation of the submucosal gland duct, which usually develops as a result of duct obstruction.

Right: At high power, the normal two-cell layer lining of the duct epithelium is seen surrounded by a rim of chronic inflammation.

General and Clinical Features. Pseudodiverticulosis is an extremely rare disorder first described by Mendl in 1960 (77). Its pathogenesis is unknown (77,78). However, it is associated with chronic inflammatory conditions of the esophagus, such as GERD, hiatus hernia, motility disorders, diabetes mellitus, candidiasis, achalasia, and chronic alcohol abuse, among others (79,80). This condition occurs in all age groups, but is more common in the elderly, with a slight male predominance (79,81). Affected patients often present with intermittent or progressive dysphagia, or in some instances, gastrointestinal bleeding (82).

Pseudodiverticulosis is normally diagnosed radiologically by the characteristic appearance in barium studies (79,83,84). The classic appearance is that of numerous flask-shaped outpouchings in the wall of the esophagus that range in size from 1 to 4 mm in length (83,84). There is a high incidence of esophageal narrowing or stricture formation, which is usually present in the upper third of the esophagus (85). Intramural tracking is detected on esophagography in up to 50 percent of patients with this condition

(83). Radiologic investigations are more sensitive than endoscopy in establishing a diagnosis, since the signature features are present in the wall and not evident to the endoscopist's eye. The orifices of pseudodiverticula are difficult to recognize, because pseudodiverticula are present deep within the submucosa and thus biopsies are usually not helpful. Due to the high association with stricture formation, the clinical, radiologic, and endoscopic appearances often simulate invasive carcinoma (86).

The outpouchings are believed to develop as a result of inflammation and periductal fibrosis, which has been proposed to lead to compression of the duct orifices, cystic dilation, and squamous metaplasia. Since the ducts may communicate with the esophageal lumen and excrete a viscous yellowish fluid that contains denuded epithelium, inflammatory cells and mucus, this feature may be seen endoscopically. Other postulated theories of pathogenesis include glandular secretory dysfunction, esophageal dysmotility, and chronic esophagitis.

Pseudodiverticulosis is a benign condition, but rare cases occur in association with

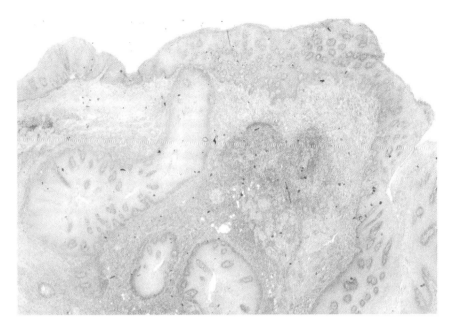

Figure 3-16

PSEUDODIVERTICULOSIS

The lamina propria and submucosa show somewhat dilated and inflamed submucosal gland ducts with extensive squamous metaplasia. The pseudodiverticula have a smooth contour and are rimmed by a dense chronic inflammatory infiltrate. The surrounding lamina propria shows inflammation and fibrosis.

squamous cell carcinoma or other infectious disorders, such as tuberculosis (80). In one study, this condition was present at a significantly higher rate in patients with carcinoma than in patients who underwent esophagography for other reasons (87).

Gross Findings. As mentioned above, pseudodiverticulosis manifests as an area of esophageal narrowing or stricture formation combined with thickening of the esophageal wall due mostly to inflammation, fibrosis, and cystic dilatation of the submucosal gland ducts. Upon tissue sectioning, tiny saccular outpouchings, as well as sinus tracts, may be evident protruding from the mucosa and extending deeper into the wall of the esophagus. Perforation is uncommon. Adjacent and overlying areas of inflammation and ulceration of the esophagus are normally present. Any portion of the esophagus may be affected by this disorder, but esophageal narrowing and stricture formation is more common in the upper third of the esophagus.

Microscopic Findings. As the name implies, the outpouchings do not represent true diverticula, but instead are dilated and inflamed submucosal esophageal gland ducts. The ducts are lined either completely or partially by metaplastic reactive-appearing squamous epithelium and are usually surrounded by a band of chronic inflammatory cells and fibrous tissue (fig. 3-16). Superinfection with *Candida* is common.

With time, the submucosal ducts and glands may become cystic or develop complex extensions, outpouchings, and sinus tracks within the wall of the esophagus. Secondary infection and accumulation of necrotic and inflammatory debris within the lumen of the ducts and cysts are common. Rarely, fistula formation occurs into adjacent organs or into the mediastinum. Despite replacement of the submucosal glands and ducts with squamous epithelium, the glands retain their normal round and smooth configuration and do not have an infiltrative appearance. The inflammation usually consists of lymphocytes, plasma cells, and occasional eosinophils. The squamous epithelium lacks the cytologic atypia that is normally associated with neoplasia, but it may show marked reactive basal changes, with increased mitoses and enlarged hyperchromatic nuclei, but without loss of polarity, overlapping nuclei, or atypical mitoses (fig. 3-17).

Differential Diagnosis. Clinically and pathologically, the most important disorder in the differential diagnosis is invasive squamous cell carcinoma. Pseudodiverticulosis lacks an infiltrative growth pattern, however, and shows an absence of cytologic features of dysplastic squamous epithelium. In addition, the pseudodiverticula are smooth, rounded structures surrounded by a cuff of inflammatory cells, unlike squamous cell carcinoma which has an irregular infiltrative appearance contains atypical

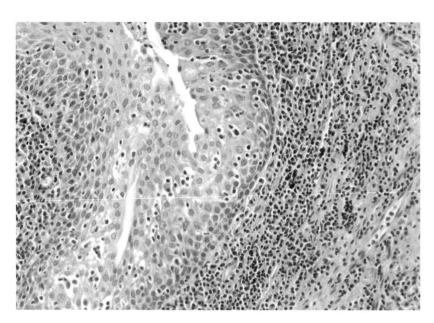

Figure 3-17

PSEUDODIVERTICULOSIS-ASSOCIATED DUCT

The duct shows reactive basal and superbasal cells, lack of maturation, periductular chronic inflammation, and intraepithelial lymphocytosis.

cells with increased N/C ratio, pleomorphism, overlapping nuclei, and atypical mitoses.

Treatment and Prognosis. Complications of pseudodiverticulosis include chronic dysmotility, fibrous stricture and fistula formation, webs, and intraluminal pseudotumor formation (79,82,85,88). Treatment is normally directed at alleviating esophageal obstruction and dealing with the underlying or associated chronic inflammatory condition (85). Some patients benefit from multiple esophageal dilatation procedures which may result in the disappearance of the saccular outpouchings with time (85). Most patients, however, show persistence of diverticula, but this may be without clinical symptoms. Conservative management usually leads to satisfactory control of symptoms in most patients, and the condition remains stable for long periods of time.

DEVELOPMENTAL CYSTS AND DUPLICATIONS

Definition. *Esophageal duplications* are cystic or tubular replicas of a segment of the gastrointestinal (GI) tract that are contiguous with the segment of the tract with which they are associated. Neuroenteric remnants include a variety of lesions that originate from the dorsal midline of the GI tract, and all are lined by normal GI layers in combination with neural tissue. Other synonyms used to describe these lesions include *dorsal enteric remnant, posterior mediastinal cyst,* *enteral cyst, neuroenteric cyst, thoracic duplication,* and *dorsal enteric cyst.*

General and Clinical Features. Esophageal malformations are classified into two broad groups: duplications and neuroenteric (dorsal enteric) remnants (89–92). Entities in both groups may, or may not, communicate with the lumen of the esophagus, and, in the latter instance, may become cystic or form an intramural nodule or mass leading to stenosis and obstruction. Ten to 15 percent of all GI tract duplications occur in the esophagus (93). They are equally common in males and females, in all age groups, and often are detected either radiologically or endoscopically in patients who are being investigated for unrelated upper GI symptoms; they may also come to clinical attention due to obstruction symptoms (90–95).

Tracheobronchial duplications are a subtype that develop from the incomplete separation of the primitive lung bud from the foregut during gestation (89,91,92). In contrast to conventional duplications, these lesions may contain mucosal and mural features of the respiratory tract, such as ciliated columnar epithelium, cartilage, and mucous glands. Depending on the location and size, cysts and duplications may cause dysphagia, bleeding, or symptoms of luminal obstruction (89–92,94). If large and present in the mediastinum, they may compress nearby respiratory or alimentary tract structures.

Neuroenteric remnants include diverticula, fistulas, fibrous cords, and cystic structures that originate from the dorsal midline of the GI tract and attach to or pass through the vertebral column and spinal cord cranial to their enteric origin. They are most common in the cervical and lumbar areas, and are usually associated with a congenital abnormality of the spinal cord or vertebrae (89,96–98).

Duplications and neuroenteric remnants have traditionally been classified by their histologic features, particularly the nature of their lining epithelium. However, since all of these conditions may be lined by any type of epithelium derived from the alimentary or respiratory tract, the histologic appearance cannot be relied upon to adequately categorize the lesions.

Gross and Microscopic Findings. Grossly, duplications are intramural or extramural, but are always attached to the esophagus in some manner. In some cases, they may be partially intramural and partially extramural, or attached to the wall of the esophagus and share muscularis propria with the involved segment of the esophagus. The lumen of the duplications may, or may not, communicate with the normal lumen of the esophagus. Extramural lesions generally attach to the adventitia or outer muscularis of the esophagus, in which case they may mimic a mediastinal mass. These lesions may occur anywhere in the esophagus, but are most common in the upper third (91,93). They may be unilocular or less commonly multilocular.

The histologic diagnostic criteria of esophageal duplications include attachment to the esophagus, typical enclosure by two muscle layers, and lining by epithelium, most often of the squamous type (93). Typically, the walls of these lesions are composed of all layers of the normal GI tract, including the inner circular and outer longitudinal muscularis propria, as well as the myenteric and submucosal nerve plexuses (fig. 3-18). Heterotopic mucosa is present in these lesions as well.

Tracheobronchial-type of duplications are typically lined by ciliated columnar or respiratory epithelium, with an underlying bland hypocellular stromal mesenchyme that may contain smooth muscle, mucous glands, cartilage, or a combination of these elements (fig. 3-19). Simple developmental retention cysts

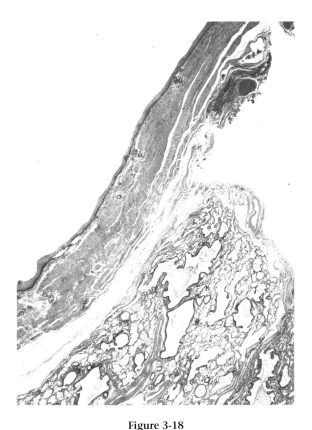

Figure 3-18

ESOPHAGEAL DUPLICATION CYST

The cyst was attached to the esophagus on one side and the lung on the other. The cyst, which communicated with the lumen of the esophagus, is composed of an inner lining of squamous epithelium and all layers of the esophageal wall, including the muscularis propria and adventitia. Multiple submucosal ducts and glands are present.

may also develop as a result of obstruction and dilation of the esophageal submucosal gland ducts (fig. 3-20). They may be lined by a simple two-layer thick ductal epithelium and rimmed by mononuclear inflammatory cells on the outer aspects of the cyst wall. These cysts are not associated with smooth muscle or cartilage.

Neuroenteric remnants are most common in the upper third of the esophagus, and grossly, may appear as a fistula, cyst, or fibrous cord-like structure (89). The walls of these lesions are similar to those of normal esophagus, and the lining epithelium may be of any type, but usually in combination with ciliated columnar epithelium. Neural or meningeal tissue and heterotopic tissue may be present as well.

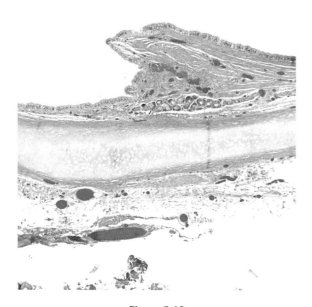

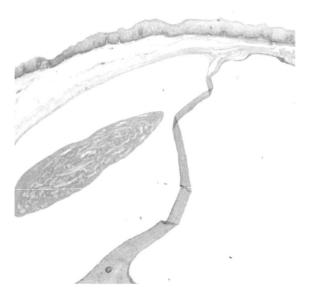

Figure 3-19

ESOPHAGEAL DUPLICATION CYST

The surface epithelium is columnar and focally has microvilli. The wall shows fibrous tissue, smooth muscle, and cartilage.

Treatment and Prognosis. These lesions are benign with minimal neoplastic potential. Rarely, adenocarcinoma, or even squamous cell carcinoma, may be associated with or develop within these lesions (99–101). The primary form of management is directed toward alleviating the symptoms, which is usually approached best by surgical resection (102).

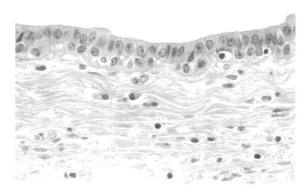

Figure 3-20

DEVELOPMENTAL RETENTION CYST

Top: This likely developed as a result of obstruction and dilatation of an esophageal submucosal gland duct.

Bottom: At high-power magnification, the epithelium is lined by simple two-layer thick ductal epithelium and rimmed by mononuclear inflammatory cells on the outer aspects of the cyst wall. These cysts are not associated with smooth muscle or cartilage.

REFERENCES

1. Tsai SJ, Lin CC, Chang CW, et al. Benign esophageal lesions: endoscopic and pathologic features. World J Gastroenterol 2015;21:1091-8.
2. Terada T. A clinicopathologic study of esophageal 860 benign and malignant lesions in 910 cases of consecutive esophageal biopsies. Int J Clin Exp Pathol 2013;6:191-8.
3. Levine MS. Benign tumors of the esophagus: radiologic evaluation. Semin Thorac Cardiovasc Surg 2003;15:9-19.
4. Nazligul Y, Aslan M, Esen R, et al. Benign glycogenic acanthosis lesions of the esophagus. Turk J Gastroenterol 2012;23:199-202.
5. Ghahremani GG, Rushovich AM. Glycogenic acanthosis of the esophagus: radiographic and pathologic features. Gastrointest Radiol 1984;9:93-8.
6. Glick SN, Teplick SK, Goldstein J, Stead JA, Zitomer N. Glycogenic acanthosis of the esophagus. AJR Am J Roentgenol 1982;139:683-8.
7. Lopes S, Figueiredo P, Amaro P, et al. Glycogenic acanthosis of the esophagus: an unusually endoscopic appearance. Rev Esp Enferm Dig 2010;102:341-2.
8. Vadva MD, Triadafilopoulos G. Glycogenic acanthosis of the esophagus and gastroesophageal reflux. J Clin Gastroenterol 1993;17:79-83.
9. Kay PS, Soetikno RM, Mindelzun R, Young HS. Diffuse esophageal glycogenic acanthosis: an endoscopic marker of Cowden's disease. Am J Gastroenterol 1997;92:1038-40.
10. Umemura K, Takagi S, Ishigaki Y, et al. Gastrointestinal polyposis with esophageal polyposis is useful for early diagnosis of Cowden's disease. World J Gastroenterol 2008;14:5755-9.
11. McGarrity TJ, Wager Baker MJ, Ruggiero FM, et al. GI polyposis and glycogenic acanthosis of the esophagus associated with PTEN mutation positive Cowden syndrome in the absence of cutaneous manifestations. Am J Gastroenterol 2003;98:1429-34.
12. Berezin S, Schwarz SM, Slim MS, Beneck D, Brudnicki AR, Medow MS. Gastrointestinal problems in a child with dyskeratosis congenita. Am J Gastroenterol 1996;91:1271-2.
13. Hizawa K, Iida M, Matsumoto T, et al. Gastrointestinal involvement in tuberous sclerosis. Two case reports. J Clin Gastroenterol 1994;19:46-9.
14. Suoglu OD, Emiroglu HH, Sokucu S, Cantez S, Cevikbas U, Saner G. Celiac disease and glycogenic acanthosis: a new association? Acta Paediatr 2004;93:568-70.
15. Terada, T. Heterotopic gastric mucosa of the gastrointestinal tract: a histopathologic study of 158 cases. Pathol Res Pract 2011;207:148-50.
16. Montalvo N, Tapia V, Padilla H, Redroban L. Heterotopic sebaceous glands in the esophagus, a very rare histopathological diagnosis: a case report and review of the literature. Clin Case Rep 2017;5:89-92.
17. Yamagiwa I, Obata K, Ouchi T, Sotoda Y, Shimazaki Y. Heterotopic pancreas of the esophagus associated with a rare type of esophageal atresia. Ann Thorac Surg 1998;65:1143-4.
18. Koval'chuk VP, Riabova MA. [A case of accessory lobe of the thyroid gland located in the area of upper esophageal narrowing.] Vestn Otorinolaringol 1997:53. [Russian]
19. Lumachi F, Zucchetta P, Varotto S, Polistina F, Favia G, D'Amico D. Noninvasive localization procedures in ectopic hyperfunctioning parathyroid tumors. Endocr Relat Cancer 1999;6:123-5.
20. Zentner J, Vogt H, Heidenreich P. A retroesophageal parathyroid adenoma detected with Tc-99m sestamibi and MRI. Clin Nucl Med 1999;24:998-9.
21. Marmuse JP, Cavillon A, Mrejen G, Toublanc M, Potet F, Benhamou G. [Congenital stenosis of the esophagus due to tracheobronchial heterotopia. Review of the literature. Apropos of a case.] Ann Chir 1993;47:190-5. [French]
22. Neumann WL, Lujan GM, Genta RM. Gastric heterotopia in the proximal esophagus ("inlet patch"): association with adenocarcinomas arising in Barrett mucosa. Dig Liver Dis 2012;44:292-6.
23. Gutierrez O, Akamatsu T, Cardona H, Graham DY, El-Zimaity HM. Helicobacter pylori and heterotopic gastric mucosa in the upper esophagus (the inlet patch). Am J Gastroenterol 2003;98:1266-70.
24. Weickert U, Wolf A, Schröder C, Autschbach F, Vollmer H. Frequency, histopathological findings, and clinical significance of cervical heterotopic gastric mucosa (gastric inlet patch): a prospective study in 300 patients. Dis Esophagus 2011;24:63-8.
25. Sanchez-Pemaute A, Hemando F, Diez-Valladares L, et al. Heterotopic gastric mucosa in the upper esophagus ("inlet patch"): a rare cause of esophageal perforation. AMJ Gastroenterol 1999;94:3047-50.
26. Ward EM, Achem SR. Gastric heterotopia in the proximal esophagus complicated by stricture. Gastrointest Endosc 2003;57:131-3.
27. Schmulewitz N, Tobias J, Singh P. Hyperplastic polyp arising from heterotopic gastric epithelium in the esophagus. Gastrointest Endosc 2007;66:1221-2; discussion, 1222

28. Bard A, Coton T, De Biasi C, Guisset M. Adenocarcinoma of the upper esophagus. Clin Res Hepatol Gastroenterol 2011;35:418-9.

29. Chatelain D, de Lajarte-Thirouard AS, Tiret E, Flejou JF. Adenocarcinoma of the upper esophagus arising in heterotopic gastric mucosa: common pathogenesis with Barrett's adenocarcinoma? Virchows Arch 2002;441:406-11.

30. Berkelhammer C, Bhagavan M, Templeton A, Raines R, Walloch J. Gastric inlet patch containing submucosally infiltrating adenocarcinoma. J Clin Gastroenterol 1997;25:678-81.

31. Suttorp AC, Heike M, Fahndrich M, Reis H, Lorenzen J. [Heterotopic sebaceous glands in the esophagus: a case report with review of the literature.] Pathologe 2013;34:162-4. [German]

32. Bhat RV, Ramaswamy RR, Yelagondahally LK. Ectopic sebaceous glands in the esophagus: a case report and review of literature. Saudi J Gastroenterol 2008;14:83-4.

33. Yüksel I, Usküdar O, Köklü S, et al. Inlet patch: associations with endoscopic findings in the upper gastrointestinal system. Scand J Gastroenterol 2008;43:910-24.

34. Nakanishi Y, Ochiai A, Shimoda T, et al. Heterotopic sebaceous glands in the esophagus: histopathological and immunohistochemical study of a resected esophagus. Pathol Int 1999;49:364-8.

35. Crighton E, Botha A. Intraductal papillary mucinous neoplasm of the oesophagus: an unusual case of dysphagia. Ann R Coll Surg Engl 2012;94:e92-4.

36. Mosca S, Manes G, Monaco R, Bellomo PF, Bottino V, Balzano A. Squamous papilloma of the esophagus: long-term follow up. J Gastroenterol Hepatol 2001;16:857-61.

37. d'Huart MC, Chevaux JB, Bressonet AM, et al. Prevalence of esophageal squamous papilloma (ESP) and associated cancer in northeastern France. Endosc Int Open 2015;3:E101-6.

38. Jideh B, Weltman M, Wu Y, Chan CHY. Esophageal squamous papilloma lacks clear clinicopathological associations. World J Clin Cases 2017;5:134-9.

39. Szanto I, Szentirmay Z, Banai J, et al. [Squamous papilloma of the esophagus. Clinical and pathological observations based on 172 papillomas in 155 patients.] Orv Hetil 2005;146:547-52. [Hungarian]

40. Lavergne D, de Villiers EM. Papillomavirus in esophageal papillomas and carcinomas. Int J Cancer 1999;80:681-4.

41. Mahajan R, Kurien RT, Joseph AJ, Dutta AK, Chowdhury SD. Squamous papilloma of esophagus. Indian J Gastroenterol 2016;35:151.

42. Lee K, Lee O, Lee S. Gastrointestinal: diffuse esophageal papillomatosis involving the entire esophagus. J Gastroenterol Hepatol 2014;29:1951.

43. Corredine TJ, Bortniker E, Birk J. A rare cause of dysphagia: squamous papillomatosis of the esophagus. Clin Gastroenterol Hepatol 2016;14:A21-2.

44. Pantham G, Ganesan S, Einstadter D, Jin G, Weinberg A, Fass R. Assessment of the incidence of squamous cell papilloma of the esophagus and the presence of high-risk human papilloma virus. Dis Esophagus 2017;30:1-5.

45. Odze R, Antonioli D, Shocket D, Noble-Topham S, Goldman H, Upton M. Esophageal squamous papillomas: clinicopathologic study of 38 lesions and analysis of human papillomavirus by the polymerase chain reaction. Am J Surg Pathol 1993;17:803-12.

46. Inomata S, Aoyagi K, Eguchi K, Sakisaka S. Giant esophageal papilloma. Gastrointest Endosc 2004;60:430.

47. Karras PJ, Barawi M, Webb B, Michalos A. Squamos cell papillomatosis of esophageal following placement of a self-expanding metal stent. Dig Dis Sci 1994;44:457-61.

48. Afonso LA, Moyses N, Cavalcanti SM. Human papillomavirus detection and p16 methylation pattern in a case of esophageal papilloma. Braz J Med Biol Res 2010;43:694-6.

49. Tiftikci A, Kutsal E, Altiok E, et al. Analyzing esophageal squamous cell papillomas for the presence of human papilloma virus. Turk J Gastroenterol 2017;28:176-8.

50. Woo YJ, Yoon HK. In situ hybridization study on human papillomavirus DNA expression in benign and malignant squamous lesions of the esophagus. J Korean Med Sci 1996;11:467-73.

51. Wong MW, Bair MJ, Shih SC, et al. Using typical endoscopic features to diagnose esophageal squamous papilloma. World J Gastroenterol 2016;22:2349-56.

52. Batra PS, Hebert RL 2nd, Haines GK 3rd, Holinger LD. Recurrent respiratory papillomatosis with esophageal involvement. Int J Ped Otorhinolaryngol 2001;58:233-8.

53. Kibria R, Akram S, Moezzi J, Ali S. Esophageal squamous papillomatosis with dysplasia. Is there a role of balloon-based radiofrequency ablation therapy? Acta Gastroenterol Belg 2009;72:373-6.

54. Attila T, Fu A, Gopinath N, Streutker CJ, Marcon NE. Esophageal papillomatosis complicated by squamous cell carcinoma. Can J Gastroenterol 2009;23:415-9.

55. Kato H, Orito E, Yoshinouchi T, et al. Regression of esophageal papillomatous polyposis caused by high-risk type human papilloma virus. J Gastroenterol 2003;38:579-83.

56. Waluga M, Hartleb M, Sliwinski ZK, Romanczyk T, Wodołazski A. Esophageal squamous cell papillomatosis complicated by carcinoma. Am J Gastroenterol 2000;95:1592-3.

57. Glickman JN, Odze RD. Epithelial neoplasms of the esophagus. In: Odze RD, Goldblum JR, Crawford JM, eds. Surgical Pathology of the GI tract, liver, biliary tract, and pancreas. Philadelphia: Saunders; 2004: 381-408.

58. Arista-Nasr J, Rivera I, Martinez-Benitez B, Bornstein-Quevedo L, Orozco H, Lugo-Guevara Y. Atypical regenerative hyperplasia of the esophagus in endoscopic biopsy: a mimicker of squamous esophagic carcinoma. Arch Pathol Lab Med 2005;129:899-904.

59. Abraham SC, Singh VK, Yardley JH, Wu TT. Hyperplastic polyps of the esophagus and esophagogastric junction: histologic and clinicopathologic findings. Am J Surg Pathol 2001;25:1180-7.

60. Singh SP, Odze RD. Multinucleated epithelial giant cell changes in esophagitis: a clinocopathologic study of 14 cases. Am J Surg Pathol 1998;22:93-9.

61. Thurberg BL, Duray PH, Odze RD. Polypoid dysplasia in Barrett's esophagus: a clinico-pathologic, immunihistochemical and molecular study of five cases. Hum Pathol 1999;30:745-52.

62. Arnold GL, Mardini HE. Barrett's esophagus-associated polypoid dysplasia: a case report and review of the literature. Dig Dis Sci 2002;47:1897-900.

63. Ahlawat SK, Ozdemirli M. Polypoid dysplasia in Barrett's esophagus: case report and qualitative systematic review of the literature. Acta Gastroenterol Belg 2012;75:49-54.

64. Asthana N, Mandich D, Ligato S. Esophageal polypoid dysplasia of gastric foveolar phenotype with focal intramucosal carcinoma associated with Barrett's esophagus. Am J Surg Pathol 2008; 32:1581-5.

65. Giblin EM, Reed CE. Diffuse esophageal polyposis: an uncommon occurrence. Ann Thorac Surg 2009;87:1258-60.

66. Rubio CA, Tanaka K, Befrits R. Traditional serrated adenoma in a patient with Barrett's esophagus. Anticancer Res 2013;33:1743-5.

67. Kushima R, Vieth M, Mukaisho K, et al. Pyloric gland adenoma arising in Barrett's esophagus with mucin immunohistochemical and molecular cytogenic evaluation. Virchows Arch 2005;446:537-41.

68. Banducci D, Rees R, Bluett MK, Sawyers JL. Pleomorphic adenoma of the cervical esophagus: a rare tumor. Ann Thorac Surg 1987;44:653-5.

69. Grimm EE, Rulyak SJ, Sekijima JH, Yeh MM. Canalicular adenoma arising in the esophagus. Arch Pathol Lab Med 2007;131:1595-7.

70. Agawa H, Matsushita M, Kusumi F, Nishio A, Takakuwa H. Esophageal submucosal gland duct adenoma: characteristic EUS and histopathologic features. Gastrointest Endosc 2003;57:983-5.

71. Lindboe CF, Matre J, Nesland JM. Adenoma of the esophagus with intracytoplasmic mucoid bodies. APMIS 2004;112:29-33.

72. Su JM, Hsu HK, Hsu PI, Wang CY, Chang HC. Sialadenoma papilliferum of the esophagus. Am J Gastroenterol 1998;93:461-2.

73. Takubo K, Esaki Y, Watanabe A, Umehara M, Sasajima K. Adenoma accompanied by superficial squamous cell carcinoma of the esophagus. Cancer 1993;71:2435-8.

74. Tsutsumi M, Mizumoto K, Tsujiuchi T, et al. Serous cystadenoma of the esophagus. Acta Pathol Jpn 1990;40:153-5.

75. Nie L, Wu HY, Shen YH, et al. Esophageal submucosal gland duct adenoma: a clinicopathological and immunohistochemical study with a review of the literature. Dis Esophagus 2016;29:1048-53.

76. Harada O, Ota H, Katsuyama T, Hidaka E, Ishazaka K, Nakayama J. Esophageal gland duct adenoma: immunohistochemical comparison with the normal esophageal gland and ultrastructural analysis. Am J Surg Pathol 2007;31:469-75.

77. Mendl K, McKay JM, Tanner CH. Intramural diverticulosis of the esophagus and Rokitansky Aschoff sinues in the gall blader. Br J Radiol 1960;33:496-501.

78. Freud E, Golinsky D, Ziv N, Mor C, Zahavi I, Zer M. Esophageal intramural pseudodiverticulosis: a congenital or acquired condition? J Ped Gastroenterol Nutr 1997;24:602-7.

79. Yamada T, Alpers DH, Kaplowitz N, Laine L, Owyang C, Powell DW, eds. Textbook of gastroenterology, 4th ed. Lippincott Williams & Wilkins; 2003.

80. Upadhyay AP, Bhatia RS, Anbarasu A, Sawant P, Rathi P, Nanivadekar SA. Esophageal tuberculosis with intramural pseudodiverticulosis. J Clin Gastroenterol 1996;22:38-40.

81. Bhattacharya S, Mahmud S, McGlinchey I, Nassar AH. Intramural pseudodiverticulosis of the esophagus. Surg Endoscop 2002;16:714-5.

82. Chen L, Walser EM, Schnadig V. Fatal hemorrhage secondary to ulcerated epiphrenic pseudodiverticulum. Arch Pathol Lab Med 2006;130:867-70.

83. Canon CL, Levine MS, Cherukuri R, Johnson LF, Smith JK, Koehler RE. Intramural tracking: a feature of esophageal intramural pseudodiverticulosis. AJR Am J Roentgenol 2000;175:371-4.

84. Brant WE, Helms CA. Fundamentals of diagnostic radiology, clinical medicine, neurology, 3rd ed. Philadelphia: Lippincott, Williams & Wilkins; 2007.

85. Teraishi F, Fujiwara T, Jikuhara A, et al. Esophageal intramural pseudodiverticulosis with esophageal strictures successfully treated with dilation therapy. Ann Thorac Surg 2006;82:1119-21.

86. Mantoo S, So J, Shabbir A, Sun LY. Pseudodiverticulosis of the gastroesophageal junction mimicking a carcinoma. Gastrointest Endosc 2011;73:1280-1.

87. Plavsic BM, Chen MY, Gelfand DW, et al. Intramural pseudodiverticulosis of the esophagus detected on barium esophagograms: increased prevalence in patients with esophageal carcinoma. AJR Am J Roentgenol 1995;165:1381-5.

88. Murakami M, Tsuchiya K, Ichakawa H, et al. Esophageal intramural pseudodiverticulosis associated with esophageal perforation. J Gastroenterol 2000;35:702-5.

89. Tubbs RS, Salter EG, Oakes WJ. Neurenteric cyst: case report and a review of the potential dysembryology. Clin Anat 2006;19:669-72.

90. Nayan S, Nguyen LH, Nguyen VH, Daniel SJ, Emil S. Cervical esophageal duplication cyst: case report and review of the literature. J Pediatr Surg 2010;45:e1-5.

91. Carachi R, Azmy A. Foregut duplications. Ped Surg Int 2002;18:371-4.

92. Wootton-Gorges SL, Eckel GM, Poulos DN, Kappler S, Milstein JM. Duplication of the cervical esophagus: a case report and review of the literature. Ped Radiol 2002;32:533-5.

93. Pianzola HM, Otino A, Canestri M. [Cystic duplication of the esophagus.] Acta Gastroenterol Latinoam 2001;31:333-8. [Spanish]

94. Overhaus M, Decker P, Zhou H, Textor HJ, Hirner A, Scheurlen C. The congenital duplication cyst: a rare differential diagnosis of retrosternal pain and dysphagia in a young patient. Scand J Gastroenterol 2003;38:337-40.

95. McNally J, Charles AK, Spicer RD, Grier D. Mixed foregut cyst associated with esophageal atresia. J Pediatr Surg 2001;36:939-40.

96. De Blasi R, Zenzola A, Lanzilotti CM, et al. An unusual association of intracranial aneurysms and esophageal duplication in a caseof Klippel-Trenaunay syndrome. Neuroradiol 2000;42:930-2.

97. Corre A, Chaudré F, Roger G, Denoyelle F, Garabédian EN. Tracheal dyskinesia associated with midline abnormality: embryological hypotheses and therapeutic implications. Pediatr Pulmonol 2001;(Suppl 23):10-2.

98. Akgur FM, Ozdemir T, Olguner M, Erbayraktar S, Ozer E, Aktug T. A case of split notochord syndrome: presence of dorsal enteric diverticulum adjacent to the dorsal enteric fistula. J Pediatr Surg 1998;33:1317-9.

99. Singh S, Lal P, Sikora SS, Datta NR. Squamous cell carcinoma arising from a congenital duplication cyst of the esophagus in a young adult. Dis Esophagus 2001;14:358-61.

100. Lee MY, Jensen E, Kwak S, Larson RA. Metastatic adenocarcinoma arising in a congenital foregut cyst of the esophagus: a case report with review of the literature. Am J Clin Oncol 1998;21:64-6.

101. Jacob R, Hawkes ND, Dallimore N, Butchart EG, Thomas GA, Maughan TS. Case report: squamous carcinoma in an esophageal foregut cyst. Br J Radiol 2003;76:343-6.

102. Cioffi U, Bonavina L, De Simone M, et al. Presentation and surgical management of bronchogenic and esophageal duplication cysts in adults. Chest 1998;113:1492-6.

4 BARRETT ESOPHAGUS AND ESOPHAGEAL ADENOCARCINOMA

Adenocarcinoma is the second most common type of esophageal cancer worldwide (1). Esophageal cancer is the eighth most common type of cancer, and the sixth most common cause of cancer-related deaths (1). In the last several decades there has been a marked shift in the epidemiology of esophageal cancer in Western populations (2,3). In North America, Australia, and Europe, adenocarcinoma has become the predominant subtype of esophageal cancer. In a 2012 analysis from the United States National Cancer Institute Surveillance Epidemiology and End Results Program (SEER), the incidence of esophageal adenocarcinoma in the United States increased at a rate of 8 percent per year up until the late 1990s, and almost 2 percent per year between 2000 and 2008 (2). The overall incidence during the period of 1993 to 2012 for adenocarcinoma was 1.8 per 100,000 person years (2).

Esophageal adenocarcinoma develops, almost exclusively, from Barrett esophagus (BE), a condition in which the normal squamous mucosa of the esophagus is replaced by columnar epithelium due to gastroesophageal reflux disease (GERD) (figs. 4-1, 4-2). BE is present in up to 15 percent of individuals with GERD and in 1 to 2 percent of the general population (4). Patients with BE have a tenfold higher risk of developing adenocarcinoma during their lifetime (5). Most (over 90 percent) patients with BE, however, die of causes other than adenocarcinoma.

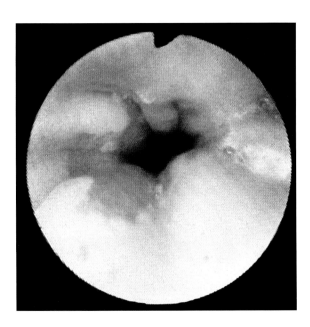

Figure 4-1

SHORT SEGMENT BARRETT ESOPHAGUS

At endoscopy, irregular tongues of gastric-appearing (erythematous) mucosa extend proximal to the gastroesophageal junction, which represents the proximal limit of the gastric folds.

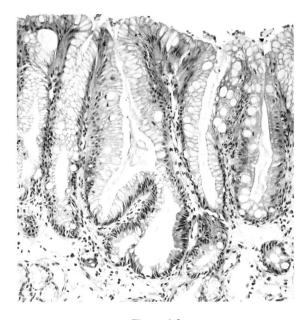

Figure 4-2

BARRETT ESOPHAGUS

The columnar epithelium is composed of a variety of cells, including goblet cells, mucinous columnar cells, distended mucinous cells (pseudogoblet cells), and a few mucous glands.

Table 4-1

RISK FACTORS FOR THE DEVELOPMENT OF BARRETT ESOPHAGUS AND ASSOCIATED NEOPLASTIC CONDITIONS

Factors	BE[a]	BE Neoplasm
Risk Factors		
Chronic GERD	√	-
Advancing age	√	√
Male gender	√	-
Central obesity (TBMI)	√	√
Caucasian race	√	-
Tobacco use	√	√
Hiatus hernia	√	√
1st degree relative of BE patient	√	-
Length of BE	√	√
Protective Factors		
NSAIDs	-	√
PPI	-	√
Statin	-	√
Equivocal Factors		
Alcohol	√	-

[a]BE = Barrett esophagus; BE Neoplasm = dysplasia or adenocarcinoma; GERD = gastroesophageal reflux disease; NSAIDs = nonsteroidal anti-inflammatory drugs; PPI = proton pump inhibitors.

Adenocarcinoma develops via a progressive sequence of histologic and molecular changes, from BE through various stages of dysplasia, to adenocarcinoma (6). Initially, BE metaplasia results from cellular reprogramming in a manner that changes the phenotypic commitment of the cells (7). Progenitor cells have been postulated to originate in either the esophagus, the proximal stomach, the bone marrow, or potentially from a variety of these organs (6,7). Recent evidence suggests that undifferentiated progenitor cells that lead to BE are located predominantly in the proximal stomach (gastric cardia); these are stimulated to differentiate into columnar epithelium as a result of ulceration (8). It is presumed that as a result of GERD-induced tissue damage, immature progenitor cells are reprogrammed to express columnar, rather than squamous, developmental transcription factors, which ultimately leads to healing with columnar epithelium, which is usually intestinalized, as an adaptive mechanism to protect the esophagus from further acid-induced injury.

The risk factors for the development of BE, and BE-associated neoplasia, have been the subject of extensive recent research (Table 4-1) (9). The known risk factors for BE include chronic (greater than 5 years) GERD symptoms, advancing patient age (particularly greater than 50 years), male gender, tobacco use, central obesity, and Caucasian race (9,10). In addition, BE is more common in first-degree relatives of patients with BE. Other reported risk factors include type II diabetes, sleep apnea, and metabolic syndrome (11–13). *Helicobacter pylori* infection (cag A+ strains) has been shown to be protective of BE in a few studies (14). No association has been noted between alcohol consumption and adenocarcinoma (15); in fact, wine consumption may be a protective factor (16). The risk factors for the development of dysplasia and adenocarcinoma are similar in some regard (9,10): advancing patient age, central obesity, and tobacco usage are known risk factors. Neoplasia is also related to increasing length of BE, lack of nonsteroidal anti-inflammatory drug (NSAID) use, lack of proton pump inhibitor (PPI) use, and lack of statin use.

There is recent evidence to suggest that risk factors vary according to patient age (17). In a recent pooled analysis from population-based case-controlled studies within the International Barrett's and Esophageal Adenocarcinoma Consortium (BEACON), which included 1,363 patients with adenocarcinoma and over 5,000 controls, body mass index (BMI), smoking status and pack-years, recurrent GERD and frequency of GERD were all associated with the development of adenocarcinoma in all patient age groups (under 50, 50 to 59, 60 to 69, and over 70 years) (17). Early onset adenocarcinoma (less than 50 years of age) is more strongly associated with GERD and BMI relative to older age groups.

The basis of cancer prevention in BE is based on surveillance of patients by endoscopy with biopsies (6,10). Morphologic demonstration of dysplasia in biopsies is the principal method of detecting an increased risk for cancer development in patients with BE, and this is discussed below.

DYSPLASIA

Definition. *Dysplasia* is defined as unequivocal intraepithelial columnar neoplasia, without evidence of invasion into the lamina propria (6). It is neoplastic-appearing epithelium that portends an increased risk of progression to adenocarcinoma.

General Features. The risk factors for dysplasia in patients with BE are similar to those for the development of adenocarcinoma. Dysplasia develops mainly in patients who have metaplastic intestinal-type epithelium, characterized by the presence of goblet cells (9,10). Some types of dysplasia, however, such as the foveolar type (see below), develop frequently in either goblet cell depleted or goblet cell absent BE (20,21).

Pathogenetically, dysplasia develops as a result of the accumulation of multiple genetic and epigenetic alterations, many of which occur even prior to the onset of morphologic dysplasia (22–24). Many of the molecular events, particularly those that occur early, are related to alterations of the cell cycle regulatory genes, apoptosis, cell signaling, and adhesion pathways (22–26); late changes are widespread genomic abnormalities, losses and gains in chromosome function, and especially, DNA instability characterized by tetraploidy, increased 4n fraction, and aneuploidy (23,24).

Advancing patient age and increasing BE segment length are risk factors specific for dysplasia (10). In one study of 309 BE patients, the risk factors for prevalent dysplasia included patient age (3.3 percent increase in dysplasia incidence per year) and BE length over 3 cm (13 percent increase in risk per centimeter of BE) (27). A variety of medications have been associated with a reduced risk of dysplasia, and these include use of PPIs, aspirin, NSAIDs, and statins (28–30).

The risk of dysplasia development in BE varies according to the type of study, the substantial intraobserver and interobserver variability in the diagnosis of dysplasia, and whether dysplasia is detected at the time of the initial (or within 1 year) diagnosis of BE ("prevalent" dysplasia) or during the course of endoscopic surveillance ("incident" dysplasia). Nevertheless, a recent meta-analysis suggests that the risk of progression to dysplasia in nondysplastic BE is lower than previously recorded (19).

Dysplasia may be detected as an isolated focus, but quite often it is present in multiple locations in the esophagus. Rarely, it is diffuse.

Clinical Features. There are no distinct clinical, radiologic, or laboratory manifestations of dysplasia in BE. The guidelines for screening and surveillance of patients with BE, and BE-associated dysplasia, are discussed in a recent publication by the American College of Gastro-enterology (ACG)(10). The guidelines are based on the fact that dysplasia is best detected by endoscopic evaluation of the mucosa, combined with biopsies of all four quadrants of the mucosa. Surveillance should be performed with the use of high-definition, high-resolution white light endoscopy, and by obtaining biopsies of all four quadrants of mucosa at 2-cm intervals in patients without dysplasia, and at 1-cm intervals in patients with dysplasia. All visible mucosal abnormalities should be sampled separately. Systematic biopsy protocols clearly detect more dysplasia, and early cancer, compared to random biopsy protocols (31–33). Mucosal abnormalities, such as ulcerations, plaques, nodules, and strictures, are associated with an increased risk of underlying cancer, and thus, these areas should all be sampled extensively (33).

In recent years, a wide variety of enhancements to endoscopic imaging with white light endoscopy have been studied. These include electronic chromoendoscopy, narrow band imaging, high definition white light endoscopy, methylene blue staining, acetic acid staining, indigo carmine staining, auto-fluorescent endoscopy, confocal laser endomicroscopy, volumetric laser endomicroscopy, spectroscopy, and molecular imaging. None of these methods, however, are recommended for clinical use at the time of this publication (10). Recently, a prospective random mixed trial of wide-area transepithelial sampling with computer-assisted three-dimensional analysis has shown marked improvements in the detection of BE (goblet cells) and dysplasia. This technique allows for greater sampling of BE mucosa and reduces sampling error.

Gross Findings. Endoscopically, dysplasia may be visibly undetectable, or appear as a flat, plaque-like or irregular area of mucosa distinct from the surrounding nondysplastic BE (6,33,34). Occasionally, dysplasia may be nodular, polypoid, or ulcerated. The endoscopic appearance has been associated with risk of progression to adenocarcinoma (35–37).

Microscopic Findings. *Grading of Dysplasia.* In most Western countries, dysplasia is classified as negative, indefinite (fig. 4-3), or positive (either low [fig. 4-4] or high grade) according to a standardized system that was developed in 1988 by Reid et al. (38). Many pathologists from

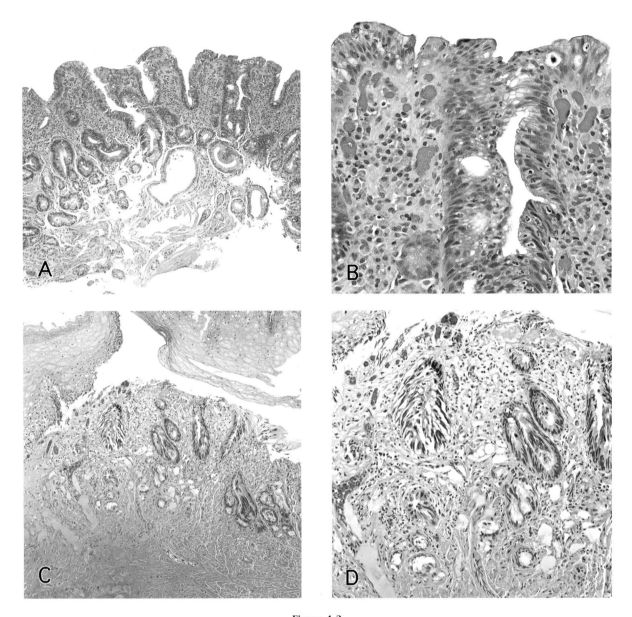

Figure 4-3

INDEFINITE FOR DYSPLASIA

A: This category is for lesions that have epithelial changes that are concerning for dysplasia, but are not diagnostic. In this case, the surface shows nuclear stratification, but there is abundant inflammation.

B: The epithelium shows nuclear stratification, but the polarity is maintained and there are numerous intraepithelial neutrophils.

C: Endoscopic mucosal resection. There are glands with hyperchromatic nuclei, but they show prominent diathermy, which interferes with interpretation.

D: Prominent diathermy/cautery artifact impedes histologic evaluation.

other countries, and particularly those from Europe and Asia, however, use the modified Vienna classification of dysplasia (Table 4-2). The Vienna system is similar to the Reid system, except that it uses the term "noninvasive neoplasia" instead of "dysplasia" and adds a separate category for lesions that are "suspicious for invasive carcinoma." The Vienna system was

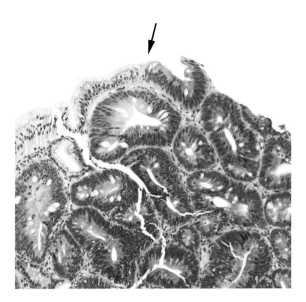 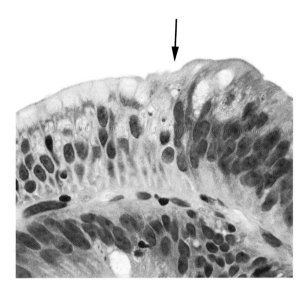

Figure 4-4

INTESTINAL-TYPE DYSPLASIA, LOW GRADE

Left: The dysplasia has an appearance similar to that of a colorectal tubular adenoma. Note the abrupt transition between an area of gastric-type epithelium and low-grade dysplasia (arrow).

Right: There is a sharp demarcation between the dysplastic and nondysplastic epithelium in this high-magnification image. The nuclei in the dysplasia are larger.

Table 4-2

VIENNA AND REID CLASSIFICATION OF DYSPLASIA IN BARRETT ESOPHAGUS

Vienna	Reid
1. Negative for neoplasia/dysplasia	Negative for dysplasia
2. Indefinite for neoplasia/dysplasia	Indefinite for dysplasia
3. Noninvasive low-grade neoplasia (low-grade adenoma/dysplasia)	Low-grade dysplasia
4. Noninvasive high-grade neoplasia High-grade dysplasia Noninvasive carcinoma (carcinoma in situ) Suspicious of invasive carcinoma	High-grade dysplasia
5. Invasive neoplasia Intramucosal adenocarcinoma Submucosal carcinoma or beyond	Adenocarcinoma Intramucosal adenocarcinoma Invasive adenocarcinoma

developed in an effort to reduce discrepancies in interpretation of dysplasia between pathologists in different countries worldwide.

Dysplasia Types. The two most common histologic types of dysplasia are *intestinal (adenoma-like)* and *nonintestinal* which is commonly referred to as *foveolar* (or *gastric*) *dysplasia* (Table 4-3) (6,40–42). Rarely, dysplasia may have a serrated pattern of growth similar to serrated neoplasia in the colon of patients with inflammatory bowel disease (43).

More often dysplasia shows a mixture of histologic types, which is most commonly a combination of intestinal and foveolar types.

Intestinal-type dysplasia is the most common. It is characterized by epithelium that resembles that of conventional adenoma of the colon, composed of columnar cells with intestinal differentiation, including goblet cells and enterocyte-like cells (6). Low-grade dysplasia (LGD) is characterized by cells with nuclear enlargement,

Table 4-3

HISTOLOGIC FEATURES OF DYSPLASIA IN BARRETT ESOPHAGUS

Histologic Feature	Intestinal		Foveolar		Serrated	
	LGD[a]	HGD	LGD	HGD	LGD	HGD
Nuclear size	2-3X	3-4X	2-3X	2-4X	1-2X	2-3X
Chromatin pattern	Dense	Dense	Dense or open	Dense or open	Dense	Dense
Nuclear stratification	Basal only	Full thickness	None	+/-	Mild	Mod
Mitoses	+	++	+	++	+	++
Atypical mitoses	+/-	+	+/-	+	+/-	+
Nuclear elongation	++	++	+/-	+/-	+	++
Round/oval nuclei	-	-	+	++	-	-
Loss of polarity	+/-	++	+/-	++	+/-	++
Pleomorphism	+/-	++	+/-	++	+/-	++
Surface involvement	- to ++	- to ++	++	++	++	++
Goblet cells	- to ++	- to ++	-	-	+/-	+/-
Mucinous cytoplasm	-	-	++	+	-	-
Hypereosinophilic cytoplasm	+/-	+/-	_	_	++	++
Prominent nucleoli	+/-	+/-	++	++	+/-	+/-
Crypt architectural irregularities[b]	- to +	- to ++	-	- to ++	-	- to ++
Luminal saw tooth	-	-	-	-	+	++

[a]LGD = low-grade dysplasia; HGD = high-grade dysplasia.
[b]Irregular size and shape of crypts, intraluminal budding, cribriforming, branching, back-to-back gland pattern

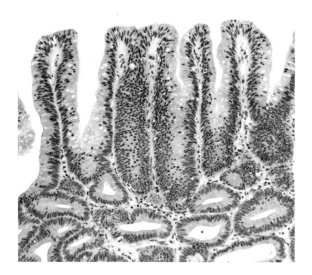

Figure 4-5

INTESTINAL-TYPE DYSPLASIA, LOW GRADE

The epithelium shows a tubulovillous proliferation of cells with hyperchromatic elongated and slightly stratified nuclei. The epithelium shows no evidence of surface maturation. There is no significant architectural distortion.

elongation (often referred to as pencil-shaped), hyperchromasia, and stratification (fig. 4-5). The cells mostly retain their nuclear polarity, with the long axis of the nucleus oriented perpendicular to the basement membrane. Mitoses are generally increased in number and more frequent in the bases of the crypts compared to the surface epithelium. The cells show nuclear stratification that is typically limited to the basal portion of the cytoplasm. The cytoplasm of dysplastic cells is generally mucin depleted and may show hypereosinophilia. Goblet cells may vary from few to numerous, but in general, decrease in number with advancing grade of dysplasia, especially compared to nondysplastic BE.

The dysplastic features of LGD are more marked in the bases of the crypts than the surface epithelium. In some cases, dysplasia is restricted completely to the bases of the crypts, and this is referred to as *crypt dysplasia* (fig. 4-6) (44,45). By definition, LGD shows little, if any, architectural crypt abnormalities. The crypts normally show visible evidence of lamina propria between them. However, as in nondysplastic BE, the bases of the crypts may show some budding or angulation, which is the normal "baseline" architecture of BE mucosa.

High-grade dysplasia (HGD) shows a greater degree of cytologic atypia but, in addition, usually shows significant architectural abnormalities of the crypts as well (fig. 4-7). Cytologically, HGD is characterized by the presence of markedly enlarged nuclei (3 to 4 times the size of lymphocytes), full-thickness nuclear stratification both in the crypt base and in the surface epithelium, mild to marked nuclear pleomorphism, irregular nuclear contours, and most significantly, loss of nuclear polarity. Mitoses are usually increased in number and may be present on the surface epithelium as well. Atypical mitoses are common. Intraluminal necrosis may be present as well. In some HGD cases, the dysplastic cells have enlarged round or irregular-shaped nuclei, with vesicular nuclei and prominent nucleoli, but this is more common in high-grade nonintestinal dysplasia. Architecturally, the crypts in HGD may vary in size and shape, appear crowded, and contain significant budding or angulation. The surface epithelium may appear villiform in contour. Back-to-back gland formation and cribriforming are common. A diagnosis of HGD is established in the presence of high-grade cytologic or architectural aberrations, but most cases show a combination of both.

Nonintestinal dysplasia resembles gastric foveolar epithelium because it contains prominent cytoplasmic mucin, and typically has few, if any, goblet cells (40,41,46). It represents about 6 to 8 percent of all BE dysplasia, but true prevalence studies have not been performed (6). Low-grade nonintestinal dysplasia consists of uniform columnar cells, usually in a single layer, containing small or slightly enlarged round to oval, basally located nuclei without stratification or significant pleomorphism (fig. 4-8). In some cases, the nuclei may be pencil-shaped and elongated, similar to intestinal-type dysplasia. In contrast to intestinal dysplasia, the degree of cytologic atypia of nonintestinal dysplasia may be more severe on the surface epithelium compared to the bases of the crypts. Mitoses are usually less common than in intestinal dysplasia. The surface epithelium may be villiform in contour.

In high-grade nonintestinal dysplasia, the epithelium shows cells with markedly increased

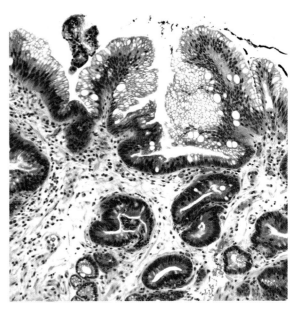

Figure 4-6

CRYPT DYSPLASIA

In this portion of mucosa, the bases of the crypts show histologic features of low-grade dysplasia: hyperchromatic elongated and slightly stratified nuclei. However, the surface epithelium shows maturation, and there is no significant inflammation.

nuclear/cytoplasmic (N/C) ratio and more irregular nuclear contours, often with an open chromatin pattern, prominent nucleoli, and increased mitoses (fig. 4-9) (46). Some cases, however, show marked stratification, of nuclei similar to intestinal-type dysplasia. Significant loss of polarity, stratification, and pleomorphism are not as common in nonintestinal dysplasia, even those that are high grade. Architecturally, HGD shows more compact and elongated crypts with increased branching and complexity, and often without intervening lamina propria.

Nonintestinal dysplasia may develop in metaplastic columnar mucosa without goblet cells (43). In one recent study by Agoston (42) of 122 patients with BE-associated adenocarcinoma, the type of dysplasia (nonintestinal versus intestinal) in the background BE mucosa correlated well with the type of adenocarcinoma (gastric versus intestinal) present in the esophagus. This suggests the possibility of multiple pathways of carcinogenesis in esophageal adenocarcinoma.

Rarely, dysplasia may appear serrated, showing a saw-tooth or jagged epithelial contour, and

Figure 4-7

INTESTINAL-TYPE DYSPLASIA, HIGH GRADE

A: The dysplasia is composed of tightly packed glands lined by cells with large hyperchromatic nuclei and loss of polarity.

B: Another example of high-grade dysplasia showing a mildly villiform contour of the epithelium.

C: Marked loss of polarity (arrows) and nuclear pleomorphism highlight this form of high-grade dysplasia.

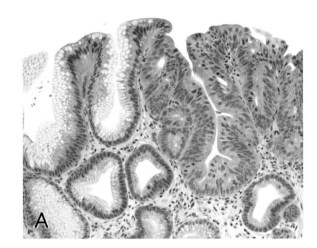

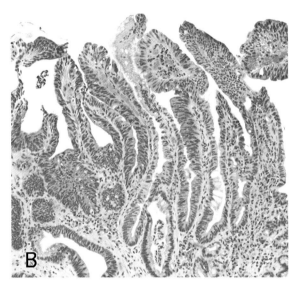

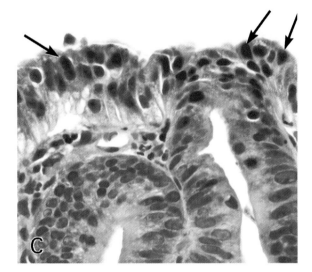

containing cells with small oval, hyperchromatic nuclei with abundant hypereosinophilic cytoplasm and few goblet cells (fig. 4-10) (43). In this type of dysplasia, the surface epithelium and superficial crypts are typically involved more severely than the bases. *High-grade serrated dysplasia* shows increased stratification, increased mitoses, atypical mitoses, more significant loss of polarity, and a more prominent intraluminal serrated growth pattern.

Immunohistochemical Findings. Dysplasia is characterized by increased Ki-67 staining, which in LGD is typically highest in the bases of the crypts compared to the surface epithelium, but it is usually high in the surface epithelium in HGD. Other markers that may be positive include PCNA, cyclin D1, p53, IGF2BP3, and AMACR (23–26,47,48). By flow cytometry, dysplasia, and in particular HGD, may show abnormal DNA content in the form of increased 4n fraction, tetraploidy, and aneuploidy (49). Some of these markers may be used as adjunctive tests to help differentiate nondysplastic from dysplastic epithelium, discussed further below.

Molecular Genetic Findings. Molecular features are discussed in the section on adenocarcinoma (47,48).

Differential Diagnosis. The main problems associated with dysplasia pathology include: 1) differentiating nondysplastic from truly dysplastic epithelium, 2) differentiating LGD from HGD, and 3) distinguishing HGD from

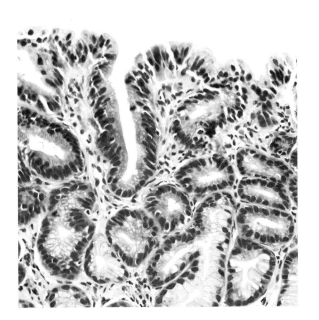
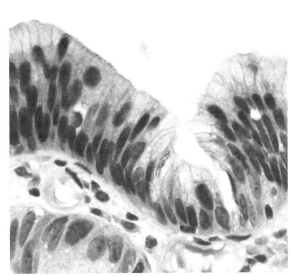

Figure 4-8

NONINTESTINAL (FOVEOLAR) DYSPLASIA, LOW GRADE

In contrast to intestinal dysplasia, nonintestinal dysplasia shows smaller, more regular nuclei that are more oval-shaped or slightly elongated, and oriented perpendicular to the basement membrane. There is less stratification than in intestinal-type dysplasia. The cytoplasm shows mucinous differentiation, without goblet cells. This particular focus arose within an area of esophageal columnar metaplasia composed of oxyntic glands, but without goblet cells.

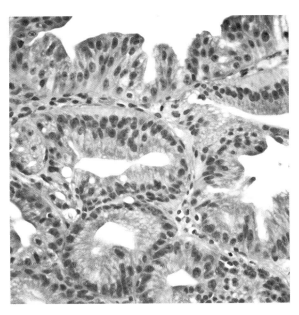
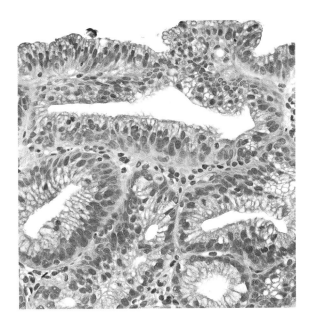

Figure 4-9

NONINTESTINAL (FOVEOLAR) DYSPLASIA, HIGH GRADE

Left: The nuclei are more round to oval shaped and show distinct loss of nuclear polarity. Nonintestinal dysplasia usually lacks the high degree of nuclear hyperchromasia that characterizes intestinal-type dysplasia.

Right: This focus shows foveolar differentiation and stratification. Many of the cells have apical mucin similar in appearance to gastric foveolar cells.

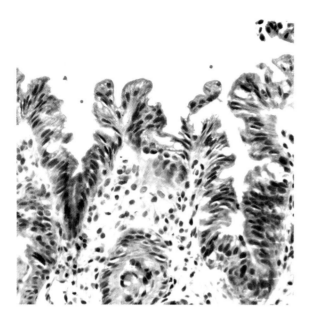

Figure 4-10

SERRATED DYSPLASIA

The epithelium shows enlarged hyperchromatic, slightly elongated and pencil-shaped nuclei with stratification. The cytoplasm is hypereosinophilic, and most significantly, shows a prominent serrated or sawtooth growth pattern.

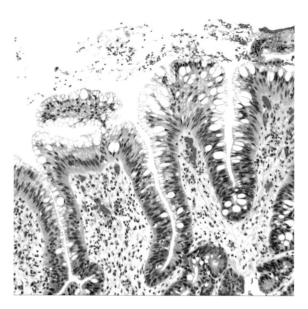

Figure 4-11

BARRETT ESOPHAGUS WITH REACTIVE CHANGES

Barrett esophagus with marked regenerative changes. The epithelium shows elongated crypts with hyperchromatic, elongated and stratified nuclei and with increased mitoses. However, the epithelium shows slight maturation of the surface and also active inflammation within the epithelium itself. This likely represents the extreme of regeneration, but if uncertain, it is appropriate to diagnose this as "indefinite for dysplasia" and have the patient rebiopsied after the inflammation subsides.

intramucosal (or invasive) adenocarcinoma. Given the subtle gradation of changes that occurs in the progression of dysplasia in BE, and the fact that neoplastic progression occurs in a linear rather than a graded scale, there continues to be a significant degree of intraobserver and interobserver variability in the diagnosis of dysplasia among general and expert pathologists (50,51). In general, the highest degree of variability occurs at the low and high ends of the spectrum of dysplasia: at the low end, separating nondysplastic from dysplastic epithelium, and at the high end, separating HGD from cancer. In an interobserver study among expert gastrointestinal pathologists, the interobserver agreement for diagnosis and grading of early and late dysplastic lesions in BE was only moderate (52). Also, there is a tendency among general pathologists to overdiagnose dysplasia. In one study of 485 BE cases diagnosed as HGD by a general pathologist, 40 percent of patients had their diagnosis downgraded to either no dysplasia (11 percent), indefinite for dysplasia (12 percent), or LGD (16 percent), after a review by an experienced gastrointestinal pathologist (53).

Distinguishing nondysplastic from dysplastic epithelium is a major problem in diagnosis because regenerative changes can be marked, particularly in areas of active inflammation or ulceration, and the histologic features may overlap significantly with LGD, and on occasion HGD (fig. 4-11). When a pathologist is uncertain whether a biopsy shows regenerative or true dysplastic features, the temporary diagnostic category of "indefinite for dysplasia" is used, with the recommendation that repeat biopsies should be considered after the patient's inflammation (or ulceration) has subsided. This diagnostic term is used most often in situations in which difficulty in interpretation is due to technical issues, the presence of atypia related to inflammation and ulceration as mentioned above, or dysplasia-like changes are present only in the bases of the crypts without evidence of surface involvement. Inflammation and ulceration cause the epithelium to show extreme regenerative changes, such as marked nuclear enlargement and stratification, hyperchromaticity, mucin depletion, and increased mitoses. In contrast to dysplasia, however, regenerating epithelium more often shows surface maturation and a gradual transition from atypical epithelium to nonatypical (background) BE, and the atypical changes usually parallel the degree and intensity of inflammation in that particular area of mucosa. Features that favor dysplasia include lack of surface maturation, an abrupt transition to adjacent nonatypical epithelium, and atypical mitoses, particularly if located at the surface. Significant architectural aberrations also favor dysplasia.

Several adjunctive, mainly immunohistochemical, markers have been investigated in order to help pathologists distinguish nondysplastic (regenerating) from dysplastic epithelium. These include cyclin D1, Ki-67, DNA content, telomerase, genetic mutations (such as *TP53*, *CDKN2A*, *APC*), beta-catenin, growth factors, apoptosis inhibitors, IMP3, and AMACR (6,47,48,54,55). Of these, Ki-67, p53, and AMACR have been most extensively studied, and each has diagnostic problems. Although Ki-67 often shows more significant staining in the base of the crypt compared to the surface epithelium, on occasion, regenerating epithelium may show marked positivity on the surface epithelium as well, similar to dysplasia. The use of p53 in the differential diagnosis of dysplasia is controversial. In general, the frequency of *p53* mutations increases from BE to LGD to HGD and adenocarcinoma (23). In some studies, however, p53 may be present in up to 10 percent of morphologically nondysplastic epithelium, and there is a high rate of false negativity and positivity (23,24,54). Some cases may show complete absence (null staining) of p53 as well (23,24,50,54). Studies have shown a high degree of specificity of AMACR for dysplasia, but low sensitivity (55,56). In one study, 0 percent of nondysplastic, 22 percent of indefinite, 18 percent of LGD, and 60 percent of HGD cases were positive for AMACR (57). Morphologic assessment of dysplasia remains the gold standard method for evaluating dysplasia. The American Gastroenterological Association (AGA) does not recommend the use of molecular biomarkers to confirm a histologic diagnosis of dysplasia (18).

Distinguishing LGD from HGD is problematic primarily because the changes in dysplasia progress in a linear, not stepwise, fashion. Also,

no consensus has been reached on how much HGD is required to be present in a biopsy in order to upgrade a biopsy from LGD to HGD (fig. 4-12); most authorities, however, believe that it is justified to establish a diagnosis of HGD when any amount of HGD (even one crypt) is present in a biopsy sample.

Distinguishing HGD from intramucosal, or even invasive, adenocarcinoma may also be problematic, particularly when glands show cribriforming or a back-to-back gland pattern, contain intraluminal necrotic debris, or are present either within or beneath muscularis mucosae fibers in biopsy samples (fig. 4-13). In one study, a kappa value of 0.30, which is fair at best, was found among several gastrointestinal pathologists for distinguishing HGD from intramucosal adenocarcinoma (58). Features that favor adenocarcinoma include an expanding glandular growth pattern, markedly irregular and angulated glands, glands that show significant variability in size and shape including small gland back-to-back profiles, and single cell infiltration.

Differentiating intramucosal from submucosally invasive adenocarcinoma may be difficult, particularly when the biopsies are tangentially sectioned, maloriented, or show duplication of the muscularis mucosae. Entrapped glands within muscularis fibers should not be overinterpreted as indicative of invasive tumor, particularly if the glands are cytologically low grade. Since most patients with BE have a duplicated muscularis mucosae, dysplastic glands present within, or even beneath, the new (superficial) muscularis mucosae, are still considered "intramucosal" for management purposes (59). On occasion, dysplastic glands are buried underneath squamous epithelium ("buried BE" or "buried dysplasia"); this is particularly common post endoscopic therapy (fig. 4-14) (60). Buried or subsquamous dysplastic glands should not be overinterpreted as invasive adenocarcinoma.

Prognosis. Reported progression rates of LGD vary between 3 and 23 percent in various studies (4,61,62). This range is undoubtedly due to interobserver variability in the diagnosis of LGD among both community and expert pathologists. In one meta-analysis of LGD, the pooled annual incidence rate of progression to adenocarcinoma alone was 0.5 percent for adenocarcinoma alone,

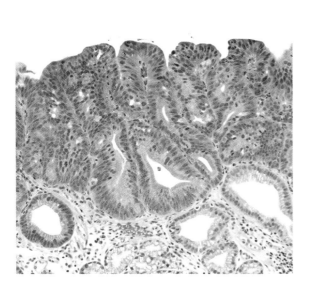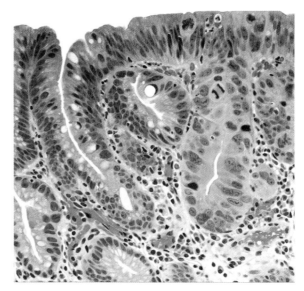

Figure 4-12

BARRETT ESOPHAGUS-ASSOCIATED DYSPLASIA, HIGH GRADE

The biopsy shows a gradiation of changes from low- to high-grade dysplasia.

Left: Low-grade dysplasia is seen on the right and high-grade on the left side of the image. Epithelium with slightly more enlarged nuclei, back-to-back gland formation, and a gland-in-gland pattern is characteristic of high-grade dysplasia. Based on the presence of at least focal high-grade dysplasia areas, this biopsy is best be diagnosed as "high-grade dysplasia."

Right: On a background of low-grade dysplasia, there are two crypts that show much more significant cytologic atypia, composed of cells with enlarged, round to irregular-shaped nuclei, with an open chromatin pattern, prominent nucleoli, distinct loss of polarity, and increased mitoses. Surface mitoses are present as well. Although these were the only two high-grade dysplastic crypts in the patient, it is best to consider a diagnosis of "high-grade dysplasia" for the patient overall.

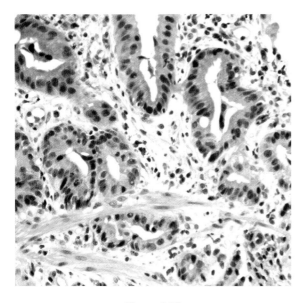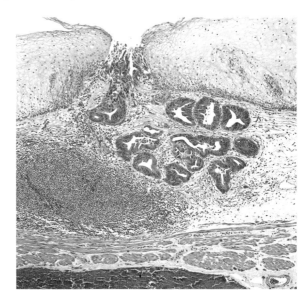

Figure 4-13

HIGH-GRADE DYSPLASIA IN BARRETT ESOPHAGUS

Dysplastic crypts are located between fibers of the muscularis mucosae, the latter of which likely represents the neo (newly developed), more luminally situated, muscularis mucosae that is often found in BE.

Figure 4-14

BURIED DYSPLASIA

Dysplastic crypts are buried underneath islands of residual, or re-epithelialized, squamous epithelium. This is common in patients who have had endoscopic ablative therapy and should not be overinterpreted as representing adenocarcinoma.

Table 4-4

UNITED STATES GUIDELINES FOR TREATMENT OF BARRETT ESOPHAGUS AND DYSPLASIA[a]

Type of Barrett Esophagus	Management Guidelines General/Surveillance	EMR	Ablation	Esophagectomy
No dysplasia	PPI Q 3-5 year endoscopy	-	-	-
Indefinite	↑ PPI Repeat biopsy after inflammation subsides, if confirmed then Q 1 year endoscopy	-	-	-
LGD	Confirm with expert pathologist ↑ PPI Repeat biopsy if confirmed Q 1 year endoscopy If 2 endoscopies normal, then Q 3-5 endoscopy	yes for mucosal nodules	+/-[b]	-
HGD	Confirm with expert pathologist ↑ PPI	yes for mucosal nodules	yes	+/-[c]

[a]Adapted from reference 10.
[b]May be preferred over surveillance.
[c]May be preferred in rare circumstances.

and 1.7 percent for HGD and adenocarcinoma combined (63). In this analysis, the incidence was 5.4 per 1000 person years (95 percent CI; 3.0-8.0). For progression to HGD or adenocarcinoma, it was 173 per 1000 person years (95 percent CI; 100-250). In a recent population-based European study, the risk of progression to adenocarcinoma was five times higher in patients with LGD than in those without dysplasia (65).

The rate of cancer development in patients with HGD is much higher, but also shows significant variability. In some studies up to 55 percent of patients with HGD progress to cancer in 5 years of follow-up (49,61,62). HGD is associated with at least a 6 percent incidence of cancer per year (64).

In a recent meta-analysis of four studies from 236 patients, a weighted annual incidence rate of cancer in patients with HGD was 7 percent (95 percent CI; 5-8) (66). However, in the AIM dysplasia trial that randomized 127 patients with dysplasia to ablation therapy compared to surveillance, a much higher yearly progression rate to cancer was noted in patients with HGD (19 percent) (67). Progression rates for both LGD or HGD have been shown to correlate with the number of pathologists who agree with the diagnosis (68).

With regard to the growth pattern of the lesion, HGD associated with a nodular abnormality at endoscopy shows an association rate with cancer of 60 percent, compared to HGD without an endoscopic abnormality (22 percent) (35). In

another study, "polypoid" dysplasia showed a higher association with adenocarcinoma, both within the polyp and in the adjacent mucosa, compared to nonpolypoid dysplasia (36). Ulceration is also associated with an increased risk of adenocarcinoma in patients with dysplasia (37). Other risk factors for progression include stricture formation, the length of the BE segment, and the presence of a hiatus hernia (69,70).

Many potential immunohistochemical and molecular biomarkers have been evaluated as markers of progression. The most common are p53 abnormalities, p16 abnormalities, and DNA content abnormalities. Several studies have shown an association between aberrant p53 expression and an increased risk of neoplastic progression (48,50,71,72). Genomic instability, such as copy number alterations and loss of heterozygosity (LOH), are useful markers of progression in BE as well (73). Some studies show that a combination of biomarkers, such as DNA content abnormalities and LOH of p53 and p16, is a more sensitive and specific indicator of progression than these markers alone (74,75).

Treatment. The management of patients with dysplasia is evolving, especially considering advancements in endoscopic and ablative therapy (Table 4-4). A recently published clinical guideline by the ACG reviews the current management scheme of dysplasia in BE (10,34). The management of patients is dependent on whether dysplasia is detected in flat columnar mucosa or whether it occurs in endoscopically visible abnormal or nodular mucosa. The type of therapies available include chemoprevention, increased surveillance, endoscopic therapy and ablation, endoscopic mucosal resection, and surgical resection. Regardless of the particular management scheme used, all diagnoses of dysplasia should be confirmed by a second pathologist with extensive experience in the interpretation of BE-associated neoplasia (10,34,51).

For patients with confirmed LGD, the treatment includes aggressive antisecretory therapy with PPIs, repeat endoscopy after optimization of acid suppressant therapy, followed by either annual endoscopic surveillance or endoscopic eradication therapy. If annual surveillance is chosen, it should be performed until two examinations in a row are negative for dysplasia, after which time surveillance intervals for nondysplastic BE can be followed. The protocol for surveillance biopsies in patients with dysplasia include four quadrant biopsies, at 1-cm intervals over the entire length of the BE. Endoscopic mucosal resection (EMR) should be performed if any mucosal abnormality is present, prior to endoscopic ablative therapy.

For pathologically confirmed HGD, endoscopic ablative therapy is warranted and highly advised over aggressive endoscopic surveillance, and this treatment should be preceded by EMR if it is associated with any form of mucosal abnormality. This is similar to the protocol recommended for stage T1a adenocarcinomas. Surgical resection is generally recommended only in patients whose EMR specimens demonstrate neoplasia at the lateral or deep margins, or if there is a T1b adenocarcinoma showing invasion into the mid or deep submucosa. For patients with T1a or early T1b (invasion into the superficial submucosa) adenocarcinoma, poor tumor differentiation, lymphovascular invasion, or incomplete EMR, surgical or multi-modality therapies including neoadjuvant chemotherapy are used.

In patients with biopsies that are indefinite for dysplasia, PPI therapy should be optimized, and a repeat endoscopy performed. Once indefinite is confirmed by a second pathologist, then the recommendation is for endoscopic surveillance similar to that recommended for patients with LGD.

The guidelines for postablation surveillance and management are controversial (10,34). For patients with HGD prior to ablation, endoscopic surveillance should be continued to detect recurrent BE and/or dysplasia, and this is recommended every 3 months for the first year following ablation, every 6 months in the second year, and then annually thereafter. For patients with LGD prior to ablation, endoscopic surveillance is recommended every 6 months in the first year, followed by every year thereafter. Treatment of recurrent dysplasia should follow similar guidelines for dysplasia detected prior to ablation.

ADENOCARCINOMA

Definition. *Esophageal adenocarcinoma* is an invasive malignant epithelial neoplasm with glandular and/or mucinous differentiation. Some adenocarcinomas are mucinous because they produce either intracellular or luminal mucin.

General Features. The World Health Organization (WHO) recognizes three rare subtypes of adenocarcinoma (76). The first is *adenoid cystic carcinoma*, a tumor histologically similar to that which arises in the salivary glands, and not associated with BE. The other two are *adenosquamous* and *mucoepidermoid carcinomas*, both of which are tumors that show a combination of glandular and squamous differentiation, and only rarely develop in patients with BE.

The epidemiology, demographics, pathogenesis, and risk factors are covered more fully in the general features section for BE and dysplasia. As mentioned above, more than 95 percent of adenocarcinomas develop in association with BE. Adenocarcinomas also develop in the submucosal glands or ducts, or from foci of heterotopic epithelium, but these are extremely rare. Adenocarcinomas may also arise from the gastroesophageal junction (GEJ) where a significant proportion are believed to develop as a result of very short segments of BE (6,77,78,79).

Clinical Features. The demographics of patients with adenocarcinoma are similar to those with BE. It affects predominantly older men (mean age, 60 years) with a male to female ratio about 3.7 to 1.0. More than 80 percent of patients are white (9,17,80). Depending on the size and location of the tumor, patients present with dysphagia, odynophagia, obstruction, or gastrointestinal bleeding (81). Dysphagia and weight loss are usually associated with advanced disease.

The most commonly used methods to diagnose and stage patients with esophageal adenocarcinoma include a combination of upper gastrointestinal tract contrast studies combined with endoscopy and biopsy (82). After an initial diagnosis is made, subsequent radiologic studies are usually performed in order to stage the cancer as accurately as possible. The first diagnostic method is usually a computerized tomography (CT) scan with oral and intravenous contrast. This method is very useful for identifying distant metastatic disease, such as in the liver and lungs. A position emission tomography (PET) scan improves staging in up to 20 percent of patients when a CT scan does not show evidence of metastatic disease (83). When the CT and PET scans fail to demonstrate metastatic disease, an endoscopic ultrasound (EUS) is typically performed in order to establish the extent of local regional disease, the depth of tumor invasion (T status), and the extent of lymph node involvement (84). EUS is less accurate for early stage lesions (T1 or T2) compared to more advanced stage tumors (85). Sometimes EUS is combined with fine-needle aspiration and this improves the sensitivity and specificity of identifying lymph node metastases (86). Upper aerodigestive endoscopy, such as bronchoscopy, is sometimes added for tumors of the upper and middle esophagus, but this is more common for squamous cell carcinoma than adenocarcinoma (82). In some instances, physicians prefer staging by a minimally invasive surgical technique, such as thoracoscopy or laparoscopy, in order to improve detection of potential metastases in the pleura or peritoneum (87).

Known specific factors increase the risk of adenocarcinoma in patients with BE. These include the presence, grade, and extent of dysplasia (49,88); DNA aneuploidy; greater lengths of BE (88,90); and the presence of a hiatus hernia (69,90).

A current area of controversy concerns the magnitude of risk of adenocarcinoma in patients without goblet cells in their metaplastic columnar mucosa (6). For most patients, adenocarcinoma arises in BE with goblet cells. In some studies, however, up to 50 percent of patients do not show goblet cells in the background columnar mucosa (91). In one study by Golden et

al. (92), the extent of goblet cell metaplasia was shown to be protective of both the development of aneuploidy and adenocarcinoma, but this was in a population of BE patients who had at least one goblet cell identified in their BE. Detailed genomic analysis of single crypts have shown that adenocarcinoma may develop from nonintestinal clones of cells (93,94). Furthermore, the background non-goblet columnar epithelium in BE has been shown to harbor genetic alterations associated with neoplastic progression (95,96). Therefore, although the magnitude of the risk of development of cancer in BE patients without goblet cells is currently unknown, current evidence suggests that this pathway accounts for a definite, albeit small, percentage of malignant tumor development (6,20,97,98).

Gross Findings. BE-associated adenocarcinomas are located predominantly in the distal third of the esophagus, and always within areas of BE. Distal tumors may extend into the proximal stomach. At early stages of development, the carcinomas appear only as an irregular mucosal abnormality, bump, nodule, or plaque. With advancing stages of growth, the tumors become ulcerated, polypoid, fungating, or stricturing (fig. 4-15). Polypoid (protruding) tumors account for 5 to 10 percent; flat tumors, 10 to 15 percent; fungating tumors, 20 to 25 percent; and diffusely infiltrative, 30 to 50 percent of cases (99,100). Large tumors may obliterate evidence of background BE, particularly those that arise in the distal esophagus and GEJ region. Patients treated with preoperative neoadjuvant chemotherapy or radiotherapy may show no gross evidence of residual tumor in up to 50 percent of cases. In these patients, an ulcerated tumor bed is usually visible (101,104).

Microscopic Findings. Histologically, esophageal adenocarcinomas are similar in many ways to gastric adenocarcinomas. Most cases are intestinal type according to the Lauren classification of gastric cancer (103). Fewer esophageal carcinomas are "diffuse." These are tumors that show discohesive or signet ring cells, with only rare gland formation. Similar to adenocarcinomas in other portions of the gastrointestinal tract, esophageal adenocarcinomas show a variable degree of neuroendocrine cell, Paneth cell, and rarely, squamous cell differentiation (104). Mucinous adenocarcinoma, defined as a tumor in which

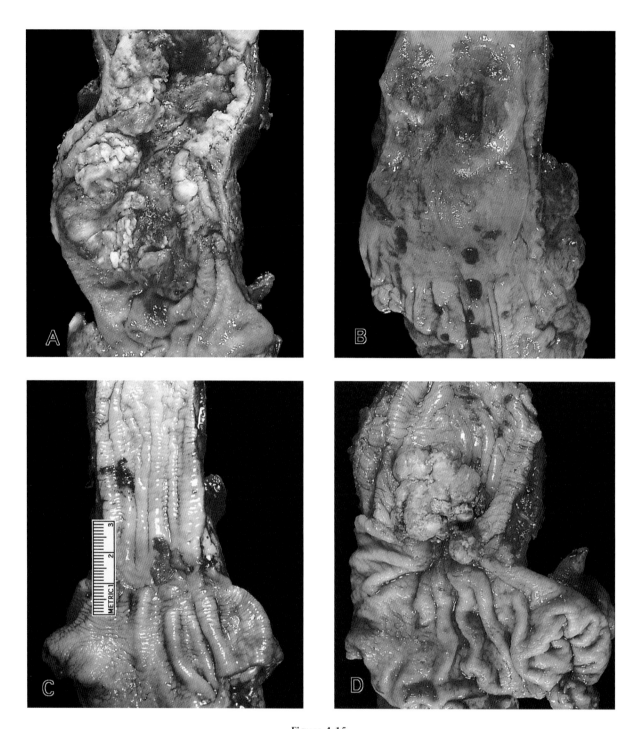

Figure 4-15

BARRETT ESOPHAGUS AND ADENOCARCINOMA

A: A large, fungating, exophytic and stricturing adenocarcinoma is seen in a patient with BE.

B: Slightly irregular and nodular adenocarcinoma shows central ulceration. It occurs within a tongue of BE located proximal to the gastroesophageal junction.

C: Small tongues of BE extend proximal to the gastroesophageal junction and contain a slightly irregular, plaque-like appearance that represents an early adenocarcinoma.

D: Distal esophageal adenocarcinoma located proximal to the gastroesophageal junction which has a nodular exophytic growth pattern.

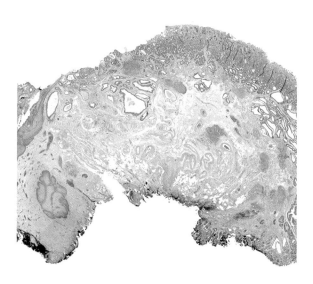

Figure 4-16

BARRETT ESOPHAGUS AND ADENOCARCINOMA

A well-differentiated adenocarcinoma composed of small tubules is invading the lamina propria, and focally into the superficial submucosa.

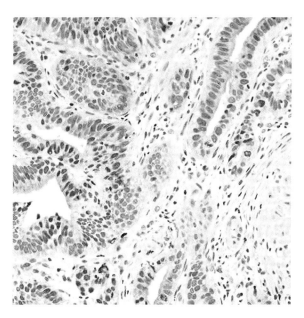

Figure 4-17

BARRETT ESOPHAGUS AND ADENOCARCINOMA

Desmoplasia is not a prominent feature in most early well-differentiated adenocarcinomas, particularly when they are superficially invasive.

greater than 50 percent of the lesion consists of intracellular and/or extracellular mucin production, accounts for only a small proportion of malignant tumors in the esophagus (76).

Esophageal adenocarcinomas are graded as well, moderately, or poorly differentiated according to the proportion of tumor composed of glands (105). Similar to colon cancer, most esophageal adenocarcinomas are moderately or well differentiated. Well-differentiated tumors are defined as those that show more than 95 percent glands, moderately differentiated are those that have 50 to 95 percent glands, and poorly differentiated are composed of less than 50 percent glands. Most moderately or well-differentiated cancers show irregularly shaped papillary or tubular profiles that infiltrate the wall of the esophagus (fig. 4-16). The tumor cells are typically columnar or less often cuboidal in shape and contain enlarged nuclei with course or vesicular chromatin, irregular nuclear membranes, often prominent and multiple nucleoli, and various amounts of eosinophilic or clear cytoplasm. As the tumors become less differentiated, the cells may be arranged in solid aggregates, cords, and irregular papillary structures, and the glandular

profiles may show microcystic change and considerable nuclear stratification (fig. 4-17).

Poorly differentiated carcinomas show sheets of cells, bizarre pleomorphic tumor cells, and discohesive and signet ring cells (fig. 4-18). Desmoplasia is common in moderately and, particularly, poorly differentiated carcinomas. Paneth cells and endocrine cells are present in up to 20 percent of carcinomas (104). Some adenocarcinomas have unusual growth patterns: micropapillary, microcystic and macrocystic, clear cell, solid, hepatoid, or simply an undifferentiated pattern of growth (figs. 4-19–4-23) (106–109). Although most of these patterns have not been studied systematically with regard to biological behavior and prognosis, preliminary studies have shown poor prognosis in tumors composed of a significant proportion of the micropapillary pattern of growth. Hepatoid tumors may produce alpha-fetoprotein and express markers of hepatic differentiation (106).

About 5 to 10 percent of adenocarcinomas are mucinous. These tumors show variable numbers and clusters of tumor cells floating within pools of extracellular mucin (fig. 4-24). Up to 5 percent show infiltrating signet ring

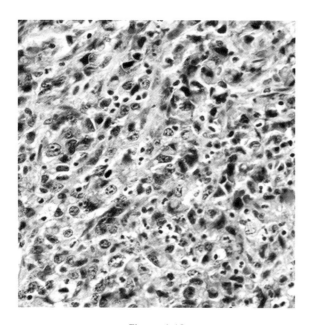

Figure 4-18

POORLY DIFFERENTIATED ADENOCARCINOMA

Highly pleomorphic and irregularly shaped cells without gland formation are present.

cells, either in isolation or in combination with extracellular mucin (101).

Preoperative (neoadjuvant) chemoradiotherapy often results in either complete, or nearly complete, destruction of the tumor, in which case the esophagus may show only acellular pools of mucin (fig. 4-25) (101,110). Post-treatment tumor cells may be present as either isolated, highly pleomorphic, irregularly shaped cells or as small clusters of cells in association with ulceration, pools of mucin, and/or densely fibrotic tissue (fig. 4-25). These cells may show extreme degrees of nuclear irregularity and enlargement, and may resemble reactive mesenchymal cells. Tumors that show only acellular mucin pools after chemoradiotherapy do not have an increased risk of recurrence or metastasis (100). In cases with only a few remaining atypical, potentially malignant epithelial cells, immunohistochemistry for broad spectrum cytokeratins may help distinguish malignant epithelial cells from reactive mesenchymal cells.

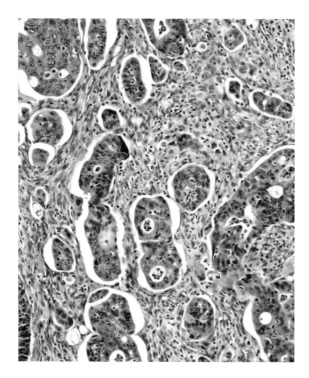
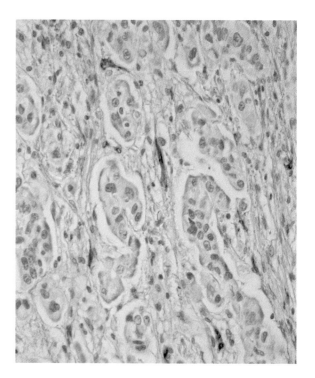

Figure 4-19

MICROPAPILLARY ADENOCARCINOMA

Small, irregularly-shaped clusters and cords of tumor cells appear to be floating within spaces that represent "reverse polarization." D2-40 stain shows that the spaces containing micropapillae are not lined by endothelial cells, but in fact, represent reverse polarization of the glandular epithelium (right).

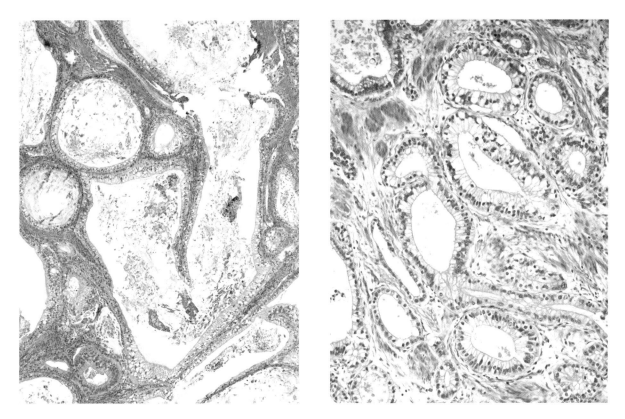

Figure 4-20

BE-ASSOCIATED ADENOCARCINOMA: MORPHOLOGIC VARIANTS

Left: Macrocystic growth pattern.
Right: Well-formed tubules contain epithelium with clear cytoplasm.

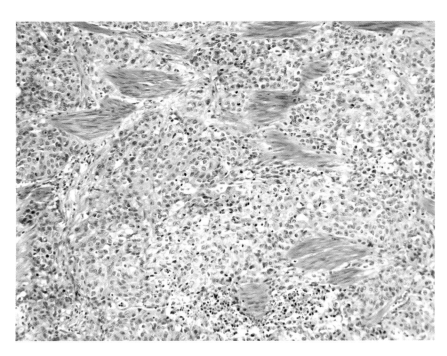

Figure 4-21

POORLY DIFFERENTIATED ADENOCARCINOMA

This malignant neoplasm consists of sheets of cells that do not form tubules.

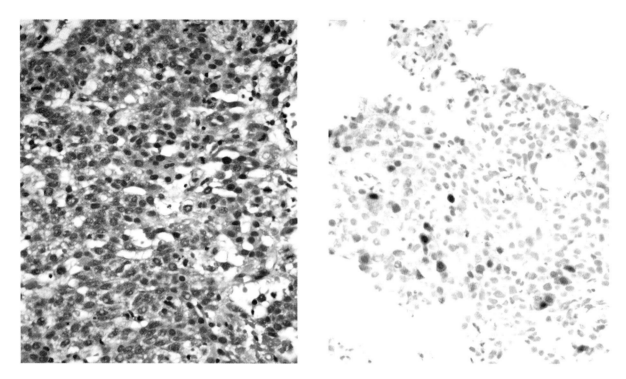

Figure 4-22

HEPATOID VARIANT OF ADENOCARCINOMA

Irregular cords and solid aggregates of small to medium-sized cells with hyperchromatic pyramidal-shaped nuclei, and hypereosinophilic cytoplasm are reminiscent of a high-grade hepatocellular carcinoma. These cells stain focally with arginase, and are positive for glypican 3 and HepPar1.

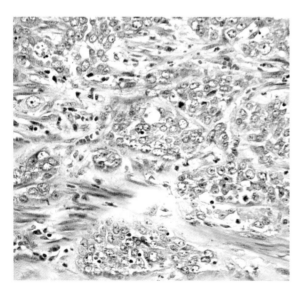

Figure 4-23

UNDIFFERENTIATED CARCINOMA IN BARRETT ESOPHAGUS

Although the malignant cells form nests suggestive of a carcinoma, in a case such as this, immunohistochemistry is needed in order to confirm a diagnosis of carcinoma.

Special studies and immunohistochemical stains are usually not necessary to establish a diagnosis of adenocarcinoma. They may be useful to distinguish primary from metastatic lesions, or in identifying residual tumor after neoadjuvant therapy. Esophageal adenocarcinomas are typically positive for mucin (including mucicarmine, periodic acid–Schiff (PAS)/diastase, alcian blue) and may be positive for MUC1, MUC2, MUC5AC, and MUC6. Most adenocarcinomas stain with broad spectrum cytokeratins, and are positive for CK7 and negative for CK20 in up to 90 percent of cases (111). CDX2 is positive in up to 70 percent of cases (112). Neuroendocrine markers are positive in some cells (up to 50 percent of cases) (113). Adenocarcinomas are typically negative for markers of lung and breast origin, including estrogen and progesterone receptors.

Mixed Adenosquamous Carcinoma. Tumor cell heterogeneity is not uncommon in BE-associated adenocarcinomas (114,115). In one study of 496 primary esophageal carcinomas, 2.2 percent showed evidence of both squamous carcinoma

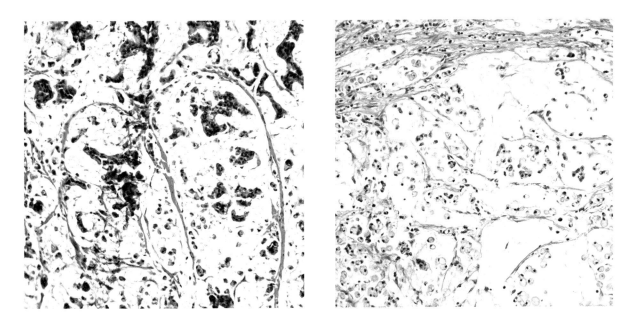

Figure 4-24

MUCINOUS ADENOCARCINOMA IN BARRETT ESOPHAGUS

Left: Irregular glands and clusters of cells appear to be floating within pools of mucin.
Right: Individual and clusters of signet ring cells float within extracellular mucin.

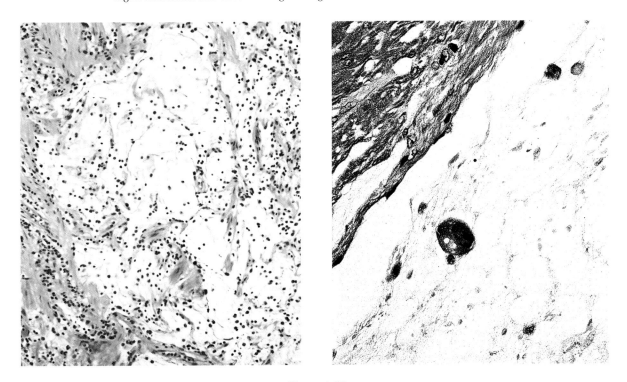

Figure 4-25

POSTNEOADJUVANT-TREATED ADENOCARCINOMA

Left: There is no evidence of residual adenocarcinoma. What remain are acellular pools of mucin, some of which show an early granulation tissue reaction.
Right: Isolated, highly atypical and pleomorphic residual carcinoma cells are present within pools of mucin.

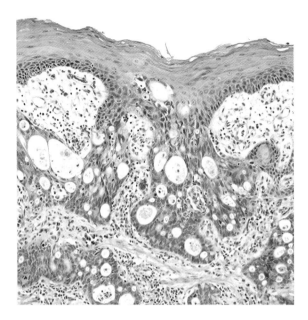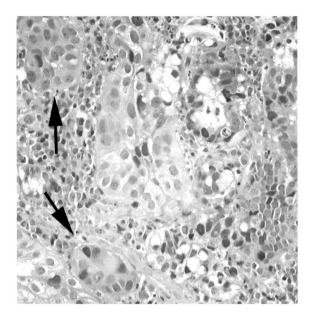

Figure 4-26

ADENOSQUAMOUS CARCINOMA

Left: This carcinoma appears to arise in association with the overlying squamous mucosa, exhibiting both squamous and adenocarcinomatous differentiation.

Right: A few squamous nests are indicated by arrows, but there are also glands and cells containing mucin.

and adenocarcinoma (115). In another study, multidirectional differentiation (showing elements of squamous, glandular, and small cell components) occurred in up to 25 percent of cases. It is presumed that these tumors develop from neoplastic transformation of a multipotential epithelial stem cell.

These tumors have been termed *mixed squamous and glandular carcinomas, adenoacanthoma, adenosquamous carcinoma,* and *mucoepidermoid carcinoma* (116,117). There are no strict histopathologic criteria to define these "mixed" tumors. Some show an intimate mixture of both squamous and mucin-secreting elements, whereas others show more discrete areas of squamous and glandular carcinomatous elements (fig. 4-26). Patients are treated like patients with pure adenocarcinoma, since the prognosis for mixed carcinomas are uncertain because of their rarity. Some studies show survival rates similar to those of pure squamous cell carcinoma, whereas others have shown slightly better survival rates (the latter may have resulted from inclusion of tumors with small size or early stage) (118).

Mixed Adenocarcinoma/Neuroendocrine Carcinoma. Mixed adenocarcinoma/neuroendocrine carcinoma, defined as a tumor that contains at least 30 percent of each of these cellular components, is uncommon. Nevertheless, in one study of 40 neuroendocrine carcinomas, 15 (37 percent) showed distinct areas of glandular differentiation (119). Survival rates are generally similar to those of patients with pure esophageal neuroendocrine carcinomas (119,120).

Cytology of Barrett Esophagus and Adenocarcinoma. *Barrett Metaplasia.* In cytologic preparations, BE is characterized by flat sheets of glandular epithelial cells with scattered goblet cells and sharply defined smooth edges (121,122). When visualized en face, the epithelium forms a honeycomb pattern (fig. 4-27). Typically, the nuclei of the glandular cells are regularly arranged and uniform in size and shape, without loss of polarity (fig. 4-28). They are round to oval in shape, have a smooth nuclear border, and have an unremarkable chromatin pattern. Reactive changes, such as a "streaming" appearance of the sheets of cells and prominent nucleoli (fig. 4-28), may be observed. Background features are normally "clean," but inflammatory cells and necrosis may be present in ulcerated cases. The goblet cells are defined by the presence of a single, large, apical mucin

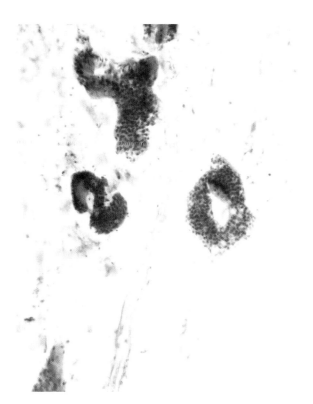

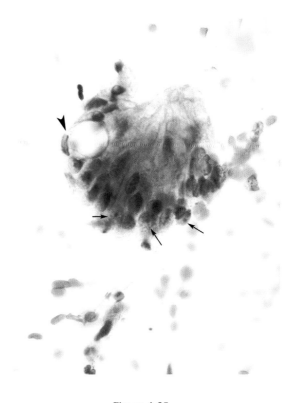

Figure 4-27

BARRETT METAPLASIA: CYTOLOGY

Three fragments of glandular epithelium are present in the field. Part of the one in the upper center field has a "Swiss cheese" appearance due to the presence of goblet cells (Papanicolaou stain of direct smear of esophageal brushings).

Figure 4-28

BARRETT METAPLASIA: CYTOLOGY

This small fragment of glandular epithelium shows small, but prominent, nucleoli (arrows) and a goblet cell (arrowhead), with a single large vacuole and a crescent-shaped nucleus (Papanicolaou stain on direct smear of esophageal brushings).

vacuole that distends the lateral cytoplasmic borders and compresses the nucleus into a flattened, or crescent, shape (fig. 4-28).

The type of preparation influences the size of the sheets of cells. Variably sized sheets and cell groups are normally present on direct smears, but small flat sheets and groups of cells, and even single cells (fig. 4-29), are more likely to be present on liquid-based cytology samples.

Isolated goblet cells need to be distinguished from signet ring cell carcinoma. Although the nuclei in goblet cells may have a crescent shape, they have characteristic round edges and smooth nuclear borders (fig. 4-29). Although the N/C ratio may be low in signet ring carcinoma cells, the degree of nuclear atypia is often easily apparent. The nuclei show pointed and sharp edges, membrane irregularity, and hyperchromasia (fig. 4-30).

Recognition of goblet cells on histology relies, in part, on the presence of a faint blue color of the cytoplasmic mucin. Unfortunately, this feature is lost in the processing of cytologic specimens during Papanicolaou staining: both acid mucin and neutral mucin appear clear with this stain. Therefore, goblet cells cannot be reliably distinguished from distended foveolar cells on cytology samples (fig. 4-31) (123,124), although distension of the cytoplasmic vacuoles in foveolar cells is typically not as marked as that normally seen in goblet cells. Consequently, the correlation of histology and cytology in the identification of goblet cells is suboptimal (Table 4-5) (124,125). Two studies used histology as the gold standard to evaluate cytology/histology correlation of BE on consecutive unselected patients undergoing upper gastrointestinal endoscopy. These studies demonstrated a sensitivity

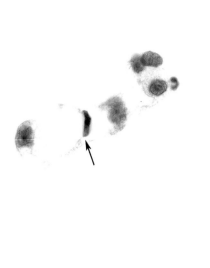

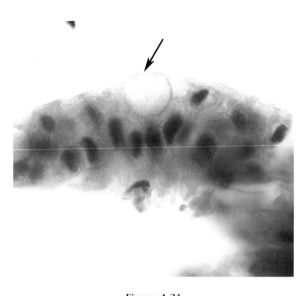

Figure 4-29

BARRETT METAPLASIA: CYTOLOGY

A few glandular cells with one goblet cell. The crescent-shaped nucleus (arrow) has a round edge (Papanicolaou stain on ThinPrep of esophageal brushings).

Figure 4-31

VACUOLATED COLUMNAR CELL

The vacuole (arrow) distended with neutral mucin in goblet-appearing surface foveolar cells appears the same as the vacuole in intestinal-type goblet cells on a Papanicolaou-stained cytology specimen.

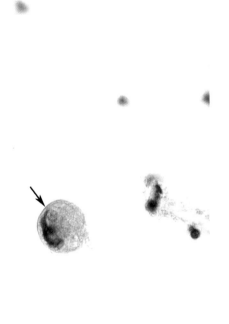

Figure 4-30

ADENOCARCINOMA: CYTOLOGY

In contrast to the goblet cell in figure 4-29, the crescent-shaped nucleus in a tumor cell from a signet ring cell carcinoma has a pointed edge (arrow) and irregular nuclear border (Papanicolaou stain on ThinPrep of esophageal brushings).

of cytology preparations of 41 to 60 percent and a specificity of 84 to 91 percent (124,125). The degree of cytohistologic agreement for BE is much higher in patients who have endoscopic evidence of columnar epithelium in the distal esophagus than it is for those patients who lack such evidence (Table 4-6).

In addition to routine cytology, cytologic samples can be analyzed by molecular markers for diagnosis and risk stratification (126). Specific intestinal immunocytochemical markers, such as villin and hepatocyte antigen (HepPar1), may be used. Villin expression in esophageal brush specimens is 81 percent sensitive and 100 percent specific for BE (127). Hepatocyte antigen was found to be virtually 100 percent sensitive and specific for intestinal metaplasia, more sensitive and specific than other markers such as CK7, CK20, and MUC2 (128). Both help identify intestinal epithelium characteristic of BE on cytologic specimens (127,129,130). Immunohistochemical staining for Trefoil factor 3 (TFF3) in cell block preparations of materials obtained with a nonendoscopic capsule sponge results in an overall sensitivity of detecting BE of 80 percent and specificity of 92 percent (131,132). For patients with a greater than 3 cm

Table 4-5

CORRELATION OF HISTOCYTOLOGIC EVIDENCE OF GOBLET CELLS (n=147)[a]

Histologic Evidence of Goblet Cells	Cytologic Evidence of Goblet Cells			
	Definite	Probable	Negative	Total
Yes	6 (46%)	7 (39%)	19 (16%)	32 (22%)
Negative	7 (54%)	11 (61%)	97 (84%)	115 (78%)
Total	13	18	113	147

[a]Data from reference 4.

Table 4-6

CORRELATION OF HISTOCYTOLOGIC EVIDENCE OF GOBLET CELLS BY ENDOSCOPIC EVIDENCE OF COLUMNAR EPITHELIUM IN THE DISTAL ESOPHAGUS (n=146)[a]

Histologic Evidence of Goblet Cells	Cytologic Evidence of Goblet Cells			
	Definite	Probable	Negative	Total
Patients with definite endoscopic evidence of columnar epithelium in the distal esophagus				
Yes	5	5	2	12
Negative	1	1	6	8
Total	6	6	8	20
Patients without definite endoscopic evidence of columnar epithelium in the distal esophagus				
Yes	1	2	17	20
Negative	6	10	90	106
Total	7	12	107	126

[a]Data from reference 4.

circumferential BE, the sensitivity increases to 90 percent.

Dysplasia. Cytology is potentially useful in screening for dysplasia in BE (122,124,125,133,134), since it has the advantage of sampling a wide area and can detect dysplasia that is not apparent endoscopically. Recent data suggest that a combination of a molecular biomarker panel (including three protein biomarkers (p53, C-MYC, and Aurora kinase A), two methylation markers (MYOD1 and RUNX3), glandular atypia, and *TP53* mutation status, applied to materials collected with a nonendoscopic Cytosponge is useful for risk stratification of patients with BE in order to triage management (135). In a cohort study of more than 500 patients with BE, 35 to 38 percent fell into the low-risk category, with a probability over 96 percent for having a truly nondysplastic lesion. Of those who fell into the moderate-risk group, 22 percent had HGD, while all 5 patients who fell into the high-risk group had HGD. It appears that endoscopy can be avoided in low-risk patients with BE.

The degree of atypia depends on the grade of dysplasia, although well-accepted criteria for diagnosing LGD and HGD on cytology have not been established (136). In fact, diagnosing LGD is difficult, with sensitivity up to 31 percent (125,134). Fortunately, a cytologic diagnosis of HGD is more accurate and is comparable to that seen with mucosal biopsy samples, with a sensitivity up to 82 percent and specificity up to 95 percent (125,134). Cytologically, dysplasia has some, but not all, of the "atypical" features of malignancy, such as cellular dyshesion, haphazard arrangement of cells, increased N/C ratio, nuclear enlargement, hyperchromasia, nuclear membrane irregularities, and chromatin aberration (either clumping or clearing).

In a background of glandular epithelial cells with goblet cells, LGD resembles "adenomatous" epithelium and is characterized by the presence of cohesive three-dimensional groups of crowded and overlapping cells with elongated stratified nuclei (fig. 4-32) (124,125). The cells are regular in appearance and the nuclear size and shape are typically uniform (fig. 4-32). A mild to moderate increase in the N/C ratio of the cells, and nuclear hyperchromasia with either absent or only small inconspicuous nucleoli, are normally

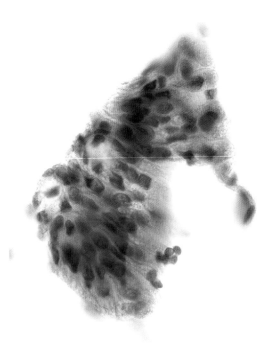

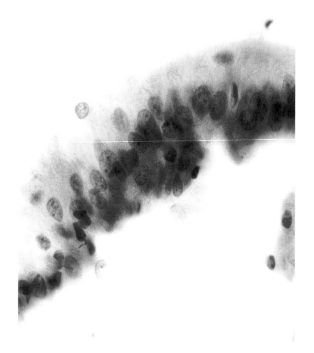

Figure 4-32

LOW-GRADE DYSPLASIA: CYTOLOGY

High magnification shows the stratified elongated nuclei in another fragment (Papanicolaou stain on direct smear of esophageal brushings).

Figure 4-33

LOW-GRADE DYSPLASIA: CYTOLOGY

In this cytology specimen of biopsy-proven low-grade dysplasia, the nuclei are oval with small nucleoli. Focal molding of nuclei is seen in the center of the field (Papanicolaou stain on ThinPrep of esophageal brushings).

present (fig. 4-33). The latter feature is helpful to separate LGD from reactive epithelium, which is normally characterized by the presence of prominent nucleoli.

Unfortunately, sampling and processing artifacts, such as folding of sheets of cells, can mimic LGD on cytology samples. In general, increased N/C ratio and nuclear enlargement define dysplasia, whereas cells with abundant cytoplasm, usually apparent at the periphery of artifactually crowded groups of non-neoplastic cells, is a feature of artifactual crowding. Thus, examination of the periphery of cell groups may be helpful in distinguishing dysplasia from reactive or nonspecific changes. Diagnostic features helpful in differentiating benign/reactive changes from LGD are listed in Table 4-7. The existence of the category of "indefinite for dysplasia" is evidence of this difficulty. No cytologic equivalent of this category has been described as it lacks specific morphologic criteria or known biologic significance, and is grouped with LGD into one cytologic category for practical purposes (134).

The features of HGD are usually more obvious than those of LGD and are manifested mainly by the presence of dyscohesive atypical cells with a high N/C ratio and moderately to markedly enlarged atypical nuclei (fig. 4-34) (124,125). Previously described atypical nuclear features of malignancy, such as haphazard arrangement, are more apparent in HGD than in LGD, albeit they are not as fully developed as in invasive adenocarcinoma. Thus, it can be difficult, if not impossible, to distinguish HGD from invasive carcinoma on cytology samples. However, samples from HGD are not usually as cellular as that from carcinoma, and the background is often "clean." Diagnostic features helpful in differentiating HGD and invasive carcinoma are listed in Table 4-7.

At one end of the spectrum, it may be difficult to separate LGD from regenerative/reactive changes even on biopsy specimens. At the other end of the spectrum, it is often difficult to distinguish HGD from early intramucosal carcinoma. Cytology cannot do better than histology in this regard.

Despite its low sensitivity and limitation regarding grading/classification of dysplasia, cytology may provide valuable prognostic information for the development of adenocarcinoma as a screening method in large populations. In 1983, esophageal balloon cytology was used to screen a high-risk population in Linxian, China (137,138). Follow-up data were collected prospectively through 1991. The columnar cell diagnoses (normal versus "hyperplasia" versus "dysplasia") in 1983 were found to be significantly associated with the subsequent risk of both esophageal and gastric cardiac carcinoma.

In order to increase the sensitivity and specificity of detecting dysplasia and adenocarcinoma, image cytometry DNA analysis (ICDA) and fluorescence in situ hybridization (FISH) have been applied to brush cytology specimens (139–141). Using FISH with probes for 8q24 (C-MYC), 9p21 (p16), 17p13.1 (p53), 17q12 (HER2), 20q13, and chromosome Y on brush cytology specimens, Fritcher (139) found the sensitivity of cytology, ICDA, and FISH for HGD to be 32 percent, 25 percent, and 82 percent, respectively; and for adenocarcinoma, 45 percent, 45 percent, and 100 percent, respectively. The specificity among

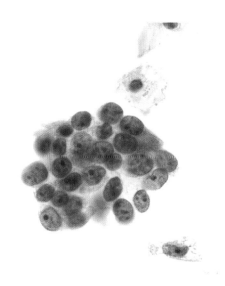

Figure 4-34

HIGH-GRADE DYSPLASIA: CYTOLOGY

A crowded group of atypical epithelial cells is present in this biopsy-proven high-grade glandular dysplasia cytology specimen. Although the nuclei appear uniform, they show a high nuclear/cytoplasmic ratio, hyperchromasia, large prominent nucleoli, and focal nuclear membrane irregularities (Papanicolaou stain on ThinPrep of esophageal brushings).

Table 4-7

COMPARISON OF CYTOLOGIC FEATURES OF REACTIVE GLANDULAR CHANGES, LOW-GRADE DYSPLASIA, HIGH-GRADE DYSPLASIA, AND ADENOCARCINOMA

Cytologic Feature	Reactive	Low-Grade Dysplasia	High-Grade Dysplasia	Adenocarcinoma
Tight 3-D clusters	Absent to rare	A few	Few to moderate	Moderate to many
Loose clusters	Absent to rare	Absent to rare	Few to moderate	Moderate to many
Single atypical cells	None to rare	None to rare	Few to moderate	Moderate to many
Mitoses	Present	Present	Present	Present
Atypical mitoses	None	None to rare	None to rare	Present
Chromatin	Vesicular	Slight to moderate hyperchromasia	Hyperchromatic and coarsely granular or hypochromatic	Hyperchromatic and coarsely granular or hyperchromatic
Nucleoli	Prominent but regular and few	Absent or inconspicuous	Variable	Variable
Nuclear pleomorphism	Absent to slight	Slight	Moderate	Moderate to marked
Nuclear stratification	Absent to slight	Prominent	Variable	Variable
Irregular nuclear spacing within tight clusters	Absent to slight	Slight	Moderate	Moderate to marked

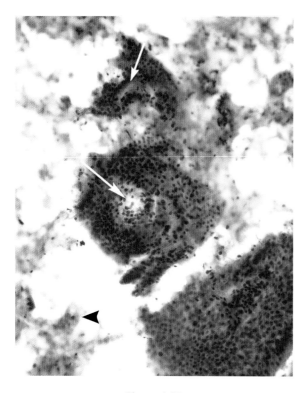

Figure 4-35

ADENOCARCINOMA: CYTOLOGY

Three fragments of crowded glandular cells from a well-differentiated adenocarcinoma of esophagus. White arrows point to the lumens of malignant glands, while the black arrowhead points to the tumor diathesis in the background (Papanicolaou stain on direct smear of esophageal brushings).

patients with benign squamous mucosa of cytology, ICDA, and FISH was 93 percent, 86 percent, and 100 percent, respectively (139). Similarly, using FISH with peri-centromeric probes for chromosomes 7 and 17, Rygiel (140) found sensitivity of 75 percent for indefinite/LGD and 85 percent for HGD/adenocarcinoma, which is superior to that of cytology or image cytometry DNA analysis.

Immunostaining for cell cycle marker cyclin A has been applied to brush cytology specimens for risk stratification of BE surveillance (142). The sensitivity, specificity, positive predictive value, and negative predictive value of this technique for any dysplasia (low and high grade) versus nondysplastic BE are 88 percent, 64 percent, 76 percent, and 82 percent, respectively; they are 98 percent, 59 percent, 63 percent, and 97 percent for HGD/adenocarcinoma, respectively.

Adenocarcinoma. Adenocarcinomas of the esophagus have no specific cytologic features. In fact, they resemble adenocarcinomas from other parts of the gastrointestinal tract, and goblet cells may or may not be present in the background. In contrast to dysplasia, cytology samples of adenocarcinoma contain a higher number of atypical cells which are arranged singly or in crowded clusters. The background of adenocarcinoma is variable, and ranges from clean to dirty depending on the presence and degree of tumor necrosis. Tumor diathesis, a diagnostic feature of invasive carcinomas, is characterized by old, lysed red blood cells and ghost tumor cells on direct smears (fig. 4-35), and by acellular granular materials on liquid-based preparations (fig. 4-36).

Well-differentiated adenocarcinomas consist of groups of cohesive cells that often have recognizable glands characterized by the presence of a central lumen surrounded by polarized tumor cells with elongated nuclei (fig. 4-35). Glands may not be as apparent on liquid-based preparations compared to direct smears, in which case tumor cells appear as crowded groups of cohesive cells (fig. 4-37). Tumor cells as well as their nuclei are fairly uniform in size and shape. However, some degree of nuclear atypia, such as chromatin clearing and clumping, and irregular nuclear membranes, may be seen upon high-power examination.

Moderately differentiated adenocarcinomas show a combination of the features described above and those described below for poorly differentiated adenocarcinomas. Poorly differentiated adenocarcinomas typically consist of single tumor cells or groups of dyscohesive cells. The malignant nature of the cells is usually apparent because of the high N/C ratio, marked chromatin aberration (either hyperchromasia or hypochromasia), and sharp nuclear membrane indentations (fig. 4-38). In contrast to round to oval and uniform nucleoli as seen in reactive changes (fig. 4-39), nucleoli in malignant tumors may be small but prominent, or numerous and very large (up to one quarter of the size of the nucleus), with sharp angles (fig. 4-40). The mere presence of nucleoli does not necessarily indicate malignancy, but their appearance may distinguish a reactive lesion from a malignant one.

Signet ring cell carcinomas, one variant of poorly differentiated adenocarcinoma, show

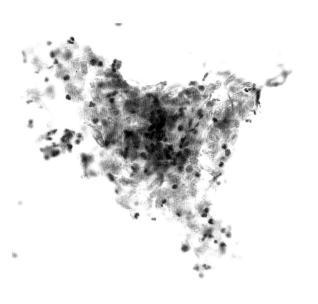

Figure 4-36

ADENOCARCINOMA: CYTOLOGY

Appearance of tumor diathesis using Papanicolaou stain on ThinPrep of esophageal brushings.

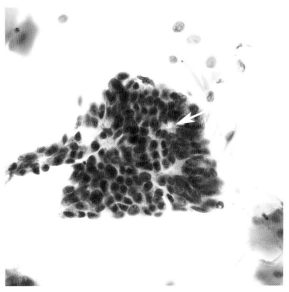

Figure 4-37

ADENOCARCINOMA: CYTOLOGY

The appearance of a well-differentiated adenocarcinoma on ThinPrep preparation of esophageal brushings. The lumen is difficult to appreciate (white arrow) (Papanicolaou stain on ThinPrep of esophageal brushings).

a range of morphologic appearances. In fact, one type mimics histiocytes and thus may be difficult to recognize as a malignant tumor. In these instances, the cells have moderate finely vacuolated cytoplasm and small nuclei. When these cells are present in large numbers and contain no phagocytized material, signet ring carcinoma should be suspected. In this scenario, these cells should be scrutinized more carefully with the use of high magnification for nuclear atypia, such as subtle nuclear membrane irregularities (see fig. 4-30). Since signet ring cell carcinoma is typically covered by normal epithelium, the tumor cells may be difficult to sample with a brush. The use of endoscopic fine-needle aspirations, with or without ultrasound guidance, increases the diagnostic yield of signet ring cell carcinomas (143).

Endoscopic ultrasound-guided fine-needle aspiration of celiac axis lymph nodes in patients with esophageal cancer has been reported to increase the staging accuracy from 90 to 100 percent compared to endoscopic ultrasound alone (144,145). When interpreting endoscopic, transluminal fine-needle aspirations of lymph nodes, the needle may become contaminated with normal or dysplastic/malignant cells that

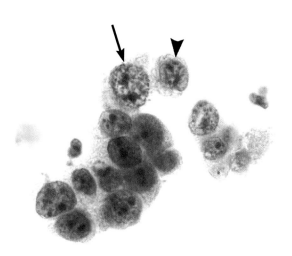

Figure 4-38

ADENOCARCINOMA: CYTOLOGY

The malignant nature of the lesion is apparent in this group of cells from a poorly differentiated adenocarcinoma arising in BE. The arrow highlights the abnormal chromatin and the arrowhead points to the highly irregular nuclear membrane (Papanicolaou stain on ThinPrep of esophageal brushings).

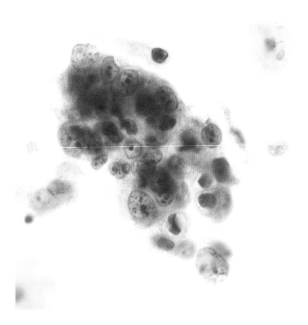

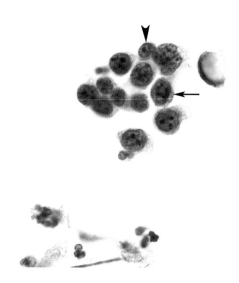

Figure 4-39

REACTIVE CHANGE: CYTOLOGY

This is a group of highly reactive epithelial cells from an esophageal ulcer with no evidence of malignancy. Although prominent nucleoli are seen, abnormal chromatin and irregular nuclear membranes are absent (Papanicolaou stain on ThinPrep of esophageal brushings).

Figure 4-40

POORLY DIFFERENTIATED ADENOCARCINOMA

A dyscohesive group of highly atypical epithelial cells from a poorly differentiated adenocarcinoma of the esophagus shows scant cytoplasm with fine vacuoles. The arrow points to a nucleus with at least five nucleoli and the arrowhead shows a nucleolus that occupies almost a quarter of a nucleus (Papanicolaou stain on ThinPrep of esophageal brushings).

originate within the lumen of the organ (145). Knowledge of image-study findings and the transmural path of the needle are essential to avoid the pitfall of overinterpreting a lymph node as positive for metastasis.

Molecular Genetic Findings. During the progression from BE to adenocarcinoma, the cells acquire multiple molecular abnormalities in several major oncogene and tumor suppressor gene categories. Inactivation of tumor suppressor genes, such as *TP53, CDKN2A, p15, p27,* and *APC* are early mutations (6,23,24,25). Alterations of genes that control cell cycle regulation and proliferation such as *MYC* and *cyclins D1, B1,* and *E* are implicated in oncogenesis as well. *ERBB2* mutations are detected in adenocarcinoma by exome and genome sequencing (26). Micro RNA expression profiles characterize progression from BE to adenocarcinoma (146). Members of the tumor necrosis factor receptor superfamily have been found in progression from BE to adenocarcinoma, and *FASL* has been reported in both esophageal

adenocarcinomas and metastases (147–150). Proapoptotic and antiapoptotic proteins, such as BCL2 and BCLX1, are involved in the molecular pathogenesis of adenocarcinoma as well (151,152). As BE cells progress to cancer, they typically show early inactivation of p53, and then later, the cancer cells typically manifest aneuploidy which is a marker of genomic instability (23,153). Genomic instability is a useful marker to predict progression to cancer (33,49).

In a comprehensive molecular analysis of 164 carcinomas of the esophagus, molecular features differentiated squamous cell carcinomas from adenocarcinomas. Esophageal adenocarcinomas resembled the chromosomally unstable variant of gastric adenocarcinoma, but DNA hypermethylation occurred disproportionately in esophageal adenocarcinomas. Significant mutations were found in *TP53, CDKN2A, ARID1A, SMAD4,* and *ERBB2* (25).

Differential Diagnosis. The diagnosis of adenocarcinoma is usually straightforward, but on occasion, it may be difficult to distinguish from proximal gastric cancer that extends into the distal esophagus (GEJ cancer), or from metastases (Table 4-8). In contrast to proximal gastric adenocarcinoma, adenocarcinoma of the esophagus is usually associated with a background of BE, is typically CK7 positive and CK20 negative, and occurs in patients who have a history of GERD and are usually *H. pylori* negative (111,154–157). An absence of chronic gastritis and intestinal metaplasia supports an esophageal origin for tumors in the distal esophagus/GEJ area. Proximal gastric adenocarcinomas have a similar immunohistochemical profile as esophageal carcinomas, but show a more frequent association with chronic gastritis, gastric metaplasia (and lack of BE), *H. pylori*, and autoimmune gastritis (156,157). Gastric adenocarcinomas occur in a slightly younger population and show a more even male to female ratio.

Metastases, particularly from the stomach, lung, or breast, may simulate a primary esophageal adenocarcinoma. The presence of BE and dysplastic epithelium is convincing evidence for a primary adenocarcinoma. In addition, esophageal adenocarcinomas do not stain for TTF1, napsin-A, or other markers of breast and lung differentiation (154).

Spread and Metastases. Esophageal adenocarcinomas initially spread locally and deeply within the esophageal wall, and then eventually into paraesophageal or even celiac lymph nodes. Distal esophageal tumors may spread into the proximal stomach and present as a GEJ carcinoma. Early cancers (superficial adenocarcinomas) spread through the newly developed (superficial) muscularis mucosae, but are still considered intramucosal since they remain in the area above the original (deep) muscularis mucosa of the native esophagus. Submucosal cancers have a higher frequency of lymphatic and lymph node invasion compared to tumors that infiltrate the original laminal propria (158,159).

As the tumors grow, they spread deeper into the wall of the esophagus into the adventitia and adjacent organs or tissues. Common sites of local spread include the mediastinum, tracheobronchial tree, lung, aorta, pericardium, heart, and spinal column. Spread to paraesophageal and paracardiac lymph nodes, those of the lesser curvature of the stomach, and celiac nodes, are common in distal esophageal tumors. Distant

Table 4-8

DISTINGUISHING DISTAL ESOPHAGEAL FROM PROXIMAL GASTRIC ADENOCARCINOMA

Feature	BE[a]-Associated Adenocarcinoma	Gastric Adenocarcinoma
Gender	M>>F	M=F
Age	>60	40-60
GERD symptoms	++	+/-
Hiatus hernia	++	+/-
Background BE	++	+/-
Helicobacter pylori infection	+/-	++
Autoimmune gastritis	+/-	++
Midpoint of tumor	Proximal to GEJ	Distal to GEJ
Intestinal type cancer	++	+
Diffuse type cancer	+	++

[a]BE = Barrett esophagus; GERD = gastroesophageal reflux disease; GEJ = gastroesophageal junction.

metastasis, such as to the lung, liver, bone, and brain, occur late in the progression of disease.

Prognosis. The most important prognostic factor in esophageal adenocarcinoma is based on the pathologic American Joint Committee on Cancer (AJCC) TNM staging system. Patients with tumors limited to the mucosa or submucosa have an 80 to 100 percent 5-year survival rate, compared to 10 to 20 percent for those with tumors that extend into or through the muscularis propria (91,105,160). Metastasis to regional lymph nodes are present in about 50 to 60 percent of patients overall (161). The likelihood of lymph node metastases is directly related to tumor depth (104,162). Superficial submucosal tumors show a lymph node metastasis rate of about 7.5 percent, compared to 45 percent for tumors that penetrate into the deep submucosa (104). Only 1 to 2 percent of intramucosal adenocarcinomas metastasize to lymph nodes (162). In some studies, submucosally invasive tumors are separated into superficial, mid, and deep submucosal invasion (SM1, SM2, and SM3), and there is an increased risk of lymph node metastases with each deeper level of penetration (fig. 4-41) (165). Lymph node micrometastases are present in up to 30 percent of patients, but it is controversial whether this finding results in a worse prognosis compared to node negative patients (164,165).

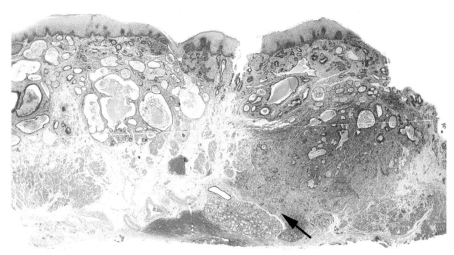

Figure 4-41

ENDOSCOPIC MUCOSAL RESECTION

There is an adenocarcinoma invading into the submucosa. A submucosal gland is located at the deep portion of the invasive front (arrow).

Other factors that have shown to have prognostic significance in esophageal carcinoma include tumor type, such as mucinous, signet ring cell, or micropapillary type; tumor grade; lymphovascular invasion; circumferential margin involvement (166); and various molecular abnormalities such as *TP53* mutations, loss of p27, amplifications (*ERBB2/HER2, MET, EGFR*), and DNA ploidy (102,167,168). Overexpression or amplification of *ERBB2* occurs in up to 70 percent of cancers, whereas *EGFR* overexpression or mutation occurs in 30 to 60 percent (169–171).

After preoperative chemoradiotherapy, prognostic factors include the histologic degree of tumor regression, which is scored in a three-tiered classification system (complete tumor regression, subtotal or partial tumor regression, and no tumor regression: 0 percent, 1 to 50 percent, and over 50 percent residual tumor) (172,173). Complete tumor regression after neoadjuvant therapy and an absence of lymph node involvement are the strongest prognostic factors and are associated with a greater than 50 percent 5-year survival rate (174).

The overall 5-year survival rate for patients with adenocarcinoma is less than 20 percent (18), which is a significant improvement over the 5 percent rate of the early 1970s (82). Up to 40 percent of patients are diagnosed with distant metastasis at the time of diagnosis, however, and among these patients, the 5-year survival rate is less than 3 percent. Five-year survival rates are lower for blacks than whites.

Survival for esophageal cancer patients remains poor despite an overall improving trend (82). Unfortunately, most patients present with either locally advanced disease (32 percent) or metastatic disease (50 percent) at the time of their initial diagnosis (176).

Treatment. The treatment strategies should follow guideline recommendations and are dependent on the stage of disease at the time of diagnosis. Often they are developed after multidisciplinary evaluation (82).

Patients with superficial cancers are treated by either local mucosal ablation or surgery (82,177). Patients with T1a N0 tumors are usually treated by endoscopic mucosal resection (EMR) combined with radiofrequency ablation (RFA), cryotherapy, or photodynamic therapy, followed by close surveillance (82,177). Patients with slightly deeper penetrating tumors (T1b N0) are best treated with surgery without induction therapy, since about 50 percent of these patients have occult lymph node involvement (178,179).

The treatment of patients with T2 N0 tumors is somewhat controversial (180). There is an increasing trend toward the use of induction therapy followed by surgical resection; however, there are insufficient data at present to show that there is a survival benefit to this method. Some even advocate induction therapy followed by surgery and adjuvant therapy for patients with T2 N0 tumors. Reliable data are variable as well for patients with either local regional (T3 or T4 N0 M0) or locally advanced disease (T1-4a N1

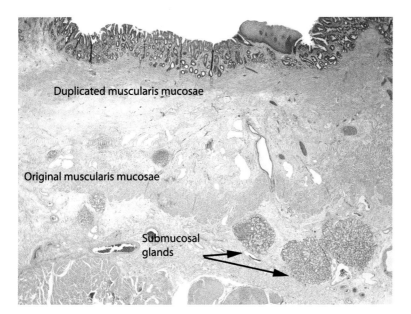

Duplicated muscularis mucosae

Original muscularis mucosae

Submucosal glands

Figure 4-42

**ENDOSCOPIC
MUCOSAL RESECTION**

BE showing a prominent duplicated muscularis mucosae. If submucosal glands are present, they serve as a helpful guide, but the vessels in the true (original) submucosa are also larger than those in the lamina propria.

M0) (181,182). Many studies show conflicting results. Induction chemoradiotherapy, followed by surgery, is one form of optimal therapy for T3-T4a tumors, either with or without nodal disease. One recent large randomized and controlled trial showed a definite survival benefit for patients with neoadjuvant chemoradiation followed by surgery, compared to surgery alone.

For patients with unresectable disease (T4b), chemoradiotherapy is the preferred method of treatment, and in some instances, this can lead to an increased chance of surgical resectability. The treatment of patients with metastatic or unresectable disease is individualized. Potential possibilities include chemotherapy, clinical trial enrollment if any are available, or simply supportive care.

Endoscopic Mucosal Resection. EMR serves as both a diagnostic and potentially therapeutic procedure. Diagnostically, EMR specimens enable pathologists to provide more accurate pathologic diagnostic and staging information (183,184). More accurate reporting of dysplasia has been reported in EMR specimens compared to biopsy specimens (184). In EMR specimens, pathologists should determine the grade and type of dysplasia; the type, grade, and depth of invasive cancer if present; the presence or absence of lymphovascular invasion; and the status of the lateral and deep tissue margins, all of which are factors that have implications with regard to further treatment and outcome (6).

When evaluating EMR specimens, one must be aware that most BE patients have a duplicated muscularis mucosae (185) (figs. 4-42, 4-43). One study showed that up to 71 percent of patients with BE show moderate or extensive duplication of the muscularis mucosae (186). The rate of lymph node metastasis has been shown to correlate with depth of infiltration of the true lamina propria, whether it involves the inner (neo) lamina propria, the inner (neo) muscularis mucosae, the outer (native) lamina propria, or the deep (native) muscularis mucosae (fig. 4-42) (187,188).

Orientation of EMR specimens is important in order to adequately evaluate the pathologic information, and this includes mounting specimens cleanly on a wax block, fixing for at least 12 hours, and proper inking of the lateral and deep margins. Tissue sections should be obtained at not more than 2-mm intervals (189).

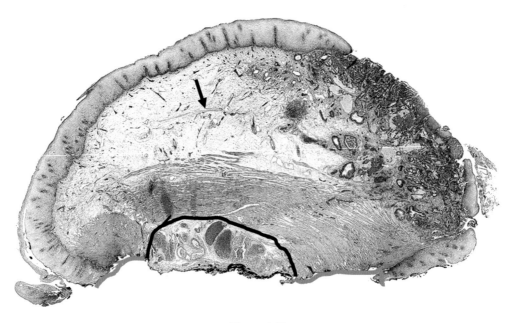

Figure 4-43

ENDOSCOPIC MUCOSAL RESECTION

Adenocarcinoma showing invasion into and through the duplicated muscularis mucosae (indicated by an arrow) and into the original (deep) muscularis mucosae. When such samples are not pinned adequately, they tend to curl, which can result in an artifact in which lateral margins can mimic the deep margins. In this specimen, the interface between the muscularis mucosae and the submucosa is delineated by a black line. The lateral mucosal margins, which consist of epithelium, lamina propria, and muscularis mucosae, are indicated by green lines.

REFERENCES

1. Ferlay J, Soerjomataram I, Ervik M, et al. GLOBO-CAN 2012 v1.1, Cancer Incidence and Mortality Worldwide: IARC CancerBase No. 11 [Internet]. Lyon, France: International Agency for Research on Cancer. (2014). Available from: http://globocan.iarc.fr.

2. Thrift AP, Whiteman DC. The incidence of esophageal adenocarcinoma continues to rise: analysis of period and birth cohort effects on recent trends. Ann Oncol 2012;23:3155-62.

3. Edgren G, Adami HO, Weiderpass E, Nyren O. A global assessment of the oesophageal adenocarcinoma epidemic. Gut 2013;62:1406-14.

4. Ronkainen J, Aro P, Storskrubb T, et al. Prevalence of Barrett's esophagus in the general population: an endoscopic study. Gastroenterology 2005;129:1825-31.

5. Hvid-Jensen F, Pedersen L, Drewes AM, Sorensen HT, Funch-Jensen P. Incidence of adenocarcinoma among patients with Barrett's esophagus. N Engl J Med 2011;365:1375-83.

6. Naini BV, Souza RF, Odze RD. Barrett's esophagus: a comprehensive and contemporary review for pathologists. Am J Surg Pathol 2016;40:e45-66.

7. Burke ZD, Tosh D. Barrett's metaplasia as a paradigm for understanding the development of cancer. Curr Opin Genet Dev 2012;22:494-9.

8. Wang X, Ouyang H, Yamamoto Y, et al. Residual embryonic cells as precursors of a Barrett's-like metaplasia. Cell 2011;145:1023-35.

9. Thrift AP. The epidemic of oesophageal carcinoma: where are we now? Cancer Epidemiol 2016;41:88-95.

10. Shaheen NJ, Falk GW, Iyer PG, Gerson LB, American College of Gastroenterology. ACG clinical guideline: diagnoses and management of Barrett's esophagus. Am J Gastroentrol 2016; 111:30-50.

11. Leggett CL, Nelsen EM, Tian J, et al. Metabolic syndrome as a risk factor for Barrett esophagus: a population-based case-control study. Mayo Clin Proc 2013;88:157-65.

12. Iyer PG, Borah BJ, Heien HC, Das A, Cooper GS, Chak A. Association of Barrett's esophagus with type II diabetes mellitus: results from a large population-based case-control study. Clin Gastroenterol Hepatol 2013;11:1108-14.
13. Leggett CL, Gorospe EC, Calvin AD, et al. Obstructive sleep apnea is a risk factor for Barrett's esophagus. Clin Gastroenterol Hepatol 2014;12:583-8.
14. Rubenstein JH, Inadomi JM, Scheiman J, et al. Association between Helicobacter pylori and Barrett's esophagus, erosive esophagitis, and gastroesophageal reflux symptoms. Clin Gastroenterol Hepatol 2014;12:239-45.
15. Anderson LA, Cantwell MM, Watson RG, et al. The association between alcohol and reflux esophagitis, Barrett's esophagus, and esophageal adenocarcinoma. Gastroenterol 2009;136:799-805.
16. Kubo A, Levin TR, Block G, et al. Alcohol types and sociodemographic characteristics as risk factors for Barrett's esophagus. Gastroenterol 2009;136:806-15.
17. Drahos J, Xiao Q, Risch H, et al. Age-specific risk factor profiles of adenocarcinomas of the esophagus: A pooled analysis from the international BEACON consortium. Int J Cancer 2016;138:55-64.
18. Spechler SJ, Sharma P, Souza RF, et al. American Gastroenterological Association medical position statement on the management of Barrett's esophagus. Gastroenterology 2011;140:1084-91.
19. Desai TK, Krishnan K, Samala N, et al. The incidence of oesophageal adenocarcinoma in non-dysplastic Barrett's oesophagus: a meta-analysis. Gut 2012;61:970-6.
20. Bhat S, Coleman HG, Yousef F, et al. Risk of malignant progression in Barrett's esophagus patients: results from a large population-based study. J Natl Cancer Inst 2011;103:1049-57.
21. Bennett C, Moayyedi P, Corley DA, et al. BOB CAT: a large-scale review and delphi consensus for management of Barrett's esophagus with no dysplasia, indefinite for, or low-grade dysplasia. Am J Gastroenterology 2015;110:662-82.
22. Weaver JM, Ross-Innes CS, Shannon N, et al. Ordering of mutations in preinvasive disease stages of esophageal carcinogenesis. Nat Genet 2014;46:837-43.
23. Stachler MD, Camarda ND, Deitrick C, et al. Somatic TP53 mutations distinguish non-dysplastic Barrett's esophagus lesions that progresses to cancer. Gastroenterology 2018;155:156-67.
24. Stachler MD, Taylor-Weiner A, Peng S, et al. Paired exome analysis of Barrett's esophagus and adenocarcinoma. Nat Genet 2015:47:1047-55.
25. The Cancer Genome Atlas Research Network, Analysis Working Group, Asan University, et al. Intergrated genomic characterization of oesophageal carcinoma. Nature 2017;541:169-75.
26. Dulak AM, Stojanov P, Peng S, et al. Exome and whole-genome sequencing of esophageal adenocarcinoma identifies recurrent driver events and mutational complexity. Nat Genet 2013;45:478-86.
27. Gopal DV, Lieberman DA, Margaret N, et al. Risk factors for dysplasia in patients with Barrett's esophagus (BE): results from a multicenter consortium. Dig Dis Sci 2003;48:1537-41.
28. Singh S, Garg SK, Singh PP, Iyer PG, El-Serag HB. Acid-suppressive medications and risk of oesophageal adenocarcinoma in patients with Barrett's oesophagus: a systematic review and meta-analysis. Gut 2014;63:1229-37.
29. Zhang S, Zhang XQ, Ding XW, et al. Cyclooxygenase inhibitors use is associated with reduced risk of esophageal adenocarcinoma in patients with Barrett's esophagus: a meta-analysis. Br J Cancer 2014;110:2378-88.
30. Singh S, Singh AG, Singh PP, Murad MH, Iyer PG. Statins are associated with reduced risk of esophageal cancer, particularly in patients with Barrett's esophagus: a systematic review and meta-analysis. Clin Gastroenterol Hepatol 2013;11:620-9.
31. Fitzgerald RC, Saeed IT, Khoo D, Farthing MJ, Burnham WR. Rigorous surveillance protocol increases detection of curable cancers associated with Barrett's esophagus. Dig Dis Sci 2001;46:1892-8.
32. Abela JE, Going JJ, Mackenzie JF, McKernan M, O'Mahoney S, Stuart RC. Systematic four-quadrant biopsy detects Barrett's dysplasia in more patients than nonsystematic biopsy. Am J Gastroenterol 2008;103:850-5.
33. Reid BJ, Blount PL, Feng Z, Levine DS. Optimizing endoscopic biopsy detection of early cancers in Barrett's high-grade dysplasia. Am J Gastroenterol 2000;95:3089-96.
34. Eluri S, Shaheen NJ. Barrett's esophagus: diagnosis and management. Gastrointest Endosc 2017;85:889-903.
35. Buttar NS, Wang KK, Sebo TJ, et al. Extent of high-grade dysplasia in Barrett's esophagus correlates with risk of adenocarcinoma. Gastroenterology 2001;120:1630-9.
36. Thurberg BL, Duray PH, Odze RD. Polypoid dysplasia in Barrett's esophagus: a clinicopathologic, immunohistochemical, and molecular study of five cases. Hum Pathol 1999;30:745-52.
37. Montgomery E, Bronner MP, Greenson JK, et al. Are ulcers a marker for invasive carcinoma in Barrett's esophagus? Data from a diagnostic variability study with clinical follow-up. Am J Gastroenterol 2002;97:27-31.
38. Reid BJ, Haggitt RC, Rubin CE, et al. Observer variation in the diagnosis of dysplasia in Barrett's esophagus. Hum Pathol 1988;19:166-78.

39. Schlemper RJ, Riddell RH, Kato Y, et al. The Vienna classification of gastrointestinal epithelial neoplasia. Gut 2000;47:251-5.
40. Rucker-Schmidt RL, Sanchez CA, Blount PL, et al. Nonadenomatous dysplasia in barrett esophagus: a clinical, pathologic, and DNA content flow cytometric study. Am J Surg Pathol 2009;33:886-93.
41. Brown IS, Whiteman DC, Lauwers GY. Foveolar type dysplasia in Barrett esophagus. Mod Pathol 2010;23:834-43.
42. Agoston AT, Srivastava A, Zheng Y, et al. Prevalence and concordance of subtypes of dysplasia in patients with Barrett's esophagus-associated adenocarcinoma. Mod Pathol 2013;27:162a.
43. Srivastava A, Sanchez CA, Cowan DS, et al. Foveolar and serrated dysplasia are rare high-risk lesions in Barrett's esophagus: a prospective outcome analysis of 214 patients. Mod Pathol 2010;23:168a.
44. Lomo LC, Blount PL, Sanchez CA, et al. Crypt dysplasia with surface maturation: a clinical, pathologic, and molecular study of a Barrett's esophagus cohort. Am J Surg Pathol 2006;30:423-35.
45. Zhang X, Huang Q, Goyal RK, Odze RD. DNA ploidy abnormalities in basal and superficial regions of the crypts in Barrett's esophagus and associated neoplastic lesions. Am J Surg Pathol 2008;32:1327-35.
46. Mahajan D, BennettAE, Liu X, Bena J, Bronner MP. Grading of gastric foveolar-type dysplasia in Barrett's esophagus. Mod Pathol 2010;23:1-11.
47. Varghese S, Lao-Sirieix P, Fitzgerald RC. Identification and clinical implementation of biomarkers for Barrett's esophagus. Gastroenterology 2012;142:435-441.
48. Zeki S, Fitzgerald RC. The use of molecular markers in predicting dysplasia and guiding treatment. Best Pract Res Clin Gastroenterol 2015;29:113-24.
49. Reid BJ, Levine DS, Longton G, Blount PL, Rabinovitch PS. Predictors of progression to cancer in Barrett's esophagus: baseline histology and flow cytometry identify low- and high-risk patient subsets. Am J Gastroenterol 2000;95:1669-76.
50. Kaye PV, Haider SA, Ilyas M, et al. Barrett's dysplasia and the Vienna classification: reproducibility, prediction of progression and impact of consensus reporting and p53 immunohistochemistry. Histopathology 2009;54:699-712.
51. Montgomery E, Bronner MP, Goldblum JR, et al. Reproducibility of the diagnosis of dysplasia in Barrett esophagus: a reaffirmation. Hum Pathol 2001;32:368-78.
52. Coco DP, Goldblum JR, Hornick JL, et al. Interobserver variability in the diagnosis of crypt dysplasia in Barrett esophagus. Am J Surg Pathol 2011;35:45-54.
53. Kerkhof M, van Dekken H, Steyerberg EW, et al. Grading of dysplasia in Barrett's oesophagus: substantial interobserver variation between general and gastrointestinal pathologists. Histopathology 2007;50:920-7.
54. Younes M, Lebovitz RM, Lechago LV, Lechago J. p53 protein accumulation in Barrett's metaplasia, dysplasia, and carcinoma: a follow-up study. Gastroenterol 1993;105:1637-42.
55. Dorer R, Odze RD. AMACR immunostaining is useful in detecting dysplastic epithelium in Barrett's esophagus, ulcerative colitis, and Crohn's disease. Am J Surg Pathol 2006;30:871-7.
56. Lisovsky M, Falkowski O, Bhuiya T. Expression of alpha-methylacyl-coenzyme A racemase in dysplastic Barrett's epithelium. Hum Pathol 2006;37:1601-6.
57. Sonwalkar SA, Rotimi O, Scott N, et al. A study of indefinite for dysplasia in Barrett's oesophagus: reproducibility of diagnosis, clinical outcomes and predicting progression with AMACR (alpha-methylacyl-CoA-racemase). Histopathology 2010;56:900-7.
58. Downs-Kelly E, Mendelin JE, Bennett AE, et al. Poor interobserver agreement in the distinction of high-grade dysplasia and adenocarcinoma in pretreatment Barrett's esophagus biopsies. Am J Gastroenterol 2008;103:2333-40.
59. Stein HJ, Siewert JR. Barrett's esophagus: pathogenesis, epidemiology, functional abnormalities, malignant degeneration, and surgical management. Dysphagia 1993;8:276-88.
60. Chennat J, Ross AS, Konda VJ, et al. Advanced pathology under squamous epithelium on initial EMR specimens in patients with Barrett's esophagus and high-grade dysplasia or intramucosal carcinoma: implications for surveillance and endotherapy management. Gastrointest Endosc 2009;70:417-21.
61. Sharma P, Falk GW, Weston AP, Reker D, Johnston M, Sampliner RE. Dysplasia and cancer in a large multicenter cohort of patients with Barrett's esophagus. Clin Gastroenterol Hepatol 2006;4:566-72.
62. Weston AP, Sharma P, Topalovski M, Richards R, Cherian R, Dixon A. Long-term follow-up of Barrett's high-grade dysplasia. Am J Gastroenterol 2000;95:1888-93.
63. Singh S, Manickam P, Amin AV, et al. Incidence of esophageal adenocarcinoma in Barrett's esophagus with low-grade dysplasia: a systematic review and meta-analysis. Gastrointest Endosc 2014;79:897-909.
64. Spechler SJ. Barrett esophagus and risk of esophageal cancer: a clinical review. JAMA 2013;310:627-36.
65. de Jonge PJ, van Blankenstein M, Looman CW, Casparie MK, Meijer GA, Kuipers EJ. Risk of malignant progression in patients with Barrett's oesophagus: a Dutch nationwide cohort study. Gut 2010;59:1030-6.

66. Rastogi A, Puli S, El-Serag HB, Bansal A, Wani S, Sharma P. Incidence of esophageal adenocarcinoma in patients with Barrett's esophagus and high-grade dysplasia: a meta-analysis. Gastrointest Endosc 2008;67:394-8.
67. Shaheen NJ, Sharma P, Overholt BF, et al. Radiofrequency ablation in Barrett's esophagus with dysplasia. N Engl J Med 2009;360:2277-88.
68. Srivastava A, Hornick JL, Li X, et al. Extent of low-grade dysplasia is a risk factor for the development of esophageal adenocarcinoma in Barrett's esophagus. Am J Gastroenterol 2007;102:483-93.
69. Weston AP, Sharma P, Mathur S, et al. Risk stratification of Barrett's esophagus: updated prospective multivariate analysis. Am J Gastroenterol 2004;99:1657-66.
70. Anaparthy R, Gaddam S, Kanakadandi V, et al. Association between length of Barrett's esophagus and risk of high-grade dysplasia or adenocarcinoma in patients without dysplasia. Clin Gastroenterol Hepatol 2013;11:1430-6.
71. Kastelein F, Biermann K, Steyerberg W, et al. Aberrant p53 protein expression is associated with an increased risk of neoplastic progression in patients with Barrett's oesophagus. Gut 2013;62:1676-83.
72. Skacel M, Petras RE, Rybicki LA, et al. p53 expression in low grade dysplasia in Barrett's esophagus: correlation with interobserver agreement and disease progression. Am J Gastroenterol 2002;97:2508-13.
73. Fitzgerald RC, di Pietro M, Ragunath K, et al. British Society of Gastroenterology guidelines on the diagnosis and management of Barrett's oesophagus. Gut 2014;63:7-42.
74. Wang JS, Guo M, Montgomery EA, et al. DNA promoter hypermethylation of p16 and APC predicts neoplastic progression in Barrett's esophagus. Am J Gastroenterol 2009;104:2153-60.
75. di Pietro M, Boerwinkel DF, Shariff MK, et al. The combination of autofluorescence endoscopy and molecular biomarkers is a novel diagnostic tool for dysplasia in Barrett's oesophagus. Gut 2015;64:49-56.
76. Flejou JF, Odze RD, Montgomery E, et al. Adenocarcinoma of the oesophagus. In: Bosman T, ed. WHO classification of tumours of the digestive system, 4th ed. Lyon: IARC Press; 2010:25-31.
77. Goldstein NS, Karim R. Gastric cardia inflammation and intestinal metaplasia: associations with reflux esophagitis and Helicobacter pylori. Mod Pathol 1999;12:1017-24.
78. Morales TG, Sampliner RE, Bhattacharyya A. Intestinal metaplasia of the gastric cardia. Am J Gastroenterol 1997;92:414-8.
79. Ruol A, Parenti A, Zaninotto G, et al. Intestinal metaplasia is the probable common precursor of adenocarcinoma in Barrett esophagus and adenocarcinoma of the gastric cardia. Cancer 2000;88:2520-8.
80. Brown LM, Devesa SS, Chow WH. Incidence of adenocarcinoma of the esophagus among white Americans by sex, stage, and age. J Natl Cancer Inst 2008;100:1184-7.
81. Daly JM, Fry WA, Little AG, et al. Esophageal cancer: results of an American College of Surgeons Patient Care Evaluation Study. J Am Coll Surg 2000;190:562-72.
82. Berry MF. Esophageal cancer: staging system and guidelines for staging and treatment. J Thorac Dis 2014;6(Suppl 3):S289-97.
83. Luketich JD, Schauer PR, Meltzer CC, et al. Role of positron emission tomography in staging esophageal cancer. Ann Thorac Surg 1997;64:765-9.
84. Choi J, Kim SG, Kim JS, et al. Comparison of endoscopic ultrasonography (EUS), positron emission tomography (PET), and computed tomography (CT) in the preoperative locoregional staging of resectable esophageal cancer. Surg Endosc 2010;24:1380-6.
85. Pech O, Gunter E, Dusemund F, Origer J, Lorenz D, Ell C. Accuracy of endoscopic ultrasound in preoperative staging of esophageal cancer: results from a referral center for early esophageal cancer. Endosc 2010;42:456-61.
86. Vazquez-Sequeiros E, Wiersema MJ, Clain JE, et al. Impact of lymph node staging on esophageal carcinoma therapy. Gastroenterol 2003;125:1626-35.
87. Krasna MJ, Flowers JL, Attar S, McLaughlin J. Combined thoracoscopic/laparoscopic staging of esophageal cancer. J Thorac Cardiovasc Surg 1996;111:800-6.
88. Thomas T, Abrams KR, De Caestecker JS, Robinson RJ. Meta analysis: cancer risk in Barrett's oesophagus. Aliment Pharmacol Ther 2007;26:1465-77.
89. Rastogi A, Puli S, El-Serag HB, Bansal A, Wani S, Sharma P. Incidence of esophageal adenocarcinoma in patients with Barrett's esophagus and high-grade dysplasia: a meta-analysis. Gastrointest Endosc 2008;67:394-8.
90. Avidan B, Sonnenberg A, Schnell TG, Chejfec G, Metz A, Sontag SJ. Hiatal hernia size, Barrett's length, and severity of acid reflux are all risk factors for esophageal adenocarcinoma. Am J Gastroenterol 2002;97:1930-6.
91. Takubo K, Aida J, Naomoto Y, et al. Cardiac rather than intestinal-type background in endoscopic resection specimens of minute Barrett adenocarcinoma. Hum Pathol 2009;40:65-74.
92. Srivastava A, Golden KL, Sanchez CA, et al. High goblet cell count is inversely associated with ploidy abnormalities and risk of adenocarcinoma in patients with Barrett's esophagus. PLoS One 2015;10:e0133403.

93. Khan S, McDonald SA, Wright NA, et al. Crypt dysplasia in Barrett's oesophagus shows clonal identity between crypt and surface cells. J Pathol 2013;231:98-104.

94. Lavery DL, Martinez P, Gay LJ, et al. Evolution of oesophageal adenocarcinoma from metaplastic columnar epithelium without goblet cells in Barrett's oesophagus. Gut 2016;65:907-13.

95. Bandla S, Peters JH, Ruff D, et al. Comparison of cancer-associated genetic abnormalities in columnar-lined esophagus tissues with and without goblet cells. Ann Surg 2014;260:72-80.

96. Liu W, Hahn H, Odze RD, Goyal RK. Metaplastic esophageal columnar epithelium without goblet cells shows DNA content abnormalities similar to goblet cell-containing epithelium. Am J Gastroenterol 2009;104:816-24.

97. Desai TK, Krishnan K, Samala N, et al. The incidence of oesophageal adenocarcinoma in non-dysplastic Barrett's oesophagus: a meta-analysis. Gut 2012;61:970-6.

98. Westerhoff M, Hovan L, Lee C, Hart J. Effects of dropping the requirement for goblet cells from the diagnosis of Barrett's esophagus. Clin Gastroenterol Hepatol 2012;10:1232-6.

99. Bosman FT, Carneiro F, Hruban RH, Thiese ND, eds. WHO classification of tumours of the digestive system. Lyon: IARC Press; 2010.

100. Torres C, Turner JR, Wang HH, et al. Pathologic prognostic factors in Barrett's associated adenocarcinoma: a follow-up study of 96 patients. Cancer 1999;85:520-8.

101. Donahue JM, Nichols FC, Li Z, et al. Complete pathologic response after neoadjuvant chemoradiotherapy for esophageal cancer is associated with enhanced survival. Ann Thorac Surg 2009;87:392-8.

102. Yoon HH, Shi Q, Sukov WR, et al. Association of HER2/ErbB2 expression and gene amplification with pathologic features and prognosis in esophageal adenocarcinomas. Clin Cancer Res 2012;18:546-54.

103. Sarbia M. The histological appearance of oesophageal adenocarcinoma- an analysis based on 215 resection specimens. Virchow Arch 2006;448:532-8.

104. Raja S, Rice TW, Goldblum JR, et al. Esophageal submucosa: the watershed for esophageal cancer. J Thorac Cardiovasc Surg 2011;142:1403-11.

105. Edge SB, Byrd DR, Compton CC, et al, eds. AJCC Cancer staging manual, 7th ed. New York: Springer; 2010.

106. Chiba N, Yoshioka T, Sakayori M, et al. AFP-producing hepatoid adenocarcinoma in association with Barrett's esophagus with multiple liver metastasis responding to paclitaxel/CDDP: a case report. Anticancer Res 2005;25:2965-8.

107. Kuroda N, Onishi K, Lee GH. Combined tubular adenocarcinoma and hepatoid adenocarcinoma arising in Barrett esophagus. Ann Diagn Pathol 2011;15:450-3.

108. Setia N, Agoston A, Shen J, et al. Clinicopathologic significance of macrocystic change in esophageal adenocarcinoma. Lab Invest 2014:828A.

109. Shen J, Tippayawong M, Agoston A, et al. Prevalence and Clinicopathologic Significance of Micropapillary Differentiation in Esophageal Adenocarcinomas. Lab Invest 2014:831A.

110. Hornick JL, Farraye FA, Odze RD. Prevalence and significance of prominent mucin pools in the esophagus post neoadjuvant chemoradiotherapy for Barrett's-associated adenocarcinoma. Am J Surg Pathol 2006;30:28-35.

111. Taniere P, Borghi-Scoazec G, Suarin JC, et al. Cytokeratin expression in adenocarcinomas of the esophagogastric junction: a comparative study of adenocarcinomas of the distal esophagus and of the proximal stomach. Am J Surg Pathol 2002;26:1213-21.

112. Werling RW, Yaziji H, Bacchi CE, Gown AM. CDX2, a highly sensitive and specific marker of adenocarcinomas of intestinal origin: an immunohistochemical survey of 476 primary and metastatic carcinomas. Am J Surg Pathol 2003;27:303-10.

113. Koppert LB, Wijnhoven BP, Tilanus HW, Stijnen T, Van Dekken H, Dinjens WN. Neuroendocrine in Barrett's mucosa and adenocarcinomas of the gastroesophageal junction. Int J Surg Pathol 2004;12:117-25.

114. Wilson CI, Summerall J, Willis I, Lubin J, Inchausti BC. Esophageal collision tumor (large cell neuroendocrine carcinoma and papillary carcinoma) arising in a Barrett esophagus. Arch Pathol Lab Med 2000;124:411-5.

115. Lam KY, Dickens P, Loke SL, Fok M, Ma L, Wong J. Squamous cell carcinoma of the oesophagus with mucin-secreting component (muco-epidermoid carcinoma and adenosquamous carcinoma): a clinicopathologic study and a review of literature. Eur J Surg Oncol 1994;20:25-31.

116. Ter RB, Govil YK, Leite L, et al. Adenosquamous carcinoma in Barrett's esophagus presenting as pseudoachalasia. Am J Gastroenterol 1999;94:268-70.

117. Chen S, Chen Y, Yang J, et al. Primary mucoepidermoid carcinoma of the esophagus. J Thorac Oncol 2011;6:1426-31.

118. Yachida S, Nakanishi Y, Shimoda T, et al. Adenosquamous carcinoma of the esophagus: clinicopathologic study of 18 cases. Oncology 2004;66:218-25.

119. Maru DM, Khurana H, Rashid A, et al. Retrospective study of clinicopathologic features and prognosis of high-grade neuroendocrine carcinoma of the esophagus. Am J Surg Pathol 2008;32:1404-11.
120. Lu J, Xue LY, Lu N, Zou SM, Liu XY, Wen P. Superficial primary small cell carcinoma of the esophagus: clinicopathological and immunohistochemical analysis of 15 cases. Dis Esophagus 2010;23:153-9.
121. Robey SS, Hamilton SR, Gupta PK, Erozan YS. Diagnostic value of cytopathology in Barrett esophagus and associated carcinoma. Am J Clin Pathol 1988;89:493-8.
122. Wang HH, Doria MI, Purohit-Buch S, Schnell T, Sontag S, Chejfec G. Barrett's esophagus. The cytology of dysplasia in comparison to benigh and malignant lesions. Acta Cytol 1992;36:60-4.
123. Genta RM, Huberman RM, Graham DY. The gastric cardia in Helicobacter pylori infection. Hum Pathol 1994;25:915-9.
124. Wang HH, Sovie S, Zeroogian JM, Spechler SJ, Goyal RK, Antonioli DA. Value of cytology in detecting intestinal metaplasia and associated dysplasia at the gastroesophageal junction. Hum Pathol 1997;28:465-71.
125. Saad RS, Mahood LK, Clary KM, Liu Y, Silverman JF, Raab SS. Role of cytology in the diagnosis of Barrett's esophagus and associated neoplasia. Diagn Cytopathol 2003;29:130-5.
126. di Pietro M, Chan D, Fitzgerald RC, Wang KK. Screening for Barrett's esophagus. Gastroenterology 2015;148:912-23.
127. MacLennan AJ, Orringer MB, Beer DG. Identification of intestinal-type Barrett's metaplasia by using the intestine-specific protein villin and esophageal brush cytology. Mol Carcinog 1999;24:137-43.
128. Chu PG, Jiang Z, Weiss LM. Hepatocyte antigen as a marker of intestinal metaplasia. Am J Surg Pathol 2003;27:952-9.
129. Lee W, Liu YL, Cho P, Tung MT, Silverman JF. Diagnostic value of Hep-Par 1 immunocytochemistry in detecting Barrett's esophagus in esophageal brushing cytology [abstract]. Mod Pathol. 2004;17(Suppl 1):74A.
130. Zhang J, Parwani AV, Ali SZ. Hepatocyte paraffin 1 immunoexpression in esophageal brush samples. Cancer 2005;105:304-9.
131. Lao-Sirieix P, Boussioutas A, Kadri SR, et al. Non-endoscopic screening biomarkers for Barrett's oesophagus: from microarray analysis to the clinic. Gut 2009;58:1451-9.
132. Ross-Innes CS, Debiram-Beecham I, O'Donovan M, et al. Evaluation of a minimally invasive cell sampling device coupled with assessment of trefoil factor 3 expression for diagnosing Barrett's esophagus: a multi-center case-control study. PLoS Med 2015;12:e1001780.
133. Geisinger KR, Teot LA, Richter JE. A comparative cytopathologic and histologic study of atypia, dysplasia, and adenocarcinoma in Barrett's esophagus. Cancer 1992;69:8-16.
134. Kumaravel A, Lopez R, Brainard J, Falk GW. Brush cytology vs. endoscopic biopsy for the surveillance of Barrett's esophagus. Endoscopy 2010;42:800-5.
135. Ross-Innes CS, Chettouh H, Achilleos A, et al. Risk stratification of Barrett's oesophagus using a non-endoscopic sampling method coupled with a biomarker panel: a cohort study. Lancet Gastroenterol Hepatol 2017;2:23-31.
136. Hughes JH, Cohen MB. Is the cytologic diagnosis of esophageal glandular dysplasia feasible? Diagn Cytopathol 1998;18:312-6.
137. Shen O, Liu SF, Dawsey SM, et al. Cytologic screening for esophageal cancer: results from 12,877 subjects from a high-risk population in China. Int J Cancer 1993;54:185-8.
138. Liu SF, Shen Q, Dawsey SM, et al. Esophageal balloon cytology and subsequent risk of esophageal and gastric-cardia cancer in a high-risk Chinese population. Int J Cancer 1994;57:775-80.
139. Fritcher EG, Brankley SM, Kipp BR, et al. A comparison of conventional cytology, DNA ploidy analysis, and fluorescence in situ hybridization for the detection of dysplasia and adenocarcinoma in patients with Barrett's esophagus. Hum Pathol 2008;39:1128-35.
140. Rygiel AM, Milano F, Ten Kate FJ, et al. Assessment of chromosomal gains as compared to DNA content changes is more useful to detect dysplasia in Barrett's esophagus brush cytology specimens. Genes Chromosomes Cancer 2008;47:396-404.
141. Fahmy M, Skacel M, Gramlich TL, et al. Chromosomal gains and genomic loss of p53 and p16 genes in Barrett's esophagus detected by fluorescence in situ hybridization of cytology specimens. Mod Pathol 2004;17:588-96.
142. Lao-Sirieix P, Lovat L, Fitzgerald RC. Cyclin A immunocytology as a risk stratification tool for Barrett's esophagus surveillance. Clin Cancer Res 2007;13(Pt 1):659-65.
143. Baloch Z, Lyle S, Hoda RS, Gupta PK. Ultrasound-guided fine-needle aspiration diagnosis of adenocarcinoma of esophagus with signet-ring cell features arising in Barrett's esophagus: a case report. Diagn Cytopathol 1998;19:51-4.
144. Parmar KS, Zwischenberger JB, Reeves AL, Waxman I. Clinical impact of endoscopic ultrasound-guided fine needle aspiration of celiac axis lymph nodes (M1a disease) in esophageal cancer. Ann Thorac Surg 2002;73:916-20.

145. Jhala NC, Jhala DN, Chhieng DC, Eloubeidi MA, Eltoum IA. Endoscopic ultrasound-guided fine-needle aspiration. A cytopathologist's perspective. Am J Clin Pathol 2003;120:351-67.

146. David S, Meltzer SJ. MicroRNA involvement in esophageal carcinogenesis. Curr Opin Pharmacol 2011;11:612-6.

147. Tselepis C, Perry I, Dawson C, et al. Tumour necrosis factor-alpha in Barrett's oesophagus: a potential novel mechanism of action. Oncogene 2002;21:6071-81.

148. van der Woude CJ, Jansen PL, Tiebosch AT, et al. Expression of apoptosis-related proteins in Barrett's metaplasia-dysplasia-carcinoma sequence: a switch to a more resistant phenotype. Hum Pathol 2002;33:686-92.

149. Hughes SJ, Nambu Y, Soldes OS, et al. Fas/APO-1 (CD95) is not translocated to the cell membrane in esophageal adenocarcinoma. Cancer Res 1997;57:5571-8.

150. Younes M, Schwartz MR, Ertan A, Finnie D, Younes A. Fas ligand expression in esophageal carcinomas and their lymph node mestatases. Cancer 2000;88:524-8.

151. Rioux-Leclercq N, Turlin B, Sutherland F, et al. Analysisof Ki-67, p53 and Bcl-2 expression in the dysplasia-carcinoma sequence of Barrett's esophagus. Oncol Rep 1999;6:877-82.

152. Katada N, Hinder RA, Smyrk TC, et al. Apoptosis is inhibited early in the dysplasia-carcinoma sequence of Barrett esophagus. Arch Surg 1997;132:728-33.

153. Fritcher EG, Brankley SM, Kipp BR, et al. A comparison of conventional cytology, DNA ploidy analysis, and fluorescence in situ hybridization for the detection of dysplasia and adenocarcinoma in patients with Barrett's esophagus. Hum Pathol 2008;39:1128-35.

154. Tot T. The role of cytokeratins 20 and 7 and estrogen receptor analysis in separation of metastatic lobular carcinoma of the breast and metastatic signet ring cell carcinoma of the gastrointestinal tract. APMIS 2000;108:467-72.

155. Shen B, Ormsby AH, Shen C, et al. Cytokeratin expression patterns in noncardia, intestinal metaplasia-associated gastric adenocarcinoma: implication for the evaluation of intestinal metaplasia and tumors at the esophagogastric junction. Cancer 2002;94:820-31.

156. Driessen A, Nafteux P, Lerut T, et al. Identical cytokeratin expression pattern CK7+/CK20– in esophageal and cardiac cancer: etiopathological and clinical implications. Mod Pathol 2004;17:49-55.

157. van Lier MG, Bomhof FJ, Leendertse I, Flens M, Balk AT, Loffeld RJ. Cytokeratin phenotyping does not help in distinguishing oesophageal adenocarcinoma from cancer of the gastric cardia. J Clin Pathol 2005;58:722-4.

158. Abraham SC, Krasinskas AM, Correa AM, et al. Duplication of the muscularis mucosae in Barrett esophagus: an underrecognized feature and its implication for staging of adenocarcinoma. AM J Surg Pathol 2007;31:1719-25.

159. Mandal RV, Forcione DG, Brugge WR, Nishioka NS, Mino-Kenudson M, Lauwers GY. Effect of tumor characteristics and duplication of the muscularis mucosae on the endoscopic staging of superficial Barrett esophagus-related neoplasia. Am J Surg Pathol 2009;33:620-5.

160. Talsma K, van Hagen P, Grotenhuis BA, et al. Comparison of the 6th and 7th editions of the UICC-AJCC TNM Classification for Esophageal Cancer. Ann Surg Oncol 2012;19:2142-8.

161. Eloubeidi MA, Desmond R, Arguedas MR, Reed CE, Wilcox CM. Prognostic factors for the survival of patients with esophageal carcinoma in the U.S.: the importance of tumor length and lymph node status. Cancer 2002;95:1434-43.

162. Dunbar KB, Spechler SJ. The risk of lymph-node metastases in patients with high-grade dysplasia or intramucosal carcinoma in Barrett's esophagus: a systematic review. Am J Gastroenterol 2012;107:850-62.

163. Estrella JS, Hofstetter WL, Correa AM, et al. Duplicated muscularis mucosae invasion has similar risk of lymph node metastasis and recurrence-free survival as intramucosal esophageal adenocarcinoma. Am J Surg Pathol 2011;35:1045-53.

164. Glickman JN, Torres C, Wang HH, et al. The prognostic significance of lymph node micrometastasis in patients with esophageal carcinoma. Cancer 1999;85:769-78.

165. Heeren PA, Kelder W, Blondeel I, van Westreenen HL, Hollema H, Plukker JT. Prognostic value of nodal micrometastases in patients with cancer of the gastro-oesophageal junction. Eur J Surg Oncol 2005;31:270-6.

166. Verhage RJ, Zandvoort HJ, ten Kate FJ, van Hillegersberg R. How to define a positive circumferential resection margin in T3 adenocarcinoma of the esophagus. Am J Surg Pathol 2011;35:919-26.

167. Marx AH, Zielinski M, Kowitz CM, et al. Homogeneous EGFR amplification defines a subset of aggressive Barrett's adenocarcinomas with poor prognosis. Histopathology 2010;57:418-26.

168. Lennerz JK, Kwak EL, Ackerman A, et al. MET amplification identifies a small and aggressive subgroup of esophagogastric adenocarcinoma with evidence of responsiveness to crizotinib. J Clin Oncol 2011;29:4803-10.

169. Lagarde SM, ten Kate FJ, Richel DJ, Offerhaus GJ, van Lanschot JJ. Molecular prognostic factors in adenocarcinoma of the esophagus and gastroesophageal junction. Ann Surg Oncol 2007;14:977-91.

170. Langer R, Von Rahden BH, Nahrig J, et al. Prognostic significance of expression patterns of c-erbB-2, p53, p16INK4A, p27KIP1, cyclin D1 and epidermal growth factor receptor in esophageal adenocarcinoma: a tissue microarray study. J Clin Pathol 2006;59:631-4.

171. Kwak EL, Jankowski J, Thayer SP, et al. Epidermal growth factor receptor kinase domain mutations in esophageal and pancreatic adenocarcinomas. Clin Cancer Res 2006;12:4283-7.

172. Mandard AM, Dalibard F, Mandard JC, et al. Pathologic assessment of tumor regression after preoperative chemoradiotherapy of esophageal carcinoma. Clinicopathologic correlations. Cancer 1994;73:2680-6.

173. Chirieac LR, Swisher SG, Ajani JA, et al. Posttherapy pathologic stage predicts survival in patients with esophageal carcinoma receiving preoperative chemoradiation. Cancer 2005;103:1347-55.

174. Berger AC, Farma J, Scott WJ, et al. Complete response to neoadjuvant chemoradiotherapy in esophageal carcinoma is associated with significantly improved survival. J Clin Oncol 2005;23:4330-7.

175. Howlader N, Noone AM, Krapcho M, et al. SEER Cancer Statistics Review, 1975-2011, National Cancer Institute, Bethesda, MD, 2013. based on November 2013 SEER data submission, posted to the SEER web site, April 2014 http://seer.cancer.gov/csr/1975_2011/.

176. Enzinger PC, Mayer RJ. Esophageal Cancer. N Engl J Med 2003;349:2241-52.

177. Soetikno R, Kaltenbach T, Yeh R, Gotoda T. Endoscopic mucosal resection for early cancers of the upper gastrointestinal tract. J Clin Oncol 2005;23:4490-8.

178. Nigro JJ, Hagen JA, DeMeester TR, et al. Prevalence and location of nodal metastases in distal esophageal adenocarcinoma confined to the wall: implications for therapy. J Thorac Cardiovasc Surg 1999;117:16-23.

179. Rice TW, Zuccaro G Jr, Adelstein DJ, Rybicki LA, Blackstone EH, Goldblum JR. Esophageal carcinoma: depth of tumor invasion is predictive of regional lymph node status. Ann Thorac Surg 1998;65:787-92.

180. Kountourakis P, Correa AM, Hofstetter WL, et al. Combined modality therapy of cT2N0M0 esophageal cancer: the University of Texas M. D. Anderson Cancer Center experience. Cancer 2011;117:925-30.

181. Smith GL, Smith BD, Buchholz TA, et al. Patterns of care and locoregional treatment outcomes in older esophageal cancer patients: the SEER-Medicare Cohort. Int J Radiat Oncol Biol Phys 2009;74:482-9.

182. Ajani JA, Barthel JS, Bentrem DJ, et al. Esophageal and esophagogastric junction cancers. J Natl Compr Canc Netw 2011;9:830-87.

183. Wani S, Mathur SC, Curvers WL, et al. Greater interobserver agreement by endoscopic mucosal resection than biopsy samples in Barrett's dysplasia. Clin Gastroenterol Hepatol 2010;8:783-8.

184. Mino-Kenudson M, Hull MJ, Brown I, et al. EMR for Barrett's esophagus-related superficial neoplasms offers better diagnostic reproducibility than mucosal biopsy. Gastrointest Endosc 2007;66:660-6.

185. Abraham SC, Krasinskas AM, Correa AM, et al. Duplication of the muscularis mucosae in Barrett esophagus: an underrecognized feature and its implication for staging of adenocarcinoma. AM J Surg Pathol 2007;31:1719-25.

186. Lewis JT, Wang KK, Abraham SC. Muscularis mucosae duplication and the musculo-fibrous anomaly in endoscopic mucosal resections for barrett esophagus: implications for staging of adenocarcinoma. Am J Surg Pathol 2008;32:566-71.

187. Vieth M, Stolte M. Pathology of early upper GI cancers. Best Pract Res Clin Gastroenterol 2005;19:857-69.

188. Estrella JS, Hofstetter WL, Correa AM, et al. Duplicated muscularis mucosae invasion has similar risk of lymph node metastasis and recurrence-free survival as intramucosal esophageal adenocarcinoma. Am J Surg Pathol 2011;35:1045-53.

189. Kumarasinghe MP, Brown I, Raftopoulos S, et al. Standardised reporting protocol for endoscopic resection for Barrett oesophagus associated neoplasia: expert consensus recommendations. Pathology 2014;46:473-80.

5 ESOPHAGEAL SQUAMOUS CELL CARCINOMA

Squamous cell carcinoma of the esophagus and its precursors are, globally, more common than esophageal columnar lesions discussed in chapter 4. In common with patients with adenocarcinomas, most patients with esophageal squamous cell carcinoma are male and at least in their fifties; however, at least in the United States, adenocarcinomas typically affect white males, while squamous cell carcinomas are most common in African-American males (1). Although recent advances have resulted in some improvement in detecting and treating esophageal adenocarcinomas, this has not been the case for squamous cell carcinomas, at least not in the United States (2), although cytologic screening programs in Southeast Asia, particularly in China, as discussed below, have resulted in some advances.

In the United States, the incidence of esophageal squamous cell carcinoma is decreasing in comparison to adenocarcinoma, but there is still a high incidence in developing countries, including those in southern Africa and in China. In Southeast Asia, polymorphisms in *ALDH*, the gene that encodes aldehyde dehydrogenase, are associated with esophageal squamous cell cancer (3,4). These polymorphisms are synergistic with alcohol use and smoking in promoting esophageal squamous cell carcinoma and its precursors. Acetaldehyde accumulates, prompting flushing upon ingestion of alcohol ("Asian flush") in up to a third of East Asians (Chinese, Japanese, and Koreans).

SQUAMOUS INTRAEPITHELIAL NEOPLASIA/DYSPLASIA AND OTHER PRECURSOR LESIONS

Definition. The terms *intraepithelial neoplasia* (IEN) and *dysplasia* are roughly equivalent but the former term is preferred in Europe and Asia and the latter is used in the United States. Most data on squamous precursor lesions are derived from Southeast Asia, where the IEN terminology is preferred (5). The World Health Organization (WHO) has defined IENs as "lesions that display cytologic or architectural alterations perceived to reflect underlying molecular abnormalities that may lead to invasive carcinoma" (5). In the case of squamous precursors, these processes are composed of altered squamous cells that lack tissue invasion.

General Features. The development of esophageal squamous cell carcinoma, similar to squamous cell carcinoma in other sites, is believed to reflect a multistep progression from unremarkable squamous epithelium to invasive carcinoma. Squamous IEN/dysplasia is an intermediate step that has not yet acquired the ability to metastasize (6).

Clinical Features. Squamous IEN/dysplasia of the esophagus is often invisible endoscopically and is generally asymptomatic. It is usually only detected on screening, which has been of value in high risk countries (7,8).

Gross Findings. Although difficult to detect grossly, endoscopic detection can be enhanced by using Lugol iodine (the lesions loose uptake of iodine, which is normally striking for squamous epithelium, resulting in a brown appearance) (fig. 5-1) or advanced imaging methods such as narrow band imaging as opposed to white light endoscopy (9).

Microscopic Findings. Esophageal squamous IEN/dysplasia has the same appearance as it does in other anatomic sites, although since it is less frequently driven by human papillomavirus (HPV), ancillary techniques that are used to confirm this lesion are not as readily applicable. Essentially, the diagnosis rests on finding epithelial changes that involve some or all of the epithelium. If the alterations involve the bottom half of the epithelium, the findings are regarded as low grade, whereas higher extension is considered high grade. In the upcoming WHO classification,

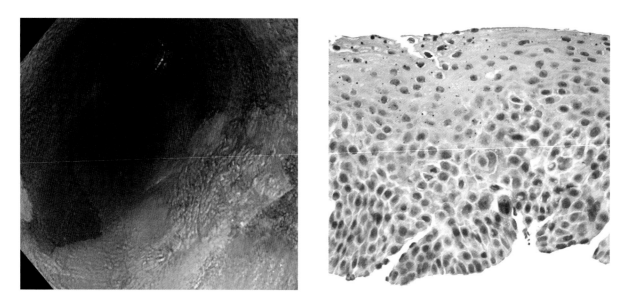

Figure 5-1

HIGH-GRADE SQUAMOUS INTRAEPITHELIAL NEOPLASIA/DYSPLASIA: LUGOL IODINE PREPARATION

Left: The nondysplastic squamous epithelium has a brown color whereas the areas that do not take up the solution are those targeted for biopsies. This inexpensive method can be a powerful screening tool. This image was from the esophagus of an elderly woman with longstanding mucocutaneous lichen planus, a condition that places patients at risk for esophageal neoplasia. (Courtesy of Dr. M. I. Canto, Baltimore, MD.)

Right: This image is from the area that did not take up Lugol iodine solution. There are enlarged hyperchromatic nuclei that involve over half the thickness of the epithelium. The inflammatory changes of lichen planus vanish once intraepithelial neoplasia supervenes.

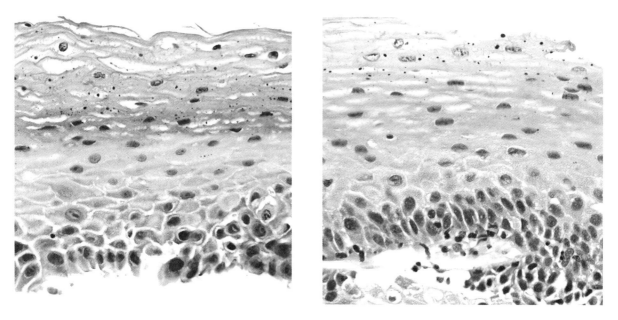

Figure 5-2

LOW-GRADE SQUAMOUS INTRAEPITHELIAL NEOPLASIA/DYSPLASIA

Left: The cells in the lower third of the sample contain enlarged nuclei that are hyperchromatic and have irregular nuclear membranes.

Right: The nuclei in the basal area are jumbled.

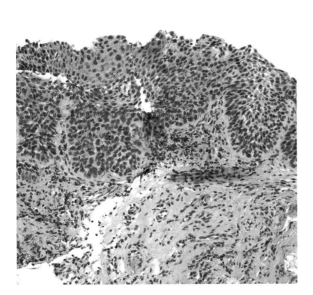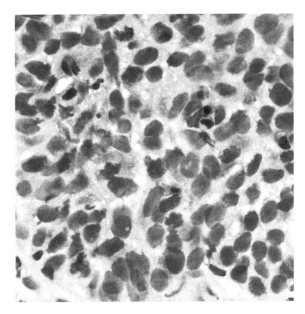

Figure 5-3

HIGH-GRADE SQUAMOUS INTRAEPITHELIAL NEOPLASIA/DYSPLASIA

Left: The lesion shown here involves the full thickness of the epithelium and contains hyperchromatic nuclei
Right: Nucleoli are inconspicuous in this high magnification image.

high grade is also defined by high-grade cytology without more than 50 percent involvement of epithelium (figs. 5-2–5-4). These alterations consist of nuclear enlargement and nuclear hyperchromasia. While intercellular bridges are prominent in reactive conditions, they are often less conspicuous in squamous IEN/dysplasia.

Basal cell hyperplasia is also believed to be a precursor of squamous cell carcinoma (fig. 5-5). It is defined as a proliferation of basal cells that comprises more than 15 percent of the epithelial thickness (5) and it lacks uptake of Lugol iodine.

Another probable precursor lesion to esophageal squamous cell carcinoma is *epidermoid metaplasia*. It is similar to lesions that have been termed "orthokeratotic dysplasia" in the head and neck but essentially consists of esophageal squamous epithelium that has a granular cell layer similar to that in the skin (fig. 5-6) (10,11). Patients tend to have the risk factors associated with squamous carcinoma and IEN/dysplasia (discussed below). Epidermoid metaplasia is an isolated finding or associated with IEN/dysplasia and squamous cell carcinoma, but follow-up studies demonstrating progression from epidermoid metaplasia to neoplasia do not exist at this point (fig. 5-7) (12,13).

Immunohistochemical Findings. Although many antigens have been studied in the evaluation of IEN/dysplasia, these are seldom used in clinical practice. TP53 immunolabeling is sometimes suggested, but since basal squamous cells normally label, it is difficult to use TP53 to confirm IEN/dysplasia. Similarly, Ki-67 does not allow separation between reactive processes and IEN/dysplasia. Although p16 is useful in anatomic sites for which HPV is the typical inciting agent, its role is not clear in Western populations; a stepwise increase in p16 labeling has been reported during esophageal squamous carcinogenesis in a high-risk Chinese population (14). There is also increasing expression of TP53, carcinoembryonic antigen (CEA), and CA19-9 protein during the progression from normal squamous epithelium to IEN/dysplasia and squamous cell carcinoma (15).

Molecular Genetic Findings. The molecular findings in esophageal IEN/dysplasia as well as squamous cell carcinoma consist mainly of mutations in *TP53* and *CDKN2A* and copy number alterations in 11q (contains *CCND1*), 3q (contains *SOX2*), 2q (contains *NFE2L2*), and 9p (contains *CDKN2A*) as the driver alterations (16). Other alterations involve methylation of

Figure 5-4

**HIGH-GRADE SQUAMOUS
INTRAEPITHELIAL NEOPLASIA/DYSPLASIA**

A: The changes that encompass the entire epithelial thickness are striking.

B: The epithelial changes involve 50 to 75 percent of the thickness of the epithelium.

C: When samples are tangentially embedded and superficial, as in this case, it can be difficult to assure that no superficial invasion is present.

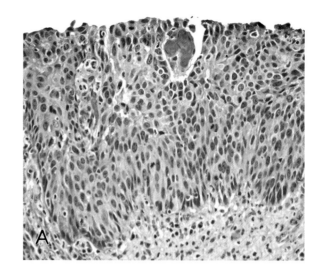

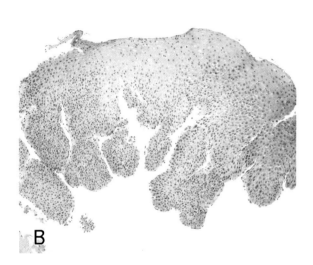

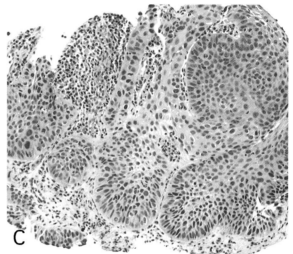

p16INK4a and mutations in *NOTCH1*, *NOTCH3*, and *FBXW7* (7).

The molecular findings in epidermoid metaplasia mirror those of IEN/dysplasia and carcinomas with which they are associated; key involved genes in one study were *TP53*, *PIK3CA*, *EGFR*, *MYCN*, and *HRAS* (13).

Cytologic Classification. The cytologic features of squamous precancerous lesions of the esophagus are based primarily upon data from regions of the world at high risk for this type of cancer, such as China. Instruments used to sample these lesions have been primarily nonendoscopic, such as balloons, sponges, or sponge-meshes (17,18) (see chapter 1 for details).

The terminology and classification of esophageal squamous IEN/dysplasia have evolved over the years. Based on esophageal balloon cytology, Chinese pathologists originally classified lesions as normal, esophagitis, hyperplasia, dysplasia 1, dysplasia 2, suspicious for cancer ("near"-cancer), or cancer (19–23). Subsequently, a United States classification system was developed which uses the following nomenclature: normal, reactive, mild dysplasia, moderate dysplasia, and severe dysplasia. The diagnostic criteria and relative risks (RR) of developing squamous cell carcinoma for each diagnostic category are described in Table 5-1. This scheme provides more statistically significant RR values compared to the Chinese system. When cytology results are compared to the final endoscopic biopsy diagnosis (Table 5-2), the Chinese system is more sensitive but less specific than the United

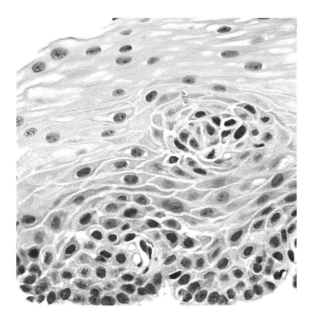

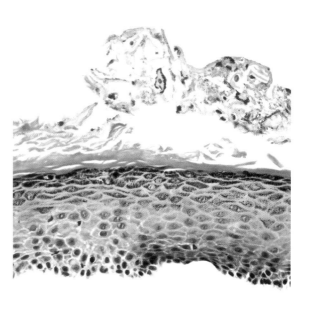

Figure 5-5

BASAL CELL HYPERPLASIA

This sample was from an area that lacked Lugol iodine solution uptake. The patient had a history of esophageal squamous cell carcinoma and was undergoing surveillance. The epithelial changes are less prominent than those in figure 5-3, but the distinction is subtle and open to observer variation. The changes involve over 15 percent of the epithelial thickness.

Figure 5-6

EPIDERMOID METAPLASIA

This biopsy was taken from the esophagus but a granular cell layer is present as in the skin. There is also orthokeratosis. This pattern shares molecular alterations with squamous intraepithelial neoplasia/dysplasia and carcinoma, although the progression rate is unknown.

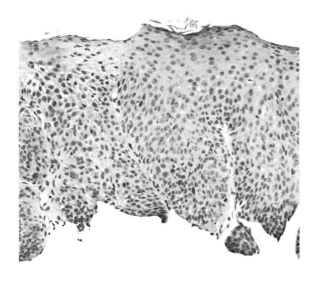

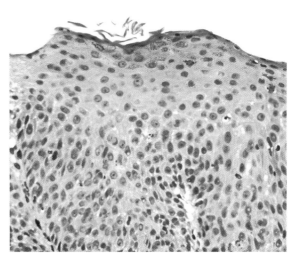

Figure 5-7

EPIDERMOID METAPLASIA OVERLYING HIGH-GRADE SQUAMOUS INTRAEPITHELIAL NEOPLASIA/DYSPLASIA

Left: The zone of granular cells is subtle at low magnification.
Right: At high magnification, the granular layer is apparent.

Table 5-1

CYTOLOGIC GRADING SYSTEMS OF ESOPHAGEAL SQUAMOUS PRECURSOR LESIONS[a]

Category	Chinese Criteria	United States Criteria	RR[b]
Normal (Chinese & US)	Mostly intermediate cells with 10-15% superficial cells and rare parabasal cells	Mostly single intermediate cells with no atypia	US: 1.00 Chinese: 1.00
Reactive (US) Hyperplasia (Chinese)	Mildly hyperchromatic and enlarged nuclei (2-3 times that of nuclei in normal intermediate cells)	Degenerating cells: normal or enlarged nuclei with smooth nuclear membrane without abnormal chromatin or nucleoli. Regenerating cells: cells in flat sheets with abundant cytoplasm, variably enlarged nuclei, prominent nucleoli, even chromatin, and smooth nuclear membrane	US: 0.68 (0.08-6-1) Chinese: 2.81 (0.38-21)
Mild dysplasia (US) Dysplasia 1 (Chinese)	Hyperchromatic nuclei with finely granular and even chromatin and a size of 3-4 times the size of the nuclei of normal intermediate cells; one cell is sufficient	Single cells with variably enlarged nuclei, finely granular and evenly distributed increased chromatin, smooth or mildly irregular nuclear membrane and mildly increased N/C ratio with no nucleoli	US: 0.85 (0.11-6.4) Chinese: 6.8 (0.92-51)
Moderate dysplasia (US) Dysplasia 2 (Chinese)	Similar to dysplasia 1 except the nuclear size is 4-5 times that of nuclei of intermediate cells; one cell is sufficient	Similar to mild dysplasia but with increased increased nuclear size, amount and coarseness of chromatin, and increased N/C ratio	US: 1.7 (0.22-13) Chinese: 7.0 (0.94-52)
Severe dysplasia (US) Near cancer (Chinese)	Similar to dysplasia 2 except the nuclear size is >5 times that of the nuclei of the normal intermediate cells; one cell is sufficient	Similar to moderate dysplasia with further increased nuclear size, amount and coarseness of chromatin, and increased N/C ratio	US: 2.8 (0.39-21) Chinese: 25 (3-2-190)

[a]Modified from reference 19.
[b]Relative risks based on US and Chinese category/criteria.

States scheme. Other studies have shown that the majority (over 60 percent) of patients with a diagnosis of "dysplasia" based on the Chinese classification scheme, including those with a diagnosis of "suspicious for cancer," did not develop cancer after a follow-up ranging from 7.5 to 15.0 years (20–22).

More recently, Roth et al. (24) used a modified version of the diagnostic categories and criteria of the Bethesda System (25), originally designed for the uterine cervix, to classify esophageal squamous cell carcinoma and precursor lesions. Since the publication of the paper by Roth et al., the Bethesda System has been revised twice (26,27). There is no significant change in diagnostic terminology or morphologic criteria for epithelial abnormalities between the 2001 and 2014 Bethesda System publications. The diagnostic criteria of the original and the two revisions are shown in Table 5-3. In the study by Roth et al., comparison of the cytologic diag-

nosis with the histologic findings showed that a cytologic diagnosis of high-grade squamous intraepithelial lesions (HSIL) or carcinoma is highly specific (greater than 99 percent) in predicting HSIL or carcinoma on histology, but the sensitivity was low (16 percent for balloon sampler and 4 percent for sponge sampler). Using a liquid-based preparation (AutoCyte PREP®) with balloon sampler cytology and taking the presence of atypical squamous cells of undetermined significance (ASCUS) as favoring neoplasia and a positive screening test for detecting any esophageal dysplasia or cancer, improved the sensitivity to 39 and 46 percent for the mechanical and inflatable balloons, respectively (28). The specificity, however, decreased to 85 percent. When lower-grade lesions such as ASCUS and low-grade squamous intraepithelial lesion (LSIL) were included, the sensitivity of cytology to detect histologic HSIL or carcinoma increased significantly. Unfortunately, the

Table 5-2

ACCURACY OF ESOPHAGEAL BALLOON CYTOLOGY RESULTS COMPARED TO ENDOSCOPIC BIOPSY DIAGNOSES (GOLD STANDARD) FOR DYSPLASIA AND MORE SERIOUS LESIONS[a,b]

	Chinese Scheme	US Scheme
Sensitivity	92%	73%
Specificity	14%	64%
Positive predictive value	24%	37%
Negative predictive value	86%	89%

[a]This includes dysplasia, near cancer, and cancer.
[b]Modified from reference 19.

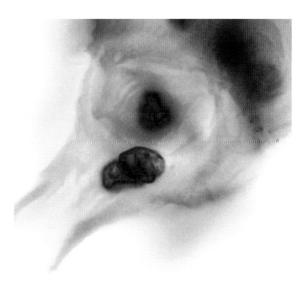

Figure 5-8

LOW-GRADE SQUAMOUS INTRAEPITHELIAL LESION

Binucleation and mildly irregular nuclear membranes are seen in these cells on esophageal balloon cytology (Papanicolaou stain). (Courtesy of Dr. Mark Roth, Bethesda, MD.)

biologic significance of the Bethesda System of classification has not been verified in long-term follow-up studies.

Cytologic Findings. The Bethesda System classifies precancerous squamous epithelial cell abnormalities into atypical squamous cells (ASC), LSIL, and HSIL (Table 5-3) (24,26,27). In the 2001 and 2014 Bethesda System classifications, ASC is divided into two subcategories: "of undetermined significance (ASC-US)"; and "cannot exclude HSIL (ASC-H)" (26,27). ASC refers to cytologic changes suggestive of a squamous intraepithelial lesion (SIL), but qualitatively or quantitatively insufficient for a definitive diagnosis of SIL. ASC-US refers to cells that are suggestive of LSIL and show nuclear enlargement up to three times the area of the nucleus of a normal intermediate squamous cell (approximately 35 μm²), slightly increased nuclear/cytoplasmic (N/C) ratio, minimal nuclear hyperchromasia and irregularity in chromatin distribution or nuclear shape, occasional binucleation or multinucleation, and perinuclear halo with a rim of condensed cytoplasm. ASC-US includes atypical parakeratosis (the above nuclear abnormalities associated with dense orangeophilic cytoplasm). The appearance of ASC-US in smears and liquid-based cytology is similar, although the cells may appear larger and flatter on smears. ASC-H refers to cells that are suggestive of HSIL and includes metaplastic-type squamous cells with nuclear enlargement up to two and a half times normal, with a N/C ratio approaching that of HSIL. On liquid-based preparations, ASC-H cells may appear small, with nuclei only two to three times the size of the neutrophil nuclei.

LSIL refers to enlarged cells with abundant, well-defined cytoplasm, nuclear enlargement more than three times the area of normal intermediate nuclei (thus slightly increased N/C ratio), variable nuclear hyperchromasia, common binucleation and multinucleation, and slightly irregular nuclear contours. Chromatin ranges from smudged or densely opaque to coarsely granular. Perinuclear cavitation, consisting of a sharply delineated clear zone and a peripheral rim of densely stained cytoplasm, is characteristic but not required for a diagnosis of LSIL. Significant nuclear hyperchromasia may not be apparent on liquid-based preparations.

HSIL refers to cells with a markedly increased N/C ratio and irregular nuclear contours with prominent indentations or grooves. Cellular and nuclear size as well as the chromatin pattern and cytoplasmic appearance may vary. Abnormal cells tend to be more dispersed and fewer in number on liquid-based preparations than on smears.

The cytologic features of squamous, preinvasive neoplastic lesions of the esophagus are similar to those in the cervix. Images considered LSIL on esophageal balloon cytology in a high-risk Chinese population show hyperchromasia and irregular nuclear membranes (fig. 5-8), multinucleation (fig. 5-8), and even perinuclear

Table 5-3

THE BETHESDA SYSTEM

Category	Modified 1993 Bethesda System (24,25)	2001/2014 Bethesda System (26,27)
Reactive	Monolayer sheets or single cells with maintained nuclear polarity and typical mitotic figures with any of the following features: minimal nuclear enlargement (2.5 times that of a normal intermediate squamous cell nucleus); occasional bi- and multinucleation; mild hyperchromasia with uniformly fine granular chromatin; smooth, rounded, and uniform nuclear outline; prominent nucleoli	Same as in 1993 Bethesda System; nucleoli may be more prominent in liquid-based preparations
Atypical squamous cells (ASC)	Atypical squamous cells of undetermined significance (ASCUS): nuclear enlargement (2.5–3 times that of a normal intermediate squamous cell nucleus) with a slight increase in the N/C[a] ratio; variation in nuclear size and shape; binucleation; mild hyperchromasia with evenly distributed chromatin; smooth and regular nuclear outlines with very limited irregularities	Atypical squamous cells of undetermined significance (ASC-US): same as in the 1993 Bethesda System Atypical squamous cells, cannot exclude HSIL (ASC-H): metaplastic type cells with nuclear enlargement to 1.5–2.5 times that of normal; N/C ratio approximates that of HSIL
Low-grade squamous intraepithelial lesion (LSIL)	Nuclear enlargement to at least 3 times that normal intermediate nuclei with increased N/C ratio; moderate variation in nuclear size and shape; bi- or multinucleation; hyperchromasia with either uniformly distributed chromatin or degenerated/smudged chromatin; slightly irregular or inapparent nuclear membrane; well-defined, optically clear perinuclear cavity with a peripheral dense rim of cytoplasm in cells with the above nuclear features	Same as in 1993 Bethesda System
High-grade squamous intraepithelial lesion (HSIL)	Nuclear enlargement to at least 3 times that of normal intermediate nuclei with decreased cytoplasmic area, leading to a marked increase in the N/C ratio; evident hyperchromasia with finely or coarsely granular and evenly distributed chromatin; irregular nuclear outlines	Same as in 1993 Bethesda System
Suspicious for carcinoma[b]	Changes similar to those seen in HSIL, but with occasional visible nucleoli and a suggestion of tumor diathesis (necrotic debris and old blood)	
Carcinoma	Nonkeratinizing type: changes similar to those seen in HSIL, but with prominent macronucleoli and markedly irregular distribution of chromatin and associated tumor diathesis Keratinizing type: marked variation in cellular size and shape with caudate and spindle cells containing dense orangeophilic cytoplasm; marked variation in nuclear size and shape with numerous dense opaque nuclear forms; coarsely granular and irregularly distributed chromatin with parachromatin clearing; occasional macronuclei and tumor diathesis	Same as in 1993 Bethesda System

[a]N/C = nuclear/cytoplasmic.
[b]Added by Roth et al. (25) for esophagus and not in the Bethesda System.

halos (fig. 5-9). HSIL demonstrates cells with an increased N/C ratio, hyperchromasia, an uneven chromatin pattern, and sharper and deeper nuclear irregularities (fig. 5-10). SILs tend to shed only small numbers of atypical cells, usually on a clean background, unless inflammation and ulceration coexist.

The distinction between HSIL and squamous cell carcinoma of the esophagus requires clini-cocytologic correlation. Based on morphology, the presence of abundant abnormal cells and a background showing changes of tumor diathesis (necrotic tumor cells, debris, and old blood) strongly suggest an invasive carcinoma. In addition, clinical evidence of a mass lesion helps to solidify the diagnosis in this setting. Due to the difficulty in this differential diagnosis, Roth et al. (24) added a category of "suspicious for

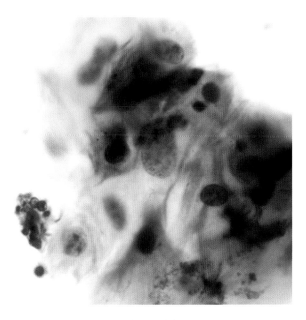

Figure 5-9

LOW-GRADE SQUAMOUS INTRAEPITHELIAL LESION

A vague perinuclear halo is seen in these cells on esophageal balloon cytology (Papanicolaou stain). (Courtesy of Dr. Mark Roth, Bethesda, MD.)

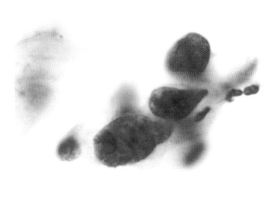

Figure 5-10

HIGH-GRADE SQUAMOUS INTRAEPITHELIAL LESION

A markedly increased nuclear/cytoplasmic ratio, hyperchromasia, and angulated nuclear membranes are seen on esophageal balloon cytology (Papanicolaou stain). (Courtesy of Dr. Mark Roth, Bethesda, MD.)

carcinoma" in their application of the Bethesda System (see Table 5-3), which refers to changes similar to those seen in HSIL but with occasional visible nucleoli and probable tumor diathesis.

Molecular Genetic Findings. The methylation status of four genes (*AHRR, CDKN2A, MT1G,* and *CLDN3*), as assessed by quantitative polymerase chain reaction (PCR) techniques applied on esophageal balloon cytology specimens resulted in sensitivity and specificity for esophageal severe squamous dysplasia of 50 and 68 percent, respectively (29). Although not particularly impressive, these results demonstrate the feasibility of the application of molecular markers on nonendoscopic cytologic specimens.

Using endoscopic brushing cytology specimens from surgery samples from patients with esophageal squamous cell carcinoma, Huang et al. (30) showed immunohistochemical staining for minichromosome maintenance protein 2 (MCM2), proliferating cell nuclear antigen (PCNA), and Ki-67 in 93, 65, and 39 percent of precancerous cells per high-power field while in no normal cells. MCM2 was found to be more sensitive and specific than PCNA and Ki-67 for the detection of dysplasia and is potentially use-

ful in screening patients at high risk of cancer in mass surveys.

Differential Diagnosis. In both cytologic preparations and biopsies, the differential diagnosis is primarily with reparative conditions. Since eosinophilic esophagitis often features intense basal zone hyperplasia, it is sometimes interpreted as low- or high-grade IEN/dysplasia (fig. 5-11). Similarly, epithelial changes associated with radiation or chemotherapy can be misinterpreted as IEN/dysplasia. An example of taxane-associated injury is shown in figure 5-12 (31).

Occasionally, invasive carcinomas in a separate or adjoining site in the mucosa proliferate in the space between the basement membrane and the normal epithelium, termed *intraepithelial cancerization.* This results in striking epithelial changes that fill less than half of the thickness of the epithelium, a pattern that would meet criteria for low-grade IEN/dysplasia. This has been referred to as a lateral spread pattern of squamous cell carcinoma (fig. 5-13).

Treatment and Prognosis. Endoscopic mucosal resection and endoscopic submucosal dissection as well as radiofrequency ablation

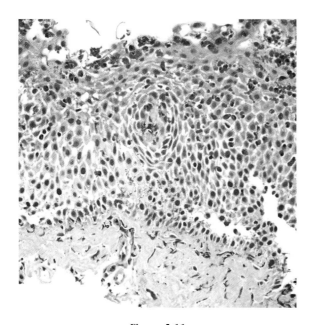

Figure 5-11

**EOSINOPHILIC ESOPHAGITIS WITH
STRIKING BASAL CELL HYPERPLASIA**

This is not a preneoplastic lesion but can result in a diagnostic pitfall. One clue is the striking amount of edema that results in prominent intracellular bridges.

have been used in high resource countries to treat squamous dysplasia, with certain caveats (the performance of multiple biopsies to assure that an invasive component is absent) (32). Before the development of radiofrequency ablation, other ablative methods (multipolar electrocoagulation, argon plasma coagulation) were used. These methods are expensive for high-risk areas and optimized protocols remain under development (7).

The natural history of esophageal squamous dysplasia is not fully known, but in one large Chinese study with 13.5 years of follow-up of untreated squamous IEN/dysplasia there was progression to squamous cell carcinoma in 14 percent of mild, 50 percent of moderate, and 74 percent of severe dysplasia cases at the 13.5 year mark. At an intermediate point of 3.5 years, carcinoma was detected in 5, 27, and 64 percent of patients, respectively (33). These findings suggest an overall prolonged progression time even in a high-risk population, with ample opportunities for intervention. In another Chinese study, screening and intervention with endoscopic mucosal resections and argon plasma coagulation treatments resulted in reduction

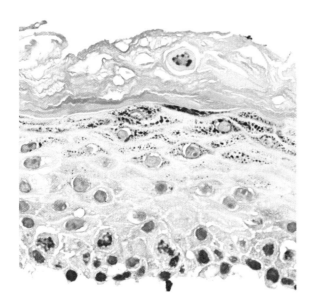
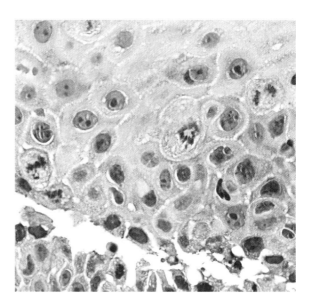

Figure 5-12

TAXANE EFFECT

Left: There is epidermoid metaplasia in this example, but the key to the diagnosis is the presence of a ring mitosis. Taxanes are administered for several types of carcinoma and result in mitotic arrest and the formation of ring mitoses and apoptotic bodies in the proliferative compartment, which, in the esophagus, is the basal layer.

Right: A ring mitosis is present. The adjacent nuclei are not hyperchromatic.

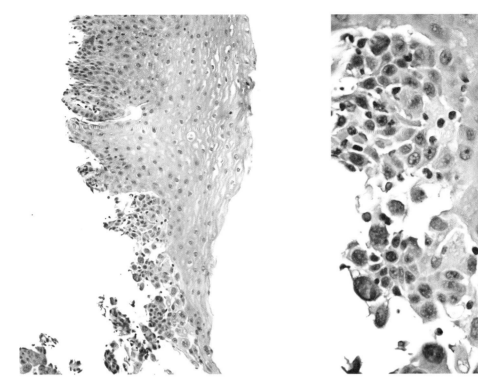

Figure 5-13

LATERAL SPREAD PATTERN

Left: The epithelial changes on the left only involve half the thickness of the epithelium, but they are in excess of low-grade intraepithelial neoplasia/dysplasia. This pattern is concerning for an adjoining, but unsampled, invasive carcinoma, and can be seen in resection specimens in the vicinity of an invasive squamous cell carcinoma.

Right: High magnification view.

of mortality compared to screening and simple clinical observation (8). Data for untreated Western patients are not available.

SQUAMOUS CELL CARCINOMA

Definition. *Esophageal squamous cell carcinoma* is a malignant epithelial neoplasm with squamous differentiation often in the form of intercellular bridges or keratinization.

General Features. Esophageal squamous carcinoma has a striking male predominance and is usually is found in middle-aged men, often in low-resource countries or low-resource settings in high-resource countries. In parts of the world with the highest risk of esophageal carcinoma overall, including northern Iran, central Asia, and north-central China, 90 percent of esophageal carcinomas are squamous cell compared to only 26 percent in whites from the United States (34). In eastern Asia, as of 2012, there were nearly 22 cases of esophageal carcinoma per 100,000 persons (34).

Esophageal squamous cell carcinoma is associated with mucosal injury: essentially any factor resulting in chronic irritation and inflammation of the esophageal mucosa. For example, skin diseases affecting the esophagus, such as lichen planus, can progress to dysplasia/carcinoma (see figs. 5-1–5-3). Heavy alcohol intake, especially combined with tobacco smoking, substantially increases the risk of squamous cell carcinoma (but not adenocarcinoma), and is believed to account for most squamous cell carcinomas of the esophagus in the developed world. The synergy of smoking and alcohol abuse is also associated with an increased risk of head and neck cancer. Squamous cell carcinoma of the esophagus is discovered incidentally in 1 to 2 percent of patients with head and neck cancers (35). Intake of hot beverages has been linked to esophageal squamous cell cancer, as well as intake of fresh fruits and vegetables (5).

Although squamous cell carcinoma is strongly associated with alcohol and tobacco use in developed countries, in areas where the incidence of squamous cell carcinoma is highest (eastern and central Asia, southern Africa), risk factors differ dramatically. For example, the Taihang mountain region of China has a staggering incidence of esophageal squamous cell carcinoma with gender parity. Most women in this region do not drink or smoke. Areas of Iran have high rates of esophageal squamous cell carcinoma, but few individuals drink alcohol. Risk factors in these latter areas of the world revolve around opium use, poor nutrition, thermal damage from drinking hot beverages, and exposure to carcinogens (7).

Other causes of esophageal irritation that are linked to esophageal squamous cell carcinoma include achalasia and esophageal diverticula. In these conditions, retained food decomposes and releases chemical irritants. Persons with a history of caustic ingestion (such as of lye) require lifelong monitoring for the development of cancer (36).

Patients with nonepidermolytic palmoplantar keratoderma (tylosis), a rare autosomal dominant disorder defined by *RHBDF2* mutations on chromosome 17q25 (37) have an inherited predisposition for esophageal squamous cell carcinoma. Tylosis is characterized by hyperkeratosis of the palms and soles and thickening of the oral mucosa (38), and confers up to a 95 percent risk of squamous cell carcinoma of the esophagus by 70 years of age.

Nutritional deficiency syndromes associated with this type of cancer, such as the Plummer-Vinson syndrome (dysphagia, iron-deficiency anemia, and esophageal webs), have become increasingly rare in the developed world as nutrition improves. The role of HPV in the development of esophageal squamous cell carcinoma is unclear. HPV DNA detection rates are minimal (0 to 2 percent) in studies from low incidence areas (39,40), whereas higher rates are reported in high incidence areas such as China and Iran (up to 35 percent) (41,42). A Mexican study (low tumor incidence population) noted the presence of high-risk HPV DNA in 25 percent of patients with esophageal squamous cell

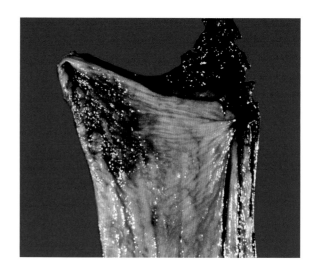

Figure 5-14

EARLY/SUPERFICIAL SQUAMOUS CELL CARCINCOMA

This lesion was resected years ago, when endoscopic treatments were under development, but it is an early superficially invasive carcinoma that would be managed endoscopically in the present era. It conforms to a Japanese type 0 lesion.

carcinomas (43), and rates of up to 50 percent are known. In the United States, the rate is about 10 percent (44), and some have suggested a role for HPV vaccination in preventing this type of cancer (as well as others) (45).

Gross Findings. Squamous cell carcinomas are most common in the middle third of the esophagus. On imaging studies, the presence of an esophageal mass in the middle third of the esophagus suggests squamous cell carcinoma. Multifocality has been reported in 14.6 percent of cases in one study (46). Since esophageal squamous cell carcinomas tend to be diagnosed at a high stage, they are often large bulky masses that invade adjacent structures, but early lesions can be quite subtle (fig. 5-14).

Squamous cell carcinomas are firm and white, and may be configured in several patterns outlined below (figs. 5-14, 5-15) (47).

Type 0. Superficial type: tumor invasion is limited to the submucosa. These tumors can be managed endoscopically.

Type 1. Protruding type: localized protruding lesion. Protruding lesions commonly have an erosive surface. The lesion is occasionally covered by intact squamous epithelium.

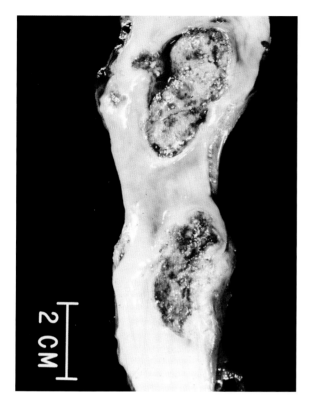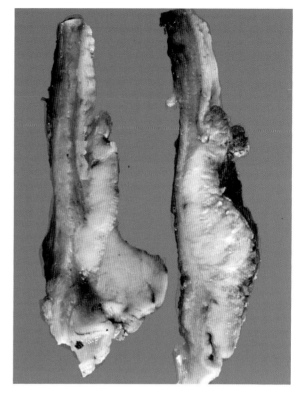

Figure 5-15

SQUAMOUS CELL CARCINCOMA

Left: This esophagectomy specimen shows two separate primaries. The one at the top represents a type 2 carcinoma in the Japanese classification system, whereas the one on the bottom is type 3. Regardless, these lesions are not amenable to endoscopic treatment.

Right: This carcinoma is bulky and deeply invasive.

Type 2. Ulcerative and localized type: the lesion has a well-demarcated surrounding ridge.

Type 3. Ulcerative and infiltrative type: the lesion has a circumferential or semicircumferential ill-demarcated surrounding ridge.

Type 4. Diffusely infiltrative type: lesion with wide intramural invasion, and generally without conspicuous ulceration or protrusion. Even if the lesion has an ulcerative and/or protruding component, it is defined as type 4.

Type 5. Unclassifiable type: the lesion has a complicated macroscopic appearance which is unclassifiable.

Microscopic Findings. On biopsies, the findings in squamous cell carcinomas of the esophagus mirror those of squamous carcinomas elsewhere. Most are well differentiated, with prominent keratinization (figs. 5-16, 5-17), but they may be basaloid (fig. 5-18), sarcomatoid/ spindled (figs. 5-19–5-21), papillary (fig. 5-22),

or verrucous (fig. 5-23). A variant of verrucous carcinoma that is composed of a highly differentiated carcinoma featuring macroscopic cysts and sinuses has been termed *esophageal carcinoma cuniculatum*, and was unassociated with HPV in a small series (48). The sarcomatoid type tends to have an exophytic gross appearance (fig. 5-18). Additionally, lympho-epithelioma-like carcinomas are occasionally reported in the esophagus (fig. 5-24) (49,50) and a subset of these is associated with Epstein-Barr virus (EBV) (49).

Tumors are described as well differentiated, moderately differentiated, or poorly differentiated. Well-differentiated tumors display prominent keratinization, few basaloid type cells, keratin pearls, and a low mitotic count. Moderately differentiated tumors feature areas of basaloid-appearing cells, but others show overt keratinization with a lack of squamous

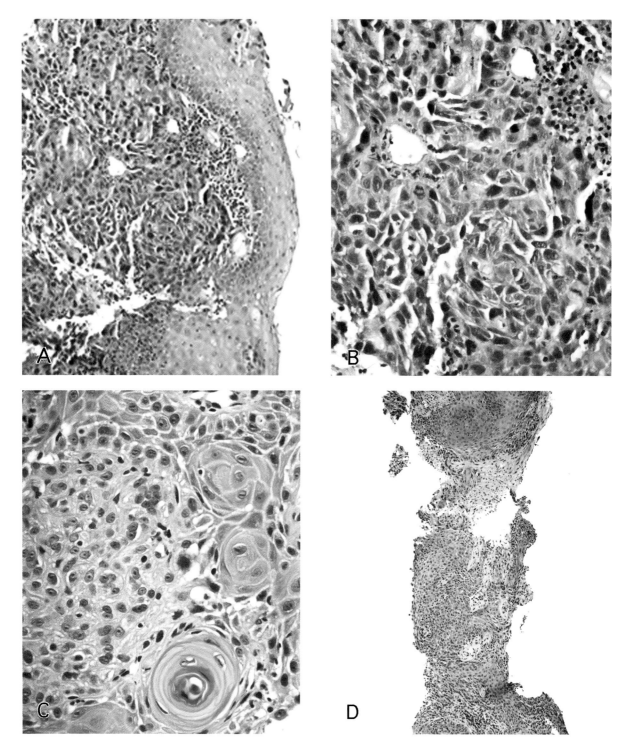

Figure 5-16

SQUAMOUS CELL CARCINCOMA

A: This lesion displays overt squamous differentiation with keratinization.

B: At high magnification, squamous carcinoma cells are separated by spaces that separate individual cells (the intercellular bridges).

C: In addition to squamous bridges between cells, there is a squamous pearl at the lower right.

D: This carcinoma arose in a patient who had esophageal lichen planus.

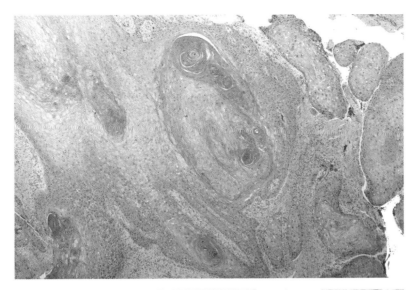

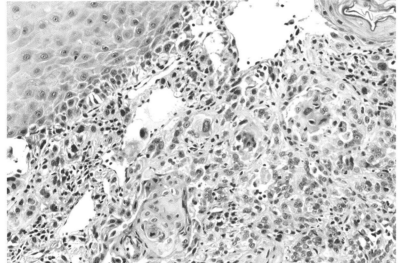

Figure 5-17

SQUAMOUS CELL CARCINCOMA

Top: This very well-differentiated carcinoma is from a patient who had ingested lye in the form of a household product. Patients who are status postcaustic ingestion are at lifelong risk for esophageal squamous cell carcinoma.

Bottom: This moderately differentiated squamous cell carcinoma shows focal keratinization.

Figure 5-18

BASALOID SQUAMOUS CELL CARCINOMA

Some squamous cell carcinomas have a basaloid pattern. These can be difficult to distinguish from neuroendocrine carcinomas but, in these instances, immunolabeling is helpful.

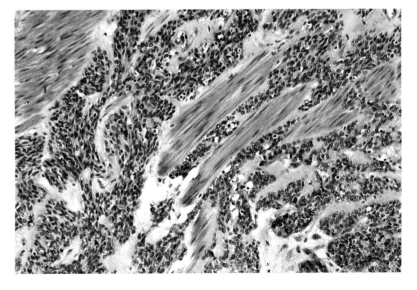

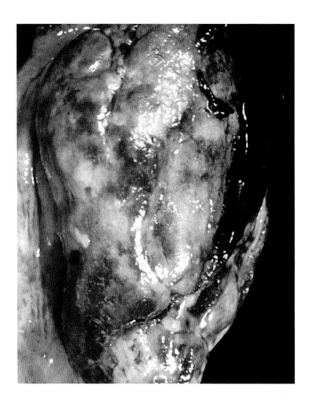
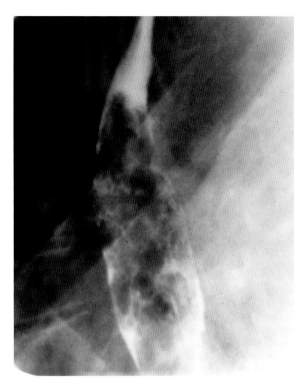

Figure 5-19

SARCOMATOID SQUAMOUS CELL CARCINOMA

Left: This sarcomatoid carcinoma has an exophytic appearance.
Right: Barium highlights the exophytic appearance of this sarcomatoid squamous cell carcinoma.

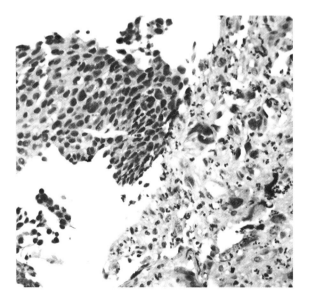
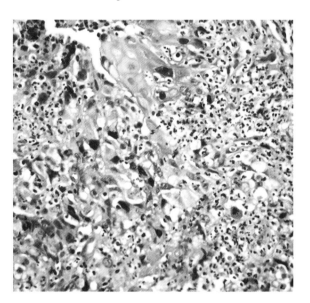

Figure 5-20

SARCOMATOID SQUAMOUS CELL CARCINOMA

Left: A dysplastic component on the left is a clue to the diagnosis of a high-grade sarcomatoid squamous cell carcinoma on the right; this sample was from an endoscopic biopsy of an exophytic lesion.
Right: Most of the lesion is sarcoma-like, but a cluster at the top shows squamous differentiation.

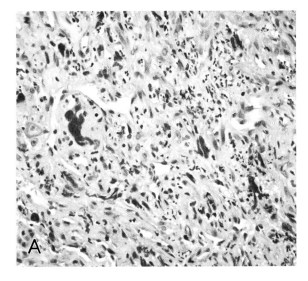

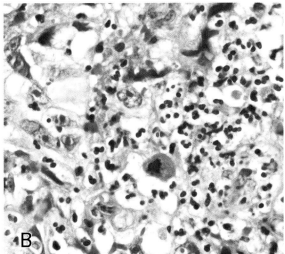

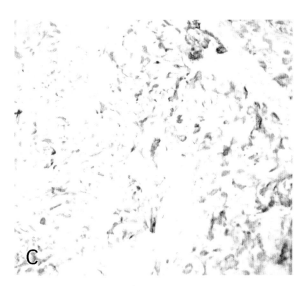

Figure 5-21

SARCOMATOID SQUAMOUS CELL CARCINOMA

A: This sarcomatoid squamous cell carcinoma is indistinguishable from a pleomorphic sarcoma or melanoma.

B: The keratinized eosinophilic cell is a clue to the diagnosis of sarcomatoid squamous cell carcinoma.

C: Sarcomatoid carcinomas label with CAM5.2.

pearls. Poorly differentiated tumors have basaloid-like cells in large and small nests with frequent necrosis, and occasional cells with overt keratinization (see Basaloid Carcinoma below). Undifferentiated carcinomas lack features of squamous differentiation; immunolabeling shows expression of squamous markers and absence of neuroendocrine ones.

Variants. Esophageal squamous cell carcinoma variants are shown in Table 5-4 and discussed below.

Verrucous Carcinoma. This subtype is rare and has been associated with various forms of chronic esophagitis as well as with esophageal diverticula, achalasia, and reflux disease. Macroscopically, it tends to have an exophytic wart-like appearance with prominent papillary projections. The lesion features a pushing pattern of invasion.

Verrucous carcinoma is difficult to diagnose on mucosal biopsies and thus should be diagnosed in association with the clinical findings. Often, several sets of biopsies are required to establish a diagnosis. These lesions are likely to have superinfection with *Candida*, further adding to the difficulty in diagnosis. Verrucous carcinomas are generally reported as single case studies, but in small series, the prognosis seems more indolent than that of classic squamous cell carcinomas (51). It only occasionally metastasizes. Early lesions are amenable to endoscopic treatment (52).

Spindle Cell Squamous Carcinoma. This type accounts for about 2 percent of all esophageal

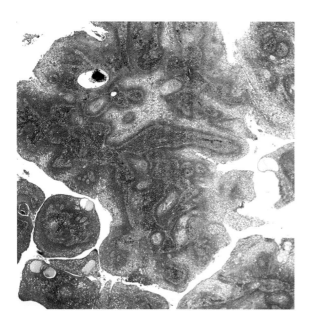
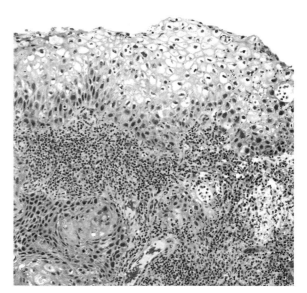

Figure 5-22

SQUAMOUS CELL CARCINOMA

Left: Papillary features are striking in this case.
Right: High magnification view of the papillary lesion shown at left.

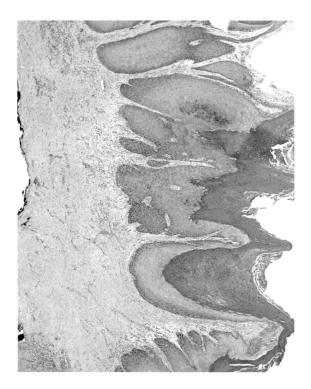
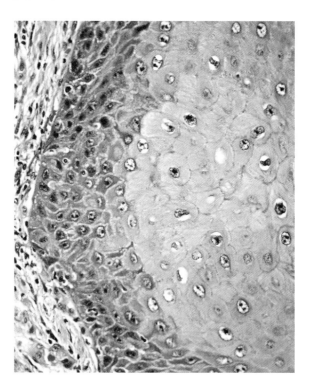

Figure 5-23

VERRUCOUS SQUAMOUS CELL CARCINOMA

Left: Verrucous carcinomas have bland cytologic features, a pushing border, and an overall good prognosis.
Right: High magnification of the base of the tumor.

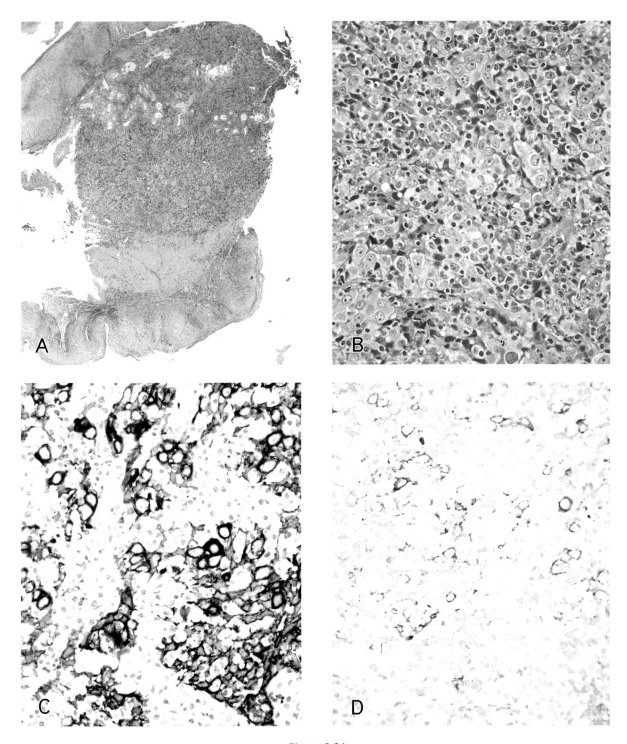

Figure 5-24

LYMPHOEPITHELIOMA-LIKE SQUAMOUS CELL CARCINOMA

A: Rare examples of esophageal squamous cell carcinoma have a lymphoepithelioma-like appearance.

B: At high magnification, the appearance is lymphoma-like, but the presence of abundant, slightly eosinophilic cells bathed in a sea of small lymphocytes is a clue to the diagnosis.

C: CAM5.2 stain.

D: CK5/6 stain.

Table 5-4

ESOPHAGEAL SQUAMOUS CELL CARCINOMA VARIANTS

Variant	Gross Findings	Microscopic Findings	Differential Diagnosis
Conventional squamous cell carcinoma	Firm whitish mass, often flat	Cytologically malignant cells with prominent keratinization, squamous pearls	Reactive conditions
Verrucous carcinoma	Polypoid papillary mass	Bland overtly squamous lesions with abundant keratinization and frequent superimposed *Candida* organisms	Reactive conditions
Spindle cell squamous carcinoma	Exophytic polypoid mass with a smooth surface	Overtly malignant spindle cells with a variable admixture of conventional squamous cell carcinoma or an in situ squamous lesion	Spindle cell melanoma, sarcoma
Basaloid squamous cell carcinoma	Firm whitish mass, often flat	Small malignant cells with scant cytoplasm in nests or sheets	High-grade neuroendocrine carcinoma, adenoid cystic carcinoma

squamous cell carcinomas. It is also termed *carcinosarcoma, sarcomatoid carcinoma, pseudosarcomatous squamous cell carcinoma, polypoid carcinoma, metaplastic carcinoma*, and *carcinoma with mesenchymal stroma* (5). Some of these terms are confusing since they suggest that the lesion is a sarcoma instead of a carcinoma that has changed its phenotype.

Most cases arise in the middle third of the esophagus, and form a polypoid mass with a smooth surface. Microscopically, there is a high-grade spindle cell component. Extensive searching may be required to demonstrate a typical squamous cell carcinoma component or dysplasia. If only the spindle cell component is detected, such a tumor is still more likely to represent a sarcomatoid carcinoma than a sarcoma. The spindle cell component can reveal osteosarcomatous, chondrosarcomatous, or even rhabdomyosarcomatous differentiation. The lesion is, essentially, a high-grade carcinoma.

Spindle cell squamous carcinoma often presents at an early stage based on its proclivity to be exophytic, which has resulted in studies that have noted a favorable prognosis (53). This favorable prognosis tends to disappear in large studies with long follow-up. In one Chinese study, spindle cell carcinoma of the esophagus was associated with a slightly better outcome than conventional squamous cell carcinoma, but this advantage was of borderline statistical significance (54).

These tumors can appear identical to sarcomas, but in the esophagus, a diagnosis of primary sarcoma is rare, and thus should be made with great caution. Even gastrointestinal stromal tumors are rare in the tubular esophagus (55). Many spindle cell carcinomas of the esophagus express keratins, or even p63 or p40, similar to such tumors in the head and neck (56), which can be of value in diagnosis, but submitting numerous sections to detect a conventional squamous cell carcinoma component or dysplasia is important.

Basaloid Squamous Cell Carcinoma. This variant of squamous cell carcinoma differentiates along the lines of basal squamous cells, but parallels conventional squamous cell carcinoma on clinical and pathologic grounds despite its unusual morphologic features (57). It is, essentially, a poorly differentiated squamous cell carcinoma (5). It tends to arise in older men who are drinkers and smokers, similar to conventional squamous cell carcinomas in high resource countries.

Basaloid squamous cell carcinoma consists of small basaloid cells with scant cytoplasm, arranged in sheet-like growth or in nests, often with dense desmoplasia. The differential diagnosis is with high-grade neuroendocrine carcinoma of the small cell type and adenoid cystic carcinoma. Immunochemistry helps separate these lesions: synaptophysin, chromogranin, and INSM1 confirm neuroendocrine differentiation (58). Although adenoid cystic carcinomas can show some expression of p40, it tends to be far more focal than in basaloid squamous cell carcinomas, at least in the head and neck (59).

Figure 5-25

WELL-DIFFERENTIATED SQUAMOUS CELL CARCINOMA

Tumor diathesis is seen as clumps of amorphous materials and isolated keratinized tumor cells (Papanicolaou stain).

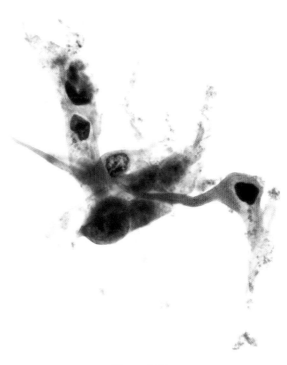

Figure 5-26

WELL-DIFFERENTIATED SQUAMOUS CELL CARCINOMA

A keratinized spindle-shaped tumor cell with triangular-shaped pyknotic nucleus and a few nonkeratinized tumor cells with sharp cell borders, increased nuclear/cytoplasmic ratios, uneven chromatin pattern, prominent nucleoli, and irregular nuclear membranes are seen (Papanicolaou stain).

Immunohistochemical Findings. Squamous cell carcinomas of the esophagus, like squamous carcinomas elsewhere, express p63, p40, CK5/6, and a host of other epithelial markers.

Molecular Genetic Findings. Mutations in *TP53* and *CDKN2A* and copy number alterations in 11q (contains *CCND1*), 3q (contains *SOX2*), 2q (contains *NFE2L2*), and 9p (contains *CDKN2A*) are the driver alterations (16). Other important genes include *NOTCH1* and *MTOR* (mutations) and amplification of *AKT2, EGFR, ERBB2* (*HER2*), *FGFR1, KRAS, MDM2,* and *PIK3CA* (60). Numerous other alterations are also reported, and some have used deep sequencing techniques in peripheral blood to detect tumors (61).

Cytologic Findings. The cytologic features of squamous cell carcinomas depend on the degree of differentiation. Well-differentiated tumors shed abundant keratinaceous debris. In addition, the tumor cells may be scant in number and bland in appearance (fig. 5-25). On liquid-based preparations, tumor diathesis appears as clumps of amorphous material (fig. 5-25). Most of the tumor cells have keratinized cytoplasm and pyknotic nuclei (fig. 5-26). Nuclear atypia, such as an increased N/C ratio and irregular nuclear contours, are usually present focally. The distinction between an infection and a well-differentiated squamous cell carcinoma is based primarily on the relatively small number or lack of inflammatory cells in the debris in carcinoma.

Moderately differentiated squamous cell carcinomas show a variable degree of keratinization. The cellular elements are more abundant than those seen in well-differentiated squamous cell carcinomas and include both keratinized and nonkeratinized tumor cells (fig. 5-27). The nonkeratinized tumor cells show dense cytoplasm and enlarged centrally-located nuclei (fig. 5-27, right). Nucleoli may or may not be present. Although squamous cell carcinomas

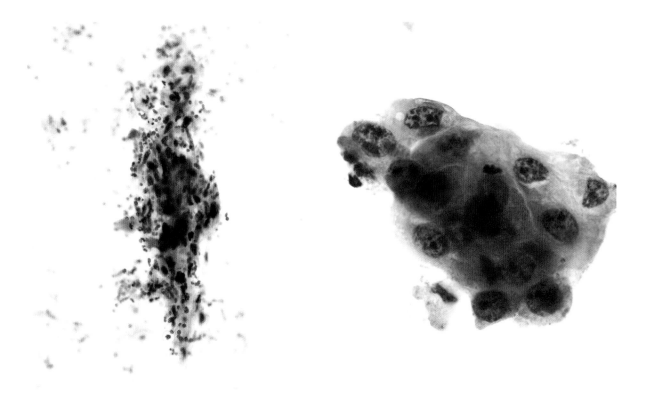

Figure 5-27

MODERATELY DIFFERENTIATED SQUAMOUS CELL CARCINOMA

Left: A clump of keratinized and nonkeratinized tumor cells with pyknotic nuclei are seen in a background of some debris on this direct smear (Papanicolaou stain).

Right: Nonkeratinized tumor cells show sharp cell borders, dense cytoplasm, central nuclei with chromatin clumping/clearing, and prominent nucleoli (Papanicolaou stain).

are more likely to shed single tumor cells than adenocarcinomas, they may appear as sheets of uniform tumor cells that are not readily recognizable as malignant, or even squamous in origin. A search for single atypical cells, especially keratinized cells, and nuclear atypia, may be necessary to establish a correct diagnosis.

Poorly differentiated squamous cell carcinomas show a high N/C ratio, enlarged atypical nuclei with an aberrant chromatin pattern, and prominent nucleoli (fig. 5-28). However, poorly differentiated squamous cell carcinomas may show only a few keratinized tumor cells, or even none at all, which makes determination of the squamous differentiation of the tumor difficult (fig. 5-29). On occasion, it is not possible to distinguish, with certainty, between a poorly differentiated squamous cell carcinoma and a poorly differentiated adenocarcinoma. These tumors may only be recognized as "large cell" carcinoma.

Clinical findings, such as location and presence or absence of Barrett esophagus, and immunohistochemical stains on cell block preparations may help to determine the specific line of differentiation of the tumor cells.

Differential Diagnosis. Most squamous cell carcinoma of the esophagus pose no diagnostic problems. However, when these carcinomas have spindle cell features, melanoma and sarcomas must be excluded. This is best accomplished by extensive sampling of the overlying squamous mucosa to detect dysplasia or a focus of conventional-appearing squamous cell carcinoma. S-100 protein (which should be negative) and various keratins can sometimes confirm a diagnosis of sarcomatoid carcinoma (see fig. 5-21C). Primary sarcomas of the esophagus are extremely rare, although occasionally sarcomas secondarily invade the esophagus. It is important not to confuse pseudoepitheliomatous changes associated with granular cell tumors with squamous cell carcinoma (fig. 5-30). Similarly, pseudosarcomatous changes in ulcers should not be mistaken for sarcomatoid carcinomas (fig. 5-31) (62,63).

At the opposite end of the spectrum, verrucous carcinoma may be impossible to distinguish from reparative processes on superficial samples. Often, the diagnosis is made simply by correlation with the clinical findings.

Treatment and Prognosis. Chemoradiation is the usual treatment, sometimes with esophagectomy. This treatment is usually palliative, however, rather than curative. Those lesions that are detected early in screening programs are often amenable to endoscopic treatment, such as mucosal ablation, endoscopic mucosal resection, and endoscopic submucosal dissection (fig. 5-32).

Squamous cell carcinomas often present late, after extension into periesophageal soft tissue is already present. Local bulky disease resulting in esophageal obstruction, with extension of carcinoma into mediastinal and intrathoracic

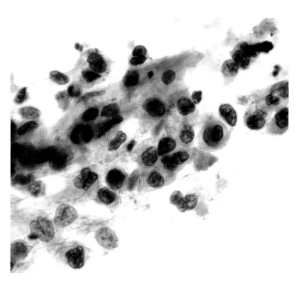

Figure 5-28

POORLY DIFFERENTIATED SQUAMOUS CELL CARCINOMA

Tumor cells show aberrant, highly uneven chromatin and irregular nuclear membranes. The dense cytoplasm with concentric rings in one cell hints at squamous differentiation (Papanicolaou stain).

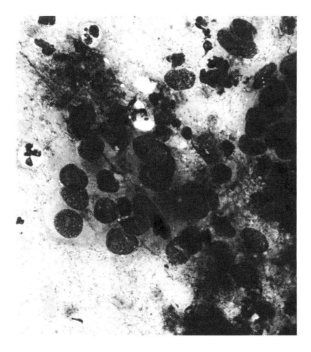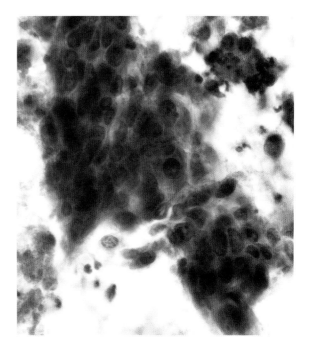

Figure 5-29

POORLY DIFFERENTIATED SQUAMOUS CELL CARCINOMA

Left: The malignant nature of these tumor cells and their stripped nuclei is apparent; however squamous differentiation is not obvious (DiffQuik stain).

Right: Squamous differentiation is difficult, if not impossible, to discern in these crowded groups of haphazardly arranged cells (Papanicolaou stain). (Courtesy of Dr. Graziella Abu-Jawdeh, Salem, MA.)

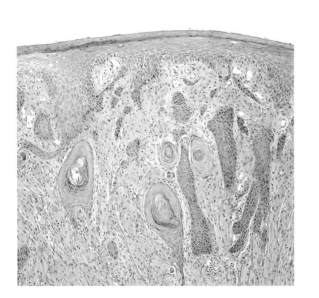
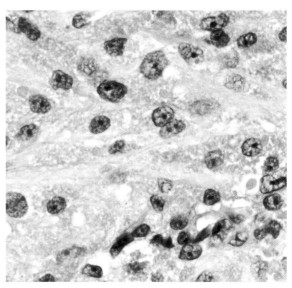

Figure 5-30

GRANULAR CELL TUMOR WITH STRIKING PSEUDOEPITHELIOMATOUS HYPERPLASIA

Left: This phenomenon can lead to misinterpretation as squamous cell carcinoma on superficial biopsies.
Right: The cytoplasm is granular.

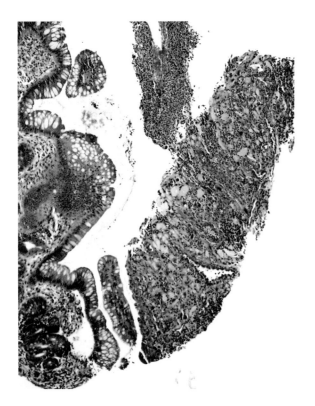
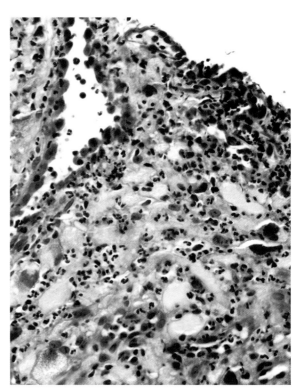

Figure 5-31

PSEUDOSARCOMATOUS REACTIVE CHANGES IN EROSIVE ESOPHAGITIS

Left: Even at low magnification, the reactive fibroblasts have a low nuclear/cytoplasmic ratio.
Right: The nuclei have a degenerative appearance.

structures (tracheobronchial tree, aorta, and lung), and mediastinal lymph node metastases are more typical clinical problems than distant metastases. Squamous carcinomas that assume a prominent spindle cell appearance tend to present as a polypoid exophytic mass. Short-term survival from such tumors is better than that for typical carcinomas, but long-term follow-up is similar to other tumor types.

The prognosis is poor: the 5-year survival rate is 15 to 20 percent, with about an 88 percent mortality rate, owing mainly to late detection (45). Patients with early lesions detected in surveillance have a favorable prognosis, on the order of 90 percent 5-year survival rate. Lifestyle adjustment (alcohol cessation) has been shown to reduce the likelihood of developing metachronous lesions in a high-risk population with *ALDH* polymorphisms using flushing as a surrogate marker for these genetic alterations (64).

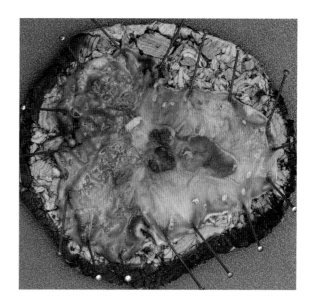

Figure 5-32

ENDOSCOPIC SUBMUCOSAL DISSECTION SPECIMEN

A superficially invasive carcinoma was resected and pinned to a corkboard for fixation. (Courtesy of Professor M. Vieth, Bayreuth, Germany.)

REFERENCES

1. Brown LM, Hoover R, Silverman D, et al. Excess incidence of squamous cell esophageal cancer among US Black men: role of social class and other risk factors. Am J Epidemiol 2001;153:114-22.
2. Njei B, McCarty TR, Birk JW. Trends in esophageal cancer survival in United States adults from 1973 to 2009: a SEER database analysis. J Gastroenterol Hepatol 2016;31:1141-6.
3. Brooks PJ, Enoch MA, Goldman D, Li TK, Yokoyama A. The alcohol flushing response: an unrecognized risk factor for esophageal cancer from alcohol consumption. PLoS Med 2009;6:e50.
4. Cui R, Kamatani Y, Takahashi A, et al. Functional variants in ADH1B and ALDH2 coupled with alcohol and smoking synergistically enhance esophageal cancer risk. Gastroenterology 2009;137:1768-75.
5. Bosman F, Carneiro F, Hruban R, Theise N, eds. WHO Classification of Tumours of the Digestive System. Lyon: IARC; 2010. Bosman F, Jaffee E, Lakhani S, Ohgaki H, eds. World Health Organization Classification of Tumours.
6. Voltaggio L, Cimino-Mathews A, Bishop JA, et al. Current concepts in the diagnosis and pathobiology of intraepithelial neoplasia: a review by organ system. CA Cancer J Clin 2016;66:408-36.
7. Taylor PR, Abnet CC, Dawsey SM. Squamous dysplasia—the precursor lesion for esophageal squamous cell carcinoma. Cancer Epidemiol Biomarkers Prev 2013;22:540-52.
8. Wei WQ, Chen ZF, He YT, et al. Long-term follow-up of a community assignment, one-time endoscopic screening study of esophageal cancer in China. J Clin Oncol 2015;33:1951-7.
9. Morita FH, Bernardo WM, Ide E, et al. Narrow band imaging versus lugol chromoendoscopy to diagnose squamous cell carcinoma of the esophagus: a systematic review and meta-analysis. BMC Cancer 2017;17:54.
10. Singhi AD, Arnold CA, Crowder CD, Lam-Himlin DM, Voltaggio L, Montgomery EA. Esophageal leukoplakia or epidermoid metaplasia: a clinicopathological study of 18 patients. Mod Pathol 2014;27:38-43.
11. Taggart MW, Rashid A, Ross WA, Abraham SC. Oesophageal hyperkeratosis: clinicopathological associations. Histopathology 2013;63:463-73.

12. Cottreau J, Gruchy S, Kamionek M, Lauwers GY, Arnason T. Prevalence of oesophageal epidermoid metaplasia in 1048 consecutive patients and 58 patients with squamous neoplasms. Histopathology 2016;68:988-95.

13. Singhi AD, Arnold CA, Lam-Himlin DM, et al. Targeted next-generation sequencing supports epidermoid metaplasia of the esophagus as a precursor to esophageal squamous neoplasia. Mod Pathol 2017. [Epub ahead of print]

14. Bai P, Xiao X, Zou J, et al. Expression of p14(ARF), p15(INK4b), p16(INK4a) and skp2 increases during esophageal squamous cell cancer progression. Exp Ther Med 2012;3:1026-32.

15. Zhang H, Li H, Ma Q, Yang FY, Diao TY. Predicting malignant transformation of esophageal squamous cell lesions by combined biomarkers in an endoscopic screening program. World J Gastroenterol 2016;22:8770-8.

16. Liu X, Zhang M, Ying S, et al. Genetic alterations in esophageal tissues from squamous dysplasia to carcinoma. Gastroenterology 2017;153:166-77.

17. Muriithi RW, Muchiri LW, Lule GN. Esophageal cytology sponge diagnostic test results in Kenyatta National Referral Hospital, Kenya. Acta Cytol 2014;58:483-488.

18. Sepehr A, Razavi P, Saidi F, Salehian P, Rahmani M, Shamshiri A. Esophageal exfoliative cytology samplers. A comparison of three types. Acta Cytol 2000;44:797-804.

19. Dawsey SM, Shen Q, Nieberg RK, et al. Studies of esophageal balloon cytology in Linxian, China. Cancer Epidemiol Biomarkers Prev 1997;6:121-30.

20. Dawsey SM, Yu Y, Taylor PR, et al. Esophageal cytology and subsequent risk of esophageal cancer. A prospective follow-up study from Linxian, China. Acta Cytol 1994;38:183-92.

21. Liu SF, Shen Q, Dawsey SM, et al. Esophageal balloon cytology and subsequent risk of esophageal and gastric-cardia cancer in a high-risk Chinese population. Int J Cancer 1994;57:775-80.

22. Wang LD, Yang HH, Fan ZM, et al. Cytological screening and 15 years' follow-up (1986-2001) for early esophageal squamous cell carcinoma and precancerous lesions in a high-risk population in Anyang County, Henan Province, Northern China. Cancer Detect Prev 2005;29:317-22.

23. Yang H, Berner A, Mei Q, et al. Cytologic screening for esophageal cancer in a high-risk population in Anyang County, China. Acta Cytol 2002;46:445-52.

24. Roth MJ, Liu SF, Dawsey SM, et al. Cytologic detection of esophageal squamous cell carcinoma and precursor lesions using balloon and sponge samplers in asymptomatic adults in Linxian, China. Cancer 1997;80:2047-59.

25. Kurman RJ, Soloman D, eds. The Bethesda System for reporting cervical/vaginal cytologic diagnosis: definitionns, criteria and explanatory notesfor terminology and specimen adequacy. New York: Springer-Verlag; 1994.

26. Nayar R, Wilbur D, eds. The Bethesda system for reporting cervical cytology—definitions, criteria, and explanatory notes, 3rd ed. New York: Springer; 2015.

27. Solomon D, Nayar R, eds. The Bethesda system for reporting cervical cytology, 2nd ed. New York: Springer-Verlag; 2004.

28. Pan QJ, Roth MJ, Guo HQ, et al. Cytologic detection of esophageal squamous cell carcinoma and its precursor lesions using balloon samplers and liquid-based cytology in asymptomatic adults in Llinxian, China. Acta Cytol 2008;52:14-23.

29. Adams L, Roth MJ, Abnet CC, et al. Promoter methylation in cytology specimens as an early detection marker for esophageal squamous dysplasia and early esophageal squamous cell carcinoma. Cancer Prev Res (Phila) 2008;1:357-61.

30. Huang B, Hu B, Su M, et al. Potential role of minichromosome maintenance protein 2 as a screening biomarker in esophageal cancer high-risk population in China. Hum Pathol 2011;42:808-16.

31. Daniels JA, Gibson MK, Xu L, et al. Gastrointestinal tract epithelial changes associated with taxanes: marker of drug toxicity versus effect. Am J Surg Pathol 2008;32:473-77.

32. Chen WC, Wolfsen H. Role of radiofrequency ablation in esophageal squamous dysplasia and early neoplasia. Gastrointest Endosc 2017;85: 330-1.

33. Wang GQ, Abnet CC, Shen Q, et al. Histological precursors of oesophageal squamous cell carcinoma: results from a 13 year prospective follow up study in a high risk population. Gut 2005;54:187-192.

34. Torre LA, Bray F, Siegel RL, Ferlay J, Lortet-Tieulent J, Jemal A. Global cancer statistics, 2012. CA Cancer J Clin 2015;65:87-108.

35. Erkal HS, Mendenhall WM, Amdur RJ, Villaret DB, Stringer SP. Synchronous and metachronous squamous cell carcinomas of the head and neck mucosal sites. J Clin Oncol 2001;19:1358-62.

36. Csikos M, Horvath O, Petri A, Petri I, Imre J. Late malignant transformation of chronic corrosive oesophageal strictures. Langenbecks Arch Chir 1985;365:231-8.

37. Blaydon DC, Etheridge SL, Risk JM, et al. RHBDF2 mutations are associated with tylosis, a familial esophageal cancer syndrome. Am J Hum Genet 2012;90:340-6.

38. Ellis A, Risk JM, Maruthappu T, Kelsell DP. Tylosis with oesophageal cancer: diagnosis, management and molecular mechanisms. Orphanet J Rare Dis 2015;10:126.

39. Turner JR, Shen LH, Crum CP, Dean PJ, Odze RD. Low prevalence of human papillomavirus infection in esophageal squamous cell carcinomas from North America: analysis by a highly sensitive and specific polymerase chain reaction-based approach. Hum Pathol 1997;28:174-8.

40. Poljak M, Cerar A, Seme K. Human papillomavirus infection in esophageal carcinomas: a study of 121 lesions using multiple broad-spectrum polymerase chain reactions and literature review. Hum Pathol 1998;29:266-71.

41. Chang F, Syrjanen S, Shen Q, et al. Human papillomavirus involvement in esophageal carcinogenesis in the high-incidence area of China. A study of 700 cases by screening and type-specific in situ hybridization. Scand J Gastroenterol 2000;35:123-30.

42. Farhadi M, Tahmasebi Z, Merat S, Kamangar F, Nasrollahzadeh D, Malekzadeh R. Human papillomavirus in squamous cell carcinoma of esophagus in a high-risk population. World J Gastroenterol 2005;11:1200-3.

43. Herrera-Goepfert R, Lizano M, Akiba S, Carrillo-Garcia A, Becker-D'Acosta M. Human papilloma virus and esophageal carcinoma in a Latin-American region. World J Gastroenterol 2009;15:3142-7.

44. Syrjanen K. Geographic origin is a significant determinant of human papillomavirus prevalence in oesophageal squamous cell carcinoma: systematic review and meta-analysis. Scand J Infect Dis 2013;45:1-18.

45. Liyanage SS, Rahman B, Ridda I, et al. The aetiological role of human papillomavirus in oesophageal squamous cell carcinoma: a meta-analysis. PloS One 2013;8:e69238.

46. Kuwano H, Ohno S, Matsuda H, Mori M, Sugimachi K. Serial histologic evaluation of multiple primary squamous cell carcinomas of the esophagus. Cancer 1988;61:1635-8.

47. Japan Esophageal Society. Japanese classification of esophageal cancer, 11th edition: part II and III. Esophagus 2017;14:37-65.

48. Landau M, Goldblum JR, DeRoche T, et al. Esophageal carcinoma cuniculatum: report of 9 cases. Am J Surg Pathol 2012;36:8-17.

49. Chen PC, Pan CC, Hsu WH, Ka HJ, Yang AH. Epstein-Barr virus-associated lymphoepithelioma-like carcinoma of the esophagus. Hum Pathol 2003;34:407-11.

50. Nakasono M, Hirokawa M, Suzuki M, et al. Lymphoepithelioma-like carcinoma of the esophagus: report of a case with non-progressive behavior. J Gastroenterol Hepatol 2007;22:2344-47.

51. Sweetser S, Jacobs NL, Wong Kee Song LM. Endoscopic diagnosis and treatment of esophageal verrucous squamous cell cancer. Dis Esophagus 2014;27:452-6.

52. Abe T, Kato M, Itagaki M, et al. Endoscopic submucosal dissection for an atypical small verrucous carcinoma: a case report. J Med Case Rep 2016;10:74.

53. Raza MA, Mazzara PF. Sarcomatoid carcinoma of esophagus. Arch Pathol Lab Med 2011;135:945-8.

54. Zhang B, Xiao Q, Yang D, et al. Spindle cell carcinoma of the esophagus: a multicenter analysis in comparison with typical squamous cell carcinoma. Medicine (Baltimore) 2016;95(37):e4768.

55. Miettinen M, Sarlomo-Rikala M, Sobin LH, Lasota J. Esophageal stromal tumors: a clinicopathologic, immunohistochemical, and molecular genetic study of 17 cases and comparison with esophageal leiomyomas and leiomyosarcomas. Am J Surg Pathol 2000;24:211-22.

56. Bishop JA, Montgomery EA, Westra WH. Use of p40 and p63 immunohistochemistry and human papillomavirus testing as ancillary tools for the recognition of head and neck sarcomatoid carcinoma and its distinction from benign and malignant mesenchymal processes. Am J Surg Pathol 2014;38:257-64.

57. Sato-Kuwabara Y, Fregnani JH, Jampietro J, et al. Comparative analysis of basaloid and conventional squamous cell carcinomas of the esophagus: prognostic relevance of clinicopathological features and protein expression. Tumour Biol 2016;37:6691-6699.

58. Rooper LM, Sharma R, Li QK, Illei PB, Westra WH. INSM1 demonstrates superior performance to the individual and combined use of synaptophysin, chromogranin and CD56 for diagnosing neuroendocrine tumors of the thoracic cavity. Am J Surg Pathol 2017. [Epub ahead of print]

59. Tilson MP, Bishop JA. Utility of p40 in the Differential Diagnosis of Small Round Blue Cell Tumors of the Sinonasal Tract. Head Neck Pathol 2014;8:141-5.

60. Yang JW, Choi YL. Genomic profiling of esophageal squamous cell carcinoma (ESCC)-Basis for precision medicine. Pathol Res Pract 2017;213:836-41.

61. Ueda M, Iguchi T, Masuda T, et al. Somatic mutations in plasma cell-free DNA are diagnostic markers for esophageal squamous cell carcinoma recurrence. Oncotarget 2016;7:62280-91.

62. Jessurun J, Paplanus SH, Nagle RB, Hamilton SR, Yardley JH, Tripp M. Pseudosarcomatous changes in inflammatory pseudopolyps of the colon. Arch Pathol Lab Med 1986;110:833-6.

63. Shekitka KM, Helwig EB. Deceptive bizarre stromal cells in polyps and ulcers of the gastrointestinal tract. Cancer 1991;67:2111-7.

64. Yokoyama A, Katada C, Yokoyama T, et al. Alcohol abstinence and risk assessment for second esophageal cancer in Japanese men after mucosectomy for early esophageal cancer. PloS One 2017;12:e0175182.

6 MISCELLANEOUS TUMORS OF THE ESOPHAGUS

NEUROENDOCRINE TUMORS

Definition. *Neuroendocrine neoplasms* of the esophagus, and elsewhere in the body, are heterogeneous neoplasms that are grouped together mainly for historic reasons. Low-grade tumors are termed *well-differentiated neuroendocrine (carcinoid) tumors*, and high-grade tumors are termed *high-grade neuroendocrine carcinomas* and further subdivided into small cell and large cell types. Low-grade and high-grade tumors have common differentiation, but high-grade tumors usually arise in association with columnar or squamous precursors, whereas low-grade lesions arise de novo. The rare *mixed adenoneuroendocrine carcinoma* (MANEC), as the name indicates, contains a mixture of a conventional adenocarcinoma and high-grade neuroendocrine carcinoma.

A neuroendocrine tumor is a neoplasm that displays neuroendocrine differentiation (1). These tumors express chromogranin A and synaptophysin, as well as newer neuroendocrine antigens (2). They have a lower proliferation rate than neuroendocrine carcinoma. They display characteristic nuclear features and low mitotic activity.

Neuroendocrine carcinoma is a poorly differentiated high-grade carcinoma that shows evidence of endocrine cell differentiation. These tumors have a characteristic nuclear morphology and a high proliferative index using either mitotic counts or MIB1/Ki-67 labeling index.

General Features. Both low- and high-grade neuroendocrine tumors are extremely rare in the esophagus, but common in the stomach, particularly in patients with autoimmune gastritis, who are prone to develop well-differentiated neuroendocrine (carcinoid) tumors of enterochromaffin-like (ECL) cell type (3). In a large analysis using Surveillance, Epidemiology, and End Results (SEER) data, carcinoid (well-differentiated neuroendocrine) tumors of the esophagus

accounted for under 1 percent of all carcinoids (4), and high-grade tumors (neuroendocrine carcinomas) accounted for fewer than 1 percent of all esophageal carcinomas.

Clinical Features. While low-grade tumors arise de novo, columnar and squamous dysplasia can be precursors to high-grade neuroendocrine carcinomas. Esophageal well-differentiated neuroendocrine (carcinoid) tumors are generally an incidental finding in adults, whereas MANECs and high-grade neuroendocrine carcinomas are symptomatic lesions of adult males aged 60 to 70 years; the median age in one series was 69 years (5). Patients with high-grade tumors present with chest pain and hematemesis or hematochezia, and their tumors are usually at an advanced stage at presentation (1).

Gross Findings. Well-differentiated neuroendocrine tumors manifest grossly as small polyps. They are often received as small endoscopic samples of tiny lesions in the area of the gastroesophageal junction. Sometimes such lesions are incidentally sampled during surveillance of patients with Barrett esophagus.

In contrast, neuroendocrine carcinomas and MANEC have a protuberant or ulcerated endoscopic appearance (5). Resected tumors are bulky large masses that usually infiltrate deeply into the esophageal muscularis propria.

Microscopic Findings. Neuroendocrine (carcinoid) tumors of the esophagus, like those elsewhere in the body, are composed of small cells with scant cytoplasm arranged in an insular growth pattern consisting of solid and cribriform structures (fig. 6-1). The nuclei are round with stippled ("salt and pepper") chromatin. Neuroendocrine tumors are usually graded as grade 1 or grade 2 based on mitotic counts, or the Ki-67 proliferation index: grade 1 tumors have less than 2 mitotic figures in 10 high-power fields and less than 3 percent Ki-67 nuclear labeling; grade 2

121

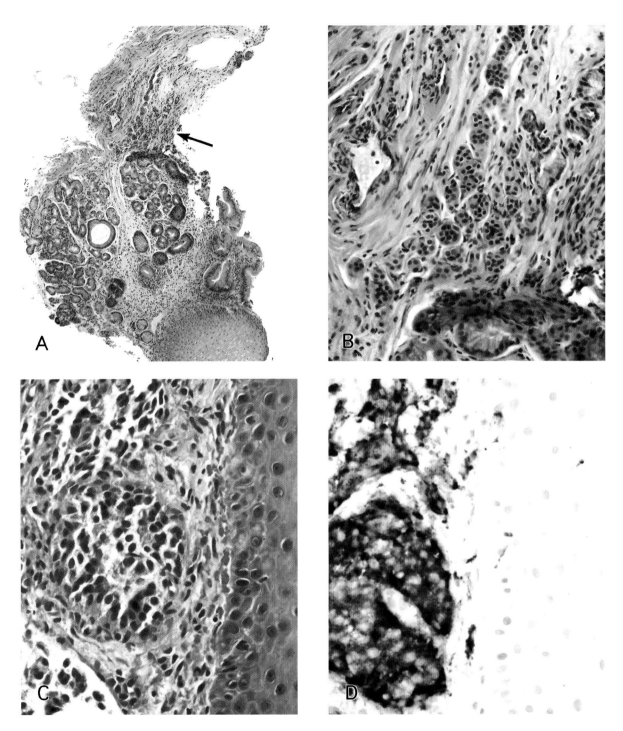

Figure 6-1

WELL-DIFFERENTIATED NEUROENDOCRINE (CARCINOID) TUMOR OF THE ESOPHAGUS

A: This lesion presented as a small nodule at the gastroesophageal junction. There is squamous epithelium. The arrow indicates a well-differentiated neuroendocrine (carcinoid) tumor in a zone of cardio-oxyntic mucosa.

B: Nests of cells show round nuclei.

C: This neoplasm formed a nodule in the mid esophagus. It is composed of nests of cells with nuclei, smaller than those of the overlying squamous epithelium.

D: Chromogranin A stain from the neoplasm seen in C.

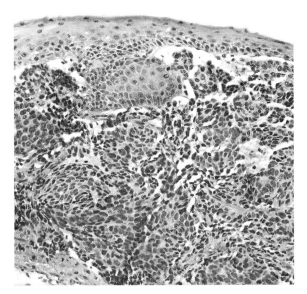

Figure 6-2

NEUROENDOCRINE CARCINOMA OF THE ESOPHAGUS, SMALL CELL TYPE

The nuclei are small and show nuclear molding.

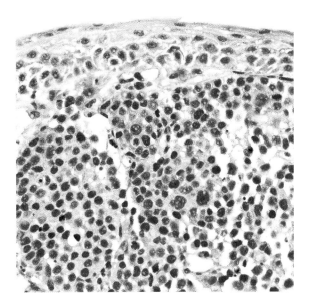

Figure 6-3

NEUROENDOCRINE CARCINOMA OF THE ESOPHAGUS, LARGE CELL TYPE

The malignant cells are arranged in organoid nests and have prominent nucleoli.

tumors have 2 to 20 mitoses in 10 high-power fields or a Ki-67 labeling index between 3 and 20 percent. These tumors are usually so small that the Ki-67 labeling index is more practical to use.

Some tumors have the morphology of a well-differentiated neuroendocrine (carcinoid) tumor, but the proliferation index of a high-grade neuroendocrine tumor. These are considered grade 3 neuroendocrine tumors (as opposed to carcinomas). There are no large studies of these tumors in the esophagus, but in the pancreas, these are associated with a better outcome than high-grade neuroendocrine carcinomas (6).

Neuroendocrine carcinomas are highly aggressive, and are either of the large cell or small cell type; their microscopic appearance is similar to neuroendocrine tumors elsewhere in the body (figs. 6-2, 6-3). They sometimes arise in association with squamous or columnar epithelial dysplasia (figs. 6-4–6-6). Large cell neuroendocrine carcinomas have an organoid pattern, with solid nests of cells with identifiable cytoplasm. Poorly formed acini are sometimes present. Many of the cells show nucleoli (fig. 6-3). Small cell neuroendocrine carcinomas have cells that are not small, but the nuclear to cytoplasmic (N/C)

ratio is high and they have dense dark nuclear chromatin. The nuclei tend to mold against one another in solid sheets and nests (fig. 6-2). Using mitotic rates and Ki-67 labeling indices, they display over 20 mitoses per 10 high-power fields and a proliferation index over 20 percent (usually more than 50 percent.

MANEC of the esophagus is rare (figs. 6-7, 6-8). This tumor consists of two types of differentiation: adenocarcinoma and high-grade neuroendocrine carcinoma. This combination is vastly more common than the combination of squamous cell carcinoma and high-grade neuroendocrine carcinoma, at least in a Western population (7); but squamous precursors are more commonly encountered in series from southeast Asia where they are detected in about half of cases (8). For a tumor to be classified as MANEC, there must be at least 30 percent of each of the components, i.e., adenocarcinoma and neuroendocrine carcinoma. In some examples, the zones with neuroendocrine differentiation are intimately admixed with the adenocarcinoma component, whereas in other tumors, these components collide. The columnar precursor lesions can contain Kulchitsky cells (fig. 6-5) (9).

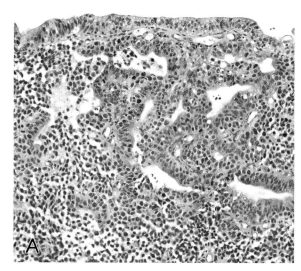

Figure 6-4

NEUROENDOCRINE CARCINOMA OF THE ESOPHAGUS, SMALL CELL TYPE

A: This tumor developed in association with high-grade columnar epithelial dysplasia, which can be seen on the surface and within the invasive carcinoma.

B: Synaptophysin stain labels the neuroendocrine carcinoma, but not the high-grade columnar epithelial dysplasia.

C: This synaptophysin stain shows dot-like labeling (arrow).

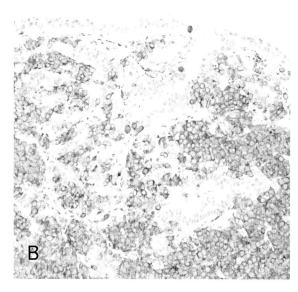

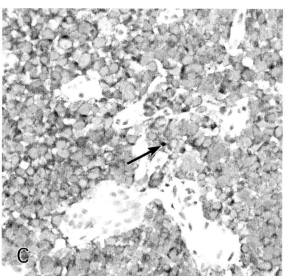

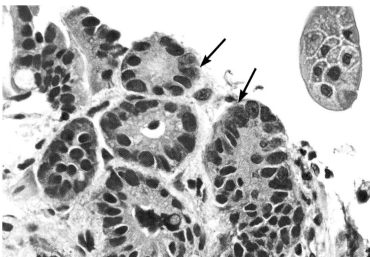

Figure 6-5

HIGH-GRADE EPITHELIAL DYSPLASIA WITH NEUROENDOCRINE CELLS

Kulchitsky cells with delicate eosin-ophilic granules oriented toward the base of the cells (facing the lamina propria vascular supply rather than the lumen) are indicated by the arrows and presumably are precursors to invasive neuroendocrine carcinoma of the esophagus. The gland at the left center of the field has several cells with neuroendocrine granules.

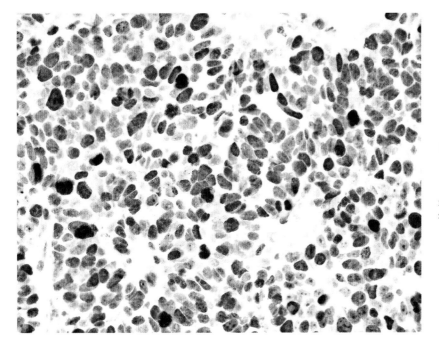

Figure 6-6

NEUROENDOCRINE CARCINOMA OF THE ESOPHAGUS, SMALL CELL TYPE

Ki-67 labels nearly every malignant cell. (This is from the same lesion depicted in figure 6-4.)

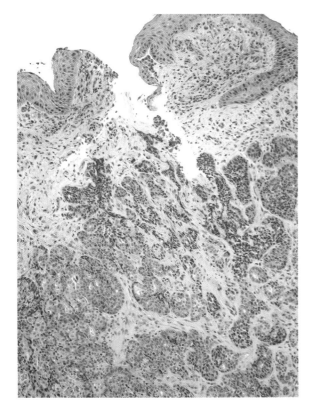
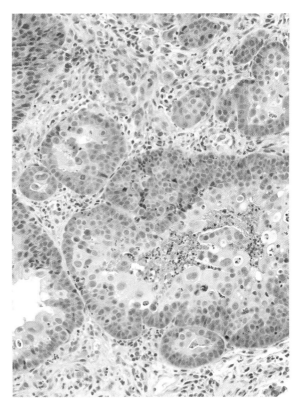

Figure 6-7

MIXED ADENONEUROENDOCRINE CARCINOMA (MANEC) OF THE ESOPHAGUS

Left: There is squamous epithelium on the left. The carcinoma forms nests with focal lumens.

Right: Although the large nest at the right displays necrosis reminiscent of that seen in colorectal adenocarcinoma, the cells at the periphery of the nest have a more solid appearance.

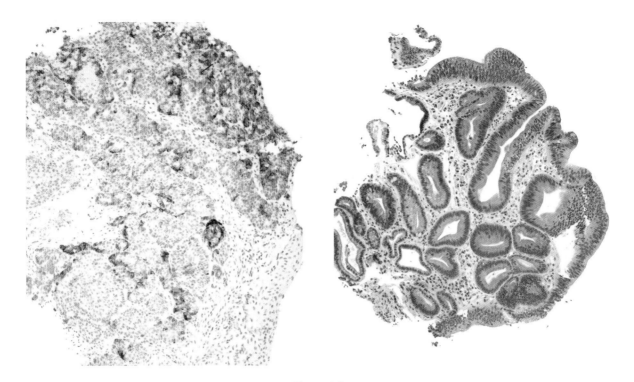

Figure 6-8

MIXED ADENONEUROENDOCRINE CARCINOMA (MANEC) OF THE ESOPHAGUS

Left: Synaptophysin labels some cells, but not others.
Right: The tumor was associated with columnar dysplasia, shown here.

Immunohistochemical Findings. Neuroendocrine tumors typically express chromogranin A and synaptophysin; the carcinomas are defined by expression of either synaptophysin, chromogranin A, or CD56 (1). Although TTF1 and KIT labeling may be encountered in neuroendocrine carcinomas, this does not correlate with either the site of origin or *KIT* mutational status (5).

Molecular Genetic Findings. Since esophageal neuroendocrine neoplasms are rare, there is little information regarding the molecular profile of these tumors.

Differential Diagnosis. The differential diagnosis of neuroendocrine tumors of the esophagus depends on the grade. For grade 1 and grade 2 neuroendocrine tumors, lymphoid aggregates and low-grade lymphomas as well as benign nerve sheath lesions (10) are in the differential diagnosis. All of these are readily separated with the use of a limited immunolabeling panel that includes a hematopoietic marker, such as CD45, and S-100 protein to address nerve sheath lesions together with synaptophysin or chromogranin

A. Synaptophysin is not as specific for neuroendocrine tumors as chromogranin A, and it can be reactive in other types of neoplasms.

The differential diagnosis is broader for neuroendocrine carcinoma and includes high-grade lymphomas, other high-grade carcinomas, melanoma, and round cell sarcomas. Esophageal lymphoma, melanoma, and sarcoma are even rarer than neuroendocrine carcinomas but any high-grade malignant neoplasm can be initially evaluated using a panel of S-100 protein (to address melanoma), a pankeratin, and a broad hematopoietic marker such as CD45. Generally, keratin expression suggests poorly differentiated squamous cell carcinoma or adenocarcinoma while a "dot-like" keratin expression suggests neuroendocrine carcinoma, small cell type.

Treatment and Prognosis. Most well differentiated neuroendocrine tumors of the esophagus are easily managed by endoscopic removal. Radiolabeled somatostatin analogue treatment has been useful for advanced lesions. Lutetium-177 (177Lu)-dotatate has been tested in patients with advanced, progressive, somatostatin receptor–positive midgut neuroendocrine tumors with promising results, but there are no data on such treatment in esophageal tumors (11).

Neuroendocrine carcinomas of the esophagus tend to be managed by surgery because of obstructive symptoms; neoadjuvant chemoradiation is often used for MANEC prior to surgery. However, there are no well-defined treatment protocols. In some studies, there is some benefit from chemotherapy (12).

The prognosis for patients with incidental well-differentiated neuroendocrine tumors is good, but it is poor for those with primary neuroendocrine carcinoma. In one study of 126 patients, the median survival time was about 1 year, and the 5-year survival rate was about 12 percent (12). Data are fewer for large cell neuroendocrine carcinomas, but case reports describe an aggressive course. Good outcomes are generally a reflection of tumors that are detected at an early stage.

ESOPHAGEAL MELANOMA

Definition. *Esophageal melanoma* is defined as a melanoma that has arisen in the esophagus. As such, it is regarded as a mucosal melanoma.

Clinical Features. Primary esophageal melanoma is extremely rare, accounting for only 0.2 percent of esophageal neoplasms, and less than 0.05 percent of all melanomas (13). These are tumors of adults and there is a male predominance (13–17). Esophageal melanomas tend to arise in the mid- or distal esophagus. At presentation, the tumors are usually bulky polypoid masses, and many are pigmented (1).

Gross Findings. In resected samples, the neoplasm is polypoid and the cut surface is frequently pigmented. Early lesions can display the appearance of a nevus (18).

Microscopic Findings. Esophageal melanomas have the same appearances as those in other anatomic sites (fig. 6-9). An in situ component is detected in some cases, half in one small series (13). Pigment is frequently identified. The growth pattern can be solid or spindled. As per melanomas in other sites, the spindle or epithelioid cells can show macronucleoli.

Immunohistochemical Findings. Similar to melanomas in other sites, esophageal melanomas express S-100 protein and SOX10, and frequently label with melanoma markers such as HMB-45, Melan-A, and tyrosinase. One caveat is that spindle cell melanomas tend to lose their immunolabeling with HMB-45 and Melan-A. KIT expression is common in esophageal melanomas and was present, at least focally, in all cases in one small series, but it is occasionally diffuse (13).

Molecular Genetic Findings. Studies of esophageal melanoma are limited since these neoplasms are rare. Similar to mucosal melanomas in other sites, a subset of esophageal melanomas harbors *KIT* mutations (13,19–24). *KIT* mutations are detected in 20 to 30 percent of mucosal melanomas from all mucosal sites, a figure mirrored in the esophagus. A small subset of esophageal melanomas harbors *BRAF* and *KRAS* mutations but *PDGFR* and *NRAS* mutations have not been detected to date (13).

Differential Diagnosis. The differential diagnosis is primarily with gastrointestinal stromal tumor based on the proclivity of melanoma to express KIT, especially in spindle cell tumors. If pigment is not present, the differential diagnosis is with any high-grade neoplasm, including lymphomas and carcinomas, especially neuroendocrine carcinoma, which is also likely to show KIT expression.

Treatment and Prognosis. Treatment has traditionally been surgical, with some success with radiation (14,25). With the availability of therapy to target mucosal melanomas with alterations in *KIT* (13,19–24) and *BRAF*, the treatment for esophageal melanoma will, no doubt, change. These tumors should also be amenable to modern anti-PD-1 and anti-CTLA4 drugs, which harness the body's immune system to target malignant cells (26–29), but specific data for esophageal melanoma are presently not available.

Except in rare cases in which lesions are identified early, the prognosis for patients with esophageal melanoma is dismal (14). Although specific data are not yet available for esophageal melanoma, targeting the molecules noted above may improve the outcome in coming years.

HEMATOPOIETIC TUMORS

Primary esophageal hematopoietic lesions are exceedingly rare. Most reported lesions are extranodal lymphomas. *Esophageal lymphoma* is an extranodal lymphoma arising in the esophagus, in contrast to extension into the

Figure 6-9

ESOPHAGEAL MELANOMA

A: The tumor is pigmented and has an in situ component so it is easy to recognize as a melanoma despite the spindled appearance of the deeper portion on the tumor.

B: The in situ and epithelioid component consists of cells with large nucleoli, whereas nucleoli are inconspicuous in the deeper area.

C: This spindle cell component is easy to mistake for a gastrointestinal stromal tumor, a mistake that could be compounded by KIT expression. Like esophageal melanoma, esophageal gastrointestinal stromal tumor is rare.

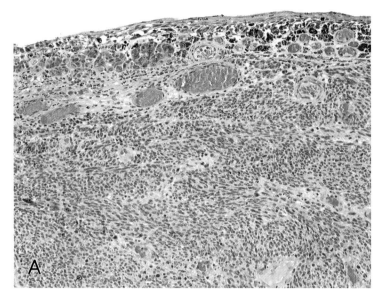

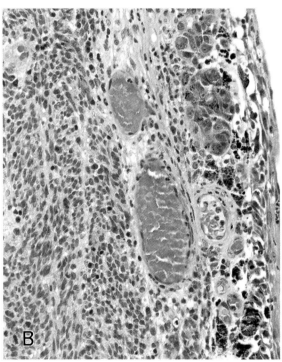

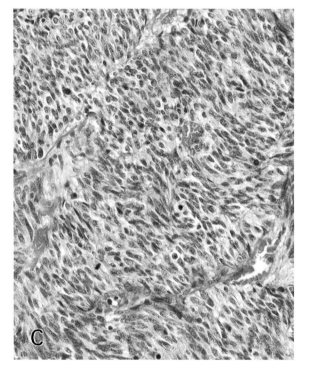

esophagus from the mediastinum, stomach, or a contiguous lymph node. Rare cases are typically large B-cell lymphomas or mucosa-associated lymphoid tissue (MALT) lymphomas. A granulocytic sarcoma and a diffuse large B-cell lymphoma of the esophagus are shown in figures 6-10–6-12.

Any type of lymphoma can, theoretically, be detected in the esophagus, and a discussion of every type is beyond the scope of this book (30). The reader is referred to Tumors of the Lymph Nodes and Spleen (31) from this series.

OTHER NEOPLASMS THAT INVOLVE THE ESOPHAGUS

A small percentage (up to 3 percent) of esophageal neoplasms spread from other sites (1), either directly (such as from lung or thyroid

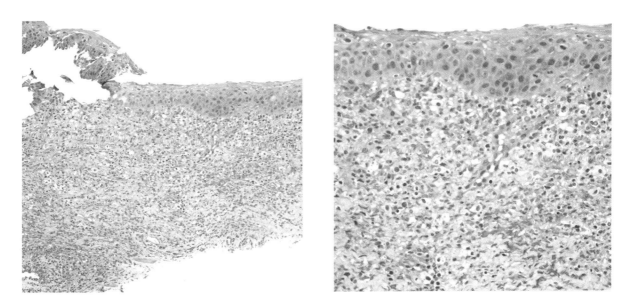

Figure 6-10

ESOPHAGEAL GRANULOCYTIC SARCOMA

Left: The appearance is similar to that of an inflammatory lesion.
Right: The malignant cells are small in comparison to the endothelial cells in the lamina propria capillary in the center of the image.

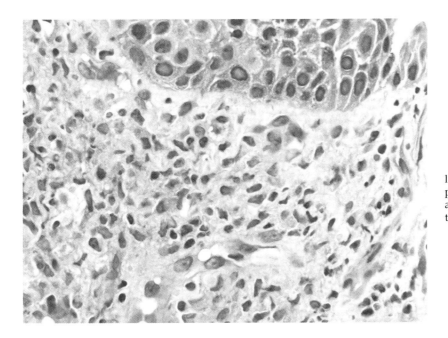

Figure 6-11

ESOPHAGEAL GRANULOCYTIC SARCOMA

This diagnosis required correlation with immunolabeling. The patient manifested overt leukemia a few months after presenting with this esophageal mass.

carcinoma) or hematogenously (such as breast carcinoma). Such lesions are often located in the middle third of the esophagus. Examples of

metastatic breast carcinoma and thyroid carcinoma that have directly invaded the esophagus are shown in figures 6-13 and 6-14.

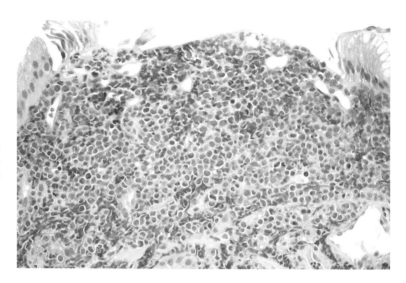

Figure 6-12

**ESOPHAGEAL DIFFUSE
LARGE B-CELL LYMPHOMA**

This tumor was associated with cardiac type mucosa in the distal esophagus. The appearance is the same as that of diffuse large B-cell lymphoma elsewhere in the body.

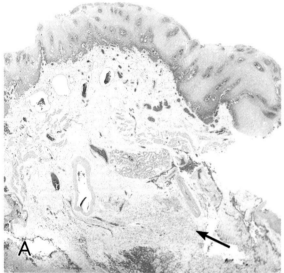

Figure 6-13

**BREAST LOBULAR CARCINOMA
METASTATIC TO THE ESOPHAGUS**

A: The tumor is very subtle (indicated by the arrow).

B: The malignant cells proliferate around blood vessels and esophageal submucosal glands.

C: This high magnification image shows mucin within the malignant cells, which contain nuclei that are larger than those of lymphocytes in the image. An esophageal submucosal gland is present at the upper left.

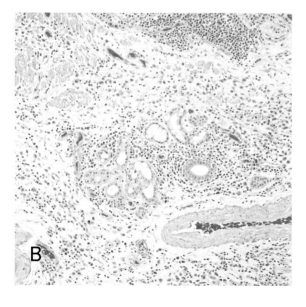

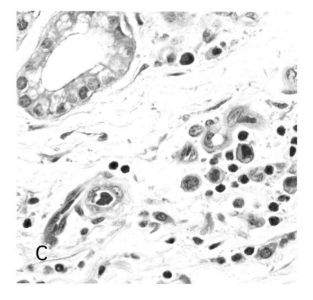

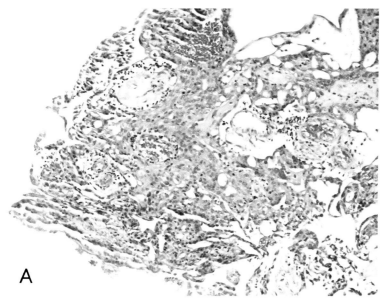

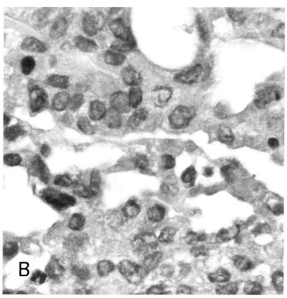

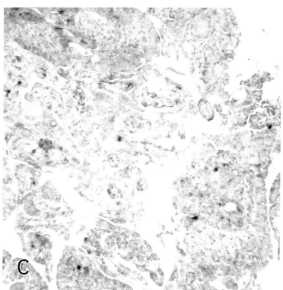

Figure 6-14

THYROID PAPILLARY CARCINOMA DIRECTLY INVADING THE ESOPHAGUS

A: The nuclei are smaller than those typically encountered in esophageal adenocarcinoma.

B: Nuclear grooves and inclusions are present.

C: This is a thyroglobulin stain, which labels the carcinoma.

REFERENCES

1. Bosman F, Carneiro F, Hruban R, Theise N, eds. WHO classification of tumours of the digestive system. In: Bosman F, Jaffee E, Lakhani S, Ohgaki H, eds. World Health Organization Classification of Tumours. Lyon: IARC; 2010.
2. Rooper LM, Sharma R, Li QK, Illei PB, Westra WH. INSM1 demonstrates superior performance to the individual and combined use of synaptophysin, chromogranin and CD56 for diagnosing neuroendocrine tumors of the thoracic cavity. Am J Surg Pathol 2017. [Epub ahead of print]
3. Park JY, Cornish TC, Lam-Himlin D, Shi C, Montgomery E. Gastric lesions in patients with autoimmune metaplastic atrophic gastritis (AMAG) in a tertiary care setting. Am J Surg Pathol 2010;34:1591-8.
4. Modlin IM, Lye KD, Kidd M. A 5-decade analysis of 13,715 carcinoid tumors. Cancer 2003;97:934-59.

5. Egashira A, Morita M, Kumagai R, et al. Neuro-endocrine carcinoma of the esophagus: clinico-pathological and immunohistochemical features of 14 cases. PloS One 2017;12:e0173501.

6. Basturk O, Yang Z, Tang LH, et al. The high-grade (WHO G3) pancreatic neuroendocrine tumor category is morphologically and biologically het-erogenous and includes both well differentiated and poorly differentiated neoplasms. Am J Surg Pathol 2015;39:683-90.

7. Maru DM, Khurana H, Rashid A, et al. Retro-spective study of clinicopathologic features and prognosis of high-grade neuroendocrine carcinoma of the esophagus. Am J Surg Pathol 2008;32:1404-11.

8. Huang Q, Wu H, Nie L, et al. Primary high-grade neuroendocrine carcinoma of the esophagus: a clinicopathologic and immunohistochemical study of 42 resection cases. Am J Surg Pathol 2013;37:467-83.

9. Vieth M, Montgomery EA, Riddell RH. Observa-tions of different patterns of dysplasia in barretts esophagus—a first step to harmonize grading. Cesk Patol 2016;52:154-63.

10. Celeiro-Munoz C, Huebner TA, Robertson SA, et al. Tactile corpuscle-like bodies in gastrointesti-nal-type mucosa: a case series. Am J Surg Pathol 2015;39:1668-72.

11. Strosberg J, El-Haddad G, Wolin E, et al. Phase 3 trial of ^{177}Lu-Dotatate for midgut neuroendocrine tumors. N Engl J Med 2017;376:125-35.

12. Lv J, Liang J, Wang J, et al. Primary small cell carcinoma of the esophagus. J Thorac Oncol 2008;3:1460-5.

13. Langer R, Becker K, Feith M, Friess H, Hofler H, Keller G. Genetic aberrations in primary esopha-geal melanomas: molecular analysis of c-KIT, PDGFR, KRAS, NRAS and BRAF in a series of 10 cases. Mod Pathol 2011;24:495-501.

14. Li B, Lei W, Shao K, et al. Characteristics and prognosis of primary malignant melanoma of the esophagus. Melanoma Res 2007;17:239-42.

15. Takubo K, Kanda Y, Ishii M, et al. Primary malig-nant melanoma of the esophagus. Hum Pathol 1983;14:727-30.

16. Volpin E, Sauvanet A, Couvelard A, Belghiti J. Primary malignant melanoma of the esophagus: a case report and review of the literature. Dis Esophagus 2002;15:244-9.

17. Yoo CC, Levine MS, McLarney JK, Lowry MA. Primary malignant melanoma of the esophagus: radiographic findings in seven patients. Radiol-ogy 1998;209:455-9.

18. Kang MJ, Yi SY. Nevus-like appearance of primary malignant melanoma of the esophagus. Gastro-enterol Res Pract 2009;2009:285753.

19. Antonescu CR, Busam KJ, Francone TD, et al. L576P KIT mutation in anal melanomas correlates with KIT protein expression and is sensitive to specific kinase inhibition. Int J Cancer 2007;121:257-64.

20. Carvajal RD, Antonescu CR, Wolchok JD, et al. KIT as a therapeutic target in metastatic mela-noma. JAMA 2011;305:2327-34.

21. Curtin JA, Busam K, Pinkel D, Bastian BC. So-matic activation of KIT in distinct subtypes of melanoma. J Clin Oncol 2006;24:4340-6.

22. Debiec-Rychter M, Dumez H, Judson I, et al. Use of c-KIT/PDGFRA mutational analysis to predict the clinical response to imatinib in patients with advanced gastrointestinal stromal tumours en-tered on phase I and II studies of the EORTC Soft Tissue and Bone Sarcoma Group. Eur J Cancer 2004;40:689-95.

23. Quintas-Cardama A, Lazar AJ, Woodman SE, Kim K, Ross M, Hwu P. Complete response of stage IV anal mucosal melanoma expressing KIT Val560Asp to the multikinase inhibitor sorafenib. Nature clinical practice. Nat Clin Pract Oncol 2008;5:737-40.

24. Satzger I, Schaefer T, Kuettler U, et al. Analysis of c-KIT expression and KIT gene mutation in human mucosal melanomas. Br J Cancer 2008;99:2065-9.

25. Wayman J, Irving M, Russell N, Nicoll J, Raimes SA. Intraluminal radiotherapy and Nd:YAG laser photoablation for primary malignant mel-anoma of the esophagus. Gastrointest Endosc 2004;59:927-9.

26. Inadomi K, Kumagai H, Arita S, et al. Bi-cytope-nia possibly induced by anti-PD-1 antibody for primary malignant melanoma of the esophagus: a case report. Medicine 2016;95:e4283.

27. Schachter J, Ribas A, Long GV, et al. Pembrolizum-ab versus ipilimumab for advanced melanoma: final overall survival results of a multicentre, randomised, open-label phase 3 study (KEYNOTE-006). Lancet 2017. [Epub ahead of print]

28. Shoushtari AN, Friedman CF, Navid-Azarbaijani P, et al. Measuring toxic effects and time to treatment failure for Nivolumab plus Ipilimumab in mela-noma. JAMA Oncol 2017. [Epub ahead of print]

29. Topalian SL, Hodi FS, Brahmer JR, et al. Safety, ac-tivity, and immune correlates of anti-PD-1 antibody in cancer. N Engl J Med 2012;366:2443-54.

30. Swerdlow SH, Campo E, Pileri SA, et al. The 2016 revision of the World Health Organization classification of lymphoid neoplasms. Blood 2016;127:2375-90.

31. Medeiros L, O'Malley DP, Caraway, NP, Vega F, Elenitoba-Johnson, KS, Lim MS. Tumors of the lymph nodes and spleen. AFIP Atlas of Tumor Palthology, 4th Series, Fascicle 25. Washington DC: American Registry of Pathology; 2017.

7 THE NORMAL STOMACH

The anatomy, physiology, and histology of the stomach are much more complicated than the esophagus. Instead of a homogeneous muscular tube whose only role is to transport food, the stomach coordinates the physical and chemical breakdown of food. Exactly where the esophagus ends and the stomach begins has become a hotly debated topic. A brief review of the embryology, anatomy, and normal histology of the stomach is provided below.

EMBRYOLOGY

The stomach begins as a dilatation of the caudal foregut at 5 weeks' gestation (1). Over the course of several weeks, it grows and rotates, so that the left side faces anteriorly and the right side faces posteriorly. This results in the left vagus nerve innervating the anterior gastric wall and the right vagus nerve innervating the posterior gastric wall (1). The posterior wall grows faster than the anterior wall, leading to the formation of the greater and lesser curvatures. As the stomach continues to develop and grow, the pyloric region moves upward and to the right while the gastroesophageal junction (GEJ) moves downward and to the left (1).

Many of the genes and molecular pathways involved in esophageal embryology are also involved in the histogenesis of the stomach (2). The sonic hedgehog and BMP pathways are critical and the genes *SOX2*, *GATA4*, and *PDX1* seem to be important in the differentiation of the different mucosal types in the stomach (2).

ANATOMY

The stomach normally lies in the central and left anterior abdomen. The traditional view has been that the stomach begins as the cardia, a narrow 1- to 2-cm cuff that starts distal to the lower esophageal sphincter and then opens into the more dilated body or corpus (fig. 7-1) (3). More recently, however, some investigators have proposed that the cardia is not a normal anatomic structure, but rather is columnar metaplasia of the distal esophagus secondary to gastroesophageal reflux (4,5). While it is clear that cardiac-type mucosa develops as a result of reflux, whether the entire cardia is the result of metaplasia remains controversial (6–8).

The proximal part of the body of the stomach extends cephalad to the diaphragm, forming a bulge known as the fundus. From here the body extends distally, with a broad curve along the left side known as the greater curvature. The right side is much shorter and is referred to as the lesser curvature. Distally, the body tapers gradually and takes a sharp turn to the right, which is called the angulus. The angulus is the dividing line between the body and antrum (9).

The antrum comprises the lower third of the stomach. It is narrower than the body and tapers to end at the pylorus. The pylorus represents the last centimeter of the stomach that overlies the muscular ridge of the internal layer of the muscularis propria, known as the pyloric sphincter. This is the dividing line between the stomach and duodenum.

The external surface of the stomach is largely covered by peritoneum. The greater curvature is attached to the omentum and transverse mesocolon, while the lesser curvature is attached to the liver via the gastrohepatic ligament.

The mucosal surfaces of the body and fundus consist of coarse folds or rugae. Rugae are composed of both mucosa and submucosa, and tend to flatten out when the stomach is distended. The mucosa in the antrum is flatter and more firmly attached to the muscularis propria. The lesser curvature typically has a more flattened appearance (fig. 7-2).

HISTOLOGY

The stomach is similar to the rest of the more distal gastrointestinal tract in that it has mucosa, muscularis mucosae, submucosa, two layers of muscularis propria, and subserosa.

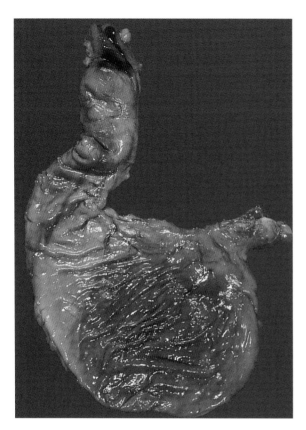 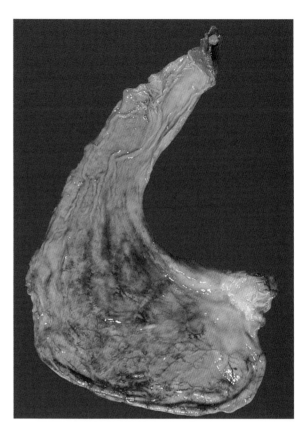

Figure 7-1

NORMAL STOMACH (AUTOPSY MATERIAL)

Left: External view prior to opening the specimen.

Right: Internal view of the posterior wall opened. In both views, the distal esophagus is the short narrow tube at the upper center. It enters the stomach at the first 1 to 2 cm of the cardia. The body extends distally from the cardia to the bend on the left, the angularis. Distal to the angularis is the antrum, which terminates at the pylorus. The outpouching on the upper right is the fundus.

Figure 7-2

MUCOSAL VIEW OF STOMACH

Mucosal view of a whole stomach opened along the greater curvature, with the esophagus on the left (tongues of Barrett mucosa are seen above the gastroesophageal junction). The parallel folds in the middle of the specimen run along the lesser curvature. The two wings at either side are the fundus. The entire fundus and body are covered by thick, often serpentine, folds or rugae. They flatten distally in the antrum. The bulge at the bottom is the pyloric sphincter.

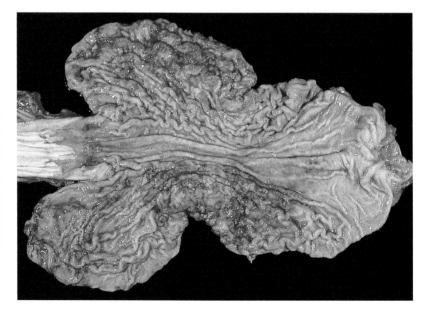

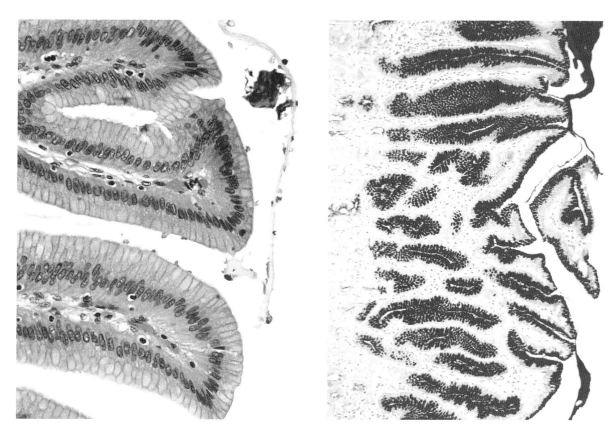

Figure 7-3

NORMAL SUPERFICIAL AND PIT EPITHELIUM

Apical mucin stains pink with hematoxylin and eosin (H&E), red with periodic acid-Schiff (PAS), and does not stain with alcian blue. (Left: H&E stain; right: alcian blue, PAS combination stain.)

Mucosa

The stomach has several types of epithelium that imperfectly correlate with gross anatomic locations. Generally, the mucosa in the gastric cardia resembles the mucosa in the antrum, while the epithelia in the body and fundus are identical to each other, but are different than the cardia and antrum.

Regardless of site, the gastric mucosa has two compartments: the superficial foveolar compartment (or pit compartment) and the deep glandular compartment. The foveolar epithelium extends down into the pits which connect to the gland lumens. The superficial epithelium is composed of tall columnar cells with apical mucin vacuoles. These neutral mucin vacuoles stain pale pink with hematoxylin and eosin (H&E), dark red/magenta with periodic acid–Schiff (PAS), and do not stain with alcian blue or mucicarmine (fig. 7-3). While the surface epithelium is the same throughout the stomach, the depth of the pits varies, being shorter in the body and longer in the cardia and antrum (figs. 7-4–7-6).

The deep glandular compartment of the mucosa differs not only in thickness, but also in cell type, depending upon location. The deep glands of the cardia and antrum are similar in that they are arranged in tightly packed clusters surrounded by fine septa of collagen and smooth muscle (fig. 7-7). Although the cytoplasm of these deep gland cells are more granular than the surface cells, they make similar mucins: neutral mucins. While a rare parietal cell may be present, chief cells are not normally found in the antrum or cardia.

The deep glands of the fundus and body are different, since the epithelium here is composed of parietal and chief cells, which make gastric acid and digestive enzymes (pepsinogen),

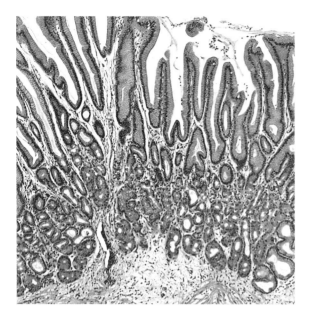

Figure 7-4

NORMAL CARDIAC-TYPE MUCOSA

The pit and the glandular compartments are approximately equal in height.

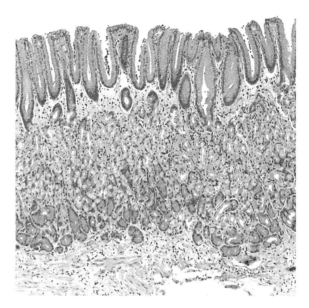

Figure 7-5

NORMAL BODY (CORPUS, FUNDIC) MUCOSA

The pit compartment is about one fourth of the entire mucosal thickness, resulting in a pit to gland ratio of 1 to 3. The glands are tightly clustered. The superficial lamina propria contains few cells.

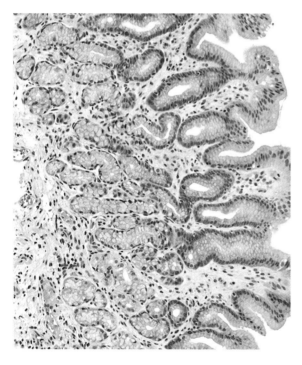

Figure 7-6

NORMAL ANTRAL (PYLORIC) MUCOSA

The pit and glandular compartments are about the same length. The glands are clustered and less densely packed than in the body.

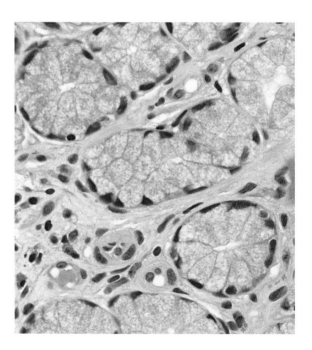

Figure 7-7

MUCOUS GLANDS

Mucous glands of the type that occur in normal cardiac and antral mucosae.

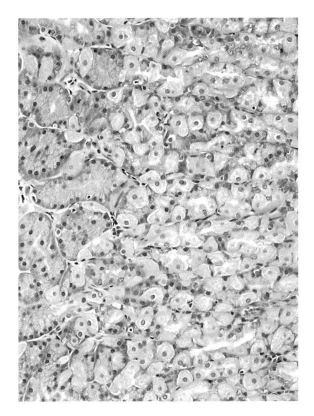

Figure 7-8

GLANDULAR COMPARTMENT OF BODY MUCOSA

The glands are tightly packed. The top two thirds is predominated by parietal cells (right) with pink granular cytoplasm. At the bottom left, several glands containing chief cell are present. Chief cells have cyanophilic cytoplasm and more basally oriented nuclei.

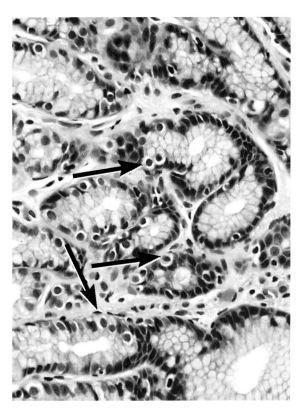

Figure 7-9

NECK REGION OF ANTRAL MUCOSA

This high-power view shows the proliferative zone of the gastric mucosa. The mucus-containing epithelium is slightly more hyperchromatic. The paler cells with a small halo surrounding the nucleus and fine gray granular cytoplasm are the gastrin-producing G cells (arrows).

respectively (fig. 7-8). In H&E-stained sections, the parietal cells have granular pale pink cytoplasm while the chief cells appear darker. Parietal cells are more numerous in the upper part of the glandular compartment while chief cells are more common at the base (fig. 7-8).

Endocrine cells are another vital component of the gastric mucosa that varies depending upon site (10). Gastrin-producing G cells are the predominant endocrine cell in the antrum. In the body, histamine-producing enterochromaffin-like (ECL) cells are more common, while G cells are rare. Endocrine cells are normally located in the lower third of the glands near the chief cells, and while they can be seen on H&E-stained sections, they are most easily visualized with immunoperoxidase stains for chromogranin, synaptophysin, and gastrin (figs. 7-9, 7-10).

The junction between the antrum and body contains a transition zone where the epithelium has features of both types of mucosa. The overall architecture of this transitional mucosa resembles antral mucosa, however, clusters of parietal and chief cells are present in the deeper glands. As people age, the transitional mucosa seems to move more proximally, especially along the lesser curvature (11).

The proliferative zone of the gastric mucosa is in the neck region (fig. 7-9). The cells in this region are called mucous neck cells. Mitotic figures may be seen here, and when these cells become crushed in endoscopic biopsy specimens, they can become disaggregated and resemble signet ring cell carcinoma cells. This same area bears the brunt of damage in graft versus host disease (12).

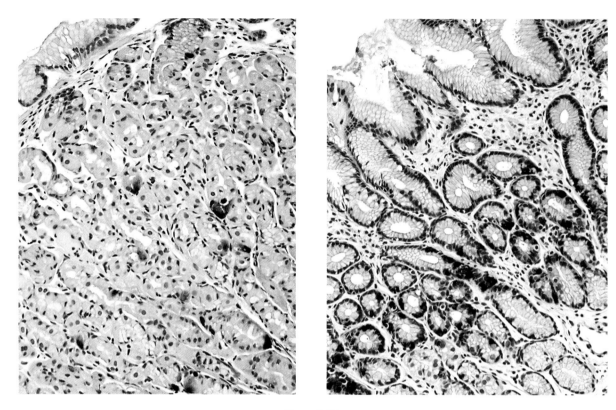

Figure 7-10

ENDOCRINE CELLS IN GASTRIC MUCOSA

Left: Immunoperoxidase stain for chromogranin shows scattered positivity in enterochromaffin-like (ECL) cells in the gastric body.

Right: Immunoperoxidase stain for gastrin showing numerous G cells in the gastric antrum.

Lamina Propria

The lamina propria is very sparse throughout the normal stomach. Body-type mucosa contains little stroma between glands, and almost no inflammatory cells (fig. 7-5). A fine reticulin meshwork supports the glands. Antral and cardiac mucosae have a few collagen and smooth muscle fibers. Arterioles, venules, and capillaries are present at all levels of the lamina propria, whereas lymphatics are normally found only in the deepest regions. Lymphatics have been reported higher up in the lamina propria in cases of atrophic gastritis (11).

There are few inflammatory cells in the normal stomach. Only rare lymphocytes, plasma cells, and macrophages may be present. Small lymphoid aggregates are thought by some to be "normal," however, this is somewhat controversial (fig. 7-11A,B) (13–15). It is clear that large lymphoid aggregates with germinal centers are

largely due to *Helicobacter pylori* infection (fig. 7-11C,D) (13). The author's experience with otherwise normal-appearing gastric biopsies in young children suggests that small lymphoid aggregates are normal and occur without antecedent *H. pylori* gastritis (fig. 7-11A,B).

Muscularis Mucosae

The muscularis mucosae consists of a thin double layer of smooth muscle (inner circular and outer longitudinal) that defines the base of the mucosa and separates it from the submucosa. Muscle fibers extend from the muscularis mucosae up to the basement membrane near the pylorus.

Submucosa

The submucosa is a layer of loose connective tissue containing adipose tissue, blood vessels, lymphatics, nerves, and ganglion cells (Meissner plexus).

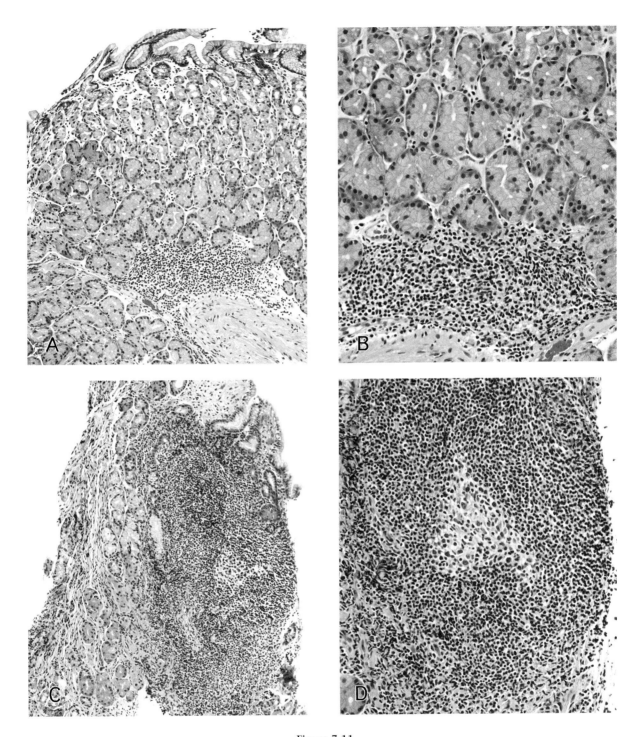

Figure 7-11

LYMPHOID AGGREGATES IN LAMINA PROPRIA

A: Low-power view of normal body-type mucosa with a small lymphoid aggregate. This biopsy came from a 12-month-old child with no other histologic abnormalities.

B: Higher-power view of the same "normal" lymphoid aggregate.

C: Low-power view of a large lymphoid aggregate with a well-formed germinal center arising in active chronic *Helicobacter pylori* gastritis.

D: High-power view of the lymphoid follicle.

Figure 7-12

ARTERIAL AND LYMPHATIC SUPPLY OF STOMACH

A schematic diagram of the arteries of the stomach illustrates: aorta (A); left gastric artery (LG); hepatic artery (H); right gastric artery (RG); gastroduodenal artery (GI); right gastroepiploic artery (RGE); splenic artery (S); left gastroepiploic artery (LGE); and superior pancreaticoduodenal artery (SD). The lymph nodes are situated along the arteries and consist of six groups: paracardiac nodes, superior gastric nodes, subpyloric nodes, inferior gastric nodes, splenic nodes, and pancreatic nodes.

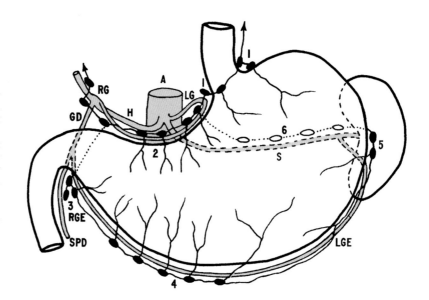

Muscularis Propria

The stomach is unique in that it has three layers of smooth muscle: the inner oblique, the middle circular, and the outer longitudinal. The circular layer gives rise to the pyloric sphincter whereas the fibers of the longitudinal layer are contiguous with the longitudinal muscle layer of the esophagus. The myenteric plexus (Auerbach) runs between the outer two muscle layers.

Subserosa and Serosa

The subserosa consists of a thin layer of collagen covered by a single layer of flat mesothelium, the serosa proper, part of the visceral peritoneum.

BLOOD SUPPLY

The blood is supplied to the gastric cardia by the celiac axis via the left gastric artery (fig. 7-12) (15,16). The right gastric artery and the right gastroepiploic artery, both branches of the hepatic artery, supply the lesser and greater curvatures, respectively. The left gastroepiploic artery and the short gastric arteries arise from the splenic artery and supply blood to the proximal greater curvature (15). There is an extensive anastomotic network of these vessels which allows for excellent collateral circulation (15). These arteries are accompanied by veins that, with the exception of the proximal stomach, drain into the portal venous system. The proximal stomach drains via the esophageal venous system.

LYMPHATIC DRAINAGE

The lymphatics follow the major blood vessels, with lymph nodes located along the main arteries (fig. 7-12) (15,16). The lesser curvature, from the cardia distally, drains to lymphatics along the left gastric vessels to the left gastric nodes. Part of the cardia is also drained by the paracardiac lymph nodes. The antral part of the lesser curvature drains to the right gastric and hepatic nodes. The proximal portion of the greater curvature drains to lymph nodes in the splenic hilum, while lymphatics from the distal greater curvature drain to the right gastroepiploic and pyloric/subpyloric nodes.

NERVES

The anterior and posterior vagus nerves provide parasympathetic innervation to the stomach, mostly via subserosal connections along the lesser curvature (15). The celiac plexus and the phrenic nerves supply sympathetic innervation.

REFERENCES

1. Langman J. Medical embryology: human development—normal and abnormal. Baltimore: Williams & Wilkins; 1975:282-4.
2. Willet SG, Mills JC. Stomach organ and cell lineage differentiation: from embryogenesis to adult homeostasis. Cell Mol Gastroenterol Hepatol 2016;2:546-59.
3. Lewin KJ, Appelman HD. Tumors of the Esophagus and Stomach. AFIP Atlas of Tumor Pathology, 3rd Series, Fascicle 18. Washington DC: American Registry of Pathology; 1996:175-82.
4. Chandrasoma PT, Der R, Ma Y, Dalton P, Taira M. Histology of the gastroesophageal junction: an autopsy study. Am J Surg Pathol 2000;24:1171-4.
5. Chandrasoma P. Controversies of the cardiac mucosa and Barrett's oesophagus. Histopathology 2005;46:361-73.
6. Glickman JN, Fox V, Antonioli DA, Wang HH, Odze RD. Morphology of the cardia and significance of carditis in pediatric patients. Am J Surg Pathol 2002;26:1032-9.
7. Kilgore SP, Ormsby AH, Gramlich TL, et al. The gastric cardia: fact or fiction? Am J Gastroenterol 2000;95:921-4.
8. Odze RD. Unraveling the mystery of the gastro-esophageal junction: a pathologist's perspective. Am J Gastroenterol 2005;100:1853-67.
9. Toner PG, Watt PC, Boyd SM. The gastric mucosa. In: Whitehead R, ed. Gastrointestinal and oesophageal pathology. Edinburgh: Churchill Livingstone, 1989:13-28.
10. Dayal Y, Wolfe HJ. Hyperplastic proliferations of the gastroduodenal endocrine cells. In: Dayal Y, ed. Endocrine pathology of the gut and pancreas. Boca Raton: CRC Press, 1991:36-42.
11. Kimura K. Chronological transition of the fundic-pyloric border determined by stepwise biopsy of the lesser and greater curvatures of the stomach. Gastroenterology 1972;63:584-92.
12. Washington K, Bentley RC, Green A, Olson J, Treem WR, Krigman HR. Gastric graft-versus-host disease: a blinded histologic study. Am J Surg Pathol 1997;21:1037-46.
13. Genta RM, Hammer HW, Graham DY. Gastric lymphoid follicles in Helicobacter pylori infection: frequency, distribution and response to triple therapy. Hum Pathol 1993;24:577-83.
14. Isaacson PG, Spencer J. Is gastric lymphoma an infectious disease? Hum Pathol 1993;24:569-70.
15. Owen DA. Normal histology of the stomach. Am J Surg Pathol 1986;10:48-61.
16. Ming SC. Tumors of the esophagus and stomach. AFIP Atlas of Tumor Pathology, 2nd Series, Fascicle 7. Washington, DC: American Registry of Pathology; 1973:84-5.

141

8 GASTRIC PRECURSOR LESIONS AND POLYPS

GASTRIC DYSPLASIA (AND ADENOMAS)

Definition. *Gastric dysplasia* is defined as unequivocal neoplastic changes of the gastric epithelium without invasion.

General Features. Gastric dysplasia is a neoplastic alteration that represents the first stage of the multistep carcinogenetic sequence leading to gastric adenocarcinoma (1). Establishing a diagnosis of gastric dysplasia is not only important for predicting the risk of malignant transformation, but it is also critical for determining the risk of synchronous and metachronous gastric cancer. Endoscopic surveillance of gastric dysplasia is, currently, the only effective preventative strategy to control the development of advanced carcinoma (2).

The diagnosis and grading of gastric dysplasia are controversial, particularly regarding nomenclature and classification. There are significant differences in interpretation of the histologic changes of dysplasia in Asian and Western countries. There is also controversy regarding the pathogenesis and terminology of "adenomas" of the stomach (3): some authorities suggest that virtually all gastric adenomas that develop outside of the setting of a genetic polyposis syndrome represent a polypoid form of dysplasia, rather than a "sporadic" adenoma, whereas others prefer to use the term "adenoma" for all nodular or polypoid dysplastic lesions regardless of the presence or absence of chronic gastritis, atrophy, or intestinal metaplasia of the background mucosa, all of which are risk factors for the development of dysplasia and carcinoma (4,5). Nevertheless, the term *gastric adenoma* is usually used for lesions that are well-circumscribed polyps, whereas the term dysplasia is reserved for endoscopically undetectable or nonadenoma-like (flat) lesions. The term *polypoid dysplasia* is used here for intestinal or foveolar-type dysplastic polyps (5–8).

Both polypoid and flat dysplasia of the stomach usually develop in patients with long-standing chronic gastritis (most often related to either *Helicobacter pylori* infection or autoimmune gastritis), mucosal atrophy, and multifocal intestinal metaplasia. Whenever a diagnosis of dysplasia (or adenoma) is made, it is prudent to reexamine the patient endoscopically for a synchronous, potentially occult, gastric cancer (7,9,10).

The prevalence of gastric dysplasia mirrors that of gastric cancer. It is higher in high-risk regions of the world such as Korea and China, where it ranges from 9 to 20 percent. The prevalence is lower in North America, Europe, India, and Australia (0.6 to 8.0 percent) (10–12). Dysplasia is usually detected late in life, with a mean patient age about a decade younger than those with gastric cancer (61 versus 70 years) (11). In patients with syndrome-related dysplasia, the mean age of occurrence of dysplasia is even younger. Some recent Western series report dysplasia in older age groups, but this may be a reflection of the aging population in general (10). There is a male predominance, but similar to gastric cancer, that finding has not been consistently found in all series (7,10–13).

Gastric dysplasia (and adenomas) share similar pathogenetic risk factors to gastric adenocarcinoma. These include chronic *H. pylori* infection, atrophic gastritis, and intestinal metaplasia (see chapter 9) (14). Dysplasia also develops in other epithelial polyps, such as fundic gland and hyperplastic polyps. It also develops in patients with a variety of polyposis syndromes (15–18): in juvenile polyposis syndrome, gastric dysplasia is noted in up to 14 percent of cases (19). In this disorder, there is a mixture of intestinal and pyloric gland differentiation, admixed with foveolar-type dysplastic epithelium (19). Polyps in familial hyperplastic gastric polyposis, which is characterized by marked foveolar hyperplasia, also show evidence of dysplasia that may precede the development of poorly cohesive gastric cancer (20). Polyps detected in gastric adenocarcinoma and proximal polyposis of stomach (GAPPS), which resemble sporadic fundic gland polyps, are frequently associated with dysplasia (21–23).

Clinical Features. Most patients with dysplasia (or adenomas) are asymptomatic. Symptoms or signs relate to the underlying inflammatory disorder, such as *H. pylori* gastritis. Ulcerating lesions can lead to gastrointestinal bleeding or hematemesis.

A diagnosis of dysplasia is usually made on random biopsies from mucosa that may show only slight endoscopic abnormalities. Neoplastic epithelium appears to be more susceptible to peptic-type erosions and superficial ulcerations. Gastric adenomas and flat dysplasia are usually diagnosed during upper endoscopic examination performed for unrelated reasons. The situation is different in Korea and Japan. In these countries, an overall higher incidence rate of cancer dictates more frequent upper endoscopic examinations, which are designed to detect and eradicate early gastric cancer.

Historically, correlation between endoscopy and histology in diagnosing gastric premalignant lesions has been poor, mainly because of the nonspecific macroscopic findings of dysplasia. In the West, lack of experience of gastroenterologists in recognizing suspicious subtle mucosal changes also leads to poor correlation between endoscopy and histology. Special, more advanced techniques, such as magnification endoscopy, chromoendoscopy, and narrow band imaging, have improved detection rates, and improved correlation with histology (14,24). One report claims that the specific phenotype of gastric dysplasia (see below) is predicted better with the use of magnifying endoscopy: round pit or tubular patterns indicate intestinal-type dysplasia and a papillary pattern indicates gastric (foveolar)-type dysplasia (7,25,26).

Gross Findings. The most common location of gastric dysplasia, either flat or polypoid, is the anterior wall of the antrum and the lesser curvature of the stomach (11,13). This is especially true for the gastric (foveolar) subtype of dysplasia, which most commonly presents as a depressed/flat reddish lesion (27). Polypoid lesions (adenomas) are sessile or pedunculated, and often display a lobulated surface. They are usually solitary (with the exception of patients

with familial adenomatous polyposis [FAP]), and commonly measure less than 2 cm in diameter (28). Large adenomas can be ulcerated and actively bleed. The surrounding gastric epithelium usually shows evidence of chronic gastritis and atrophy (29).

Flat dysplasia is rarely detected macroscopically. It is usually inconspicuous, but it may appear as a slightly raised, thickened, and erythematous area of mucosa or as an area of ill-defined nodularity (features commonly characteristic of low-grade dysplasia), or as a slightly depressed or eroded lesion (commonly noted with high-grade dysplasia) (11,13,26).

Microscopic Findings. Dysplasia in the stomach is categorized as either intestinal or gastric (foveolar) type. Some cases show a mixture of both types. Most dysplasias (and adenomas) display an intestinal phenotype, which usually, shows features that resemble colonic adenomas. Cytologically, the nuclei in intestinal-type dysplasia are enlarged, elongated, stratified, and hyperchromatic, and show increased mitoses and eosinophilic cytoplasm (30,31). Absorptive cells and goblet cells, as well as endocrine and Paneth cells, are common (32). Some authorities use the presence of an intestinal brush border (highlighted by CD10 immunostain) to define this type of dysplasia, even in the absence of goblet cells, endocrine cells, and Paneth cells (30).

Architecturally, dysplastic glands may be crowded, branched, or show cribriforming or luminal infolding. They grow in tubular, tubulovillous, or villous/papillary configurations. Pedunculated adenomas, measuring less than 1 cm in diameter, are usually tubular and show only low-grade dysplasia. The same is true for sessile adenomas, in which the dysplastic changes are usually confined to the superficial zone. Larger pedunculated adenomas are frequently villous and show high-grade dysplasia (33).

Dysplasia, regardless of the type, is graded as either low or high grade (figs. 8-1, 8-2). The grade is based on the degree of nuclear crowding, hyperchromasia, stratification, mitotic activity, cytoplasmic differentiation, and architectural distortion (7,34,35).

Low-grade intestinal-type dysplasia is characterized by mild to moderate nuclear hyperchromasia, little or no pleomorphism, and maintenance of basal polarity (fig. 8-1). Atypical

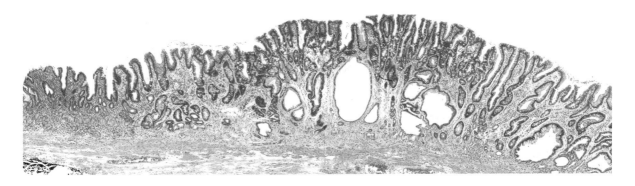

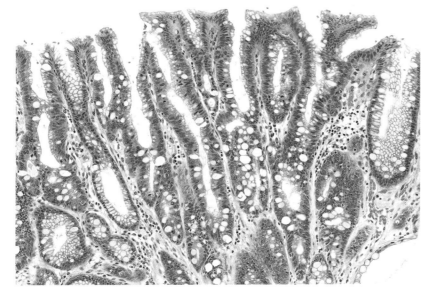

Figure 8-1

LOW-GRADE DYSPLASIA, INTESTINAL TYPE

Above: Low-power view of a specimen removed by endoscopic submucosal dissection (ESD) shows low-grade dysplasia. Hyperchromatic tubular glands are seen at the superficial part of the mucosa; dilated nondysplastic glands are observed in the deeper zone of the mucosa.

Left: High-power view shows preservation of the glandular architecture. There is mild to moderate nuclear hyperchromasia, little pleomorphism, and maintenance of basal polarity of the nuclei. Goblet cells are also present.

mitoses are generally absent. Preservation of the glandular architecture is characteristic. A biopsy diagnosis of low-grade dysplasia is upgraded to either high-grade dysplasia or carcinoma in approximately 19 percent of endoscopic resections. An upgraded diagnosis is more common in lesions that measure greater than 2 cm (37.5 versus 18.7 percent), and ones that show an absence of whitish discoloration on endoscopy (36–38).

High-grade intestinal-type dysplasia shows prominent cytologic atypia, amphophilic cytoplasm, and large cuboidal-shaped nuclei with a high nuclear to cytoplasmic (N/C) ratio (fig. 8-2). Nuclei tend to be large and contain prominent nucleoli. Mitoses (including atypical forms) are frequently detected. Irregularities of the nuclear membrane and clumping of chromatin are characteristic of high-grade dysplasia as well. There is usually significant loss of nuclear polarity and extension of atypical nuclei to the luminal surface. The mucosal architecture is usually complex, showing marked distortion, including back-to-back glands. Marked glandular crowding, budding, and intraluminal bridges should suggest intramucosal adenocarcinoma (5,7,39).

The cytoarchitectural abnormalities of dysplasia may involve the superficial, foveolar, and neck zones of the gastric pit, and often occur in association with cystic dilatation of the underlying specialized glands (fig. 8-1, above). Low-grade sessile tubular adenomas and flat dysplasia usually display abnormalities limited to the superficial half of the mucosa; the lower half is composed of distorted and cystically dilated glands lined by non-neoplastic gastric gland cells (35).

Grading. One of the most challenging aspects of gastric dysplasia is establishing a classification system that is both reproducible and clinically significant. Up until the early 1980s, the grading system was three-tiered (mild, moderate, and severe). In 1995, Rugge et al. (40,41) demonstrated that only moderate or severe

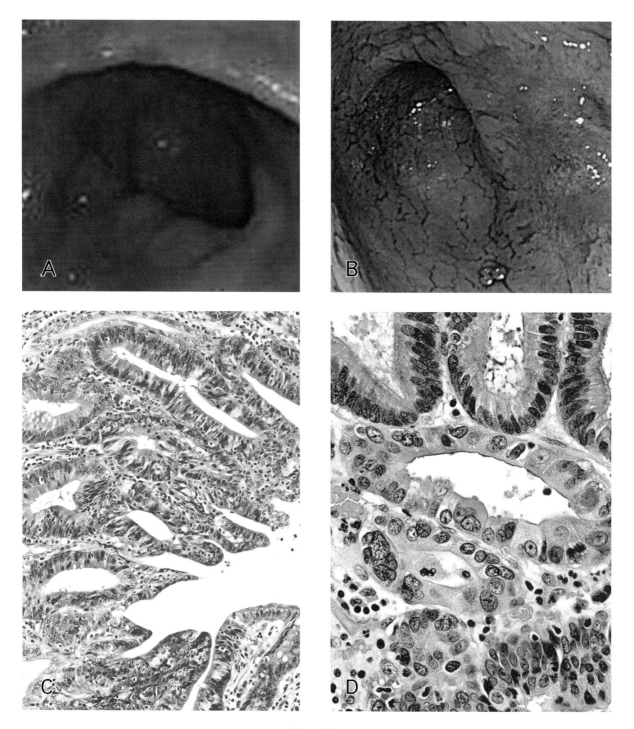

Figure 8-2

HIGH-GRADE DYSPLASIA, INTESTINAL TYPE

A: A reddish, shallow mucosal depression is seen by white conventional endoscopy.

B: Chromoendoscopy shows a well-demarcated mucosal depression.

C: Well-developed high-grade dysplastic glands with glandular crowding and complex architecture, including back-to-back glands limited to the lamina propria.

D: High-power view of another example of high-grade dysplasia shows prominent cytologic atypia, amphophilic cytoplasm, large nuclei, high nuclear/cytoplasmic (N/C) ratio, and prominent nucleoli.

Table 8-1

COMPARISON OF THE DIFFERENT CLASSIFICATION SYSTEMS FOR GASTRIC DYSPLASIA

Japanese (2011) (44)	New Vienna Classification (2003) (46)	World Health Organization (WHO) Classification (2010) (34)
Group 1: Normal tissue or nonneoplastic lesion	Category 1: No neoplasia	Negative for intraepithelial neoplasia/dysplasia
Group 2: Benign with atypia/indefinite for neoplasia	Category 2: Indefinite for neoplasia	Indefinite for intraepithelial neoplasia/dysplasia
Group 3: Adenoma	Category 3: Low-grade adenoma/dysplasia	Low-grade intraepithelial neoplasia/dysplasia (low-grade adenoma/dysplasia)
Group 4: Suspicious for carcinoma	Category 4: High-grade neoplasia 4.1: High-grade adenoma/dysplasia 4.2: Noninvasive carcinoma 4.3: Suspicious for invasive carcinoma 4.4: Intramucosal carcinoma	High-grade intraepithelial neoplasia/dysplasia (high-grade adenoma/dysplasia Intramucosal invasive neoplasia (intramucosal carcinoma)
Group 5: Carcinoma	Category 5: Submucosal invasive carcinoma (carcinoma with invasion of the submucosa or deeper)	Invasive neoplasia

dysplasia were significantly associated with an increased risk of developing carcinoma, and he therefore proposed a two-tiered system, which is still in effect today. The two-tiered classification of low- and high-grade dysplasia improves interobserver variability and clinically relevant risk stratification of affected patients (40,41).

There are significant differences between Japan and Western countries when evaluating gastric dysplasia. In Japan, architectural complexity and nuclear atypia are considered of paramount importance in establishing a diagnosis of carcinoma. In the West, disruption of the basement membrane and invasion into the lamina propria are considered cardinal characteristics of adenocarcinomas (7,25). It is well recognized that noninvasive intramucosal neoplastic lesions with high-grade cellular or architectural atypia are more often diagnosed as intramucosal carcinoma in Japan, whereas similar appearing lesions are more commonly classified as high-grade dysplasia by Western pathologists.

The Japanese Society for Research on Gastric Cancer (JSRGC) classification is stratified into the following groups: normal tissue or non-neoplastic lesion (group 1), benign (non-neoplastic) lesions with atypia/indefinite for neoplasia (group 2), adenoma (group 3), strongly suspected of carcinoma (group 4), and definite carcinoma (group 5). The Japanese classification system does

not employ the terms "low" and "high-grade dysplasia." Low-grade dysplasia corresponds to group 3 and high-grade dysplasia corresponds to a part of group 4 in the Japanese system (42–44).

In 1996, a group of Japanese and Western pathologists attempted to bridge differences in interpretation. Pathologists from Asia, North America, Europe, and Australia gathered to develop an international classification in Vienna, later termed the "Vienna classification" (2000) (25,45), for which a revision was proposed in 2003 (46). The World Health Organization (WHO) classification (2010) is similar to the Vienna classification; in the WHO classification, intraepithelial neoplasia and dysplasia are considered synonymous terms (34). The relationship between these classification systems is explained in further detail in Table 8-1.

Differential Diagnosis. The diagnosis and grading of gastric dysplasia can be challenging because of technical limitations (insufficient material, poor orientation) and the presence of active inflammation which often leads to regenerative changes that mimic dysplasia. As a result, the category of "indefinite for intraepithelial neoplasia (dysplasia)" is used for lesions in which regeneration cannot be differentiated from true dysplasia with certainty. It includes regenerative changes that arise near gastric erosions or ulcerations, in areas of inflamed

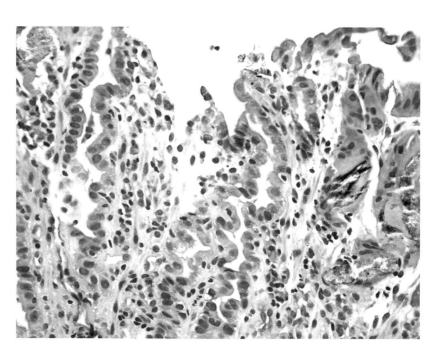

Figure 8-3

**REGENERATIVE CHANGES
ASSOCIATED WITH AN EROSION**

There are striking reactive changes associated with iron pill gastritis in this biopsy. The regenerative cells show nucleoli, but they have smooth nuclear membranes. The iron pigment has a golden brown color.

mucosa, and in areas of reactive or chemical gastropathy, among others (30). This term can also be used when the biopsy is limited in material, and when the degree of architectural or cytologic atypia is insufficient for establishing a definite diagnosis of dysplasia. When this diagnosis is rendered, it should indicate to the clinician that re-endoscopy, with additional tissue sampling (sometimes after medical therapy), should be considered in order to provide better, or more, material to the pathologist.

Regenerative changes can be quite severe. Appreciation of a few key features help differentiate regeneration from true dysplasia. First, dysplasia should always be diagnosed cautiously in the presence active inflammation and in areas of erosions (fig. 8-3) or ulcers. Preservation of the glandular architecture and maturation of the epithelium toward the mucosal surface heavily favor regeneration. The nuclei of regenerative epithelium, although often hyperchromatic, are usually rounder and more basally oriented, and show only mild or no pseudostratification. Nucleoli can be prominent, but they are usually small and regular in shape. Vascular congestion and a gradual rather than an abrupt transition between the atypical epithelium and adjacent normal mucosa are suggestive of a regenerative process.

Degenerating glands in the vicinity of gastric erosions or ulcers can also mimic dysplasia, or

even frank carcinoma. Recognition that the atypical glands are embedded in eosinophilic fibrin or granulation tissue may be helpful. Degenerated epithelium does not show mitoses. Recognition that proliferative activity, when evaluated by Ki-67, is confined to the deep foveolar zone, combined with the absence of atypical mitoses and the presence of maturation toward the luminal surface, are all important features for diagnosing regenerating rather than dysplastic epithelium (6,47–51).

Another lesion to be considered in the differential diagnosis is reactive dysplasia-like epithelial atypia (47), secondary to chemoradiotherapy (fig. 8-4) (47) or hepatic arterial infusion chemotherapy (50,51). Reactive changes are seen in the foveolar and glandular epithelium. Foveolar changes consist of slightly elongated pits containing pseudostratified cells with mucin depletion, hypereosinophilic cytoplasm, normal or slightly low N/C ratio, and hyperchromatic oval to pencil-shaped enlarged nuclei. Affected glands reveal atrophic features, such as irregular microcystic change lined by attenuated epithelium. The lumens of the glands occasionally show neutrophilic and cellular debris. The cells of the reactive glands may show elongated and bubbly cytoplasm with enlarged round to oval nuclei with an open chromatin pattern and inconspicuous or small

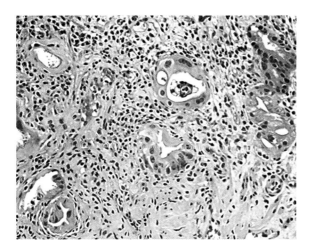

Figure 8-4

DYSPLASIA-LIKE EPITHELIAL CHANGES ASSOCIATED WITH CHEMORADIOTHERAPY FOR ESOPHAGEAL CANCER

Above: Medium-power view of the mucosa shows abundant inflammatory stroma. Affected glands reveal atrophic features and irregular cystic change. The lumen of one of the glands shows cellular debris. The nuclei are round to oval with inconspicuous or small nucleoli. Some cells in the glandular epithelium have eosinophilic cytoplasm.

Right: High-power view shows an elongated gland lined by cells with flattened cytoplasm with focal microvacuolization. The other glands show hyperchromatic nuclei and eosinophilic cytoplasm.

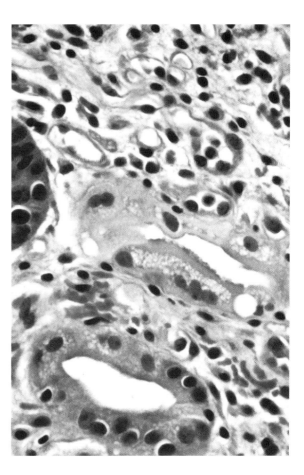

eccentrically located nucleoli. Some cells in the glandular epithelium show hypereosinophilic cytoplasm similar to that seen in the foveolar epithelium. The N/C ratio of affected glandular cells, however, is either normal or low. The glandular changes may cause diagnostic confusion with adenocarcinoma (47).

The presence of dysplasia-like basal atypia ("pit dysplasia") is another challenging issue (see below.) This is noted commonly in cases of incomplete intestinal metaplasia. Closely packed metaplastic glands in the deep mucosa are lined by enlarged cells with hyperchromatic pseudostratified nuclei with frequent mitoses, similar to low-grade dysplasia in some cases (fig. 8-5A,B) and high grade in others (fig. 8-5C,D). Surface maturation is, by definition, present, and there is no inflammation or ulceration that can explain these changes as regenerative in nature. The low-grade form can be considered a very early stage of neoplasia.

Polypoid dysplasia (adenomas) are usually easily distinguished from other types of epithelial

polyps histologically (fig. 8-6). The main criterion of differentiation is the presence or absence of epithelial dysplasia, but sometimes this distinction is difficult, especially in large, eroded or inflamed polyps, and when regenerative changes are present. In addition to the features discussed above, the presence of intraglandular necrosis and intestinal-type differentiation, which is usually inconspicuous in non-neoplastic polyps, is important to diagnose neoplasia (52).

Intramucosal carcinoma can be difficult to differentiate from high-grade dysplasia. Although there should be, by definition, evidence of invasion of the lamina propria in intramucosal carcinoma, desmoplasia at that stage of development is often minimal or absent. Features helpful to establish a diagnosis (in the absence of desmoplasia) include: 1) excessive architectural disarray with irregular jagged budding of neoplastic epithelium into the surrounding loose connective tissue, including glandular budding, branching, or crowding, manifested by the presence of small abortive glands or back-to-back small,

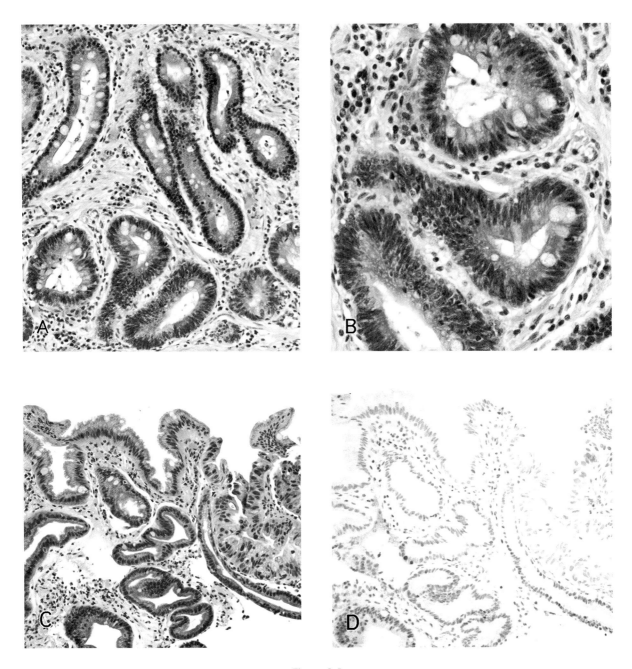

Figure 8-5

PIT DYSPLASIA

A: Low-power view of an area of intestinal metaplasia displaying, in the deep mucosa, metaplastic glands lined by cells with hyperchromatic pseudostratified nuclei similar to low-grade dysplasia. There is mild inflammation and surface maturation.

B: High-power view of the basal dysplastic glands seen in A.

C: The surface epithelium in this lesion is nondysplastic, but beneath the surface is a focus of dysplasia that has cytologic features of high-grade dysplasia. There is incomplete intestinal metaplasia in the surrounding mucosa.

D: This is a p53 stain showing a so-called null pattern that is in keeping with biallelic inactivation of the *TP53* gene. The p53 protein is a normal molecule found in proliferating cells to serve its tumor suppressor function. It has a short half-life such that immunolabeling shows light staining (wild-type pattern) in normal proliferating nuclei at the bases of the pits. There is usually very little p53 labeling in the surface nuclei since they are no longer proliferating. When the *TP53* gene is mutated, it produces a protein with a long half-life that results in intense nuclear labeling in the *TP53* mutated cells. Alternatively, as in this case, if both *TP53* alleles are mutated or lost, there is complete absence of the protein in the dysplastic cells.

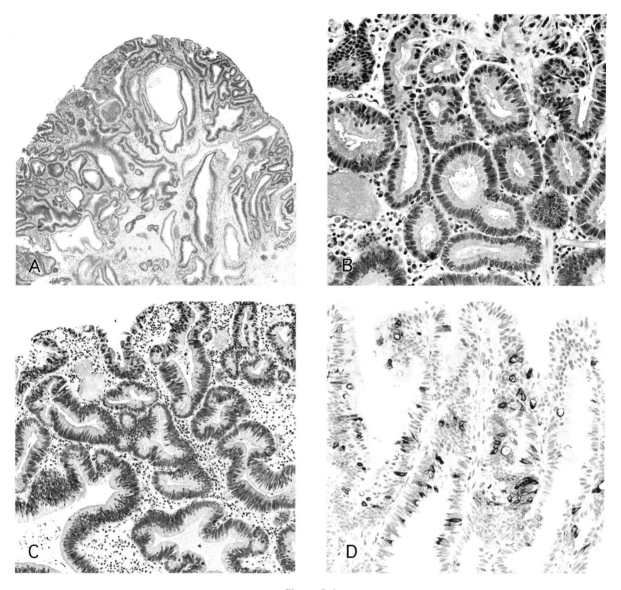

Figure 8-6

POLYPOID DYSPLASIA (ADENOMA), INTESTINAL TYPE

A: Low-power view of a polypoid lesion with dysplastic features.

B: At high power, the glands are tubular and the nuclei are cigar-shaped, localized at the basal compartment of the cells (features of low-grade dysplasia).

C: In another area of the polyp, the dysplastic glands are tortuous but display the cytologic features of low-grade dysplasia.

D: Expression of MUC2 in the dysplastic epithelium confirms intestinal differentiation.

round tubules with cribriforming (fig. 8-7, left); 2) detection of single infiltrating cells; and 3) presence of intraluminal necrotic debris within the atypical glands (fig. 8-7, right).

Subtypes of Dysplasia. As mentioned above, dysplasia is categorized as either intestinal or gastric (foveolar) on the basis of its morphologic (and in some cases immunohistochemical) char-

acteristics (32,53). In one large series that evaluated endoscopic mucosal material combined with immunohistochemistry, intestinal-type dysplasia was the most frequent, seen in 45 percent of cases. This was followed by gastric (foveolar) dysplasia in 21.7 percent of cases and hybrid (mixed) cases in 33.3 percent (53). A second series reported similar results (54).

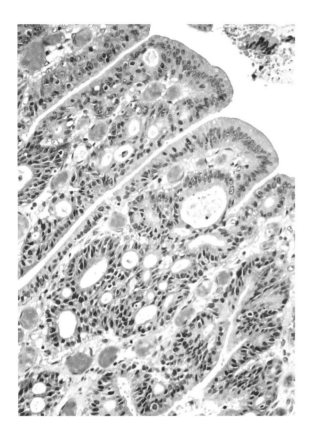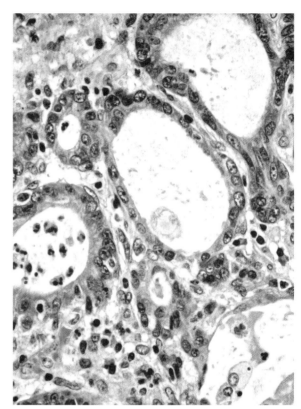

Figure 8-7

INTRAMUCOSAL CARCINOMA

Left: Back-to-back tubules with cribriform structures. The lesion is associated with foveolar-type dysplasia (see figures 8-8 and 8-9).

Right: Presence of intraluminal necrotic debris within atypical glands, budding of tubules, and small glands in the loose connective tissue.

Gastric-type (foveolar) dysplasia is composed of glands of different size and shape, and with occasional cystification. Papillary infolding and gland serration are common. The lining epithelium, which is foveolar (mucinous) in nature, ranges from low cuboidal to low columnar in shape. It shows pale to clear cytoplasm due to the presence of apical mucin. The distinction from intestinal-type dysplasia is based, in part, on the nuclear features. Gastric (foveolar) dysplasia generally does not show pencillate, or pseudostratified, nuclei as in intestinal-type dysplasia. Instead, the nuclei are round to oval, contain variably prominent nucleoli, and display minimal nuclear overlapping.

There is poor interobserver agreement in separating low-grade foveolar dysplasia from reactive gastric mucosa and the criteria for separating low- (fig. 8-8) from high-grade (fig. 8-9) foveolar dysplasia are not well established. In general, high-grade dysplasia shows architectural complexity, with more crowded and irregular glandular architecture. The nuclei are more enlarged and have prominent nucleoli (55). Nevertheless, interobserver variation, even among expert gastrointestinal pathologists, remains high (7,55). Although some studies have suggested that this form of dysplasia is almost always low grade, at least two series presented different opinions in this regard (53,54). Foveolar dysplasia is more commonly associated with poorly differentiated adenocarcinoma (31,56).

There are no validated criteria for establishing a "hybrid" phenotype of dysplasia (cases with both intestinal and foveolar differentiation). Immunohistochemical expression of MUC proteins (MUC2, MUC5AC, and MUC6), CDX2, and CD10, rather than the morphologic

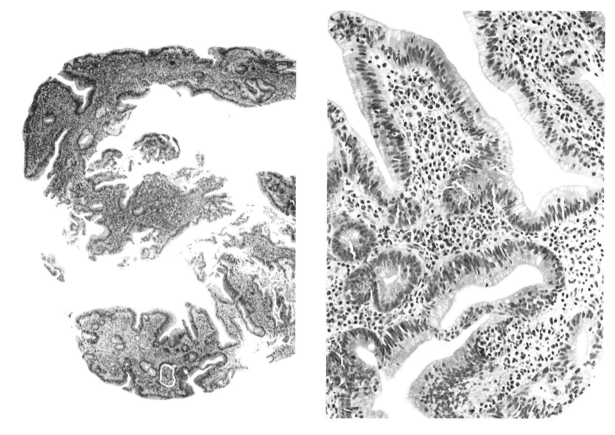

Figure 8-8

LOW-GRADE FOVEOLAR-TYPE DYSPLASIA

Left: At low power, irregular fragments of gastric mucosa are lined by dysplastic epithelium with papillary infoldings; in this case the stroma is abundant and inflammatory.

Right: At high power, the dysplastic cells are columnar, the cytoplasm is pale to eosinophilic with apical mucin, and the nuclei are round to oval with little nuclear overlapping.

appearance, have been used to establish the principle cell lineage in these instances (27,54).

Pit Dysplasia. Pit dysplasia is also referred to as *gastric pit dysplasia-like atypia (DLA)*, *intestinal metaplasia with basal gland atypia (IM-BGA)*, or simply *indefinite for dysplasia* (57). The changes of either low- or high-grade intestinal-type dysplasia are limited to the bases of the pits, without surface epithelial involvement (fig. 8-5). There is evidence that these changes represent an independent predictor of progression. Importantly, these changes have been reported adjacent to areas of traditional neoplasia in 49 (58) to 72 percent (10,59) of cases. Pit dysplasia is associated with older age, male sex, and MUC6 expression. However, different clinicopathologic features have been reported between studies in Korea and the United States: body/fundic location was more common in

the Korean study, whereas antral location and poorly differentiated histologic appearance of the cancer was more common in the US study.

Tubule Neck Dysplasia. This entity, also termed nonmetaplastic dysplasia (60–62), has been described in rare reports associated with sporadic diffuse-type gastric carcinoma, and was characterized by elongated, rigid and distorted tubular neck glands lined by cells showing an increased N/C ratio; enlarged, atypical, and hyperchromatic nuclei; irregular nuclear membranes; distinct nucleoli; and cytoplasm featuring either eosinophilia or granular neutral mucin. These cells retain expression of gastric mucin (MUC5AC) and show reduced E-cadherin expression (62). In most cases, the diagnosis can be made with certainty only in the presence of an associated diffuse-type gastric cancer.

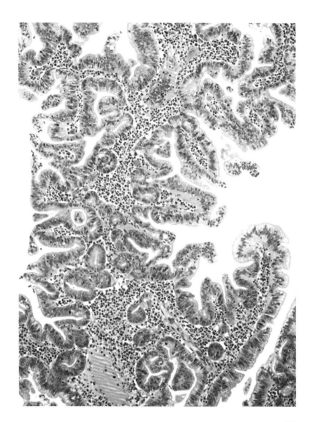 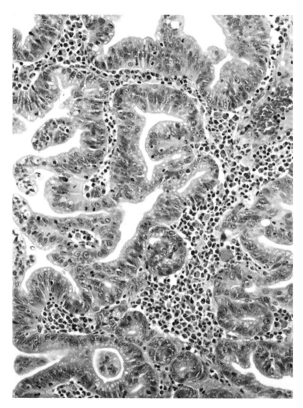

Figure 8-9

HIGH-GRADE FOVEOLAR-TYPE DYSPLASIA

Left: This high-grade foveolar-type dysplasia is characterized by architectural complexity, with crowded and irregular glandular architecture. The cytoplasm of the dysplastic cells is clear, a feature that is more evident at the apical pole of the cells.

Right: High-power view of an area with architectural complexity displaying prominent, roundish nuclei with nucleoli and high N/C ratio. Apical mucin is observed in the cytoplasm of some cells.

In the setting of hereditary diffuse gastric cancer (HDGC), as illustrated in chapter 9, precursor lesions of early intramucosal carcinoma (pT1a) encompass: 1) pagetoid spread of signet ring cells below the preserved epithelium of glands and foveolae, but within the basement membrane; and 2) in situ signet ring cell carcinoma, characterized by the presence of signet ring cells within the basement membrane, substituting for the normal epithelial cells generally with hyperchromatic and depolarized nuclei.

Immunohistochemical and Molecular Genetic Findings. The lineage of differentiation in gastric dysplasia is usually evident immunohistochemically. Immunohistochemistry, however, is not normally used to establish a diagnosis of dysplasia (55). The immunophenotypic classification of dysplasia is based primarily on the type of gastric mucins expressed. Intestinal-type dysplasia shows MUC2, CD10 (a marker of the brush border), and CDX2 positivity, whereas foveolar dysplasia shows MUC5AC or MUC6 positivity, absence of CD10, and absent or low expression of CDX2 (21,30,53). P53 expression is common in dysplasia as well: in one study, p53 expression was significantly less common in regenerative epithelium and indefinite for dysplasia compared to true dysplasia and adenocarcinoma (6.98, 20.0, 57.14, and 50.0 percent, respectively) (63).

Other markers reported to be to be positive in dysplasia include lethal giant larvae (Lgl2) and LINE-1 methylation. Loss of the normal basolateral expression of Lgl2 has been reported in low-grade (79 percent) and high-grade (83 percent) foveolar-type dysplasia (64). LINE-1 methylation (which is a marker of global methylation) is significantly lower in dysplastic epithelium compared to normal mucosa. In patients with *H. pylori* infection, microsatellite instability (MSI) correlates with reduced LINE-1 methylation, which suggests that *H. pylori* infection and MSI might be driving forces of gastric carcinogenesis (65,66). Increased expression of IMP3 has also been reported in gastric dysplasia and carcinoma compared to normal gastric epithelium. In one study, high-grade dysplasia could be distinguished from low-grade dysplasia and reactive atypia by using a combination of IMP3 and p53 immunohistochemistry (67,68).

The frequency of somatic mutations, gene fusions, and copy number variations increases from low- to high-grade dysplasia, to early cancer. Whole exome sequencing of gastric adenomas has revealed a high rate of mutations, similar to what has been reported in gastric cancer. The frequency of intratumoral mutational heterogeneity differs between MSI-high and microsatellite-stable gastric adenomas (69).

Several genes involved in the inhibition of the Wnt signaling pathway are implicated in gastric carcinogenesis. *RNF43*, which encodes a transmembrane ubiquitin ligase that downregulates surface expression of the Wnt receptor, is upregulated in low-grade dysplasia, and shows a gradual decrease in expression with neoplastic progression. *AXIN2* shows an expression pattern similar to *RNF43*. Other genes related to adhesion and extracellular matrix receptor interaction pathways are upregulated when low-grade dysplasia progresses to early gastric cancer (69,70).

APC mutations are present in 67 and 58 percent of low- and high-grade dysplasias, respectively, but are present in less than 20 percent of early cancers. Near universal APC inactivation in dysplasia suggests that it represents an initiating event in the neoplasia pathway (69,70). In contrast, mutations of *TP53* and *ARID1A* are late events. They have been noted in 64.7 and 11.8 percent of early cancers, but are not present in most low- and high-grade dysplasia cases (69,70).

Treatment. Management of flat and polypoid dysplasia (adenoma) includes complete excision of the area of mucosal irregularity, biopsy search for synchronous adenocarcinoma, assessment of the severity and extent of background gastritis, and follow-up endoscopic surveillance combined with eradication of *H. pylori* (14,21). Low-grade and high-grade dysplasias differ in their risk of synchronous and metachronous gastric cancer. Recent advances in endoscopic techniques, such as endoscopic ultrasound, chromoendoscopy, and endoscopic resection, have led to an overall decrease in the use of, and need for, surgical resection. For low-grade dysplasia, if the lesion is not endoscopically visible, immediate re-endoscopy is recommended, preferably in a specialized center with multiple biopsies in order to exclude concurrent carcinoma. This is normally followed by biannual endoscopic examinations until two negative endoscopies are achieved, and this is then decreased to yearly examinations. For high-grade dysplasia, a thorough and detailed endoscopic evaluation, and resection, is recommended (71,72).

A meticulous pathologic examination of endoscopically resected specimens is required to confirm the completeness of excision, and to identify adverse prognostic indicators if an invasive cancer is found (73,74). Annual follow-up should be performed to screen for metachronous lesions in these patients. Eradication of *H. pylori* infection is recommended, since absence of this organism causes regression of atrophic gastritis and a decreased rate of progression to advanced neoplasia.

Prognosis. The prognosis of patients with gastric dysplasia is poorly understood. The risk of progression of low-grade dysplasia to adenocarcinoma has varied significantly among studies. Prior studies have reported progression to adenocarcinoma ranging from 0 to 32.1 percent for low-grade dysplasia, with a mean interval of 10 months to 4 years, and 60 to 85 percent, with a median interval of 4 to 48 months for high-grade dysplasia. In some cases, rapid progression may be due to failure by the endoscopist to detect a synchronous adenocarcinoma (41,71,75–80). Recent studies performed with more modern endoscopic equipment have shown that there is a low risk of progression to cancer in patients with low-grade dysplasia (0 to 9 percent); the risk of malignant transformation associated with high-grade dysplasia is 4.8 to 100 percent (81,82).

In a recent study from a Western population of patients, after exclusion of cases detected during the first year of follow-up, 4.3 percent of patients with low-grade dysplasia progressed to invasive carcinoma (median follow-up interval of 2.6 years) while 4.5 percent of patients with high-grade dysplasia progressed to invasive carcinoma (median follow-up interval of 3.1 years) (10). Another study from the Netherlands reported that the annual incidence rate of gastric cancer was 0.6 percent for patients with low-grade dysplasia and 6 percent for patients with high-grade dysplasia within 5 years of diagnosis (10,12). One study from Australia reported that 15.8 percent of patients with indefinite for dysplasia developed cancer within 12 months. In that study, the authors attributed the outcome to sampling error and suggested that "indefinite for dysplasia" should be considered a surrogate marker of true dysplasia elsewhere in the stomach (83).

Although the clinical guidelines for the management of dysplasia are based on the grade of dysplasia (see below), there is evidence to suggest a role for phenotyping as well. Several studies have demonstrated a higher rate of high-grade dysplasia in patients with foveolar dysplasia compared to intestinal-type dysplasia (27,53,54). Foveolar dysplasia has also been associated with a depressed endoscopic appearance and with high-grade histologic features of the cancer (27,31,53,56,84). Foveolar dysplasia is not highly associated with intestinal metaplasia in the background stomach, so that the pathway to cancer may be different than for intestinal-type dysplasia. Foveolar dysplasia may be associated with the spasmolytic polypeptide-expressing metaplasia (SPEM) pathway of carcinogenesis in the stomach.

GASTRIC POLYPS

Polyps and tumor-like lesions of the stomach comprise a heterogeneous group of lesions. The prevalence of gastric polyps in general, and of the specific types, has shifted over the past 10 to 20 years primarily due to a decrease in the incidence of *H. pylori* infection, particularly in the Western world. This is believed to be a result of improvements in antibiotic therapy and a reflection of the increased use of proton pump inhibitors.

Most gastric polyps are asymptomatic. They are usually discovered incidentally at the time of upper endoscopy performed for other reasons (85). The prevalence rate of gastric polyps is 1 to 4 percent of endoscopies.

When evaluating gastric polyps endoscopically, relevant factors to consider include the anatomic distribution, size, color, growth pattern,

shape, and contour of the lesion. Mucosal depressions and irregular shapes are features more frequently associated with neoplasia. Even with improved endoscopic techniques, however, histologic evaluation remains the primary method of diagnosing the specific type of gastric polyp and, most importantly, excluding neoplasia. New endoscopic techniques, such as magnifying narrow band imaging, have improved the correlation with the pathologic diagnosis of polypoid lesions of the stomach (86,87).

The histopathologic diagnosis of gastric polyps helps to guide clinical management and surveillance. Effective communication with clinicians is the key. Attention to the quality of the sample is important: a diagnosis is rendered on a polypectomy pinch biopsy in only about 56 percent of specimens (88).

The epidemiology of gastric polyps reflects the type of underlying gastric pathology and the presence or absence of *H. pylori* infection and chronic gastritis. A large German study (89) that evaluated the prevalence rate of gastric polyps collected between 1969 and 1989 found 47 percent were fundic gland polyps and 28.3 percent were hyperplastic polyps; in the same cohort, adenomas and adenocarcinomas represented only 7.2 percent of lesions. In a recent study of 200,000 patients from the United States (90), the overall prevalence rate of gastric polyps was 3.75 percent. Most lesions were fundic gland polyps (77.2 percent), followed by hyperplastic polyps (14.4 percent) and gastric adenomas (0.7 percent). The prevalence rate of *H. pylori* infection was low (12.3 percent). In parts of the world, such as Asia, where *H. pylori* infection is higher than the United States, most gastric polyps are hyperplastic polyps and adenomas rather than fundic gland polyps. The former two polyps commonly arise on a background of chronic gastritis secondary to *H. pylori* infection or autoimmune gastritis.

Classification of Gastric Polyps

There are several methods of classifying gastric polyps. One simple method is to classify them as either "neoplastic" or "non-neoplastic." Most authorities prefer the classification method summarized in Table 8-2, which classifies polyps based on the major cell types that are abnormal, namely, the epithelium or the stroma.

Epithelial polyps are the most prevalent type of gastric polyp. They are further subdivided into non-neoplastic hamartomatous and neoplastic polyps. The latter includes all types of adenomas, polypoid dysplasia, and low-grade neuroendocrine tumors. Historically, fundic gland polyps were regarded as hamartomatous lesions, but recent molecular evidence suggests that they may be neoplastic in nature.

The proliferation of mesenchymal and stromal elements can give rise to nonepithelial gastric polyps. These are a heterogeneous group of lesions in which immunohistochemistry is often required to establish a final specific diagnosis. Entities in this category include inflammatory fibroid polyps, gastrointestinal stromal tumors (GIST), inflammatory myofibroblastic tumors, nerve sheath tumors (i.e., schwannomas and ganglioneuromas), and smooth muscle tumors. Tumors that do not fit into these two general categories are included in the "miscellaneous" polyp category. These include xanthomas, heterotopic pancreas, lymphoid proliferative lesions, and a variety of other rare tumors and pseudotumors.

An updated classification of gastric polyps has been recently proposed by Hackeng et al. (91), which divides gastric polyps into only two groups: 1) polyps that arise from, or show differentiation toward, the foveolar compartment (hyperplastic polyps, foveolar adenomas, and intestinal-type adenomas) and 2) polyps that arise from, or show differentiation toward, the glandular compartment (fundic gland polyp and gastric adenomas with *GNAS* mutations, the latter including oxyntic gland adenomas and pyloric gland adenomas).

Pyloric Gland Adenoma

Definition. *Pyloric gland adenoma* (PGA) is a neoplasm composed of a proliferation of pyloric-type glands that has an increased risk of malignancy (91,92).

General Features. PGAs are rare lesions. They account for less than 3 percent of all gastric polyps (29). They often develop on a background of *H. pylori* infection or autoimmune atrophic gastritis (92). PGAs also develop in patients with familial adenomatous polyposis (FAP). They occur in 6 percent of these patients, in addition to fundic gland polyps and gastric foveolar-type adenomas, which are also common in this ge-

Table 8-2

CLASSIFICATION OF GASTRIC POLYPS

Epithelial polyps	Fundic gland polyp/polyposis
	Hyperplastic polyp (and variants)
	Adenomatous polyps
	Pyloric gland adenoma
	Oxyntic gland adenoma
	Ménétrier disease-associated polyps
	Gastritis cystica profunda/polyposa
	GAPPS[a]
	Neuroendocrine tumors
	Hamartomatous polyps/polyposis
	Juvenile polyps/polyposis
	Peutz-Jeghers syndrome
	Cowden syndrome
	Cronkhite-Canada syndrome associated polyps
Nonepithelial polyps[a]	Gastrointestinal stromal tumor (GIST)
	Smooth muscle tumors
	Inflammatory myofibroblastic tumor
	Neural tumors (schwannoma/neuroma, ganglioneuroma, granular cell tumor)
	Glomus tumor
	Lipoma
	Inflammatory fibroid polyp[a]
Miscellaneous	Xanthoma
	Ectopic pancreas
	Lymphoid hyperplasia or lymphoma
	Other rare tumors and pseudotumors

[a]See chapter 9 for details of gastric adenocarcinoma and proximal polyposis of stomach (GAPPS), and chapter 12 for information on nonepithelial polyps.

netic disorder (91,93,94). PGAs have also been described in patients with Lynch syndrome, and have been reported to undergo malignant transformation in this condition (95).

The pathogenesis is unknown, but PGAs typically develop in areas of the gastrointestinal tract that undergo pyloric gland metaplasia related to chronic mucosal injury. Thus, it is presumed to develop as a result of chronic repeated injury and repair. There are differences in the frequency and distribution of PGAs in various populations worldwide, paralleling the incidence of chronic gastritis in these regions.

Clinical Features. Most PGAs are found in elderly female patients of an average age of 75 years (96). They are most common in the gastric corpus, but can develop anywhere in the stomach. They also occur in other organs, such as in association with gastric heterotopia in the duodenum, and in the pancreatobiliary

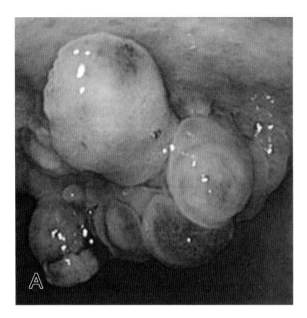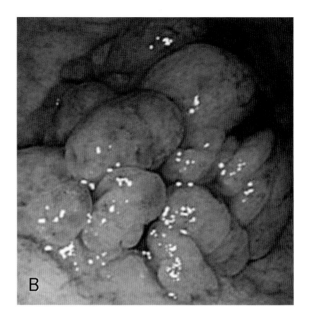

Figure 8-10

PYLORIC GLAND ADENOMA (PGA)

A: A well-demarcated multinodular polypoid lesion is seen by white conventional endoscopy.
B: Chromoendoscopy shows a well-demarcated multinodular/fungating polypoid lesion, with a smooth surface.

ducts, gallbladder, rectum, and uterine cervix (97–100). Gastric/pyloric metaplasia and heterotopia have been suggested as the precursor lesions for extragastric PGAs. Patients with PGA are usually asymptomatic. They typically come to clinical attention due to symptoms or signs related to the underlying gastritis.

Gross Findings. PGA is usually a polypoid, dome-shaped polyp, but when it grows, it can develop into a fungating mass (fig. 8-10A–C). The median diameter is 1.7 cm.

Microscopic Findings. PGAs are characterized by a proliferation of closely packed pyloric-type glands/tubules lined by a monolayer of cuboidal to low columnar epithelial cells. The latter contain round nuclei and pale to eosinophilic cytoplasm with a "ground glass" appearance (fig. 8-10D–F). Occasionally, cystic dilatation of the glands is observed (92). The nuclei are small and round to slightly ovoid in shape, and usually contain inconspicuous nucleoli and an open chromatin pattern. Periodic acid–Schiff (PAS) alcian blue stains the granular cytoplasm of the epithelial cells of PGAs.

PGAs are, by definition, neoplastic lesions, and thus all are considered to have low-grade dysplasia despite the minimal degree of nuclear atypia. PGAs with high-grade dysplasia show cells with increased cytologic atypia, enlargement of nuclei, hyperchromasia, increased N/C ratio, and mitoses. Architecturally, the glands are more complex and crowded (92).

Immunohistochemical Findings. PGAs are immunohistochemically positive for MUC6 and MUC5AC (fig. 8-11). MUC6 is expressed always at the base of the lesion, but it can also involve the entire lesion including the surface epithelium (fig. 8-11B,D). MUC5AC expression varies from case to case (fig. 8-11A,C), but coexpression of both types of mucins occurs (101,102). TFF2 is also diffusely expressed in PGAs, in keeping with the pyloric gland phenotype of these polyps. MIST-1 and pepsinogen-I are also expressed focally, suggesting that PGAs show chief cell differentiation, phenotypically resembling mucous neck cells rather than pyloric glands in some cases (103). MUC2 expression in PGAs is rare, and like CDX2, occurs only in areas of intestinal metaplasia, often in portions of mucosa adjacent to the PGA.

Molecular Genetic Findings. Mutations of *GNAS* and *RAS* genes are frequently observed in PGAs (104). In FAP-associated PGAs, *GNAS* and *RAS* mutations are present in 83 to 100 percent

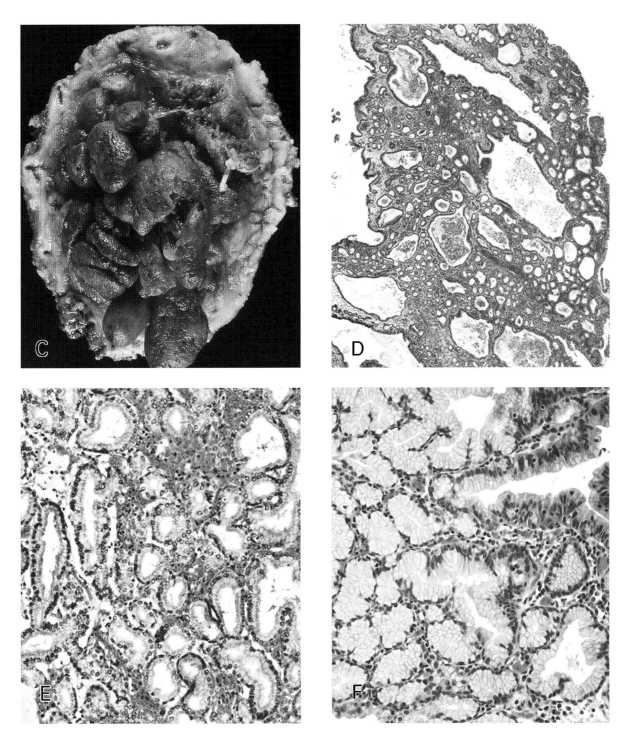

Figure 8-10, continued

C: Polyp was removed by ESD.

D: A compact arrangement of small glands with overlying foveolar type epithelium together with cystically dilated glands.

E: At higher magnification, the PGA shows mild to moderate cytologic atypia of pyloric-type glands which fulfills the criteria for low-grade dysplasia. Cystic dilatation of some glands is observed.

F: Another PGA shows a proliferation of closely packed pyloric-type glands/tubules lined by a monolayer of cuboidal to low columnar epithelial cells that contain round nuclei and pale cytoplasm. The glands have minimal cytologic atypia; however, the overlying epithelium shows enlarged hyperchromatic nuclei with stratification. (Courtesy of Dr. Tadakazu Shimoda, Japan.)

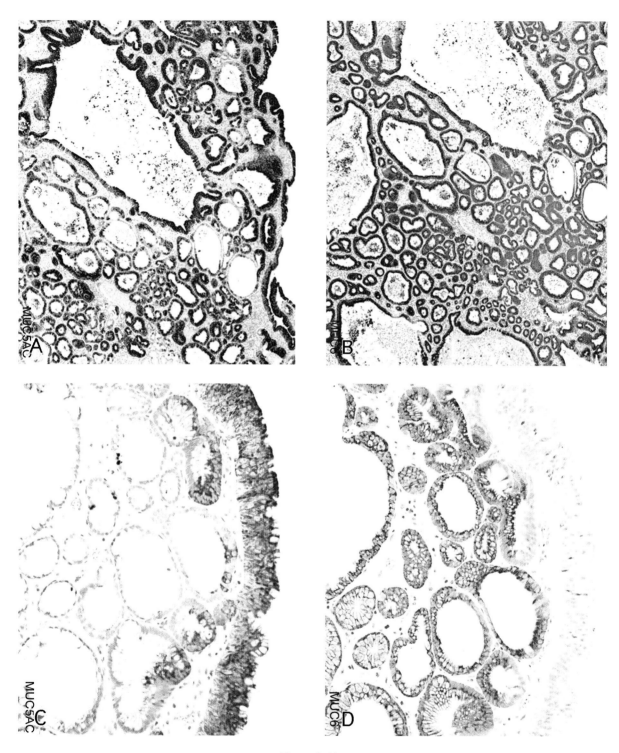

Figure 8-11

PYLORIC GLAND ADENOMAS: IMMUNOHISTOCHEMISTRY

A: Diffuse expression of MUC5AC.
B: Diffuse expression of MUC6 in the PGA shown in A. (A and B courtesy of Dr. Tadakazu Shimoda, Japan.)
C: Expression of MUC5AC in the foveolar epithelium of another polyp.
D: Expression of MUC6 in the glandular component of the PGA shown in C.

and 50 to 67 percent of the cases, respectively. Somatic truncating *APC* mutations are present in all FAP-associated PGAs (100 percent) and in 44 percent of sporadic PGAs (91,94). FAP-associated and sporadic PGAs not only show similar morphology, but also share common genetic aberrations, including mutations of the *GNAS*, *KRAS*, and *APC* genes. Oxyntic gland adenomas (OGAs) share these molecular features as well (see below), which suggests a common molecular pathogenesis for these lesions. It has been hypothesized that PGAs and OGAs are closely related tumors (91). In contrast, fundic gland polyps (FGPs) are wild type for *KRAS* and *GNAS*. At variance with sporadic PGAs, those that develop in Lynch syndrome display MSI (95).

Differential Diagnosis. PGAs may be difficult to distinguish from foveolar-type adenomas. Foveolar-type adenomas have cells that show a well-formed apical mucin cap, are positive for MUC5AC, and are negative for MUC6; PGAs do not have a well-formed apical mucin cap, and label for both MUC5AC and MUC6 (92,102). PAS/alcian blue demonstrates a bright red, uniform staining pattern of mucin in the epithelial cells of gastric foveolar-type adenomas but only granular cytoplasmic staining of the epithelial cells in PGAs. Morphologically, FAP-associated PGAs exhibit parietal cells that vary from scattered to abundant, a feature not commonly observed in sporadic PGAs (91). PGAs may also be difficult to differentiate from OGAs (see below).

Treatment. Due to the risk of malignant transformation, PGAs are treated by complete surgical excision (105). There is limited clinical data available regarding follow-up of patients with gastric PGAs, but the association of these lesions with atrophic gastritis and intestinal metaplasia suggests that their presence reflects an underlying field effect of the mucosa at risk for neoplastic change, and that regular surveillance with biopsies should be considered in affected patients.

Prognosis. Dysplasia is common in gastric PGAs. One study reported high-grade dysplasia rates in 39 percent of cases, and invasive carcinoma in up to 30 percent of cases (92,97). In another study, high-grade dysplasia was reported in 51.2 percent of cases, approximately 25 percent of which also had an associated invasive cancer (91,92). These results show that, despite its bland histologic appearance, PGAs can, and often do, evolve into invasive adenocarcinoma with pyloric gland differentiation (92).

Oxyntic Gland Adenoma

Definition. *Oxyntic gland adenoma* (OGA) is a gastric tumor characterized by an admixture of gastric gland cell types, including chief cells and parietal cells. Other terms used for this lesion are *gastric adenocarcinoma with chief cell differentiation* (GA-CCD) and *gastric adenocarcinoma of fundic gland type* (GA-FG), although the term oxyntic gland polyp is more appropriate for this type of lesion (106). Some have suggested that there is a biologic spectrum of chief cell-predominant gastric polyps, which, at one end is represented by OGA and at the opposite end by adenocarcinoma with fundic gland (chief cell) differentiation (107).

Clinical Features. Patients at diagnosis range in age from 44 to 79 years (mean, 64 years; median, 67 years) with an equal sex distribution. Patients typically present with symptoms unrelated to the tumor itself.

Gross Findings. Lesions are usually located in the upper third of the stomach. Usually they are superficially elevated, but they can also be depressed. Tumor diameter ranges from 4 to 20 mm.

Microscopic Findings. OGAs have a range of architectural and cytologic patterns. Normally, however, they are composed of clusters of solid glands with or without well-defined lumens, anastomosing cords, dilated glands with or without luminal infolding, complex glands with multiple layers of cells, and cribriform glands (fig. 8-12). Ueyama et al. (108,109) subclassified OGA into three categories: chief cell-predominant type, parietal-predominant type, and mixed type. Some show prominent nuclear atypia. A fourth category, consisting of predominantly mucous neck cells, has been suggested by Singhi et al. (106), who defined OGA as mucosal lesions composed primarily of chief cells that do not show features of malignancy (such as desmoplasia, necrosis, perineural or lymphovascular space invasion), in addition to the lack of submucosal involvement.

The cells of OGA display nuclear hyperchromasia, nucleomegaly, slight nuclear pleomorphism, anisonucleosis, and an increased N/C ratio with usually only a few mitotic figures. Architecturally, OGAs are limited to the mucosa, but

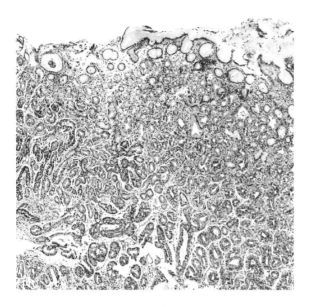

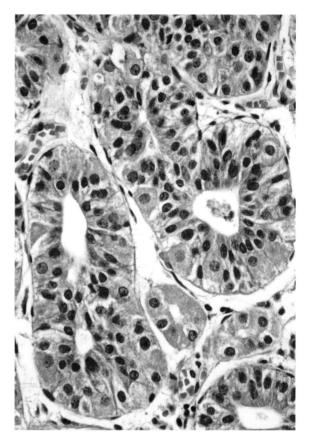

Figure 8-12

OXYNTIC GLAND ADENOMA (OGA)

Above: A compact proliferation of tubules, glands, and acini are present within the deep lamina propria of the gastric corpus.

Right: OGA is characterized by a proliferation of parietal and chief cells with scattered mucous neck cells that show a mild degree of nuclear atypia. The nuclei are slightly enlarged, hyperchromatic, and stratified.

involvement of the muscularis and submucosa occurs. Neoplastic cells express MUC6 and pepsinogen-I (gastric phenotype), and are negative for MUC5AC, MUC2, and CD10.

Molecular Genetic Findings. Constitutive activation of the Wnt/β-catenin pathway is a feature of OGA and leads to the accumulation of β-catenin. Approximately 50 percent of cases harbor at least one mutation in *CTNNB1/AXIN/APC*. *GNAS* mutations and activating mutations in *KRAS* are seen in 19.2 and 7.7 percent of cases, respectively. Mutations in the Wnt component genes and those in *GNAS* occur as an alternative mechanism of activation of the Wnt/β-catenin signaling pathway in OGA (110).

Differential Diagnosis. OGAs should be differentiated from PGAs as well as fundic gland polyps (FGPs), the latter displaying cystic glands lined by foveolar epithelium which is immunoreactive for MUC5AC. Rarely, neuroendocrine tumors should be considered in the differential diagnosis as well, but these tumors are generally diffusely and strongly positive for chromogranin or synaptophysin (111).

Prognosis. Considering that most patients have neither true recurrence nor progression of disease, these lesions are best regarded as benign. Close follow-up is recommended, however, until further larger studies are performed and more information is known regarding the natural history and potential risk of malignancy. A single report illustrated a large (44 mm) deeply invasive (pT3) case with lymphovascular invasion and negative lymph nodes (109a).

Fundic Gland Polyps

Definition. *Fundic gland polyps* (FGPs) are benign epithelial polyps composed of disordered and microcystic oxyntic glands lined by hypoplastic epithelium. They are also termed *fundic gland cyst polyps* or *Elster glandular cysts*.

General Features. There is a recent wide shift in the incidence rate of FGP, particularly related to geographic location of the patient population, and the clinical practices related to use of proton pump inhibitors (PPI). Studies performed prior to the widespread use of PPIs reported a prevalence rate between 0.8 and 1.9

percent. Recent series in Western countries that show a much lower rate of *H. pylori* infection have shown that FGPs represent as much as 77 percent of all gastric polyps (90,112,113).

FGPs arise in two general settings: sporadic and syndrome associated. Sporadic polyps often occur in patients using high dose PPIs but also occur in patients who do not use PPIs. Associated syndromes include familial and attenuated adenomatous polyposis (FAP), *MUTYH*-associated polyposis, and GAPPS (Table 8-3) (23,93,114,115). In addition, fundic gland polyposis can develop as a familial condition confined to the stomach, but without associated colorectal polyposis (116,117). Sporadic and syndromic polyps are histologically identical, but differ in their demographic distribution, molecular alterations, and risk of neoplastic transformation (23,93,114,115,118).

Sporadic FGPs are common in middle-aged individuals (119,120). They were once believed to be more frequent in females but gender difference is not detected in all studies (113). FGPs that develop on a background of normal gastric mucosa have a negative association with *H. pylori* infection. FGPs may disappear upon *H. pylori* infection and then recur after bacterial eradication (17,113,119,121,122).

PPIs are well known to be associated with the genesis of FGPs: 23 percent of patients on PPIs develop FGPs compared to 12 percent of control patients (119,123). The polyps develop in a time- and dose-dependent manner, with a mean interval 32.5 months (119,124), and have been shown to regress within as little as 3 months after cessation of therapy (119,124). PPIs can induce the development of gastric lesions with a cobblestone-like appearance, which is characterized by cystic dilation of the fundic glands (79.2 percent), parietal cell hyperplasia (75.0 percent), and cytoplasmic vacuolation (29.2 percent) (125).

In patients with FAP, the prevalence rate of FGPs varies from 51 percent (126) to 88 percent (123). The incidence in patients with attenuated FAP is reported to be even higher (93 percent) (112). In FAP patients, FGPs occur at a younger age, and a high proportion (31 percent) develops dysplasia (113). In patients with GAPPS, which is a recently described autosomal dominant inherited syndrome, multiple FGPs are common. In this syndrome, FGPs often are associated with low- and high-grade dysplasia and even adenocarcinoma (23,127). FGPs can also be detected in patients with *MUTYH*-associated polyposis. In this condition, FGPs develop in about 11 percent of patients and many also have adenomas as well (128).

Clinical Features. FGPs are typically asymptomatic. They are usually discovered incidentally at the time of endoscopy that is performed for other reasons, such as for GERD (113,120,129). FGPs are most common in adults, occur in males and females equally, but may occur in syndromic patients as young as 8 years of age (130,131).

Gross Findings. FGPs are round, sessile lesions typically covered by translucent, smooth, somewhat pale mucosa. They develop exclusively in oxyntic mucosa, and almost always in the background of normal mucosa (fig. 8-13A). They are usually small (2 to 5 mm), but "giant" FGPs, measuring as much as 8 cm in diameter, have been reported (132). Using virtual chromoendoscopy (such as narrow band imaging [NBI]), FGPs have a characteristic honeycomb appearance, with a dense vasculature (86,113).

In sporadic cases, FGPs are either single or multiple, but usually number less than 10. Syndromic patients usually have multiple polyps and some can have 50 or more. The rarely used term *fundic gland polyposis* has been arbitrarily defined as the presence of over 20 polyps (133). Patients with GAPPS have over 30, or even 100 polyps (23,127). When multiple polyps are present, they may appear confluent and coalesce into much larger polyps (fig. 8-14).

Microscopic Findings. With the exception of GAPPS, syndromic and sporadic polyps are histologically indistinguishable (23,119). They are characterized by the presence of dilated and cystic oxyntic glands lined by parietal cells, chief cells, and mucous neck cells (fig. 8-13B). The cysts may also be lined by foveolar epithelium, either in isolation or combined with oxyntic cells. Parietal cell hyperplasia, a microscopic marker of PPI therapy, is commonly present (129,134). The lamina propria is typically noninflamed, but it can show edema, hemorrhage, or congestion, particularly in polyps that are large. The surface foveolar epithelium is usually normal in appearance, but shows hypoplastic pits.

FGPs may develop dysplasia, which is usually low grade (fig. 8-13C–E). High-grade dysplasia is

Table 8-3

CHARACTERISTICS OF POLYPOSIS SYNDROMES THAT INVOLVE THE STOMACH

Mode of Syndrome	Gene	Mode of Inheritance	Clinical Criteria	Associated Gastric Polyps	Gastric Cancer Lifetime Risk; Histologic Type
GAPPS[a]	Point mutations in exon 1B of *APC*	AD	Gastric polyps restricted to the body and fundus with no evidence of colorectal or duodenal polyposis More than 100 polyps carpeting the proximal stomach in the index case or >30 polyps in a first-degree relative Predominantly fundic gland polyps, some having regions of dysplasia (or a family member with either dysplastic fundic gland polyps or gastric adenocarcinoma) Exclusion of another gastric polyposis syndrome and use of PPIs	Fundic gland polyps with antral sparing; few hyperplastic polyps and adenomas	Increased, no definite estimate; intestinal and mixed adenocarcinoma
(A)FAP	*APC* Germline *APC* mutation in one allele: somatic second hit inactivation of *APC*	AD	Colorectal polyps (>100) and duodenal polyposis	Predominantly fundic gland polyps; few gastric foveolar adenomas and pyloric gland adenoma	Not increased in Western patients
Peutz-Jeghers syndrome	*STK11 (LKB1)*	AD	WHO criteria ≥3 Peutz-Jeghers polyps ≥1 Peutz-Jeghers polyp with a positive family history Mucocutaneous melanosis with a positive family history Mucocutaneous melanosis and ≥1 Peutz-Jeghers polyp	Hamartomatous polyps (Peutz-Jeghers)	29%; intestinal adenocarcinoma
Juvenile polyposis syndrome	*SMAD4* or *BMPR1A* Codeletion of *BMPR1A* and *PTEN* is associated with severe form of JPS (JPS of infancy)	AD	WHO criteria >3-5 juvenile polyps in the colon at one time Juvenile polyps throughout GI tract ≥1 juvenile polyp with a positive family history	Hamartomatous polyps (juvenile)	11-32%; intestinal adenocarcinoma
Cowden syndrome	*PTEN* Other genes involved: *SDHx, KLLN, PIK3CA, AKT1*	AD	Mucocutaneous lesions (see Table 8-4), gastrointestinal polyps (hamartomas, adenoma, ganglioneuromas, lipomas), diffuse esophageal glycogenic acanthosis and macrocephaly	Hamartomatous polyps, ganglioneuromas	Increased, no definite estimate; intestinal and diffuse adenocarcinoma
Cronkhite-Canada syndrome	NA	Non-inherited	Ectodermal abnormalities (alopecia, onychodystrophy, and skin hyperpigmentation that may involve extremities, face, and buccal mucosa) and gastrointestinal hamartomatous polyposis associated with protein-losing enteropathy	Inflammatory/hamartomatous polyps	Not increased

[a]GAPPS = gastric adenocarcinoma and proximal polyposis of the stomach; (A)FAP = (attenuated) familial adenomatous polyposis; AD = autosomal dominant; AR = autosomal recessive; NA = not applicable; PPI = proton pump inhibitor.

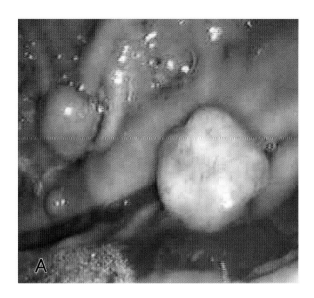

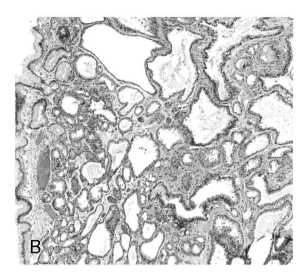

Figure 8-13

FUNDIC GLAND POLYP (FGP)

A: The well-circumscribed sessile nodule has a smooth glassy mucosal surface without ulceration.

B: Multiple cystic spaces are lined by chief cells, oxyntic cells, and mucous neck cells. The intervening lamina propria shows slight edema, but without significant inflammation. The surface foveolar epithelium is hypoplastic. A few strands of muscularis may be detected surrounding the microcysts.

C: Low-power magnification of FGP with low-grade dysplasia. The dysplasia is characterized by cells with enlarged, hyperchromatic, and slightly stratified nuclei with increased mitoses. The dysplastic epithelium involves the surface epithelium and the pits, and may involve the superficial aspect of the oxyntic glands.

D: High-power view of low-grade dysplasia in a FGP shows large nuclei with increased N/C ratio, hyperchromicity, increased mitoses, a more compact gland-in-gland pattern, and lack of surface maturation.

E: Focus of dysplasia in a FGP involving the deeper portions of the pit and deeper microcysts; hypertrophy of the oxyntic cells secondary to proton pump inhibitor therapy is shown.

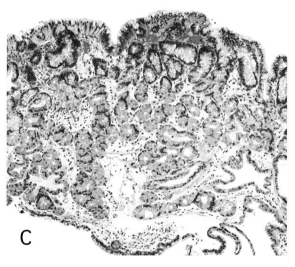

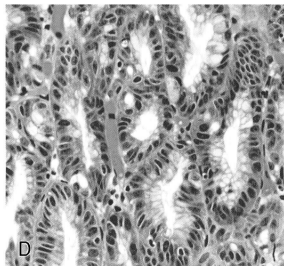

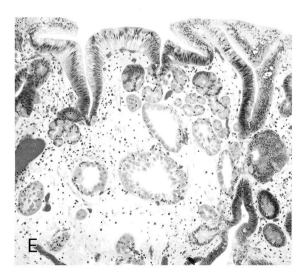

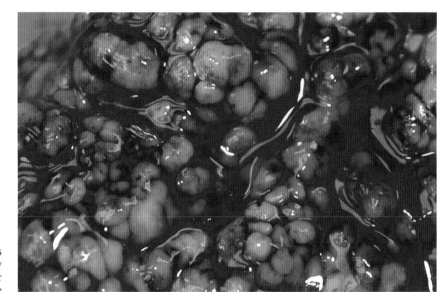

Figure 8-14

GASTRIC ADENOCARCINOMA AND PROXIMAL POLYPOSIS OF THE STOMACH (GAPPS)

Top: Diffuse gastric polyposis of the stomach shows many polyps coalescing to form larger polyps. The polyps have the classic appearance of a FGP: a smooth surface contour, well-circumscribed borders, and a glassy, slightly pale, erythematous mucosa.

Bottom: The classic histology of FGPs is seen. (Courtesy of Dr. Priyanthi Kumarasinghe and Dr. Bastiaan de Boer, Australia.)

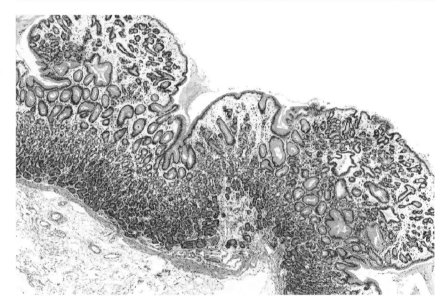

uncommon and more prevalent in patients with FAP or GAPPS. The dysplasia is usually of the foveolar type, composed of cells with enlarged hyperchromatic nuclei, slight stratification, increased mitoses, and lack of surface maturation. The dysplasia often involves the surface and pit epithelium, but deeper cyst epithelium may be involved.

Immunohistochemical Findings. FGPs are typically diffusely positive for cytokeratin (CK) 7, a marker of epithelial differentiation, which is typically absent in normal gastric epithelium (135). There is also a loss of tuberin nuclear expression, which suggests a role for deregulation of transcriptional activity in the development of these lesions (136).

Molecular Genetic Findings. Molecular analyses have demonstrated different features in sporadic versus syndromic polyps (137). FAP is caused by heterozygous mutations of the tumor suppressor gene *APC*. Mutations are detected in 67 percent of patients, and include point mutations/substitutions and insertion deletions. Mutations toward the 5' and 3' ends (codons 1982-1983) are associated with gastric polyposis (138). Somatic mutations involving codons 1554-1556 occur in 51 percent of FAP-associated FGPs and 50 percent of gastric adenomas. Rare

KRAS mutations, in codon 12, have been detected in FGPs with low-grade dysplasia (139). Mutations occur in exon 4 of the *APC* gene in gastric polyposis, and also early onset gastric carcinoma, in patients with attenuated FAP (140).

Sporadic FGPs are devoid of *APC* mutations, but instead reveal mutations in the *CTNNB1* (β-catenin) gene in 65 to 91 percent of cases (137,139,141). Different mutations may be present in FGPs when they are multiple, which confirms the somatic nature of the mutations (117,137,141). In the setting of sporadic fundic gland polyposis (SFGP), the polyps are histologically and genetically identical to sporadic FGPs, and they also reveal somatic activating mutations in exon 3 of the *CTNNB1* gene (117).

Rare cases of sporadic FGPs with dysplasia harbor *APC* mutations similar to those observed in FAP-associated FGPs, and these are also negative for β-catenin gene mutations (142). In patients with GAPPS (fig. 8-14), the presence of point mutations in the YY1 binding site of the *APC* promoter 1B have been detected (143,144). The molecular features of *MUTYH*-associated FGPs are unknown (145).

Treatment. Large FGPs should be removed, not only to confirm the diagnosis, but also to exclude dysplasia, which shows an increased prevalence rate in large polyps (85). The presence of ulceration should also prompt a more aggressive approach (22). In patients with many (over 20) FGPs, or in cases with large polyps, consideration should be given to reducing, or preferably stopping, PPIs in order to assess regression (22). Identification of multiple FGPs or concomitant dysplasia should raise suspicion for an underlying polyposis syndrome and prompt an appropriate clinical workup (146). Due to a high frequency of colonic adenomas in patients with FGP, some have recommended that a colonoscopy should be performed when multiple gastric FGPs are diagnosed (147).

When FGPs are associated with duodenal adenomas, a familial polyposis syndrome should be considered, and a colonoscopy recommended in order to exclude FAP (22). Although, there are no established surveillance guidelines for FAP patients with FGPs, most authorities suggest that it should begin at 21 to 30 years of age (148) and then continue at intervals of 3 to 5 years (149). Nonsteroidal anti-inflammatory drugs and acid

suppressive therapy are associated with regression and a reduction in the number of FGPs (150) and in the incidence of dysplasia (17).

When GAPPS is suspected in patients with FGPs and dysplasia, testing for point mutations in the *APC* promoter 1B should be performed to help decide whether a prophylactic gastrectomy should be performed. For families with *MUTYH* germline mutations, current guidelines recommend that surveillance upper endoscopy be performed between the ages of 30 and 35 years, and then subsequently at intervals of 3 to 5 years (128).

Prognosis. In FAP patients, dysplasia occurs at an incidence rate of about 25 to 44 percent (151), but it remains low in sporadic FGPs (about 1 percent) (152). The risk of developing dysplasia in syndrome-associated FGP correlates with the increased severity of duodenal polyposis and larger polyp size (17). When dysplasia is detected, it is usually low grade (15,93). High-grade dysplasia is rare (15,93,153).

FGPs are rarely associated with gastric cancer, and the risk varies geographically. A higher risk of cancer has been reported in Japan (4.5 to 13.6 percent) (154,155), but this has not been confirmed in the West, where the risk of malignancy remains very low (0.6 to 4.2 percent) (156). Korean and Japanese FAP patients are 7 to 10 times more likely to develop an adenocarcinoma, traditionally of tubular type, compared to nonsyndromic patients (157,158). Multicentric or metachronous cancers have also been described rarely (157,159). The increased risk of cancer in syndromic patients with FGPs may be related to the generalized increased rate of chronic atrophic gastritis, intestinal metaplasia, and *H. pylori* infection in these patient populations compared to Western patients.

Hyperplastic Polyps

Definition. *Hyperplastic polyps* (HPs) are benign inflammatory lesions that develop as a result of a hyperproliferative response to chronic mucosal injury. They are characterized by hyperplastic, elongated and distorted foveolar epithelium and increased inflammation in the lamina propria (160).

General Features. HPs formerly represented the most common type of gastric polyp. Prevalence rates ranged from 50 to 90 percent in regions where *H. pylori* infection and chronic gastritis are high (35,161,162). Recent studies, particularly in the Western world, show that HPs actually represent the second most common type of gastric polyp. This epidemiologic shift is due to increasing PPI use and a decrease in the prevalence rate of *H. pylori* infection, particularly in the United States and other Western populations of the world. The currently reported frequency is about 14 percent of all gastric polyps (90,163).

The role of *H. pylori* infection in the genesis of HPs is substantiated by their tendency to disappear, or regress, after *H. pylori* eradication, and to reappear in cases of reinfection (164,165). Solid organ transplantation is a risk factor as well: up to 15 percent of HPs arise in transplant patients (166, 167). Other risk factors include Billroth II antrectomy and portal hypertension gastropathy (168).

Clinical Features. HPs usually develop in adults (mean age, 60 years). They develop in males and females at approximately the same rate (160,163,169). HPs occur most commonly in the antrum, but they can develop anywhere in the stomach. When the surrounding mucosa is sampled, the background usually shows chronic inflammation (in 85 percent of cases) and mucosal atrophy, either in association with *H. pylori* infection or autoimmune gastritis (170,171). The risk of developing HP increases with the severity of mucosal atrophy, particularly in the proximal stomach.

Most patients are asymptomatic. Larger and eroded polyps may be associated with blood loss, iron deficiency anemia, and abdominal pain (160,172). Rare examples of gastric outlet obstruction have also been described for patients with large antral HPs that protrude into the duodenum (173–176). True gastric hyperplastic polyposis (50 HPs or more) is rare (177,178). A putative association between hyperplastic polyposis and colorectal cancer has also been suggested (177). One report described sporadic diffuse hyperplastic and adenomatous polyposis of the stomach (179).

Gross Findings. Most HPs are small, round, sessile lesions measuring between 0.5 and 1.5 cm (fig. 8-15A). Large HPs (usually 2 cm or larger) may become pedunculated, and often have an eroded surface. Multiple polyps are detected in about 20 percent of patients (160).

Microscopic Findings. HPs are composed of elongated, disorganized, distorted and branched foveolae; the stroma usually shows edema, congestion, and increased inflammation consisting of lymphocytes, plasma cells, neutrophils, and even eosinophils (fig. 8-15B). Intraluminal infolding and branching of the foveolae is common. Cystic dilatation is present almost invariably in the deeper portions of the polyps (180). Sparse, thin bundles of smooth muscle fibers are frequently present. Lymphoid aggregates with germinal centers can be present as well.

Most HPs are lined by a single layer of foveolar epithelium which usually contains abundant neutral mucin. The foveolar epithelium may appear regenerative, showing cells with elongated, hyperchromatic nuclei, stratification, and mucin depletion. Cuboidal cells are observed focally in areas where ulcers are being re-epithelialized (52,181). The surface epithelium can contain "globoid" cells (fig. 8-15C), which is considered a form of goblet cells. These cells should be differentiated from true signet ring cell carcinoma in situ. HPs may show pseudo-pyloric metaplasia. Oxyntic glands are uncommon, even in polyps that occur in the body of the stomach. Intestinal metaplasia may be present, usually focally, of incomplete type (169).

Dysplasia is rarely observed and is more common in polyps larger than 20 mm. The dysplasia is usually of the intestinal type, but may be foveolar. The features of dysplasia are similar to those seen in intestinal or foveolar type adenomas. Low-grade dysplasia shows enlarged, hyperchromatic, elongated nuclei, with stratification and lack of maturation, but with little or no architectural changes (fig. 8-15D–E). High-grade dysplasia shows increased cytologic and architectural changes, the latter often consisting of back-to-back glands or a gland-in-gland pattern (fig. 8-15F).

The surface of HPs, particularly large ones, may be eroded and, thus, covered by fibrinopurulent exudates (fig. 8-15G). Reactive epithelium, with mucin depletion, may be present and mimic dysplastic epithelium. These changes are usually associated with acute inflammation and granulation tissue (fig. 8-15G). In these areas, mitotically active, bizarre-appearing reactive stromal cells ("pseudosarcoma") with hyperchromatic nuclei and prominent nucleoli may be present as well (182,183).

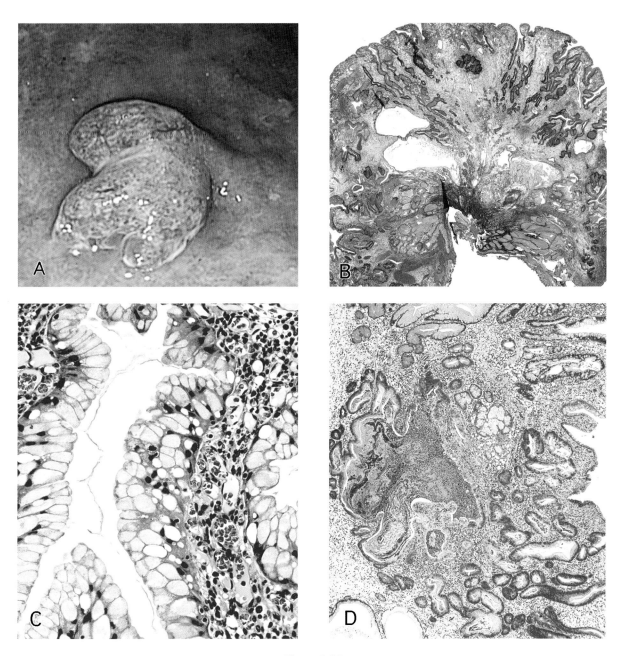

Figure 8-15

HYPERPLASTIC POLYPS (HP)

A: The typical HP is a lobulated but well-circumscribed irregular nodule with an erythematous congested appearance, with alternating areas of pallor and superficial necrosis.

B: Marked foveolar hyperplasia, elongation, tortuosity, and cystic change of the foveolar epithelium are typical of HP. Increased amount of lamina propria with edema, congestion, hemorrhage, acute and chronic inflammation, and patchy areas where strands of muscularis protrude from the deep portion of the polyp are also seen.

C: One area of the foveolar epithelium shows rows of dystrophic goblet cells, termed "globoid dysplasia." These cells, however, are not dysplastic and represent distended goblet cell-like mucinous cells that simulate signet ring cell carcinoma in situ.

D: HP with low- and high-grade dysplasia, and features bordering on intramucosal adenocarcinoma. In the superficial half of the polyp, the epithelium has markedly enlarged, hyperchromatic and stratified nuclei with focal areas of gland budding and a gland-in-gland pattern. In the deep middle portion of the polyp, the dysplasia is high grade, involving a large cystic space lined by markedly atypical cells with loss of polarity and increased N/C ratio, a gland-in-gland pattern, and intraluminal necrosis.

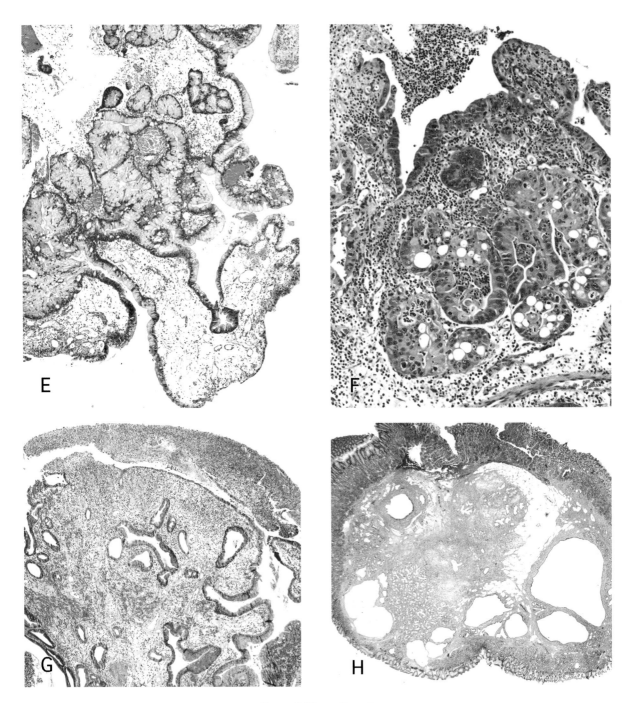

Figure 8-15, continued

E: Another focus of low-grade dysplasia shows atypical epithelium with more prominent mucinous differentiation. Both the cytologic and architectural features of this area are indicative of dysplasia.

F: Intestinal-type high-grade dysplasia and intramucosal carcinoma in a HP. The cells contain markedly enlarged nuclei, which in this focus have a more round to oval shape, irregular nuclear borders with distinct loss of polarity and pleomorphism, and intraluminal necrosis.

G: Surface ulceration and marked reactive changes of the foveolar epithelium underlying and adjacent to an ulcer. The surface of the ulcer is freshly re-epithelialized overlying an area of necrosis, granulation tissue, edema, hemorrhage, and active inflammation.

H: In an "inverted" HP, the surface mucosa is normal, but the submucosa shows multiple cystic spaces surrounded by gastric glands lined by normal or reactive epithelium, lamina propria, and muscularis hyperplasia. There is an increased amount of edema and active and chronic inflammation. This polyp shares features with gastritis cystica profunda-polyposa.

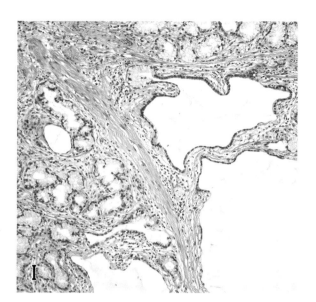
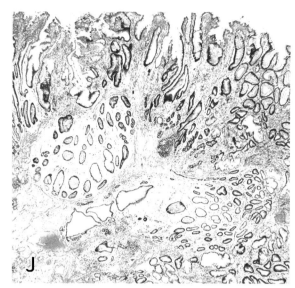

Figure 8-15, continued

I: An inverted HP shows cysts and glands in the submucosa with intervening lamina propria and strands of muscularis. The epithelium is cytologically benign or mildly reactive in appearance.

J: HP of the antral region has features of a HP, but it also shows more prominent muscularis hyperplasia in the deeper mid portions of the polyp, with prominent edema. One theory is that this HP developed from mucosal prolapse.

Variants of Hyperplastic Polyps. *Polypoid foveolar hyperplasia* is a small lesion, usually only 1 to 2 mm in size, that shows simple foveolar hyperplasia without cystic change or gland distortion. This is regarded as a precursor lesion to HP, although this has never been proven. It is commonly noted at the edges of ulcers or erosions and is also etiologically related to chronic mucosal injury and repair.

Inverted hyperplastic polyp (184) is a less common subtype of HP (fig. 8-15H,I). It is a submucosal glandular proliferation often with cystic dilatation. The inverted glands are usually surrounded by a delicate layer of smooth muscle. Inverted HPs may develop secondary to deep ulceration, or protrusion or entrapment of glands in the submucosa (184,185). They may be associated with gastritis cystica profunda (184). Some of these polyps have been termed *hamartomatous inverted polyp*. The pathogenesis of these lesions remains controversial (186) and their association with gastric cystica polyposa is unclear. Multifocal adenocarcinoma has been reported in one inverted HP (187).

The *mucosal prolapse variant* of gastric HP is more commonly sessile than typical HPs. It is also distinguished by the presence of basal glandular elements and prominent hypertrophic muscle fibers that extend perpendicularly from the muscularis mucosae into the lamina propria (fig. 8-15J), and by the presence of thick-walled blood vessels. This subtype is more common in the antrum, in a zone of pronounced peristalsis, which suggests that mucosal prolapse probably plays a role in the development of these lesions (188).

HP with extensive vascular proliferation and dilatation is another variant of HP that develops in a background of portal hypertension. This variant is characterized by a less pronounced foveolar proliferation and a greater degree of vascular dilatation. The absence of *H. pylori* infection suggests a different pathophysiologic process. The mucosal hyperplasia may be related to vascular proliferation (168).

HPs of the gastroesophageal junction usually arise in association with GERD, and often in patients with Barrett esophagus. These polyps typically occur in the absence of gastric pathology (189).

Immunohistochemical Findings. Immunohistochemistry is not needed to establish a diagnosis of HP. When performed, increased Ki-67 activity (169), and increased COX2 and p21 expression, all consistent with increased cellular turnover and proliferation, are present (169,190,191).

171

Molecular Genetic Findings. Molecular studies of HPs are limited. Of the two main genetic abnormalities associated with gastric cancer, *TP53* mutations have been frequently identified in dysplastic or malignant foci of gastric HPs. *KRAS* mutations are less common (169,192,193). Chromosomal aberrations and MSI have also been reported in HPs with dysplasia (22).

Treatment. Most HPs are biopsied, or excised, if the latter is possible endoscopically. Biopsies of HPs, and examination of the background stomach, are often helpful to determine the type of polyp and the cause of the lesion and help distinguish HPs from other polyps (see differential diagnosis section below). Polypectomy is usually reserved for large polyps (over 1 cm), ones with obstructive symptoms, and of course, those with dysplasia or cancer.

Since these polyps generally arise as a response to mucosal injury and inflammation, an examination of the surrounding mucosa is important to identify and treat associated conditions (e.g., *H. pylori* infection) (194). Caution is suggested for polyps related to portal hypertension, since there is an increased risk of hemorrhage in these patients; watchful surveillance is likely safer for these patients given the clinical risk (195).

Prognosis. Dysplasia is present in 2.0 to 3.3 percent of HPs (169,196,197). In one study, *TP53* gene mutations were common in dysplasia-associated HPs (198). Adenocarcinoma is uncommon. It occurs in large polyps in less than 2 percent of cases. Most cancers are tubular adenocarcinomas (199) but signet ring cell carcinoma (200) or papillary carcinoma (201) have been observed as well. In one family, diffuse gastric cancer developed in the setting of familial hyperplastic polyposis (20).

There is a direct correlation between the risk of neoplastic transformation and the size of the polyps. Polyps larger than 2 cm are at highest risk (169,202). Since neoplastic transformation is usually focal within the polyp, and since white light endoscopic criteria of gastric HPs with dysplasia have not been well defined, it may be missed at endoscopic examination. Magnifying endoscopy combined with NBI (ME-NBI) improves detection (203). As a consequence, some recommend removal of all HPs that measure more than 2 cm (85). Furthermore,

since HPs are associated with gastritis, atrophy, and intestinal metaplasia, all well-known risk factors for gastric cancer (171), HPs should be considered a surrogate marker for cancer elsewhere in the stomach. Indeed, associated synchronous or metachronous gastric cancer has been reported in 4 to 6 percent of patients with HPs.

H. pylori eradication may also decrease the risk of malignant transformation of HPs and the surrounding mucosa. Patients with extensive atrophy and intestinal metaplasia of the surrounding gastric mucosa should be considered at high risk for gastric cancer and benefit from watchful follow-up.

Gastritis Cystica Profunda-Polyposa

Definition. *Gastritis cystica profunda-polyposa* (GCP) is a rare benign lesion of the stomach characterized by the displacement of foveolar epithelium, glands, and often mucin, into the deeper portions of the wall of the stomach, such as the submucosa, muscularis, or even serosa.

General Features. GCP was first described by Littler and Gleibermann in 1972 (204), and since then there have been many reports of this lesion, but mostly as isolated case reports or small series (205–208). As a result, the biologic characteristics, pathogenesis, natural history, and clinical significance are still poorly understood. Although the pathogenesis is unknown, GCP is considered to develop as a result of chronic inflammation and injury to the stomach or ischemia. GCP develops most often in stomachs that have been operated on, in patients who have had a gastroenterostomy (209–211), and rarely in unoperated stomachs (206). It is presumed that the damage caused by prior surgery, combined with localized ischemia, results in herniation or displacement of mucosal elements into the wall of the stomach during the process of tissue repair. In patients who have had a partial gastrectomy, it is presumed that chronic bile reflux plays a role in its development as well. The lesion is referred to as "polyposa" when there is a prominent intraluminal polyp identified, and as "profunda" when the bulk of the lesion is located in the wall of the stomach, but without a prominent polyp.

Clinical Features. The clinical manifestations of GCP are variable and dependent on the location and type of lesion (205,209). These include abdominal pain, gastrointestinal bleeding, anemia, the presence of an abdominal mass, and occasionally, gastric outlet obstruction. GCP affects predominantly adults of both genders, but is more prominent in males. Since the lesion is mainly submucosal, diagnosis by endoscopic biopsy is usually difficult. Endoscopic ultrasound and computerized tomography (CT) play a complementary role in delineating the characteristics of the lesion, such as the size, surface contour, depth of involvement of the wall, and presence or absence of cystic change (209). In one recent study by Laratta et al. (205), a comprehensive literature review between 1972 and 2011 revealed 37 cases of GCP. Seventy-eight percent of patients were male and the mean age at diagnosis was 60.5 years. Sixty-five percent of patients had prior gastric surgery; 62 percent of lesions were located in the body, 25 percent in the fundus, 8 percent in the antrum, and 6 percent in the cardia. GCP was an incidental finding in 19 percent of patients. Most patients were treated by complete excision (73 percent), but some were treated by endoscopic resection (18 percent) or polypectomy.

Gross Findings. GCP may develop anywhere in the stomach, but it is most often located in the body or fundus, followed by the antrum and cardia (205). It usually develops on the gastric side of a gastroenteric anastomosis in patients who have had prior surgery. It appears as irregular enlarged rugal folds, with or without a polyp, which in some cases has been shown to measure 3 to 5 cm. The mucosal surface may be intact or ulcerated.

Microscopic Findings. The characteristic histologic feature of GCP is entrapment and displacement of epithelium or glands, often in a cystic configuration or mixed with mucin, into and through the muscularis mucosae and submucosa of the stomach (fig. 8-16). Rare cases involve the muscularis propria and even the serosa.

The epithelium is typically mucinous or glandular, is often cystic and present in well-organized lobules. The epithelium and the glands are usually surrounded by a rim of lamina propria-like stroma. On occasion, the cysts are entrapped and surrounded by disorganized bundles of smooth muscle that extend down from the muscularis mucosae. Adjacent stromal changes suggestive of prior injury, such as in-flammation, granulation tissue, or hemosiderin deposition, are common.

The displaced epithelium may be mature or show hyperplastic or degenerative changes. If the hyperplastic or regenerative changes are prominent, it may resemble dysplasia. When the epithelium is atrophic, the lining of the microcysts may be difficult to discern with accuracy. The overlying mucosa may show evidence of chronic gastritis, bile reflux gastritis, or prior gastric surgery. Superficial erosions and intestinal metaplasia may be present as well.

Differential Diagnosis. The main entity in the differential diagnosis of GCP is well-differentiated invasive adenocarcinoma. Invasive adenocarcinoma typically shows more marked cytologic, and in particular, architectural atypia. The glands are more irregular in shape and size and show an infiltrative pattern of growth, without a lobulated segregation of the epithelium in the wall of the stomach. The cytologic atypia, including irregularity in the size and shape of the nuclei, and increased mitoses help diagnose adenocarcinoma. Adenocarcinoma may contain desmoplasia, but when it does not, the lack of a lamina propria rim surrounding the epithelium favors adenocarcinoma over GCP. Caution should be exercised in diagnosing GCP in a patient who has no previous gastric surgery or in patients who have chronic gastritis combined with dysplasia or adenomas in the overlying or adjacent mucosa. Although immunohistochemistry is not helpful for a diagnosis, adenocarcinoma may be positive for p53 and show at a high Ki-67 proliferation rate. The presence of multiple epithelial elements within the lesion favors GCP (lesions that show a combination of foveolar epithelium, glandular epithelium, and endocrine cells).

Treatment. The treatment of GCP is complete excision, which is most often performed because of the presence of a mass or polypoid lesion that is suspected to represent malignancy. Some cases are treated by endomucosal resection or polypectomy. If the lesion has been excised in total, there is little risk of local recurrence.

Prognosis. A definite association between GCP and cancer has been reported in the literature, but the magnitude of that risk is unclear (205,211–214). Furthermore, it is unclear whether the frequency of neoplasia is equal to

Figure 8-16

GASTRITIS CYSTICA PROFUNDA-POLYPOSA

Top: The submucosa shows a proliferation of gastric epithelium and glands in a cystic and lobulated configuration. The lobules of epithelium and glands are separated by intervening fascicles of smooth muscle. There is also increased inflammation and lamina propria-like stroma surrounding the glands. The overlying mucosa shows a moderate degree of chronic gastritis.

Bottom: At high magnification, the submucosal glandular epithelium shows a minimal degree of reactive change, but no evidence of dysplasia. The intervening interglandular space shows lamina propria-like stroma.

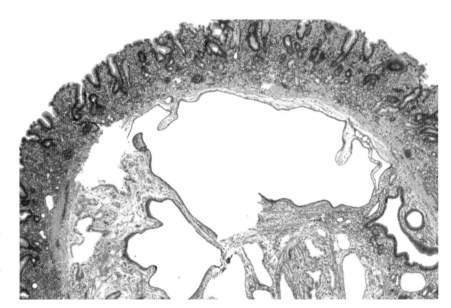

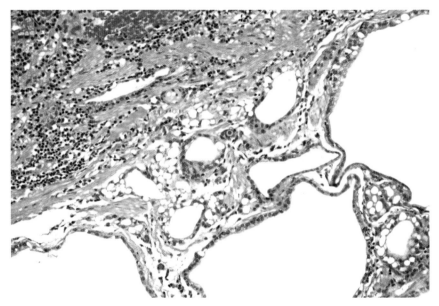

or greater than that of ordinary hyperplastic polyps or in patients who have had a Billroth II antrectomy, which itself is known to be associated with an increased risk of malignancy.

Choi et al. (210) reviewed the records of 10,728 patients with gastric cancer who underwent gastric surgery, and found 161 with GCP. The features of those patients were compared to those without GCPs. GCP was associated with older age, male gender, proximal tumor location, better differentiated histology, and Lauren intestinal-type cancer compared to non-GCP-associated malignancies. Patients with GCP presented at an earlier tumor stage, in terms of depth of invasion and lymph node metastasis, and had a lower incidence of lymphatic and neural invasion. The Epstein-Barr virus (EBV) in situ hybridization positivity rate was significantly higher in the GCP group (31.1 percent) compared to the non-GCP group (5.8 percent), which suggests a possible role for this virus as a premalignant lesion in patients with GCP. It is not clear whether GCP itself is a precancerous lesion, or if it is simply associated with stomachs that are at increased risk for malignancy because of its association with chronic and often atrophic gastritis.

Juvenile Polyps and Polyposis

Definition. *Juvenile polyps* (JP) are a benign type of hamartoma composed of disordered epithelium mixed with abundant, often edematous lamina propria and inflammation. *Juvenile polyposis syndrome* (JPS) is an autosomal dominant, diffuse gastrointestinal hamartomatous polyposis syndrome, with variable penetrance, characterized by the development of multiple JPs in the stomach and associated with an increased risk of cancer in the gastrointestinal tract (Table 8-3) (215–217).

General Features. JPS is diagnosed by fulfilling one of the following criteria: 1) presence of more than five JPs in the colorectum; 2) presence of multiple JPs throughout the gastrointestinal system; 3) any number of JPs in a patient with a known family history of JPs. JPS develops at a much earlier age than sporadic JPs and commonly presents with a more severe clinical course. Patients with JPS have a reduced life expectancy and pronounced extraintestinal manifestations. Patients with large gene deletions involving both the *BMPR1A* and *PTEN* genes often have a more severe clinical presentation.

Juvenile polyposis of infancy is believed to be a unique subtype of JPS that often shows combined features of both Cowden syndrome and Bannayan-Riley-Ruvalcaba syndrome along with JPs (219,220). These patients often show loss of both *BMPR1A* and *PTEN* genes. Some patients with JPS have mutations in *SMAD4* or *BMPR1A* and they exhibit a mixed polyposis phenotype similar to individuals with hereditary mixed polyposis syndrome (221).

Clinical Features. JPs occur in 1 of 100,000 to 160,000 population. Isolated sporadic JPs are typically asymptomatic. Occasionally, large polyps cause obstructive symptoms (216).

JPS is usually diagnosed in adults (median age, 41 years), although colorectal JPS is typically detected earlier (median age, 16 years). Patients with JPS can develop polyps isolated to the stomach, without lower gastrointestinal involvement (222–224). The gastric antrum is most frequently involved (226–228). In the antrum, large and distal polyps may be associated with symptoms of pyloric obstruction (229), iron deficiency anemia (224, 228,229), hematemesis, and hypoproteinemia (224,228, 229). This clinical presentation may mimic Ménétrier disease.

Rare patients develop *massive gastric juvenile polyposis*, which can occur in patients with or without known JPS. This disorder may mimic a variety of other disorders and other polyposis syndromes, and even Ménétrier disease (225).

Gross Findings. Most gastric JPs, regardless of whether they are sporadic or associated with JPS, are typically small, round, sessile lesions, but they may have a lobular or pedunculated appearance as they grow larger (fig. 8-17A) (230,231). Most JPs measure 0.5 to 1.0 cm, but large lesions measure up to 10 cm (225). Grossly, JPs are indistinguishable from hyperplastic polyps or other types of hamartomatous polyps.

Microscopic Findings. Sporadic and syndrome-associated JPs are histologically similar. Both are characterized by the presence of cystically dilated, elongated, and tortuous glands lined by foveolar epithelium set within a stroma with edema, congestion, and a mixed inflammatory infiltrate (fig. 8-17B,C). Most JPs show a few strands of smooth muscle fibers within the lamina propria, but this is not as well developed as it is in some hyperplastic polyps. Although most polyps show an equal distribution of epithelium and lamina propria, some are "epithelium-rich," showing prominent convoluted and hyperplastic glands with little stroma while others are "stroma-rich," showing more prominent lamina propria, inflammation, and edema, and less prominent glands (which may be flat and show only occasional dilated cystic spaces) (225,232).

The foveolar epithelium may be completely mature, with a normal complement of mucin, or reactive or degenerative depending on the presence of inflammation or ulceration. When the epithelium is reactive, the cells have elongated and hyperchromatic nuclei, pseudostratification, mucin depletion, and increased mitoses.

JPs, either sporadic or syndrome-associated, may develop dysplasia although this is far more common in the latter (19). The dysplasia shows intestinal type, foveolar type, or pyloric gland-like differentiation. Intestinal dysplasia may be low or high grade. The dysplastic epithelium shows markedly enlarged and hyperchromatic nuclei, stratification, lack of surface maturation, increased mitoses, and an abrupt transition with surrounding nondysplastic epithelium. The cells may show enterocyte-like or goblet cell differentiation. High-grade changes include

Figure 8-17

JUVENILE POLYPOSIS

A: There is complete replacement of the mucosa with a dense carpet of polyps which have a nodular, lobulated, and slightly villiform appearance.

B: Prominent cystic change, edema, active and chronic inflammation, and reactive changes are present in a juvenile polyp.

C: High-power view of the surface of a juvenile polyp shows HP-like changes with foveolar hyperplasia, edema, hemorrhage of the lamina propria, a slight increase in inflammation, and microcystic change. In biopsies, these polyps are histologically indistinguishable from a HP. (Courtesy of Prof. Paula Chaves and Dr. Gonçalo Esteves, Portugal.)

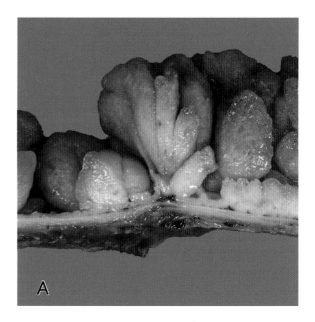

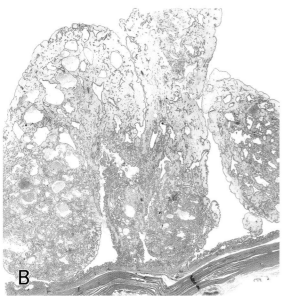

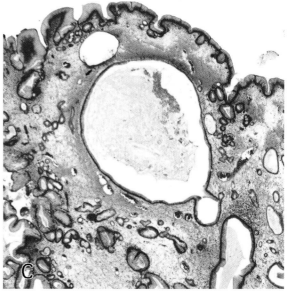

markedly enlarged nuclei with increased N/C ratio and architectural abnormalities, such as back-to-back gland formation or gland-in-gland pattern. JPs with gastric-type dysplasia show similar nuclear features, but with mucinous cytoplasmic differentiation rather than goblet cells. The epithelium may have a pyloric gland phenotype, showing smaller round to oval nuclei, with prominent nucleoli, and a mucinous type of cytoplasm that resembles pyloric glands.

Immunohistochemical Findings. Loss of SMAD4 immunostaining occurs in some gastric JPs and in some cases this can be used as a screening method. The epithelium of JPs shows decreased or absent staining compared to non-polypoid epithelium, but in some instances, the results are difficult to interpret (225,233,234). Unfortunately, retained SMAD4 expression does not exclude a germline *SMAD4* mutation. In contrast, sporadic JPs and polyps from patients with *BMPR1A* mutation carriers never show loss of SMAD4 expression (217,233).

Molecular Genetic Findings. JPS is caused by mutations in several genes. Most commonly involved are *SMAD4* and *BMPRIA*, which are two genes implicated in the TGF-β signaling pathway (219,235). *SMAD4* (18q21.2) is responsible for 20 to 40 percent of cases, and *BMPR1A* (10q23.2) for 20 to 40 percent of cases. Severe gastric polyposis develops in patients with *SMAD4* mutations, but not in those with *BMPR1A* mutations (236).

Mutations of *SMAD4* have also been detected in patients with Ménétrier disease. Since both diseases are related to deregulation of the TGF-β signaling pathway, some authors have suggested that Ménétrier disease represents a variant of JPS in which a superimposed alternative etiology (e.g., cytomegalovirus or *H. pylori* infection) results in the expression of its characteristic clinical phenotype (237).

Germline mutations in *PTEN*, which is involved in the PI3K/AKT signaling pathway, and possibly *ENG*, which encodes for endoglin, have also been associated with early childhood symptoms (238,239). Endoglin, a transforming factor-beta protein, is involved in the pathophysiology of hereditary hemorrhagic telangiectasia (HHT), which explains the occasional overlap observed between JPS and HHT. The JPS and HHT syndromes are also caused by *SMAD4* mutations (240). Consequently, it is recommended that HHT patients be screened for gastric polyposis.

Treatment. The treatment of sporadic JPs is simple biopsy or polypectomy. These patients have no risk of developing malignancy, and the polyps are typically removed for diagnostic purposes and to exclude a neoplastic lesion. These patients do not need further surveillance. Patients with JPS should receive genetic counseling and undergoing endoscopic surveillance (216,218). These patients have a propensity to develop intestinal and extraintestinal malignancies. Current guidelines recommend that upper gastrointestinal tract endoscopy, with the removal of polyps larger than 5 mm, should begin at age 12, or earlier in case of symptoms, and then repeated every 1 to 3 years for life, depending on the severity of upper gastrointestinal polyposis (216). Gastrectomy is typically reserved for patients who are symptomatic with many polyps and for those with massive gastric polyposis, high-grade dysplasia, or cancer (216).

Prognosis. Colorectal carcinoma develops in 38 percent and gastric adenocarcinoma in 21 to 32 percent of patients with JPS (225,241). In general, the risk of cancer increases proportion-

ally with the size of the polyps. Phenotypically, intestinal and diffuse type gastric cancers have been reported in association with JPS (242).

Peutz-Jeghers Polyps and Syndrome

Definition. *Peutz-Jeghers syndrome* (PJS) is an autosomal dominant disorder characterized by the development of hamartomatous polyps that develop anywhere in the gastrointestinal tract, combined with perioral pigmentation, which is termed melanocytic macule (Table 8-3). Rarely, Peutz-Jeghers type polyps develop sporadically in patients without the PJS syndrome but most cases are associated with PJS (243–245).

General Features. Sporadic Peutz-Jeghers polyps occur anywhere in the gastrointestinal tract, but are most common in the proximal small intestine, stomach, and colon (with a prevalence rate of about 90, 50, and 25 percent, respectively) (128). Gastroduodenal polyps are more prevalent in children than adults; the prevalence rate of colonic polyps is similar in children and adults. The median age of onset of gastric polyps is 16 years (246).

Most patients with sporadic polyps are asymptomatic and their polyps are detected at the time of endoscopy performed for other reasons. The prevalence of PJS is estimated at 1 in 50,000 to 200,000 (247). In up to 80 percent of cases, the PJS is caused by a germline mutation of the *STK11/LKB1* gene (248), but this is not a prerequisite for the diagnosis. In fact, PJS is diagnosed by the detection of: 1) small intestinal polyposis (at least two polyps with characteristic histologic features); 2) at least one characteristic polyp combined with hyperpigmentation of the lips, buccal mucosa, and digits (which usually fades by puberty); or 3) the presence of one histologically characteristic polyp combined with a positive family history (249).

Clinical Features. Patients with PJS present with a variety of symptoms. These include intestinal intussusception, occult bleeding with secondary iron deficiency anemia, and acute abdominal pain depending on the site and size of the polyp (250).

PJS affects multiple organ systems in which hamartomatous, metaplastic, or neoplastic lesions develop. Glandular lesions are the most common manifestation in the urinary bladder, including glandular metaplasia, lobular

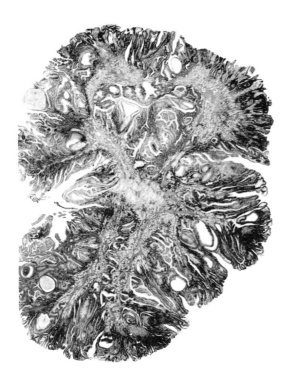 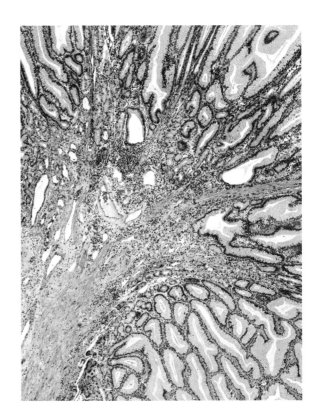

Figure 8-18

GASTRIC PEUTZ-JEGHERS POLYP

Left: The polyp has a lobulated polypoid contour. The foveolar epithelium shows elongation, tortuosity, branching, and cystic change. The lamina propria has increased inflammation, congestion, and hemorrhage. In contrast to HPs, there is a well-established arborizing tree-like network of muscularis dissecting through the polyp.

Right: Increased inflammation in the lamina propria and a tree-like branching framework of muscularis dissecting through the lobules of the mucosa.

endocervical glandular hyperplasia of the uterine cervix, mucinous metaplasia of the fallopian tube, and mucinous adenoma of the ovary. Regardless of the location of the lesions, most are associated with pyloric gland metaplasia (251).

Gross Findings. Peutz-Jeghers polyps may be small or large, and occur anywhere in the stomach but are most common in the antrum and pylorus, where they may be large and cause luminal obstruction (90). Gastric PJS polyps are sessile, in contrast to those that occur elsewhere in the gastrointestinal tract, which are more often pedunculated (252). The polyps range from a few millimeters to several centimeters in dimension.

Microscopic Findings. Peutz-Jeghers polyps are characterized by hyperplastic, elongated, tortuous and cystically dilated glands lined by foveolar epithelium with abundant lamina propria; the latter is often composed of a tree-like network of smooth muscle separating the polyps into lobules (fig. 8-18). The smooth muscle component of gastric polyps is usually less developed than in those that occur in the colon, and certainly less developed than in those that occur in the small intestine (90). Peutz-Jeghers polyps may ulcerate and cause the epithelium to have reactive changes. Those with dysplasia have features similar to those seen in hyperplastic polyps. Some polyps, particularly those that are markedly inflamed, show intestinal metaplasia.

Molecular Genetic Findings. Germline mutations of the tumor suppressor gene *STK11* (serine threonine kinase 1), also known as liver kinase B1 *(LKB1)* located on chromosome 19p13.3, are present in 70 to 80 percent of PJS patients (247,253,254). Truncating mutations tend to be associated with an earlier, and higher, frequency of gastric involvement, as well as a higher risk of neoplastic transformation than missense mutations (250). Additional genetic alterations (loss of heterozygosity [LOH] of 17p and 18q) are present in adenocarcinomas, suggesting that *STK11* may be an "initiator" mutation for the development of hamartomas, and that secondary somatic "driver" mutations underlie malignant transformation (255). Some authorities, however, suggest that Peutz-Jeghers polyps may represent an epiphenomenon to the cancer prone condition, and thus, are not obligate malignant precursors (256).

Furthermore, it was shown that PJS polyps are polyclonal cell expansions, not supporting the neoplastic nature of these polyps and the so-called hamartoma-carcinoma sequence (257). However, the exact way these polyps grow and which molecular alterations underlie this process is largely unknown. The stem cell behavior has been studied in PJS polyps and in normal appearing intestinal epithelium from PJS patients. In the latter, stem cell dynamics was increased and the progenitor zone was expanded, indicative of a protracted clonal evolution, a scenario predicting that premalignant lesions in patients with PJS will arise at an accelerated rate in comparison to the general population (258). This mechanism was pointed out as a potential explanation for the increased cancer risk in PJS (258).

PJS polyps display impaired epithelial differentiation, which affects primarily the gastric glands, foveolae, and stroma. A deficit of pepsinogen C-expressing gland cells and an increase in precursor neck cells, along with expansion of the proliferative zone and an increase in smooth muscle actin expressing myofibroblasts of the stroma, are seen.

Treatment. The treatment of sporadic polyps is simple biopsy or polypectomy, the latter of which is typically done in order to rule out a neoplastic polyp. For patients with PJS, surveillance should be initiated as early as 8 years of age. Polyps over 15 mm should be removed. Since children have smaller stomachs than adults, smaller lesions may cause obstruction or intussusception, and some authorities recommend that all pedunculated polyps, regardless of size, be removed.

The type and frequency of follow-up is usually determined on the basis of the findings at first endoscopy. Upper gastrointestinal tract surveillance is recommended to start at 8 years of age if polyps are detected and repeated at 3-year intervals; if no polyps are detected surveillance can be postponed until 18 years of age and then every 3 years, or earlier if symptoms occur (216). More rigorous surveillance (every 1 to 2 years) is recommended after the age of 50 years (218).

Medical management, intended to limit the development of polyps, has shown limited success. Since COX-2 upregulation is involved in PJS polyps, COX-2 inhibitors may be efficacious in patients with severe gastric polyposis (259). Metformin has also been used to decrease polyp burden (260). mTOR inhibition therapy has been evaluated since *mTOR* is the final downstream effector of *STK11/LKB1* inactivation (261).

Prognosis. PJS patients are predisposed to the development of neoplasms of the tubal gut, pancreas, breast, uterus, cervix, testis, ovary, and lung (262). Up to 89 percent of individuals are affected by malignancy by the age of 70 years (262). The lifetime risk for gastric cancer is estimated at 29 percent (216). The youngest reported gastric cancer patient was 12 years of age (263), but in most patients, cancer is detected after a long clinical latency period (greater than 25 years in one study [264]). In the few reported cases, the adenocarcinoma is of the intestinal phenotype (263).

Cowden Syndrome-Associated Polyps

Definition. *Cowden syndrome* is an autosomal dominant disorder that is a component of *PTEN* hamartoma tumor syndrome (PHTS), which encompasses also Bannayan-Riley-Ruvalcaba syndrome, Proteus syndrome, and all syndromes caused by germline mutations of the tumor suppressor gene *PTEN*. Following the recognition of *PTEN* (phosphatase and tensin homolog gene), a tumor suppressor gene located on 10q23.31 (265), germline mutations in individuals with *Cowden syndrome* (CS) were first reported in 1997 (266,267).

General Features. Cowden syndrome was first reported in 1963 (268). The incidence of CS has been reported as 1 in 200,000 (269), but the actual incidence is likely higher given the difficulties in establishing a clinical diagnosis (268). Patients with CS develop polyps in the gastrointestinal tract. CS is a rare autosomal dominant familial cancer syndrome.

Table 8-4

DIAGNOSTIC CRITERIA FOR THE *PTEN* HAMARTOMA TUMOR SYNDROME[a]

Major Criteria
  Breast cancer
  Endometrial cancer (epithelial)
  Thyroid cancer (follicular)
  Gastrointestinal hamartomas (including ganglio-
    neuromas, but excluding hyperplastic polyps; ≥3)
  Lhermitte-Duclos disease (adult)
  Macrocephaly (≥97 percentile: 58 cm for females,
    60 cm for males)
  Macular pigmentation of the glans penis
  Multiple mucocutaneous lesions: trichilemmomas
    (≥3, at least one biopsy proven); acral keratoses
    (≥3 palmoplantar keratotic pits and/or acral
    hyperkeratotic papules); mucocutaneous neuro-
    mas (≥3); oral papillomas (particularly on tongue
    and gingiva), multiple (≥3)

Minor Criteria
  Autism spectrum disorder
  Colon cancer
  Esophageal glycogenic acanthosis (≥3)
  Lipomas (≥3)
  Mental retardation (i.e., IQ ≤75)
  Renal cell carcinoma
  Testicular lipomatosis
  Thyroid cancer (papillary or follicular variant of
    papillary)
  Other thyroid lesions (e.g., adenoma, multinodular
    goiter)
  Vascular anomalies (including multiple intracranial
    developmental venous anomalies)

[a]Adapted from reference 268.

Diagnostic criteria for the principal *PTEN*-related disorders were first established in 1996, prior to identification of the *PTEN* gene and availability of the molecular tools that are used today to confirm the diagnosis. These "consortium" criteria were based on anecdotal clinical experience, combined with data from case reports. Although it was initially reported that approximately 85 percent of patients with CS had an identifiable germline *PTEN* mutation, recent work has shown this diagnostic criterion is not specific (270,271). Newly refined diagnostic criteria for CS were presented in 2013 (268), and include both major and minor criteria (Table 8-4). In order to establish an operational diagnosis in any particular individual, the following is required: 1) three or more major criteria, of which one must include macrocephaly, Lhermitte-Duclos disease, or gastrointestinal

hamartomas; 2) any combination of two major and three minor criteria.

Clinical Features. The *PTEN* mutation is responsible for a combination of mesodermal, endodermal, and ectodermal alterations, and results in the development of multiple hamartomas that involve many organs. In CS, upper gastrointestinal manifestations are detected in 60 percent of patients. Esophageal glycogenic acanthosis is observed in 80 percent of those patients with upper gastrointestinal manifestations (268,272,273).

Gastric polyps are usually numerous, and are present in most patients with CS (273,274). In addition, up to 95 percent of patients develop colonic polyps (268,275). There is increasing recognition that CS patients develop adenomatous, inflammatory, and ganglioneuromatous polyps in addition to intramucosal lipomas and the classic hamartomatous lesions (234,276). Ganglioneuromatous polyps, which are rare in the general population, and intramucosal lipomas, which may be unique to CS, should both prompt further evaluation for the presence of this disorder (276).

Gross Findings. Polyps generally range in size from 0.1 to 2 cm. Most are sessile, without surface erosion (274,277).

Microscopic Findings. CS-associated polyps of the stomach closely resemble hyperplastic polyps and juvenile polyps (278–280). They typically consist of cystically dilated, torturous and irregular foveolar epithelium, often combined with mucin-filled crypts, set within a lamina propria that is mildly fibrotic and shows a minimal degree of chronic inflammation. Some polyps have prominent smooth muscle fibers interspersed among the glands and cysts, and sometimes extending into the submucosa (281). These features may be present in the nonpolypoid gastric mucosa, but often to a lesser degree. In the nonpolypoid mucosa, mild architectural distortion of the crypts and slight fibrosis of the lamina propria are seen. Other polyps that occur in patients with CS, such as ganglioneuromas, fibrolipomas, lipomas, and adenomas, the latter of which are much more common in the colon, have histologic features similar to those that occur in the sporadic setting (278).

Molecular Genetic Findings. CS is linked to germline mutations of the tumor suppressor gene *PTEN* (10q23.31), in which the protein product antagonizes the PI3K/AKT and MAPK pathways (282). Although it is commonly reported that mutations of *PTEN* are responsible for most cases of CS, one prospective accrual study revealed that only 25 percent of patients had a *PTEN* mutation (282). Ten percent of patients have germline *SDHx* mutations (283), approximately 30 percent have germline *KLLN* hypermethylation (284), 9 percent carry *PIK3CA* mutations, and 2 percent display *AKT1* mutations (282). A study by Mester and Eng (285) revealed a 10 percent de novo *PTEN* mutation frequency and also demonstrated the potential for a 47 percent de novo mutation frequency. These features may still be low, given that patients without a positive family history of CS are not usually referred for genetic testing.

Treatment. Although there are no formal guidelines for surveillance of patients with CS, endoscopic surveillance is recommended every 2 to 3 years starting at 15 years of age (216). In patients with concurrent *H. pylori* infection, eradication of the bacterium has been linked to regression of the polyps. This may result in a decrease in the risk of malignancy (286).

Prognosis. CS is associated with an increased risk of breast, endometrial, thyroid gland, and brain cancer (274), as well as an increased risk for the development of benign hamartomatous lesions in mucocutaneous sites, the cerebellum, thyroid gland, and gastrointestinal tract (268). Several reports of gastric cancer in CS patients have been published (275,287,288).

Cronkhite-Canada Syndrome-Associated Polyps

Definition. *Cronkhite-Canada syndrome* is a rare noninherited disorder that shows a combination of ectodermal abnormalities and gastrointestinal hamartomatous polyps associated with protein losing enteropathy. The polyps in the stomach resemble hyperplastic polyps (Table 8-3) (289).

General Features. Most patients affected with Cronkhite-Canada syndrome are in the 6th to 7th decades of life. There is a slight male predominance (290,291). Rare cases that have been reported in pediatric patients may represent infantile juvenile polyposis (292–294). Although Cronkhite-Canada syndrome is ob-

served worldwide, with about 500 cases reported in the literature, most have been diagnosed in Japan. The largest series consists of 180 patients (295,296). The pathogenesis is unknown; recently, however, an autoimmune mechanism has been suggested (295,296).

Clinical Features. Gastrointestinal manifestations of Cronkhite-Canada syndrome typically affect the entire gastrointestinal tract, sparing only the esophagus (297,298). Patients usually present with malabsorption, diarrhea, mucus hypersecretion often with hypoproteinemia, peripheral edema, and weight loss (295,297,298). Secondary symptoms related to electrolyte imbalances also occur, such as paresthesia, tetanus, and seizures (297). Extragastrointestinal symptoms usually follow gastrointestinal manifestations by weeks to months, although they may be present at the time of diagnosis. These include ectodermal manifestations, such as alopecia, onychodystrophy, and skin hyperpigmentation, which may involve extremities, face, and buccal mucosa (299–302). Other systemic manifestations are observed as well (295).

Gross Findings. Endoscopically, patients with Cronkhite-Canada syndrome often show generalized gastric mucosal edema. The polyps are usually sessile, erythematous lesions that often have a characteristic "polyp on polyp" appearance (fig. 8-19, left) (295). The esophagus and other portions of the gastrointestinal tract may be completely spared by involvement with polyps. Rare polyps are villiform in shape, and the adjacent mucosa shows diffuse mucosal thickening or cobblestoning, particularly after medical therapy (295).

Cronkhite-Canada syndrome-associated polyps resemble sporadic hyperplastic polyps. The polyps range in size from 0.5 to 1.5 cm and are often superimposed on enlarged, diffuse and irregular rugae in the fundus and antrum. In this manner, the endoscopic appearance of the stomach resembles Ménétrier disease. In Ménétrier disease, however, the antrum is normally spared.

Microscopic Findings. The foveolar epithelium is elongated, papillary, villiform, and distorted, and associated with abundant lamina propria showing vascular proliferation, congestion, a mild degree of active and chronic inflammation and edema (fig. 8-19, right).

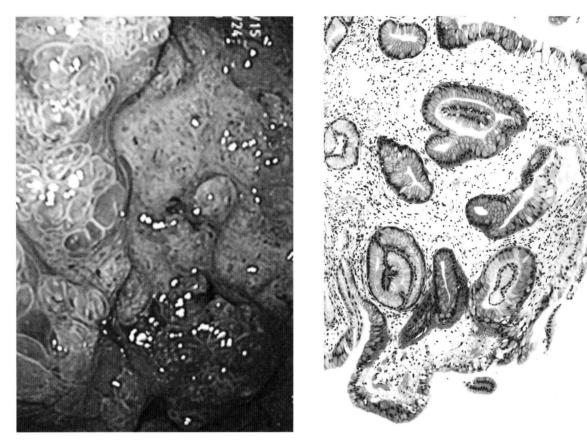

Figure 8-19

CRONKHITE-CANADA SYNDROME

Left: Multiple nodules carpet the gastric mucosa. In areas, there appears to be a "polyp-on-polyp" pattern, with smaller polyps appearing to develop on top of larger polyps.

Right: A typical Cronkhite-Canada syndrome polyp has foveolar hyperplasia and reactive changes, lamina propria edema, and increased inflammation.

Cronkhite-Canada syndrome polyps do not normally show prominent inflammation or muscularis hyperplasia to the degree that occurs in hyperplastic polyps. Some polyps show a dense eosinophilic infiltrate or abundant neutrophils with microabscesses (289,303). Polyps may show erosions and, on occasion, non-necrotizing granulomas, which may mimic inflammatory bowel disease. Rarely, IgG4 plasma cell infiltration, associated with atrophy and prominent apoptotic bodies, is present and suggests a defect in immune regulation.

The interpolypoid gastric mucosa also resembles that of Ménétrier disease (304,305). This mucosa may show marked surface and foveolar hyperplasia with cystic change and atrophy of the glands (290,305). Alternating areas of atro-phy and foveolar hyperplasia with microcystic change are characteristic.

Treatment. Treatment recommendations have not been standardized. Oral corticosteroids remain the most common form of therapy. Surgery is usually reserved for the treatment of complications, whether medical or surgical (303). Medical therapy can lead to attenuation of mucosal lesions, which then may result in the development of a nodular cobblestone mucosal appearance (295).

Prognosis. The prognosis of patients with Cronkhite-Canada syndrome is poor. The 5-year mortality rate is about 55 percent. Common causes of mortality include gastrointestinal bleeding, sepsis, and congestive heart failure. The risk of cancer is controversial, even though colorectal and gastric carcinomas seem to be more frequent than in the general population (289,303,306), with an incidence rate of approximately 5 percent (307). Gastric carcinomas typically show a gastric phenotype (308).

Differential Diagnosis of Hyperplastic and Hamartomatous Polyps

From a pathologic point of view, hyperplastic polyps are difficult to differentiate from most other benign polyps of the stomach, such as polypoid foveolar hyperplasia, gastritis cystica polyposa, Ménétrier disease, and virtually all of the gastric hamartomas including juvenile polyps, Peutz-Jeghers polyps, Cowden syndrome-associated polyps, and Cronkhite-Canada syndrome-associated polyps. The characteristics of polyposis syndromes that involve the stomach are summarized in Table 8-3.

Differentiating these polyps from one another is difficult in biopsies when the entire polyp has not been removed and in instances when the nonpolypoid gastric mucosa has not been sampled. A definite and specific diagnosis is normally made in conjunction with knowledge of the clinical and endoscopic features, combined with evaluation of the changes in the adjacent nonpolypoid gastric mucosa. Both Cronkhite-Canada syndrome-associated polyps and polyps associated with Ménétrier disease show epithelial and lamina propria abnormalities in the nonpolypoid mucosa, whereas other disorders, such as juvenile polyps and Peutz-Jeghers polyps, do not. Hyperplastic polyps generally develop on a background of chronic gastritis or in the postsurgical setting. Thus, in the absence of clinical evidence of a genetic syndrome, the presence of one or several hyperplastic-like polyps in a patient with *H. pylori* or autoimmune gastritis is almost always diagnostic of a hyperplastic polyp.

In addition to evaluation of the clinical, endoscopic, and interpolypoid gastric mucosal features, there are slight differences in the pattern of each of the major polyps that can help pathologists distinguish these lesions from each other. In contrast to hyperplastic polyps, fundic gland polyps show surface and foveolar hypoplasia, contain cystically dilated glands lined predominantly by parietal and chief cells, and show little or no inflammation

in the lamina propria. Gastritis cystica polyposa is a predominantly submucosal lesion characterized by cystically dilated, distorted, and irregularly shaped glands and acellular mucin located either within or beneath the muscularis mucosae in the submucosa. The surface mucosa and surrounding tissue usually reveal chronic gastritis and bile reflux related changes. The patient usually has a history of prior gastric surgery. Juvenile polyps may appear identical to hyperplastic polyps histologically, but the former are not usually as inflamed, and the surface mucosa is usually intact. However, definite identification would require clinical correlation. Peutz-Jeghers syndrome-associated polyps show a better developed muscularis framework, more extensive than that normally seen in hyperplastic polyps, and lack significant stromal inflammation. These polyps are also not normally associated with chronic gastritis. Cowden syndrome-associated polyps show more extensive lamina propria fibrosis and less edema and inflammation, and less conspicuous glandular distortion and cysts, compared to hyperplastic polyps. Furthermore, these polyps may be associated with ganglioneuromas and show more abundant adipose tissue in the lamina propria. Similar to Ménétrier disease, Cronkhite-Canada syndrome-associated polyps often show foveolar hyperplasia, glandular atrophy, and microcystic change in the adjacent nonpolypoid mucosa, but in Ménétrier disease, the features are much less pronounced and atrophy may not be present. Furthermore, Ménétrier disease, in contrast to Cronkite-Canada syndrome which involves the entire stomach, affects exclusively the gastric corpus.

XANTHOMA

Definition. *Gastric xanthoma* is a benign mucosal lesion that develops as a result of accumulation of PAS-negative lipid-laden foamy histiocytes in the lamina propria.

General Features. Xanthomas are detected in 1 to 7 percent of endoscopies. Gastric xanthomas develop as a result of chronic mucosal injury, such as secondary to *H. pylori* gastritis, and as a result also show an association with intestinal metaplasia and carcinoma (309–312).

The pathogenesis of xanthoma formation is unclear, but it is not considered a result of a lipid metabolic disorder (313). Xanthomas show

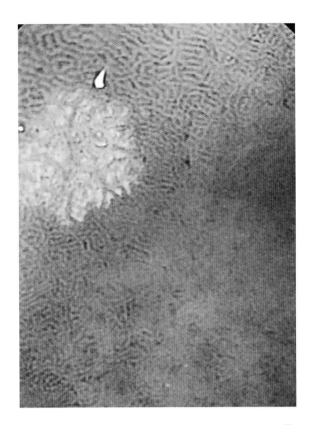
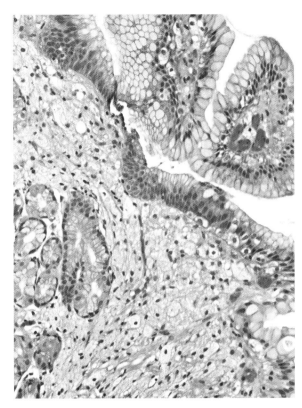

Figure 8-20

GASTRIC XANTHOMA

Left: Endoscopically, the xanthoma is an irregular patch of yellow or tan mucosa with irregular borders. The background mucosa appears normal.

Right: High-power view of a xanthoma shows an organized collection of histiocytes in the lamina propria containing pale cytoplasm. In contrast to signet ring cell carcinoma, these cells have a low N/C ratio, small round to oval and centrally located nuclei, and absence of mitoses.

a high percentage of oxidized LDL, thus, this is considered evidence that it arises secondary to chronic mucosal injury and macrophage chemotaxis (310). Various lipids (cholesterol, neutral fat, low-density lipoprotein, and oxidized low-density lipoprotein), have been detected within xanthoma cells.

Gross Findings. Gastric xanthomas are typically small (less than 1 cm), rounded, yellowish, sessile, flat to slightly elevated polypoid lesions (fig. 8-20, left) that usually occur in the antrum, along the lesser curvature. In addition, they often develop close to stomas, on the posterior wall or along the greater curvature, in patients who have had previous gastric surgery (309,313,314). Xanthomas are usually solitary. Multiple lesions are uncommon, although rare cases of gastric xanthomatosis have been reported (311,314).

Microscopic Findings. Xanthomas are composed of an organized collection of macrophages usually localized to the upper third of the mucosa (fig. 8-20, right) (310). The affected macrophages have distinct cell membranes and small, centrally located, round or oval nuclei. *H. pylori* gastritis, chronic atrophic gastritis, and intestinal metaplasia are commonly noted in the surrounding mucosa (309–311). The main use of immunohistochemistry is to confirm the histiocytic nature of the cells. They are typically CD68 positive, but negative for cytokeratins.

Differential Diagnosis. The main differential diagnosis includes signet ring cell carcinoma, clear cell variant of low-grade neuroendocrine tumors, and metastatic renal cell carcinoma. These entities are excluded by the lack of cytokeratins and neuroendocrine markers in xanthomas.

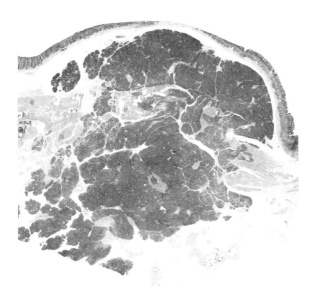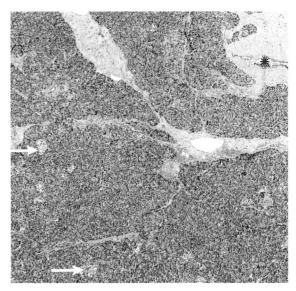

Figure 8-21

PANCREATIC HETEROTOPIA

Left: A collection of pancreatic tissue involves the submucosa, muscularis, and even the serosa. The overlying mucosa is intact.

Right: The focus of heterotopia is composed of pancreatic acinar tissue, scattered endocrine cell islets (white arrows), and a centrally located pancreatic duct (black star).

Treatment. Xanthomas have no malignancy risk and as a result, do not require any distinct form of treatment.

PANCREATIC HETEROTOPIA

Definition. *Pancreatic heterotopia* is the presence of (heterotopic) pancreatic tissue within the stomach. Heterotopic components may include one or more combinations of ductal, acinar, and endocrine cell islet tissue.

General and Clinical Features. Pancreatic heterotopia is the second most common type of pancreatic congenital abnormality after pancreas divisum. It commonly presents as a polypoid lesion located within a few centimeters of the pylorus. The submucosa is the most common area of involvement, but it can also involve the muscularis and serosa (315).

Heterotopic pancreas is present in 1 of 500 laparotomies, and tends to occur more often in males (315). A slight female predominance was observed in a series of 184 cases from China (316). The pathogenesis is unknown, but likely is related to abnormal migration or accumulation of residual rests or pancreatic buds in the stomach during embryogenesis.

Gastric heterotopic pancreas is usually asymptomatic. Large lesions may be associated with abdominal pain, vomiting, gastric outlet obstruction, or dysphagia (317–319).

Gross Findings. Endoscopically, heterotopic pancreas often appears as small (typically 0.5 to 1.0 cm) submucosal lesions often containing a central nipple-like umbilication in the mucosa on the surface. They occur most often within 5 cm of the pylorus. On endoscopic ultrasound, heterotopic pancreas appears as a hypoechoic submucosal mass with small, scattered, heterogeneous signals which correspond to adipose tissue (320). Because of its usual submucosal location, endoscopic biopsies often fail to provide a tissue diagnosis (320).

Microscopic Findings. Heterotopic pancreas may show all of the components of the normal pancreas (ducts, acinar tissue, and endocrine islets) (fig. 8-21) or only one or two components. Isolated endocrine islets are rare (317). Abundant smooth muscle may be present, especially in lesions that are associated with pancreatic ducts. This has sometimes been termed "adenomyoma" or "myoepithelial hamartoma." The surrounding gastric mucosa may show reactive changes, edema, congestion, and inflammation.

Differential Diagnosis. The differential diagnosis includes well-differentiated adenocarcinoma, gastritis cystica polyposa, and pancreatic acinar metaplasia. The presence of all three cellular components of the pancreas, i.e., ducts, acini, and endocrine islets, helps differentiate these other disorders. If either acini or islets are not present, the diagnosis is more difficult. Adenocarcinoma reveals architectural and cytologic atypia, and usually other features of malignancy, such as necrosis or desmoplasia. The ducts in pancreatic heterotopia are normally well organized or lobular, and the duct profiles are smooth (as opposed to irregular or jagged in adenocarcinoma). Smooth muscle hyperplasia is often present in heterotopia and typically surrounds the ducts in a uniform and consistent manner. Pancreatic acinar metaplasia is usually arranged in small nests or lobules, in continuity with the surrounding gastric glands, and is histologically indistinguishable from pancreatic acinar cells. The presence of ductal elements, pancreatic stroma, or well-defined islets excludes pancreatic acinar metaplasia.

Treatment. Definitive treatment is usually justified when the lesion causes symptoms or when the clinician is uncertain about the nature of the lesion (e.g., exclusion of GIST or other neoplasm). Endoscopic resection or limited surgical resection is the treatment of choice based on the size, extent, and location of the lesion.

Prognosis. Ectopic pancreatic tissue can undergo pathologic changes similar to those that occur in the normal pancreas, such as acute or chronic pancreatitis (321), pseudocysts (322), and mucinous cysts (323,324). Neoplastic transformation, including pancreatic intraepithelial neoplasia (323), ductal adenocarcinoma, acinar cell carcinoma, and pancreatic endocrine tumors, have all been reported in association with pancreatic heterotopia in the stomach, but are rare (325–327).

REFERENCES

1. Correa P. A human model of gastric carcinogenesis. Cancer Res 1988;48:3554-60.
2. Kato M, Asaka M. Recent development of gastric cancer prevention. Jpn J Clin Oncol 2012;42:987-94.
3. Vieth M, Riddell RH, Montgomery EA. High-grade dysplasia versus carcinoma: east is east and west is west, but does it need to be that way? Am J Surg Pathol 2014;38:1453-6.
4. Lewin KJ. Nomenclature problems of gastrointestinal epithelial neoplasia. Am J Surg Pathol 1998;22:1043-7.
5. Goldstein NS, Lewin KJ. Gastric epithelial dysplasia and adenoma: historical review and histological criteria for grading. Hum Pathol 1997;28:127-33.
6. Ming SC, Bajtai A, Correa P, et al. Gastric dysplasia. Significance and pathologic criteria. Cancer 1984;54:1794-1801.
7. Lauwers GY, Riddell RH. Gastric epithelial dysplasia. Gut 1999;45:784-90.
8. Zhang YC. Typing and grading of gastric dysplasia. In: Zhang YC, Kawai K, eds. Precancerous conditions and lesions of the stomach. Berlin, Heidelberg: Springer; 1993:65-84.
9. Correa P, Haenszel W, Cuello C, et al. Gastric precancerous process in a high risk population: cross-sectional studies. Cancer Res 1990;50:4731-6.
10. Li D, Bautista MC, Jiang SF, et al. Risks and predictors of gastric adenocarcinoma in patients with gastric intestinal metaplasia and dysplasia: a population-based study. Am J Gastroenterol 2016;111:1104-13.
11. Jeon SW. Endoscopic management of gastric dysplasia: cutting edge technology needs a new paradigm. World J Gastrointest Endosc 2010;2:301-4.
12. de Vries AC, van Grieken NC, Looman CW, et al. Gastric cancer risk in patients with premalignant gastric lesions: a nationwide cohort study in the Netherlands. Gastroenterology 2008;134:945-2.
13. Ahn SY, Jang SI, Lee DW, Jeon SW. Gastric endoscopic submucosal dissection is safe for day patients. Clin Endosc 2014;47:538-43.

14. Dinis-Ribeiro M, Areia M, de Vries AC, et al. Management of precancerous conditions and lesions in the stomach (MAPS): guideline from the European Society of Gastrointestinal Endoscopy (ESGE), European Helicobacter Study Group (EHSG), European Society of Pathology (ESP), and the Sociedade Portuguesa de Endoscopia Digestiva (SPED). Endoscopy 2012;44:74-94.

15. Arnason T, Liang WY, Alfaro E, et al. Morphology and natural history of familial adenomatous polyposis-associated dysplastic fundic gland polyps. Histopathology 2014;65:353-62.

16. Stolte M, Vieth M, Ebert MP. High-grade dysplasia in sporadic fundic gland polyps: clinically relevant or not? Eur J Gastroenterol Hepatol 2003;15:1153-6.

17. Bianchi LK, Burke CA, Bennett AE, Lopez R, Hasson H, Church JM. Fundic gland polyp dysplasia is common in familial adenomatous polyposis. Clin Gastroenterol Hepatol 2008;6:180-5.

18. Garrean S, Hering J, Saied A, Jani J, Espat NJ. Gastric adenocarcinoma arising from fundic gland polyps in a patient with familial adenomatous polyposis syndrome. Am Surg 2008;74:79-83.

19. Ma C, Giardiello FM, Montgomery EA. Upper tract juvenile polyps in juvenile polyposis patients: dysplasia and malignancy are associated with foveolar, intestinal, and pyloric differentiation. Am J Surg Pathol 2014;38:1618-26.

20. Carneiro F, David L, Seruca R, Castedo S, Nesland JM, Sobrinho-Simoes M. Hyperplastic polyposis and diffuse carcinoma of the stomach. A study of a family. Cancer 1993;72:323-9.

21. Alfaro EE, Lauwers GY. Early gastric neoplasia: diagnosis and implications. Adv Anat Pathol 2011;18:268-80.

22. Shaib YH, Rugge M, Graham DY, Genta RM. Management of gastric polyps: an endoscopy-based approach. Clin Gastroenterol Hepatol 2013;11:1374-84.

23. Worthley DL, Phillips KD, Wayte N, et al. Gastric adenocarcinoma and proximal polyposis of the stomach (GAPPS): a new autosomal dominant syndrome. Gut 2012;61:774-9.

24. Tsuji Y, Ohata K, Sekiguchi M, et al. Magnifying endoscopy with narrow-band imaging helps determine the management of gastric adenomas. Gastric Cancer 2012;15:414-8.

25. Schlemper RJ, Riddell RH, Kato Y, et al. The Vienna classification of gastrointestinal epithelial neoplasia. Gut 2000;47:251-5.

26. Kang DH, Choi CW, Kim HW, et al. Predictors of upstage diagnosis after endoscopic resection of gastric low-grade dysplasia. Surg Endosc 2017. [Epub ahead of print]

27. Baek DH, Kim GH, Park DY, et al. Gastric epithelial dysplasia: characteristics and long-term follow-up results after endoscopic resection according to morphological categorization. BMC Gastroenterol 2015;15:17.

28. Domizio P, Talbot IC, Spigelman AD, Williams CB, Phillips RK. Upper gastrointestinal pathology in familial adenomatous polyposis: results from a prospective study of 102 patients. J Clin Pathol 1990;43:738-43.

29. Oberhuber G, Stolte M. Gastric polyps: an update of their pathology and biological significance. Virchows Arch 2000;437:581-90.

30. Srivastava A, Lauwers GY. Gastric epithelial dysplasia: the Western perspective. Dig Liver Dis 2008;40:641-9.

31. Jass JR. A classification of gastric dysplasia. Histopathology 1983;7:181-93.

32. Abraham SC, Park SJ, Lee JH, Mugartegui L, Wu TT. Genetic alterations in gastric adenomas of intestinal and foveolar phenotypes. Mod Pathol 2003;16:786-95.

33. Ito H, Yasui W, Yoshida K, Nakayama H, Tahara E. Depressed tubular adenoma of the stomach: pathological and immunohistochemical features. Histopathology 1990;17:419-26.

34. Lauwers GY, Carneiro F, Graham DY, Curado MP, Franceschi S, Montgomery E, Tatematsu M, Hattori T. Gastric carcinoma. Lyon: IARC Press; 2010.

35. Nakamura T, Nakano G. Histopathological classification and malignant change in gastric polyps. J Clin Pathol 1985;38:754-64.

36. Cho SJ, Choi IJ, Kim CG, et al. Risk of high-grade dysplasia or carcinoma in gastric biopsy-proven low-grade dysplasia: an analysis using the Vienna classification. Endoscopy 2011;43:465-71.

37. Hull MJ, Mino-Kenudson M, Nishioka NS, et al. Endoscopic mucosal resection: an improved diagnostic procedure for early gastroesophageal epithelial neoplasms. Am J Surg Pathol 2006;30:114-8.

38. Kim YJ, Park JC, Kim JH, et al. Histologic diagnosis based on forceps biopsy is not adequate for determining endoscopic treatment of gastric adenomatous lesions. Endoscopy 2010;42:620-6.

39. Rugge M, Correa P, Dixon MF, et al. Gastric dysplasia: the Padova international classification. Am J Surg Pathol 2000;24:167-76.

40. Rugge M, Leandro G, Farinati F, et al. Gastric epithelial dysplasia. How clinicopathologic background relates to management. Cancer 1995;76:376-82.

41. Rugge M, Farinati F, Di Mario F, Baffa R, Valiante F, Cardin F. Gastric epithelial dysplasia: a prospective multicenter follow-up study from the Interdisciplinary Group on Gastric Epithelial Dysplasia. Hum Pathol 1991;22:1002-8.

42. Japanese Gastric Cancer Association. Japanese Classification of Gastric Carcinoma - 2nd English Edition. Gastric Cancer 1998;1:10-24.

43. Riddell RH, Iwafuchi M. Problems arising from eastern and western classification systems for gastrointestinal dysplasia and carcinoma: are they resolvable? Histopathology 1998;33:197-202.

44. Japanese Gastric Cancer Association. Japanese classification of gastric carcinoma: 3rd English edition. Gastric Cancer 2011;14:101-12.

45. Schlemper RJ, Itabashi M, Kato Y, et al. Differences in diagnostic criteria for gastric carcinoma between Japanese and western pathologists. Lancet 1997;349:1725-9.

46. Stolte M. The new Vienna classification of epithelial neoplasia of the gastrointestinal tract: advantages and disadvantages. Virchows Arch 2003;442:99-106.

47. Brien TP, Farraye FA, Odze RD. Gastric dysplasia-like epithelial atypia associated with chemoradiotherapy for esophageal cancer: a clinicopathologic and immunohistochemical study of 15 cases. Mod Pathol 2001;14:389-96.

48. Riddell RH, Goldman H, Ransohoff DF, et al. Dysplasia in inflammatory bowel disease: standardized classification with provisional clinical applications. Hum Pathol 1983;14:931-68.

49. Isaacson P. Biopsy appearances easily mistaken for malignancy in gastrointestinal endoscopy. Histopathology 1982;6:377-89.

50. Weidner N, Smith JG, LaVanway JM. Peptic ulceration with marked epithelial atypia following hepatic arterial infusion chemotherapy. A lesion initially misinterpreted as carcinoma. Am J Surg Pathol 1983;7:261-8.

51. Petras RE, Hart WR, Bukowski RM. Gastric epithelial atypia associated with hepatic arterial infusion chemotherapy. Its distinction from early gastric carcinoma. Cancer 1985;56:745-50.

52. Hattori T. Morphological range of hyperplastic polyps and carcinomas arising in hyperplastic polyps of the stomach. J Clin Pathol 1985;38:622-30.

53. Park DY, Srivastava A, Kim GH, et al. Adenomatous and foveolar gastric dysplasia: distinct patterns of mucin expression and background intestinal metaplasia. Am J Surg Pathol 2008;32:524-33.

54. Valente P, Garrido M, Gullo I, et al. Epithelial dysplasia of the stomach with gastric immunophenotype shows features of biological aggressiveness. Gastric Cancer 2015;18:720-8.

55. Serra S, Ali R, Bateman AC, et al. Gastric foveolar dysplasia: a survey of reporting habits and diagnostic criteria. Pathology 2017;49:391-6.

56. Murayama H, Kikuchi M, Enjoji M, Morita N, Haraguchi Y. Changes in gastric mucosa that antedate gastric carcinoma. Cancer 1990;66:2017-26.

57. Tava F, Luinetti O, Ghigna MR, et al. Type or extension of intestinal metaplasia and immature/atypical "indefinite-for-dysplasia" lesions as predictors of gastric neoplasia. Hum Pathol 2006;37:1489-97.

58. Agoston AT, Odze RD. Evidence that gastric pit dysplasia-like atypia is a neoplastic precursor lesion. Hum Pathol 2014;45:446-55.

59. Shin N, Jo HJ, Kim WK, et al. Gastric pit dysplasia in adjacent gastric mucosa in 414 gastric cancers: prevalence and characteristics. Am J Surg Pathol 2011;35:1021-9.

60. Ghandur-Mnaymneh L, Paz J, Roldan E, Cassady J. Dysplasia of nonmetaplastic gastric mucosa. A proposal for its classification and its possible relationship to diffuse-type gastric carcinoma. Am J Surg Pathol 1988;12:96-114.

61. Misdraji J, Lauwers GY. Gastric epithelial dysplasia. Semin Diagn Pathol 2002;19:20-30.

62. Kumarasinghe MP, Lim TK, Ooi CJ, Luman W, Tan SY, Koh M. Tubule neck dysplasia: precursor lesion of signet ring cell carcinoma and the immunohistochemical profile. Pathology 2006;38:468-71.

63. Dong B, Xie YQ, Chen K, et al. Differences in biological features of gastric dysplasia, indefinite dysplasia, reactive hyperplasia and discriminant analysis of these lesions. World J Gastroenterol 2005;11:3595-600.

64. Lisovsky M, Ogawa F, Dresser K, Woda B, Lauwers GY. Loss of cell polarity protein Lgl2 in foveolar-type gastric dysplasia: correlation with expression of the apical marker aPKC-zeta. Virchows Arch 2010;457:635-42.

65. Lee JR, Chung WC, Kim JD, et al. Differential LINE-1 hypomethylation of gastric low-grade dysplasia from high grade dysplasia and intramucosal cancer. Gut Liver 2011;5:149-53.

66. Kim EJ, Chung WC, Kim DB, et al. Long interspersed nuclear element (LINE)-1 methylation level as a molecular marker of early gastric cancer. Dig Liver Dis 2016;48:1093-7.

67. Wang L, Li HG, Xia ZS, Lu J, Peng TS. IMP3 is a novel biomarker to predict metastasis and prognosis of gastric adenocarcinoma: a retrospective study. Chin Med J 2010;123:3554-8.

68. Strehl JD, Hoegel J, Hornicek I, Hartmann A, Riener MO. Immunohistochemical expression of IMP3 and p53 in inflammatory lesions and neoplastic lesions of the gastric mucosa. Int J Clin Exp Pathol 2014;7:2091-101.

69. Lim CH, Cho YK, Kim SW, et al. The chronological sequence of somatic mutations in early gastric carcinogenesis inferred from multiregion sequencing of gastric adenomas. Oncotarget 2016;7:39758-67.

70. Min BH, Hwang J, Kim NK, et al. Dysregulated Wnt signalling and recurrent mutations of the tumour suppressor RNF43 in early gastric carcinogenesis. J Pathol 2016;240:304-314.

71. Lansdown M, Quirke P, Dixon MF, Axon AT, Johnston D. High grade dysplasia of the gastric mucosa: a marker for gastric carcinoma. Gut 1990;31:977-83.

72. Rugge M, Farinati F, Baffa R, et al. Gastric epithelial dysplasia in the natural history of gastric cancer: a multicenter prospective follow-up study. Interdisciplinary Group on Gastric Epithelial Dysplasia. Gastroenterology 1994;107:1288-96.

73. Lauwers GY, Ban S, Mino M, et al. Endoscopic mucosal resection for gastric epithelial neoplasms: a study of 39 cases with emphasis on the evaluation of specimens and recommendations for optimal pathologic analysis. Mod Pathol 2004;17:2-8.

74. Ono H, Kondo H, Gotoda T, et al. Endoscopic mucosal resection for treatment of early gastric cancer. Gut 2001;48:225-9.

75. Kokkola A, Haapiainen R, Laxen F, et al. Risk of gastric carcinoma in patients with mucosal dysplasia associated with atrophic gastritis: a follow up study. J Clin Pathol 1996;49:979-84.

76. Bearzi I, Brancorsini D, Santinelli A, Rezai B, Mannello B, Ranaldi R. Gastric dysplasia: a ten-year follow-up study. Pathol Res Pract 1994;190:61-8.

77. Di Gregorio C, Morandi P, Fante R, De Gaetani C. Gastric dysplasia. A follow-up study. Am J Gastroenterol 1993;88:1714-9.

78. You WC, Blot WJ, Li JY, et al. Precancerous gastric lesions in a population at high risk of stomach cancer. Cancer Res 1993;53:1317-21.

79. Saraga EP, Gardiol D, Costa J. Gastric dysplasia. A histological follow-up study. Am J Surg Pathol 1987;11:788-96.

80. Fertitta AM, Comin U, Terruzzi V, et al. Clinical significance of gastric dysplasia: a multicenter follow-up study. Gastrointestinal Endoscopic Pathology Study Group. Endoscopy 1993;25:265-8.

81. Yamada H, Ikegami M, Shimoda T, Takagi N, Maruyama M. Long-term follow-up study of gastric adenoma/dysplasia. Endoscopy 2004;36:390-6.

82. Rugge M, Cassaro M, Di Mario F, et al. The long term outcome of gastric non-invasive neoplasia. Gut 2003;52:1111-6.

83. Raftopoulos SC, Kumarasinghe P, de Boer B, et al. Gastric intraepithelial neoplasia in a Western population. Eur J Gastroenterol Hepatol 2012;24:48-54.

84. Morson BC, Sobin LH, Grundmann E, Johansen A, Nagayo T, Serck-Hanssen A. Precancerous conditions and epithelial dysplasia in the stomach. J Clin Pathol 1980;33:711-21.

85. Carmack SW, Genta RM, Graham DY, Lauwers GY. Management of gastric polyps: a pathology-based guide for gastroenterologists. Nat Rev Gastroenterol Hepatol 2009;6:331-41.

86. Omori T, Kamiya Y, Tahara T, et al. Correlation between magnifying narrow band imaging and histopathology in gastric protruding/or polypoid lesions: a pilot feasibility trial. BMC Gastroenterol 2012;12:17.

87. Wallace M, Lauwers GY, Chen Y, et al. Miami classification for probe-based confocal laser endomicroscopy. Endoscopy 2011;43:882-91.

88. Muehldorfer SM, Stolte M, Martus P, Hahn EG, Ell C, Multicenter Study Group "Gastric Polyps." Diagnostic accuracy of forceps biopsy versus polypectomy for gastric polyps: a prospective multicentre study. Gut 2002;50:465-70.

89. Stolte M, Sticht T, Eidt S, Ebert D, Finkenzeller G. Frequency, location, and age and sex distribution of various types of gastric polyp. Endoscopy 1994;26:659-65.

90. Carmack SW, Genta RM, Schuler CM, Saboorian MH. The current spectrum of gastric polyps: a 1-year national study of over 120,000 patients. Am J Gastroenterol 2009;104:1524-32.

91. Hackeng WM, Montgomery EA, Giardiello FM, et al. Morphology and genetics of pyloric gland adenomas in familial adenomatous polyposis. Histopathology 2017;70:549-57.

92. Chen ZM, Scudiere JR, Abraham SC, Montgomery E. Pyloric gland adenoma: an entity distinct from gastric foveolar type adenoma. Am J Surg Pathol 2009;33:186-93.

93. Wood LD, Salaria SN, Cruise MW, Giardiello FM, Montgomery EA. Upper GI tract lesions in familial adenomatous polyposis (FAP): enrichment of pyloric gland adenomas and other gastric and duodenal neoplasms. Am J Surg Pathol 2014;38:389-93.

94. Hashimoto T, Ogawa R, Matsubara A, et al. Familial adenomatous polyposis-associated and sporadic pyloric gland adenomas of the upper gastrointestinal tract share common genetic features. Histopathology 2015;67:689-98.

95. Lee SE, Kang SY, Cho J, et al. Pyloric gland adenoma in Lynch syndrome. Am J Surg Pathol 2014;38:784-92.

96. Vieth M, Montgomery EA. Some observations on pyloric gland adenoma: an uncommon and long ignored entity! J Clin Pathol 2014;67:883-90.

97. Vieth M, Kushima R, Borchard F, Stolte M. Pyloric gland adenoma: a clinico-pathological analysis of 90 cases. Virchows Arch 2003;442:317-21.

98. Vieth M, Kushima R, de Jonge JP, Borchard F, Oellig F, Stolte M. Adenoma with gastric differentiation (so-called pyloric gland adenoma) in a heterotopic gastric corpus mucosa in the rectum. Virchows Arch 2005;446:542-5.

99. Poeschl EM, Siebert F, Vieth M, Langner C. Pyloric gland adenoma arising in gastric heterotopia within the duodenal bulb. Endoscopy 2011;43(Suppl 2)UCTN:E336-7.

100. Kushima R, Ruthlein HJ, Stolte M, Bamba M, Hattori T, Borchard F. 'Pyloric gland-type adenoma' arising in heterotopic gastric mucosa of the duodenum, with dysplastic progression of the gastric type. Virchows Arch 1999;435:452-7.
101. Pezhouh MK, Park JY. Gastric pyloric gland adenoma. Arch Pathol Lab Med 2015;139:823-6.
102. Vieth M, Kushima R, Mukaisho K, Sakai R, Kasami T, Hattori T. Immunohistochemical analysis of pyloric gland adenomas using a series of Mucin 2, Mucin 5AC, Mucin 6, CD10, Ki67 and p53. Virchows Arch 2010;457:529-36.
103. Kushima R, Sekine S, Matsubara A, Taniguchi H, Ikegami M, Tsuda H. Gastric adenocarcinoma of the fundic gland type shares common genetic and phenotypic features with pyloric gland adenoma. Pathol Int 2013;63:318-25.
104. Matsubara A, Sekine S, Kushima R, et al. Frequent GNAS and KRAS mutations in pyloric gland adenoma of the stomach and duodenum. J Pathol 2013;229:579-87.
105. Dumoulin FL, Abel J, Zumfelde P, Hildenbrand R, Bollmann R. [Endoscopic resection of a rare gastric adenoma (pyloric gland adenoma) with transition into a well-differentiated adenocarcinoma.] Z Gastroenterol 2012;50:393-5. [German]
106. Singhi AD, Lazenby AJ, Montgomery EA. Gastric adenocarcinoma with chief cell differentiation: a proposal for reclassification as oxyntic gland polyp/adenoma. Am J Surg Pathol 2012;36:1030-5.
107. Chan K, Brown IS, Kyle T, Lauwers GY, Kumarasinghe MP. Chief cell-predominant gastric polyps: a series of 12 cases with literature review. Histopathology 2016;68:825-33.
108. Ueyama H, Matsumoto K, Nagahara A, Hayashi T, Yao T, Watanabe S. Gastric adenocarcinoma of the fundic gland type (chief cell predominant type). Endoscopy 2014;46:153-7.
109. Ueyama H, Yao T, Nakashima Y, et al. Gastric adenocarcinoma of fundic gland type (chief cell predominant type): proposal for a new entity of gastric adenocarcinoma. Am J Surg Pathol 2010;34:609-19.
109a. Ueo T, Yonemasu H, Ishida T. Gastric adenocarcinoma of fundic gland type with unusual behavior. Dig Endosc 2014;26:293-4.
110. Nomura R, Saito T, Mitomi H, et al. GNAS mutation as an alternative mechanism of activation of the Wnt/beta-catenin signaling pathway in gastric adenocarcinoma of the fundic gland type. Hum Pathol 2014;45:2488-96.
111. Lee TI, Jang JY, Kim S, Kim JW, Chang YW, Kim YW. Oxyntic gland adenoma endoscopically mimicking a gastric neuroendocrine tumor: a case report. World J Gastroenterol 2015;21:5099-104.
112. Weston BR, Helper DJ, Rex DK. Positive predictive value of endoscopic features deemed typical of gastric fundic gland polyps. J Clin Gastroenterol 2003;36:399-402.
113. Genta RM, Schuler CM, Robiou CI, Lash RH. No association between gastric fundic gland polyps and gastrointestinal neoplasia in a study of over 100,000 patients. Clin Gastroenterol Hepatol 2009;7:849-54.
114. Jasperson KW, Patel SG, Ahnen DJ. APC-associated polyposis conditions. In: Adam MP, Ardinger HH, Pagon RA, et al., eds. GeneReviews(R). Seattle (WA): University of Washington, Seattle University of Washington, Seattle. 2017.
115. Poulsen ML, Bisgaard ML. MUTYH associated polyposis (MAP). Curr Genomics 2008;9:420-35.
116. Tsuchikame N, Ishimaru Y, Ohshima S, Takahashi M. Three familial cases of fundic gland polyposis without polyposis coli. Virchows Arch A Pathol Anat Histopathol 1993;422:337-40.
117. Torbenson M, Lee JH, Cruz-Correa M, et al. Sporadic fundic gland polyposis: a clinical, histological, and molecular analysis. Mod Pathol 2002;15:718-23.
118. Talseth-Palmer BA. The genetic basis of colonic adenomatous polyposis syndromes. Hered Cancer Cin Pract 2017;15:5.
119. Jalving M, Koornstra JJ, Wesseling J, Boezen HM, De Jong S, Kleibeuker JH. Increased risk of fundic gland polyps during long-term proton pump inhibitor therapy. Aliment Pharmacol Ther 2006;24:1341-8.
120. Samarasam I, Roberts-Thomson J, Brockwell D. Gastric fundic gland polyps: a clinico-pathological study from North West Tasmania. ANZ J Surg 2009;79:467-70.
121. Shand AG, Taylor AC, Banerjee M, et al. Gastric fundic gland polyps in south-east Scotland: absence of adenomatous polyposis coli gene mutations and a strikingly low prevalence of Helicobacter pylori infection. J Gastroenterol Hepatol 2002;17:1161-4.
122. Watanabe N, Seno H, Nakajima T, et al. Regression of fundic gland polyps following acquisition of Helicobacter pylori. Gut 2002;51:742-5.
123. Ally MR, Veerappan GR, Maydonovitch CL, et al. Chronic proton pump inhibitor therapy associated with increased development of fundic gland polyps. Dig Dis Sci 2009;54:2617-22.
124. Kazantsev GB, Schwesinger WH, Heim-Hall J. Spontaneous resolution of multiple fundic gland polyps after cessation of treatment with lansoprazole and Nissen fundoplication: a case report. Gastrointest Endosc 2002;55:600-2.

125. Takahari K, Haruma K, Ohtani H, et al. Proton pump inhibitor induction of gastric cobblestone-like lesions in the stomach. Intern Med 2017;56:2699-703.

126. Vieth M, Stolte M. Fundic gland polyps are not induced by proton pump inhibitor therapy. Am J Clin Pathol 2001;116:716-20.

127. Yanaru-Fujisawa R, Nakamura S, Moriyama T, et al. Familial fundic gland polyposis with gastric cancer. Gut 2012;61:1103-4.

128. Setia N, Clark JW, Duda DG, et al. Familial gastric cancers. Oncologist 2015;20:1365-77.

129. Declich P, Bellone S, Porcellati M, et al. Parietal cell protrusions with fundic gland cysts and fundic gland polyps: are they related or simply similar but distinguishable? Hum Pathol 2000;31:1536-7.

130. Attard TM, Giardiello FM, Argani P, Cuffari C. Fundic gland polyposis with high-grade dysplasia in a child with attenuated familial adenomatous polyposis and familial gastric cancer. J Pediatr Gastroenterol Nutr 2001;32:215-8.

131. Iida M, Yao T, Itoh H, et al. Natural history of fundic gland polyposis in patients with familial adenomatosis coli/Gardner's syndrome. Gastroenterology 1985;89:1021-5.

132. Winkler A, Hinterleitner TA, Langner C. Giant fundic gland polyp mimicking a gastric malignancy. Endoscopy 2007;39(Suppl 1):E34.

133. Seow-Choen F, Ho JM, Wong J, Goh HS. Gross and histological abnormalities of the foregut in familial adenomatous polyposis: a study from a South East Asian Registry. Int J Colorectal Dis 1992;7:177-83.

134. Declich P, Ambrosiani L, Bellone S, et al. Parietal cell hyperplasia with deep cystic dilations: a lesion closely mimicking fundic gland polyps. Am J Gastroenterol 2000;95:566-8.

135. Declich P, Tavani E, Bellone S, et al. Sporadic, syndromic, and Zollinger-Ellison syndrome associated fundic gland polyps consistently express cytokeratin 7. Virchows Arch 2002;441:96-7.

136. Wei J, Chiriboga L, Yee H, et al. Altered cellular distribution of tuberin and glucocorticoid receptor in sporadic fundic gland polyps. Mod Pathol 2002;15:862-9.

137. Abraham SC, Nobukawa B, Giardiello FM, Hamilton SR, Wu TT. Sporadic fundic gland polyps: common gastric polyps arising through activating mutations in the beta-catenin gene. Am J Pathol 2001;158:1005-10.

138. Gardner RJ, Kool D, Edkins E, et al. The clinical correlates of a 3' truncating mutation (codons 1982-1983) in the adenomatous polyposis coli gene. Gastroenterology 1997;113:326-31.

139. Abraham SC, Nobukawa B, Giardiello FM, Hamilton SR, Wu TT. Fundic gland polyps in familial adenomatous polyposis: neoplasms with frequent somatic adenomatous polyposis coli gene alterations. Am J Pathol 2000;157:747-54.

140. Tao H, Shinmura K, Yamada H, et al. Identification of 5 novel germline APC mutations and characterization of clinical phenotypes in Japanese patients with classical and attenuated familial adenomatous polyposis. BMC Res Notes 2010;3:305.

141. Sekine S, Shibata T, Yamauchi Y, et al. Beta-catenin mutations in sporadic fundic gland polyps. Virchows Arch 2002;440:381-6.

142. Abraham SC, Park SJ, Mugartegui L, Hamilton SR, Wu TT. Sporadic fundic gland polyps with epithelial dysplasia: evidence for preferential targeting for mutations in the adenomatous polyposis coli gene. Am J Pathol 2002;161:1735-42.

143. Repak R, Kohoutova D, Podhola M, et al. The first European family with gastric adenocarcinoma and proximal polyposis of the stomach: case report and review of the literature. Gastrointest Endosc 2016;84:718-25.

144. Li J, Woods SL, Healey S, et al. Point mutations in Exon 1B of APC reveal gastric adenocarcinoma and proximal polyposis of the stomach as a familial adenomatous polyposis variant. Am J Hum Genet 2016;98:830-42.

145. Nielsen M, Franken PF, Reinards TH, et al. Multiplicity in polyp count and extracolonic manifestations in 40 Dutch patients with MYH associated polyposis coli (MAP). J Med Genet 2005;42:e54.

146. Cheesman AR, Greenwald DA, Shah SC. Current Management of benign epithelial gastric polyps. Curr Treat Options Gastroenterol 2017;15:676-90.

147. Lash RH, Kinsey S, Genta R, Lauwers G. Gastric Polyps. Wolters Kluwer Health Adis; 2012.

148. Attard TM, Yardley JH, Cuffari C. Gastric polyps in pediatrics: an 18-year hospital-based analysis. Am J Gastroenterol 2002;97:298-301.

149. Sawada T, Muto T. Familial adenomatous polyposis: should patients undergo surveillance of the upper gastrointestinal tract? Endoscopy 1995;27:6-11.

150. Hirata K, Okazaki K, Nakayama Y, Nagata N, Itoh H, Ohsato K. Regression of gastric polyps in Gardner's syndrome with use of indomethacin suppositories: a case report. Hepatogastroenterology 1997;44:918-20.

151. Wu TT, Kornacki S, Rashid A, Yardley JH, Hamilton SR. Dysplasia and dysregulation of proliferation in foveolar and surface epithelia of fundic gland polyps from patients with familial adenomatous polyposis. Am J Surg Pathol 1998;22:293-8.

152. Bertoni G, Sassatelli R, Nigrisoli E, et al. Dysplastic changes in gastric fundic gland polyps of patients with familial adenomatous polyposis. Italian J Gastroenterol Hepatol 1999;31:192-7.

153. Sekine S, Shimoda T, Nimura S, et al. High-grade dysplasia associated with fundic gland polyposis in a familial adenomatous polyposis patient, with special reference to APC mutation profiles. Mod Pathol 2004;17:1421-6.

154. Iwama T, Mishima Y, Utsunomiya J. The impact of familial adenomatous polyposis on the tumorigenesis and mortality at the several organs. Its rational treatment. Ann Surg 1993;217:101-8.

155. Yamaguchi T, Ishida H, Ueno H, et al. Upper gastrointestinal tumours in Japanese familial adenomatous polyposis patients. Jpn J Clin Oncol 2016;46:310-5.

156. Offerhaus GJ, Giardiello FM, Krush AJ, et al. The risk of upper gastrointestinal cancer in familial adenomatous polyposis. Gastroenterology 1992;102:1980-2.

157. Shibata C, Ogawa H, Miura K, Naitoh T, Yamauchi J, Unno M. Clinical characteristics of gastric cancer in patients with familial adenomatous polyposis. Tohoku J Exp Med 2013;229:143-6.

158. Ravoire A, Faivre L, Degrolard-Courcet E, et al. Gastric adenocarcinoma in familial adenomatous polyposis can occur without previous lesions. J Gastrointest Cancer 2014;45:377-9.

159. Nakamura K, Nonaka S, Nakajima T, et al. Clinical outcomes of gastric polyps and neoplasms in patients with familial adenomatous polyposis. Endosc Int Open 2017;5:E137-45.

160. Abraham SC, Singh VK, Yardley JH, Wu TT. Hyperplastic polyps of the stomach: associations with histologic patterns of gastritis and gastric atrophy. Am J Surg Pathol 2001;25:500-7.

161. Ming SC, Goldman H. Gastric polyps; a histogenetic classification and its relation to carcinoma. Cancer 1965;18:721-6.

162. Tomasulo J. Gastric polyps. Histologic types and their relationship to gastric carcinoma. Cancer 1971;27:1346-55.

163. Morais DJ, Yamanaka A, Zeitune JM, Andreollo NA. Gastric polyps: a retrospective analysis of 26,000 digestive endoscopies. Arq Gastroenterol 2007;44:14-7.

164. Ji F, Wang ZW, Ning JW, Wang QY, Chen JY, Li YM. Effect of drug treatment on hyperplastic gastric polyps infected with Helicobacter pylori: a randomized, controlled trial. World J Gastroenterol 2006;12:1770-3.

165. Ohkusa T, Miwa H, Hojo M, et al. Endoscopic, histological and serologic findings of gastric hyperplastic polyps after eradication of Helicobacter pylori: comparison between responder and non-responder cases. Digestion 2003;68:57-62.

166. Amaro R, Neff GW, Karnam US, Tzakis AG, Raskin JB. Acquired hyperplastic gastric polyps in solid organ transplant patients. Am J Gastroenterol 2002;97:2220-4.

167. Jewell KD, Toweill DL, Swanson PE, Upton MP, Yeh MM. Gastric hyperplastic polyps in post transplant patients: a clinicopathologic study. Mod Pathol 2008;21:1108-12.

168. Lam MC, Tha S, Owen D, et al. Gastric polyps in patients with portal hypertension. Eur J Gastroenterol Hepatol 2011;23:1245-9.

169. Murakami K, Mitomi H, Yamashita K, Tanabe S, Saigenji K, Okayasu I. p53, but not c-Ki-ras, mutation and down-regulation of p21WAF1/CIP1 and cyclin D1 are associated with malignant transformation in gastric hyperplastic polyps. Am J Clin Pathol 2001;115:224-34.

170. Di Giulio E, Lahner E, Micheletti A, et al. Occurrence and risk factors for benign epithelial gastric polyps in atrophic body gastritis on diagnosis and follow-up. Aliment Pharmacol Ther 2005;21:567-74.

171. Dirschmid K, Platz-Baudin C, Stolte M. Why is the hyperplastic polyp a marker for the precancerous condition of the gastric mucosa? Virchows Arch 2006;448:80-4.

172. Al-Haddad M, Ward EM, Bouras EP, Raimondo M. Hyperplastic polyps of the gastric antrum in patients with gastrointestinal blood loss. Dig Dis Sci 2007;52:105-9.

173. Alper M, Akcan Y, Belenli O. Large pedunculated antral hyperplastic gastric polyp traversed the bulbus causing outlet obstruction and iron deficiency anemia: endoscopic removal. World J Gastroenterol 2003;9:633-4.

174. Kosai NR, Gendeh HS, Norfaezan AR, Razman J, Sutton PA, Das S. Prolapsing gastric polyp causing intermittent gastric outlet obstruction. Int Surg 2015;100:1148-52.

175. Gencosmanoglu R, Sen-Oran E, Kurtkaya-Yapicier O, Tozun N. Antral hyperplastic polyp causing intermittent gastric outlet obstruction: case report. BMC Gastroenterol 2003;3:16.

176. Parikh M, Kelley B, Rendon G, Abraham B. Intermittent gastric outlet obstruction caused by a prolapsing antral gastric polyp. World J Gastrointest Oncol 2010;2:242-6.

177. Niv Y, Delpre G, Sperber AD, Sandbank J, Zirkin H. Hyperplastic gastric polyposis, hypergastrinaemia and colorectal neoplasia: a description of four cases. Eur J Gastroenterol Hepatol 2003;15:1361-6.

178. Seruca R, Carneiro F, Castedo S, David L, Lopes C, Sobrinho-Simoes M. Familial gastric polyposis revisited. Autosomal dominant inheritance confirmed. Cancer Genet Cytogenet 1991;53:97-100.

179. Spaziani E, Picchio M, Di Filippo A, et al. Sporadic diffuse gastric polyposis: report of a case. Surg Today 2011;41:1428-31.

180. Muller-Lissner SA, Wiebecke B. Investigations of hyperplasiogenous gastric polyps by partial reconstruction. Pathol Res Pract 1982;174:368-78.

181. Muto T, Ota K. Polypogenesis of gastric mucosa. Gan 1970;61:435-42.

182. Dirschmid K, Walser J, Hugel H. Pseudomalignant erosion in hyperplastic gastric polyps. Cancer 1984;54:2290-3.

183. Honda H, Kume K, Murakami H, Yamasaki T, Yoshikawa I, Otsuki M. Pseudomalignant erosion in hyperplastic polyp at esophago-gastric junction. J Gastroenterol Hepatol 2005;20:800-1.

184. Yamashita M, Hirokawa M, Nakasono M, et al. Gastric inverted hyperplastic polyp. Report of four cases and relation to gastritis cystica profunda. APMIS 2002;110:717-23.

185. Yun JT, Lee SW, Kim DP, et al. Gastric inverted hyperplastic polyp: A rare cause of iron deficiency anemia. World J Gastroenterol 2016;22:4066-70.

186. Mori H, Kobara H, Tsushimi T, et al. Two rare gastric hamartomatous inverted polyp cases suggest the pathogenesis of growth. World J Gastroenterol 2014;20:5918-23.

187. Kim HS, Hwang EJ, Jang JY, Lee J, Kim YW. Multifocal Adenocarcinomas Arising within a Gastric Inverted Hyperplastic Polyp. Korean J Pathol 2012;46:387-91.

188. Gonzalez-Obeso E, Fujita H, Deshpande V, et al. Gastric hyperplastic polyps: a heterogeneous clinicopathologic group including a distinct subset best categorized as mucosal prolapse polyp. The Am J Surg Pathol 2011;35:670-7.

189. Long KB, Odze RD. Gastroesophageal junction hyperplastic (inflammatory) polyps: a clinical and pathologic study of 46 cases. Am J Surg Pathol 2011;35:1038-44.

190. Kawada M, Seno H, Wada M, et al. Cyclooxygenase-2 expression and angiogenesis in gastric hyperplastic polyp—association with polyp size. Digestion 2003;67:20-4.

191. Nakajima A, Matsuhashi N, Yazaki Y, Oka T, Sugano K. Details of hyperplastic polyps of the stomach shrinking after anti-Helicobacter pylori therapy. J Gastroenterol 2000;35:372-5.

192. Lauwers GY, Wahl SJ, Melamed J, Rojas-Corona RR. p53 expression in precancerous gastric lesions: an immunohistochemical study of PAb 1801 monoclonal antibody on adenomatous and hyperplastic gastric polyps. Am J Gastroenterol 1993;88:1916-9.

193. Yao T, Kajiwara M, Kuroiwa S, et al. Malignant transformation of gastric hyperplastic polyps: alteration of phenotypes, proliferative activity, and p53 expression. Hum Pathol 2002;33:1016-22.

194. Goddard AF, Badreldin R, Pritchard DM, Walker MM, Warren B, British Society of Gastroenterology. The management of gastric polyps. Gut 2010;59:1270-6.

195. Boyd JT, Lee L. Portal hypertension-associated gastric polyps. BMJ Case Rep 2011;2011.

196. Hizawa K, Fuchigami T, Iida M, et al. Possible neoplastic transformation within gastric hyperplastic polyp. Application of endoscopic polypectomy. Surg Endosc 1995;9:714-8.

197. Orlowska J, Jarosz D, Pachlewski J, Butruk E. Malignant transformation of benign epithelial gastric polyps. Am j Gastroenterol 1995;90:2152-9.

198. Salomao M, Luna AM, Sepulveda JL, Sepulveda AR. Mutational analysis by next generation sequencing of gastric type dysplasia occurring in hyperplastic polyps of the stomach: Mutations in gastric hyperplastic polyps. Exp Mol Pathol 2015;99:468-73.

199. Markowski AR, Guzinska-Ustymowicz K. Gastric hyperplastic polyp with focal cancer. Gastroenterol Rep (Oxf) 2016;4:158-61.

200. Hirasaki S, Suzuki S, Kanzaki H, Fujita K, Matsumura S, Matsumoto E. Minute signet ring cell carcinoma occurring in gastric hyperplastic polyp. World J Gastroenterol 2007;13:5779-80.

201. Hirasaki S, Kanzaki H, Fujita K, et al. Papillary adenocarcinoma occurring in a gastric hyperplastic polyp observed by magnifying endoscopy and treated with endoscopic mucosal resection. Intern Med 2008;47:949-52.

202. Yamanaka K, Miyatani H, Yoshida Y, et al. Malignant transformation of a gastric hyperplastic polyp in a context of Helicobacter pylori-negative autoimmune gastritis: a case report. BMC Gastroenterol 2016;16:130.

203. Horiuchi H, Kaise M, Inomata H, et al. Magnifying endoscopy combined with narrow band imaging may help to predict neoplasia coexisting with gastric hyperplastic polyps. Scand J Gastroenterol 2013;48:626-32.

204. Littler ER, Gleibermann E. Gastritis cystica polyposa. (Gastric mucosal prolapse at gastroenterostomy site, with cystic and infiltrative epithelial hyperplasia). Cancer 1972;29:205-9.

205. Laratta JL, Buhtoiarova TN, Sparber LS, Chamberlain RS. Gastritis cystica profunda: a rare gastric tumor masquerading as a malignancy. Surgical Science 2012;3:158-64.

206. Bechade D, Desrame J, Algayres JP. Gastritis cystica profunda in a patient with no history of gastric surgery. Endoscopy 2007;39(Suppl 1):E80-1.

207. Itte V, Mallick IH, Moore PJ. Massive gastrointestinal haemorrhage due to gastritis cystica profunda. Cases J 2008;1:85.

208. Kurland J, DuBois S, Behling C, Savides T. Severe upper-GI bleed caused by gastritis cystica profunda. Gastrointest Endos 2006;63:716-7.

209. Machicado J, Shroff J, Quesada A, et al. Gastritis cystica profunda: Endoscopic ultrasound findings and review of the literature. Endosc Ultrasound 2014;3:131-4.

210. Choi MG, Jeong JY, Kim KM, et al. Clinical significance of gastritis cystica profunda and its association with Epstein-Barr virus in gastric cancer. Cancer 2012;118:5227-33.

211. Mukaisho K, Miwa K, Kumagai H, Bamba M, Sugihara H, Hattori T. Gastric carcinogenesis by duodenal reflux through gut regenerative cell lineage. Dig Dis Sci 2003;48:2153-8.

212. Roepke TK, Purtell K, King EC, La Perle KM, Lerner DJ, Abbott GW. Targeted deletion of Kcne2 causes gastritis cystica profunda and gastric neoplasia. PloS One 2010;5:e11451.

213. Moon SY, Kim KO, Park SH, et al. [Gastritis cystica profunda accompanied by multiple early gastric cancers.] Korean J Gastroenterol 2010;55:325-30. [Korean]

214. Tsuji T, Iwahashi M, Nakamori M, et al. Multiple early gastric cancer with gastritis cystica profunda showing various histological types. Hepatogastroenterology 2008;55:1150-2.

215. Jass JR, Williams CB, Bussey HJ, Morson BC. Juvenile polyposis—a precancerous condition. Histopathology 1988;13:619-30.

216. Syngal S, Brand RE, Church JM, Giardiello FM, Hampel HL, Burt RW. ACG clinical guideline: Genetic testing and management of hereditary gastrointestinal cancer syndromes. Am J Gastroenterol 2015;110:223-62; quiz 263.

217. Brosens LA, Langeveld D, van Hattem WA, Giardiello FM, Offerhaus GJ. Juvenile polyposis syndrome. World J Gastroenterol 2011;17:4839-44.

218. Chun N, Ford JM. Genetic testing by cancer site: stomach. Cancer J 2012;18:355-63.

219. Dahdaleh FS, Carr JC, Calva D, Howe JR. Juvenile polyposis and other intestinal polyposis syndromes with microdeletions of chromosome 10q22-23. Clin Genet 2012;81:110-6.

220. Delnatte C, Sanlaville D, Mougenot JF, et al. Contiguous gene deletion within chromosome arm 10q is associated with juvenile polyposis of infancy, reflecting cooperation between the BMPR1A and PTEN tumor-suppressor genes. Am J Hum Genet 2006;78:1066-74.

221. Cao X, Eu KW, Kumarasinghe MP, Li HH, Loi C, Cheah PY. Mapping of hereditary mixed polyposis syndrome (HMPS) to chromosome 10q23 by genomewide high-density single nucleotide polymorphism (SNP) scan and identification of BMPR1A loss of function. J Med Genet 2006;43:e13.

222. Hizawa K, Iida M, Yao T, Aoyagi K, Fujishima M. Juvenile polyposis of the stomach: clinicopathological features and its malignant potential. J Clin Pathol 1997;50:771-4.

223. Watanabe A, Nagashima H, Motoi M, Ogawa K. Familial juvenile polyposis of the stomach. Gastroenterology 1979;77:148-51.

224. Lawless ME, Toweill DL, Jewell KD, et al. Massive gastric juvenile polyposis: a clinicopathologic study using SMAD4 immunohistochemistry. Am J Clin Pathol 2017;147:390.

225. Gonzalez RS, Adsay V, Graham RP, et al. Massive gastric juvenile-type polyposis: a clinicopathological analysis of 22 cases. Histopathology 2017;70:918-28.

226. Jarvinen HJ, Sipponen P. Gastroduodenal polyps in familial adenomatous and juvenile polyposis. Endoscopy 1986;18:230-4.

227. Shikata K, Kukita Y, Matsumoto T, et al. Gastric juvenile polyposis associated with germline SMAD4 mutation. Am J Med Genet A 2005;134:326-9.

228. Yamashita K, Saito M, Itoh M, et al. Juvenile polyposis complicated with protein losing gastropathy. Intern Med 2009;48:335-8.

229. Wong-Chong N, Kidanewold WH, Kirsch R, May GR, McCart JA. Giant stomach secondary to juvenile polyposis syndrome. J Gastrointest Surg 2012;16:669-72.

230. Coffin CM, Dehner LP. What is a juvenile polyp? An analysis based on 21 patients with solitary and multiple polyps. Arch Pathol Lab Med 1996;120:1032-8.

231. Covarrubias DJ, Huprich JE. Best cases from the AFIP. Juvenile polyposis of the stomach. Armed Forces Institute of Pathology. Radiographics 2002;22:415-20.

232. van der Post RS, Carneiro F. Emerging concepts in gastric neoplasia: heritable gastric cancers and polyposis disorders. Surg Pathol Clin 2017;10:931-45.

233. Langeveld D, van Hattem WA, de Leng WW, et al. SMAD4 immunohistochemistry reflects genetic status in juvenile polyposis syndrome. Clin Cancer Res 2010;16:4126-34.

234. Brosens LA, Giardiello FM, Offerhaus GJ, Montgomery EA. Syndromic gastric polyps: at the crossroads of genetic and environmental cancer predisposition. Adv Exp Med Biol 2016;908:347-69.

235. van Hattem WA, Brosens LA, de Leng WW, et al. Large genomic deletions of SMAD4, BMPR1A and PTEN in juvenile polyposis. Gut 2008;57:623-7.

236. Friedl W, Uhlhaas S, Schulmann K, et al. Juvenile polyposis: massive gastric polyposis is more common in MADH4 mutation carriers than in BMPR1A mutation carriers. Hum Genet 2002;111:108-11.

237. Piepoli A, Mazzoccoli G, Panza A, et al. A unifying working hypothesis for juvenile polyposis syndrome and Menetrier's disease: specific localization or concomitant occurrence of a separate entity? Dig Liver Dis 2012;44:952-6.

238. Sweet K, Willis J, Zhou XP, et al. Molecular classification of patients with unexplained hamartomatous and hyperplastic polyposis. JAMA 2005;294:2465-73.

239. Jelsig AM, Brusgaard K, Hansen TP, et al. Germline variants in Hamartomatous Polyposis Syndrome-associated genes from patients with one or few hamartomatous polyps. Scand J Gastroenterol 2016;51:1118-25.

240. Jelsig AM, Torring PM, Kjeldsen AD, et al. JP-HHT phenotype in Danish patients with SMAD4 mutations. Clin Genet 2016;90:55-62.

241. Howe JR, Mitros FA, Summers RW. The risk of gastrointestinal carcinoma in familial juvenile polyposis. Ann Surg Oncol 1998;5:751-6.

242. Aretz S, Stienen D, Uhlhaas S, et al. High proportion of large genomic deletions and a genotype phenotype update in 80 unrelated families with juvenile polyposis syndrome. J Med Genet 2007;44:702-9.

243. Kantarcioglu M, Kilciler G, Turan I, et al. Solitary Peutz-Jeghers-type hamartomatous polyp as a cause of recurrent acute pancreatitis. Endoscopy 2009;41(Suppl 2):E117-18.

244. Oncel M, Remzi FH, Church JM, Goldblum JR, Zutshi M, Fazio VW. Course and follow-up of solitary Peutz-Jeghers polyps: a case series. Int J Colorectal Dis 2003;18:33-5.

245. Burkart AL, Sheridan T, Lewin M, Fenton H, Ali NJ, Montgomery E. Do sporadic Peutz-Jeghers polyps exist? Experience of a large teaching hospital. Am J Surg Pathol 2007;31:1209-14.

246. Amos CI, Keitheri-Cheteri MB, Sabripour M, et al. Genotype-phenotype correlations in Peutz-Jeghers syndrome. J Med Genet 2004;41:327-33.

247. Giardiello FM, Trimbath JD. Peutz-Jeghers syndrome and management recommendations. Clin Gastroenterol Hepatol 2006;4:408-15.

248. Volikos E, Robinson J, Aittomaki K, et al. LKB1 exonic and whole gene deletions are a common cause of Peutz-Jeghers syndrome. J Med Genet 2006;43:e18.

249. Tomlinson IP, Houlston RS. Peutz-Jeghers syndrome. J Med Genet 1997;34:1007-11.

250. Salloch H, Reinacher-Schick A, Schulmann K, et al. Truncating mutations in Peutz-Jeghers syndrome are associated with more polyps, surgical interventions and cancers. Int J Colorectal Dis 2010;25:97-107.

251. Kato N, Sugawara M, Maeda K, Hosoya N, Motoyama T. Pyloric gland metaplasia/differentiation in multiple organ systems in a patient with Peutz-Jegher's syndrome. Pathol Int 2011;61:369-72.

252. Lin J, Chen M, Lei W, Law W, Hu C. Eradication of diffuse gastric Peutz-Jeghers polyps by unsedated transnasal snare polypectomy and argon plasma coagulation. Endoscopy 2009;41(Suppl 2):E207-8.

253. Jenne DE, Reimann H, Nezu J, et al. Peutz-Jeghers syndrome is caused by mutations in a novel serine threonine kinase. Nat Genet 1998;18:38-43.

254. Hemminki A, Markie D, Tomlinson I, et al. A serine/threonine kinase gene defective in Peutz-Jeghers syndrome. Nature 1998;391:184-7.

255. Miyaki M, Iijima T, Hosono K, et al. Somatic mutations of LKB1 and beta-catenin genes in gastrointestinal polyps from patients with Peutz-Jeghers syndrome. Cancer Res 2000;60:6311-3.

256. Jansen M, de Leng WW, Baas AF, et al. Mucosal prolapse in the pathogenesis of Peutz-Jeghers polyposis. Gut 2006;55:1-5.

257. de Leng WW, Jansen M, Keller JJ, et al. Peutz-Jeghers syndrome polyps are polyclonal with expanded progenitor cell compartment. Gut 2007; 56: 1475– 6.

258. Ma H, Brosens LAA, Offerhaus GJA, et al. Pathology and genetics of hereditary colorectal cancer. Pathology. 2018; 50:49-59

259. Udd L, Katajisto P, Rossi DJ, et al. Suppression of Peutz-Jeghers polyposis by inhibition of cyclooxygenase-2. Gastroenterology 2004;127:1030-7.

260. Huang X, Wullschleger S, Shpiro N, et al. Important role of the LKB1-AMPK pathway in suppressing tumorigenesis in PTEN-deficient mice. Biochem J 2008;412:211-21.

261. Kuwada SK, Burt R. A rationale for mTOR inhibitors as chemoprevention agents in Peutz-Jeghers syndrome. Fam Cancer 2011;10:469-72.

262. Turpin A, Cattan S, Leclerc J, et al. [Hereditary predisposition to cancers of the digestive tract, breast, gynecological and gonadal: focus on the Peutz-Jeghers.] Bull Cancer 2014;101:813-22. [French]

263. Schneider C, Simon T, Hero B, et al. [18F]Fluorodeoxyglucose positron emission tomography/computed tomography-positive gastric adenocarcinoma in a 12-year-old girl with Peutz-Jeghers syndrome. J Clin Oncol 2012;30:e140-3.

264. Giardiello FM, Welsh SB, Hamilton SR, et al. Increased risk of cancer in the Peutz-Jeghers syndrome. N Engl J Med 1987;316:1511-4.

265. Nelen MR, Padberg GW, Peeters EA, et al. Localization of the gene for Cowden disease to chromosome 10q22-23. Nat Genet 1996;13:114-6.

266. Liaw D, Marsh DJ, Li J, et al. Germline mutations of the PTEN gene in Cowden disease, an inherited breast and thyroid cancer syndrome. Nat Genet 1997;16:64-7.

267. Nelen MR, van Staveren WC, Peeters EA, et al. Germline mutations in the PTEN/MMAC1 gene in patients with Cowden disease. Hum Mol Genet 1997;6:1383-7.

268. Pilarski R, Burt R, Kohlman W, Pho L, Shannon KM, Swisher E. Cowden syndrome and the PTEN hamartoma tumor syndrome: systematic review and revised diagnostic criteria. J Natl Cancer Inst 2013;105:1607-16.

269. Cauchin E, Touchefeu Y, Matysiak-Budnik T. Hamartomatous tumors in the gastrointestinal tract. Gastrointest Tumors 2015;2:65-74.

270. Pilarski R, Stephens JA, Noss R, Fisher JL, Prior TW. Predicting PTEN mutations: an evaluation of Cowden syndrome and Bannayan-Riley-Ruvalcaba syndrome clinical features. J Med Genet 2011;48:505-12.

271. Tan MH, Mester J, Peterson C, et al. A clinical scoring system for selection of patients for PTEN mutation testing is proposed on the basis of a prospective study of 3042 probands. Am J Hum Genet 2011;88:42-56.

272. Kay PS, Soetikno RM, Mindelzun R, Young HS. Diffuse esophageal glycogenic acanthosis: an endoscopic marker of Cowden's disease. Am J Gastroenterol 1997;92:1038-40.

273. Coriat R, Mozer M, Caux F, et al. Endoscopic findings in Cowden syndrome. Endoscopy 2011;43:723-6.

274. Levi Z, Baris HN, Kedar I, et al. Upper and lower gastrointestinal findings in PTEN mutation-positive Cowden syndrome patients participating in an active surveillance program. Clin Transl Gastroenterol 2011;2:e5.

275. Heald B, Mester J, Rybicki L, Orloff MS, Burke CA, Eng C. Frequent gastrointestinal polyps and colorectal adenocarcinomas in a prospective series of PTEN mutation carriers. Gastroenterology 2010;139:1927-33.

276. Shaco-Levy R, Jasperson KW, Martin K, et al. Gastrointestinal polyposis in Cowden syndrome. J Clin Gastroenterol 2017;51:e60-7.

277. Shaco-Levy R, Jasperson KW, Martin K, et al. Morphologic characterization of hamartomatous gastrointestinal polyps in Cowden syndrome, Peutz-Jeghers syndrome, and juvenile polyposis syndrome. Hum Pathol 2016;49:39-48.

278. Hizawa K, Iida M, Matsumoto T, et al. Gastrointestinal manifestations of Cowden's disease. Report of four cases. J Clin Gastroenterol 1994;18:13-8.

279. Vasovcak P, Krepelova A, Puchmajerova A, et al. A novel mutation of PTEN gene in a patient with Cowden syndrome with excessive papillomatosis of the lips, discrete cutaneous lesions, and gastrointestinal polyposis. Eur J Gastroenterol Hepatol 2007;19:513-7.

280. Campos FG, Habr-Gama A, Kiss DR, et al. Cowden syndrome: report of two cases and review of clinical presentation and management of a rare colorectal polyposis. Curr Surg 2006;63:15-9.

281. Carlson GJ, Nivatvongs S, Snover DC. Colorectal polyps in Cowden's disease (multiple hamartoma syndrome). Am J Surg Pathol 1984;8:763-70.

282. Orloff MS, He X, Peterson C, et al. Germline PIK3CA and AKT1 mutations in Cowden and Cowden-like syndromes. Am J Hum Genet 2013;92:76-80.

283. Ni Y, He X, Chen J, et al. Germline SDHx variants modify breast and thyroid cancer risks in Cowden and Cowden-like syndrome via FAD/NAD-dependant destabilization of p53. Hum Mol Genet 2012;21:300-10.

284. Nizialek EA, Mester JL, Dhiman VK, Smiraglia DJ, Eng C. KLLN epigenotype-phenotype associations in Cowden syndrome. Eur J Hum Genet 2015;23:1538-43.

285. Mester J, Eng C. Estimate of de novo mutation frequency in probands with PTEN hamartoma tumor syndrome. Genet Med 2012;14:819-22.

286. Isomoto H, Furusu H, Ohnita K, Takehara Y, Wen CY, Kohno S. Effect of Helicobacter pylori eradication on gastric hyperplastic polyposis in Cowden's disease. World J Gastroenterol 2005;11:1567-9.

287. Hamby LS, Lee EY, Schwartz RW. Parathyroid adenoma and gastric carcinoma as manifestations of Cowden's disease. Surgery 1995;118:115-7.

288. Al-Thihli K, Palma L, Marcus V, et al. A case of Cowden's syndrome presenting with gastric carcinomas and gastrointestinal polyposis. Nat Clin Pract Gastroenterol Hepatol 2009;6:184-9.

289. Takeuchi Y, Yoshikawa M, Tsukamoto N, et al. Cronkhite-Canada syndrome with colon cancer, portal thrombosis, high titer of antinuclear antibodies, and membranous glomerulonephritis. J Gastroenterol 2003;38:791-5.

290. Ward EM, Wolfsen HC, Raimondo M. Novel endosonographic findings in Cronkhite-Canada syndrome. Endoscopy 2003;35:464.

291. Cronkhite LW Jr, Canada WJ. Generalized gastrointestinal polyposis; an unusual syndrome of polyposis, pigmentation, alopecia and onychotrophia. N Engl J Med 1955;252:1011-5.

292. de Silva DG, Fernando AD, Law FM, Premarathne M, Liyanarachchi DS. Infantile Cronkhite-Canada syndrome. Indian J Pediatr 1997;64:261-6.

293. Scharf GM, Becker JH, Laage NJ. Juvenile gastrointestinal polyposis or the infantile Cronkhite-Canada syndrome. J Pediatr Surg 1986;21:953-4.

294. Kucukaydin M, Patiroglu TE, Okur H, Icer M. Infantile Cronkhite-Canada syndrome?—Case report. Eur J Pediatr Surg 1992;2:295-7.

295. Slavik T, Montgomery EA. Cronkhite-Canada syndrome six decades on: the many faces of an enigmatic disease. J Clin Pathol 2014;67:891-7.

296. Goto A. [Cronkhite-Canada syndrome; observation of 180 cases reported in Japan.] Nihon Rinsho 1991;49:221-6. [Japanese]

297. Daniel ES, Ludwig SL, Lewin KJ, Ruprecht RM, Rajacich GM, Schwabe AD. The Cronkhite-Canada Syndrome. An analysis of clinical and pathologic features and therapy in 55 patients. Medicine (Baltimore) 1982;61:293-309.

298. Ward EM, Wolfsen HC. Review article: the non-inherited gastrointestinal polyposis syndromes. Aliment Pharmacol Ther 2002;16:333-42.

299. Piraccini BM, Rech G, Sisti A, Bellavista S. Twenty nail onychomadesis: an unusual finding in Cronkhite-Canada syndrome. J Am Acad Dermatol 2010;63:172-4.

300. Ho V, Banney L, Falhammar H. Hyperpigmentation, nail dystrophy and alopecia with generalised intestinal polyposis: Cronkhite-Canada syndrome. Australas J Dermatol 2008;49:223-5.

301. Nyam DC, Ho MS, Goh HS. Progressive ectodermal changes in the Cronkhite-Canada syndrome. Aust N Z J Surg 1996;66:780-1.

302. Johnston MM, Vosburgh JW, Wiens AT, Walsh GC. Gastrointestinal polyposis associated with alopecia, pigmentation, and atrophy of the fingernails and toenails. Ann Intern Med 1962;56:935-40.

303. Yamaguchi K, Ogata Y, Akagi Y, et al. Cronkhite-Canada syndrome associated with advanced rectal cancer treated by a subtotal colectomy: report of a case. Surg Today 2001;31:521-6.

304. Bettington M, Brown IS, Kumarasinghe MP, de Boer B, Bettington A, Rosty C. The challenging diagnosis of Cronkhite-Canada syndrome in the upper gastrointestinal tract: a series of 7 cases with clinical follow-up. Am J Surg Pathol 2014;38:215-23.

305. Anderson RD, Patel R, Hamilton JK, Boland CR. Cronkhite-Canada syndrome presenting as eosinophilic gastroenteritis. Proc (Bayl Univ Med Cent) 2006;19:209-12.

306. Watanabe T, Kudo M, Shirane H, et al. Cronkhite-Canada syndrome associated with triple gastric cancers: a case report. Gastrointest Endosc 1999;50:688-91.

307. Egawa T, Kubota T, Otani Y, et al. Surgically treated Cronkhite-Canada syndrome associated with gastric cancer. Gastric Cancer 2000;3:156-60.

308. Karasawa H, Miura K, Ishida K, et al. Cronkhite-Canada syndrome complicated with huge intramucosal gastric cancer. Gastric Cancer 2009;12:113-7.

309. Gursoy S, Yurci A, Torun E, et al. An uncommon lesion: gastric xanthelasma. Turk J Gastroenterol 2005;16:167-70.

310. Kaiserling E, Heinle H, Itabe H, Takano T, Remmele W. Lipid islands in human gastric mucosa: morphological and immunohistochemical findings. Gastroenterology 1996;110:369-74.

311. Gravina AG, Iacono A, Alagia I, D'Armiento FP, Sansone S, Romano M. Gastric xanthomatosis associated with gastric intestinal metaplasia in a dyspeptic patient. Dig Liver Dis 2009;41:765.

312. Muraoka A, Suehiro I, Fujii M, et al. Type IIa early gastric cancer with proliferation of xanthoma cells. J Gastroenterol 1998;33:326-9.

313. Yi SY. Dyslipidemia and H pylori in gastric xanthomatosis. World J Gastroenterol 2007; 13:4598-601.

314. Jeong YS, Park H, Lee DY, Lee SI, Park C. Gastric xanthomatosis. Gastrointest Endosc 2004;59:399-400.

315. Lai EC, Tompkins RK. Heterotopic pancreas. Review of a 26 year experience. Am J Surg 1986;151:697-700.

316. Zhang Y, Sun X, Gold JS, et al. Heterotopic pancreas: a clinicopathological study of 184 cases from a single high-volume medical center in China. Hum Pathol 2016;55:135-42.

317. Rodriguez FJ, Abraham SC, Allen MS, Sebo TJ. Fine-needle aspiration cytology findings from a case of pancreatic heterotopia at the gastroesophageal junction. Diagn Cytopathol 2004;31:175-9.

318. Shalaby M, Kochman ML, Lichtenstein GR. Heterotopic pancreas presenting as dysphagia. The Am J Gastroenterol 2002;97:1046-9.

319. Rhim JH, Kim WS, Choi YH, Cheon JE, Park SH. Radiological findings of gastric adenomyoma in a neonate presenting with gastric outlet obstruction. Pediatr Radiol 2013;43:628-30.

320. Kim JH, Lim JS, Lee YC, et al. Endosonographic features of gastric ectopic pancreases distinguishable from mesenchymal tumors. J Gastroenterol Hepatol 2008;23(Pt 2):e301-7.

321. Hirasaki S, Tanimizu M, Moriwaki T, Nasu J. Acute pancreatitis occurring in gastric aberrant pancreas treated with surgery and proved by histological examination. Intern Med 2005;44:1169-73.

322. Lee SL, Ku YM, Lee HH, Cho YS. Gastric ectopic pancreas complicated by formation of a pseudocyst. Clin Res Hepatol Gastroenterol 2014;38:389-91.

323. Kaufman A, Storey D, Lee CS, Murali R. Mucinous cyst exhibiting severe dysplasia in gastric heterotopic pancreas associated with gastrointestinal stromal tumour. World J Gastroenterol 2007;13:5781-2.

324. Padberg BC, Schroder S. Mucus retention in heterotopic pancreas of the gastric antrum: a lesion mimicking mucinous carcinoma. Am J Surg Pathol 1995;19:1445-7.

325. Plier M, Durez P, Komuta M, Raptis A. Severe panniculitis and polyarthritis caused by acinar cell carcinoma arising from an ectopic pancreas. BMJ Case Rep 2017;2017.

326. Osanai M, Miyokawa N, Tamaki T, Yonekawa M, Kawamura A, Sawada N. Adenocarcinoma arising in gastric heterotopic pancreas: clinicopathological and immunohistochemical study with genetic analysis of a case. Pathol Int 2001;51:549-54.

327. Chetty R, Weinreb I. Gastric neuroendocrine carcinoma arising from heterotopic pancreatic tissue. J Clin Pathol 2004;57:314-7.

9 GASTRIC CARCINOMAS

Gastric carcinomas represent a biologically and genetically heterogeneous group of tumors with multifactorial etiologies, both environmental and genetic. They are characterized by broad morphologic heterogeneity with respect to patterns of architecture and growth, cell differentiation, and histogenesis.

GENERAL FEATURES

Gastric cancer is the fifth most common cancer worldwide, and the third leading cause of cancer mortality worldwide, with 952,000 new cases (7 percent of total cancer incidence) and 723,000 deaths (9 percent of total cancer mortality) in 2012 (1). Despite a declining incidence in many countries in the developed world, there is an increase in global mortality from the disease because of population growth and increasing longevity in developing countries (2,3).

Both sexes are not equally affected: rates in men are approximately double those in women (4). There is also a 9-fold international variation in stomach cancer incidence based on geographic localization. The highest age-standardized incidence rates are reported in East Asia and central and eastern Europe, while incidence rates tend to be low in Africa and in North America (4). Over the past 50 years, the incidence and mortality rates of distal gastric cancer have been uniformly decreasing in many countries of North America and Europe, and also more recently, in many Asian and Latin American countries (5). However, the absolute number of gastric cancer cases remains stable or may even be increased due to the predicted growth of the world population and increasing longevity (6). In regions of high incidence, cancers of the antrum and pylorus are the most common, whereas in countries with low incidence, neoplasms of the proximal stomach and of the esophagogastric junction (EGJ) are more predominant (6).

Esophagogastric Junction Adenocarcinoma

Esophagogastric junction adenocarcinomas share many epidemiologic characteristics with adenocarcinomas of the distal esophagus and proximal stomach. Incidence rates are higher among Caucasians, particularly men compared to women, and in older patients (7). The incidence of this type of tumor increased markedly in the second half of the 20th century in Asian populations (8,9) as well as in the United States (10,11) and Europe (12), in parallel with the rising incidence of adenocarcinomas of the lower esophagus (13,14).

Gastric Carcinoma in Young Patients (Early-Onset Gastric Cancer)

Less than 10 percent of gastric cancer patients present with the disease before 45 years of age (*early-onset gastric cancer* [EOGC]) (15,16). In this group of patients, the male to female ratio is approximately equal or even shows female predominance. Most tumors are of diffuse type (15,17–19). Once considered to be associated with a poor prognosis (20), recent studies show that young gastric cancer patients no longer present with more advanced disease than the elderly, and overall survival is better in young patients with resectable tumors (18,19).

Several studies point to a pathogenesis of EOGC different from that of sporadic adenocarcinoma occurring later in life (16,21–27). In some populations an association has been found between virulent strains of *Helicobacter pylori* and the development of early-onset cancers (28,29). Furthermore, 10 to 25 percent of young patients with gastric cancer have a positive family history, suggesting the etiologic importance of genetic factors. Among these are hereditary cancers in individuals with germline mutations of the *CDHI* (e-cadherin) gene (30). The molecular features of EOGC have been reviewed by Skierucha et al. (31).

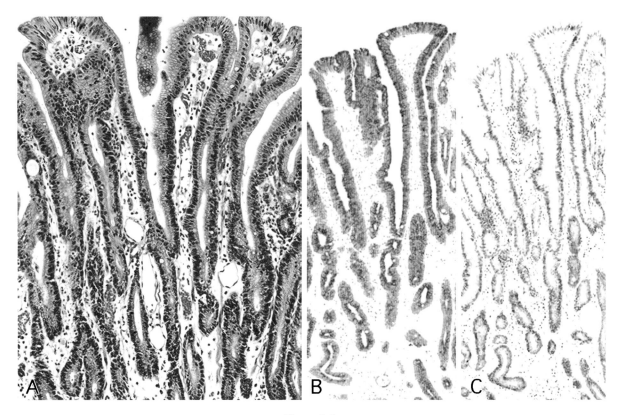

Figure 9-1

LOW-GRADE DYSPLASIA (FOVEOLAR TYPE)

A: The lining epithelium is composed of tall cells with varying amounts of apical mucin and retention of a distinctly foveolar phenotype.

B: There is strong and diffuse immunoexpression of MUC5AC.

C: There is faint immunoexpression of MUC6 in the base of the glands.

Early Gastric Cancer

Early gastric cancer is an invasive carcinoma limited to the mucosa or submucosa, regardless of nodal status. The term "early" does not imply a stage in the genesis of the cancer but means that these are gastric cancers that can often be cured (32) and the 5-year survival rate is about 95 percent (33). If untreated, however, 63 percent of EGCs progress to advanced tumors within 5 years (34). Countries with a high incidence of gastric cancer and in which asymptomatic patients are screened have a high incidence of EGCs, ranging from 30 to 50 percent in East Asia (35,36) with lower figures for the West (16 to 24 percent) (37–39).

ETIOLOGY AND PATHOGENESIS

Gastric carcinogenesis is a multistep and multifactorial process that, in many cases, appears to involve a progression from normal mucosa through chronic gastritis, atrophic gastritis, and intestinal metaplasia to dysplasia and carcinoma, a sequence that has been designated as the Correa cascade of multistep gastric carcinogenesis (40,41). The Correa model does not explain all carcinogenic steps of gastric cancer. Actually, a proportion of gastric adenocarcinomas arises in nonintestinalized mucosa and retains a gastric phenotype (and gastric differentiation is also observed in gastric dysplasia, the precursor lesion of gastric adenocarcinoma) (fig. 9-1) (4,42). Also, in the recently identified syndrome of gastric adenocarcinoma and proximal polyposis of the stomach (discussed below), gastric dysplasia and gastric adenocarcinoma develop in fundic gland polyps and are related not to intestinal metaplasia but instead to foveolar hyperplasia. Together, this evidence shows that gastric adenocarcinoma can arise in mucosa without intestinal metaplasia.

A number of precancerous conditions have been recognized, such as atrophic gastritis and intestinal metaplasia due to *H. pylori* infection or autoimmunity, pyloric metaplasia, gastric ulcers, gastric polyps, previous gastric surgery, and Menetrier disease. There also are putative associations with environmental agents such as dietary constituents and the formation of carcinogenic N-nitroso compounds within the stomach. In a minority of cases, there is good evidence for an inherited disposition.

Precancerous Conditions

Chronic Gastritis and Intestinal Metaplasia. An association has been demonstrated between chronic gastritis, particularly atrophic gastritis with intestinal metaplasia, and gastric cancer, especially in high incidence areas (40,41,43). Epidemiologically, the prevalence of chronic atrophic gastritis within populations correlates closely with the incidence and death rates from gastric cancer (41,43,44), and in follow-up studies, atrophic gastritis has been shown to precede the development of malignancy (45,46). Conditions that predispose to gastric cancer, such as pernicious anemia and the postoperative stomach, are frequently characterized by extensive atrophic gastritis and intestinal metaplasia and, less frequently, by spasmolytic polypeptide-expressing metaplasia (SPEM) (47).

Several classification schemes for chronic gastritis have been developed, although these are often used for investigational purposes rather than in daily reporting (48,49). In the Sydney classification system, several features of inflammation, atrophy, and intestinal metaplasia are assessed individually. A visual analogue scale was added to facilitate grading but agreement is limited (50–53). Four histopathology indices have been proposed to evaluate the cancer risk associated with atrophic gastritis: the Gastric Risk Index (54), the OLGA (Operative Link for Gastritis Assessment) system (55,56), the Baylor system (57), and the OLGIM (modified OLGA) system (58).

Proposed in 2005, the OLGA staging system is an instrument built on the natural history of gastric atrophy and its associated cancer risk (55,56); it ranks the histologic phenotypes of gas-

tritis along a scale (0 to IV) of increasing mucosal atrophy. The cancer risk associated with stages 0, I, and II is extremely low, while stages III and IV (with extensive atrophy of both antral and oxyntic mucosa) are associated with high risk of intestinal-type gastric adenocarcinoma. An alternative staging method proposed as a modification of the OLGA system (OLGIM) evaluates exclusively the extent of intestinal metaplasia (IM), as assessed in both antral and oxyntic biopsy samples (58). Both systems have their own limitations but may be useful in the prognostication of cancer risk by allowing the placement of patients at approximate points along the path in which chronic gastritis progresses from reversible inflammatory lesions (generally most severe in the antrum) to the extensive atrophic changes involving both antrum and corpus (59–62). In practice, sampling is usually insufficient to apply these tools effectively.

Intestinal Metaplasia. Two main types of intestinal metaplasia have been described: "complete" (that is small intestinal type or type I) and "incomplete" (types IIA/II and IIB/III) (63,64). In the Filipe classification, the typing of intestinal metaplasia (types I, II, III) was based on detection of sialomucin and sulphomucin by high iron diamine–alcian blue staining (an approach discontinued due to toxicity of the reagents). Type III intestinal metaplasia is the least common, characterized by the presence of columnar mucous cells containing sulphomucins, and is the most closely associated with gastric cancer, especially with intestinal-type adenocarcinoma (65,66). Currently used classifications take into consideration the presence of Paneth cells (complete metaplasia) or crescent architectural changes, dedifferentiation, and the absence of Paneth cells (incomplete metaplasia), as well as the pattern and type of mucin expression (67).

Complete intestinal metaplasia displays goblet cells and absorptive cells with a brush border lining the enterocytes, decreased/absent expression of gastric mucins (MUC1, MUC5AC, and MUC6), and expression of MUC2 (an intestinal mucin). In contrast, incomplete intestinal metaplasia displays goblet and columnar nonabsorptive cells without a brush border and co-expression of gastric mucins and MUC2. Incomplete intestinal metaplasia has a mixed gastric and intestinal phenotype reflecting an aberrant differentiation program (67). Some studies indicate a positive correlation between the degree of incomplete intestinal metaplasia, the extent of intestinal metaplasia, and the risk of progression to carcinoma (62,66,68–70). These associations have not been universally confirmed, however (71–73). While some authors claim that intestinal metaplasia is a "paracancerous" rather than a precancerous lesion (74), other studies provide different results regarding incomplete intestinal metaplasia. Specifically, it has been demonstrated that the high-risk gastritis stages (OLGA and OLGIM stages III and IV) feature mostly types II and III incomplete metaplasia, which incorporates the prognostic message obtainable from histochemical gastric mucin subtyping within the staging groups.

Another pattern of metaplasia, spasmolytic polypeptide-expressing metaplasia (SPEM), which expresses trefoil factor family 2 spasmolytic polypeptide, is associated with oxyntic atrophy and represents the metaplastic replacement of oxyntic glands by mucin-secreting antral-like glands. SPEM characteristically develops in the gastric body and fundus, and is strongly associated with chronic *H. pylori* infection and gastric adenocarcinoma. It is believed to represent another pathway to gastric neoplasia (47,75,76).

Autoimmune Gastritis and Pernicious Anemia. Autoimmune gastritis is associated with an increased risk of gastric dysplasia and adenocarcinoma (77–80). The magnitude of the risk is debated: it is reported by some to be around three times that of the general population (81–85), while a large population-based cohort study in the United States found an incidence of gastric cancer of only 1.2 percent, similar to that of the general population (86). In a single European study, it was observed that the cancer risk is restricted to high-risk gastritis stages (OLGA III-IV), and is associated mainly with concomitant *H. pylori* infection (87).

There is also an increased incidence of mucosal polyps in autoimmune gastritis, including pyloric gland adenoma, and some cases show adenomatous dysplasia of the glandular epithelium (88,89). Furthermore, there is a well established increased risk of development of neuroendocrine tumors (80,90,91) that arise as a result of the proliferative effect of longstanding

hypergastrinemia on gastric fundic enterochromaffin-like (ECL) cells (80,92).

The Operated Stomach and Cancer. Patients with a gastric stump after previous gastric surgery have an increased risk of developing gastric cancer compared to the general population and the risk has been estimated at 5 to 10 percent (93–95). Gastric stump carcinoma is defined as a malignancy of the stomach occurring more than 5 years after initial partial gastrectomy, to avoid confusion with cancer recurrence after initial misdiagnosis (95). The risk increases, usually after 15 to 25 years (96–99). It is higher following Billroth II gastrectomy and in those who have undergone surgery for gastric ulcer, while those operated on for duodenal ulcer are at a lower risk (100). Two categories of gastric stump carcinoma after distal gastrectomy have been suggested: one develops at the stomal area following distal gastrectomy for benign disease after a long latency period (15 to 20 years or more), caused by the duodenogastric reflux; the other develops in the remnant stomach following gastric cancer surgery during the follow-up period (10 years or less), and is correlated with *H. pylori* infection (101,102).

Peptic Ulcer Disease. It is well established that chronic duodenal ulcer is associated with a reduced risk of gastric cancer (103). The association between chronic gastric ulcer and cancer is less clear. In a study of Swedish patients with gastric ulcer who did not undergo surgery, the incidence of gastric cancer was almost twice the expected rate during an average follow-up of 9 years (104). This was particularly true for women and for patients with ulcers in the body of the stomach compared to those with prepyloric ulcers. Eradication of *H. pylori* is associated with a decreased risk of gastric cancer in patients with peptic ulcer disease (105).

Gastric Polyps and Cancer. Epithelial polyps, neoplastic and non-neoplastic, are associated with the development of gastric cancer.

Risk Factors

Helicobacter Pylori **Infection.** *H. pylori* infection plays an important role in gastric carcinogenesis. *H. pylori* infection was shown to be associated with the development of early gastric cancer in Japan (106). It is now estimated that at least 89 percent of all non-cardia gastric cancers are caused by *H. pylori* (107). In 1994, the International Agency for Research on Cancer (IARC) classified *H. pylori* as a group 1 carcinogen for gastric cancer (108-111).

A systematic review and meta-analysis to assess the prevalence of *H. pylori* infection worldwide found that more than half the world's population is infected. The geographic variation is great: among individual countries, the prevalence of *H. pylori* infection varies from as low as 18.9 percent in Switzerland to 87.7 percent in Nigeria (112). Another meta-analysis combining 12 prospective cohort studies determined an association between *H. pylori* seropositivity and non-cardia gastric cancer with an odds ratio of 2.97 (95 percent confidence interval, 2.34 to 3.77) (113). Higher risk figures have been reported, especially when more sensitive *H. pylori* detection assays are used (114–116).

The epidemiologic data that link *H. pylori* and gastric cancer have been reinforced by data obtained in animal models of infection, in particular in Mongolian gerbils (117–120). Furthermore, *H. pylori* eradication studies in humans have helped to consolidate this link by showing a reduction in the incidence of gastric cancer. A meta-analysis of six randomized eradication trials showed that *H. pylori* eradication was superior to placebo or no treatment in preventing gastric cancer, with a risk ratio of 0.66 (95 percent confidence interval, 0.46 to 0.95) (121).

The disproportion between the number of *H. pylori*-infected individuals and those who eventually develop an adenocarcinoma reflects the effects of differences in *H. pylori* virulence, host genetic susceptibility, and environmental factors (41,122,123). *H. pylori* virulence factors that show variation between strains, namely the *cag* pathogenicity island-encoded CagA and the vacuolating cytotoxin VacA, appear to influence the pathogenicity of the bacteria and the risk of gastric precancerous lesions and adenocarcinoma (124). *H. pylori* strains that harbor the CagA protein are associated with higher degrees of mucosal inflammation, gastric precancerous lesion progression, and increased risk of gastric cancer development (125,126). Variation in tyrosine phosphorylation (EPIYA) motifs of the CagA protein seems to be a likely 'actor' in these changes (127–129). More recently, it has been shown that the strain-specific sequences

in the *CagA* gene promoter region influence CagA expression, the secretion of pro-inflammatory cytokines, and gastric histopathology (130,131). Polymorphisms that impact the VacA activity include the signal- (s1 and s2), the intermediate- (i1 and i2), and the mid- (m1 and m2) region (132–134). Infection with *H. pylori* strains with the most virulent VacA s1, m1, and i1 forms is associated with the development of premalignant lesions and an increased risk for gastric adenocarcinoma (123,126,129,135). While these relationships are well established in Western countries, in East Asian countries the impact of *H. pylori* virulence factors in gastric cancer is difficult to unveil as the prevalence of virulent strains is over 95 percent (124,136).

Although the role of *H. pylori* in gastric carcinogenesis is undisputed, there is growing evidence that other microbes in the gastric niche could also affect transformation of gastric epithelial cells (137–139). *H. pylori* plays a crucial role in the initial steps of carcinogenesis by causing enhanced inflammation and progressive degradation of the architecture and function of the gastric epithelium, culminating in atrophic gastritis (140,141). Development of atrophic gastritis, which induces hypochlorhydria due to parietal cell loss, is a key step in the histologic progression to intestinal-type gastric cancer and can lead to overgrowth of non-*Helicobacter* microbiota that contribute to malignant transformation through maintenance of inflammation and conversion of nitrates into *N*-nitrosamines (139,140).

In addition to bacterial factors, host genetic susceptibility that affects the inflammatory response to *H. pylori* infection has been associated with increased gastric cancer risk. For example, polymorphisms in genes encoding interleukin (IL)-1β, IL-1 receptor antagonist, tumor necrosis factor (TNF)-α, and IL-10, all cytokines implicated in the initiation and modulation of the inflammatory response toward *H. pylori*, are shown to be associated with susceptibility to carcinogenesis (123,142–146). The role of bone marrow-derived cells (BMDCs) in the repopulation of damaged gastric mucosa has been shown to be associated with gastric carcinogenesis, both in humans in relation with *H. pylori* infection (147) and in experimental models (148,149).

H. pylori infection also has been implicated in the modification of oncogenes and tumor suppressors. These include *CTNNB1* (encoding β-catenin), *CCND1* (encoding cyclin D1), *TP73* (encoding p73), and *CDKN1B* (encoding p27) (150–152).

Diet. Food and nutrition may play an important role in the prevention and causation of gastric cancer. Diets high in salted, pickled, smoked, or poorly preserved foods; those with high meat content; and those with low fruit and vegetable content are most commonly associated with an increased risk for developing gastric cancer (153–160). An analysis of 60 relevant studies suggests a potential 50 percent higher risk of gastric cancer associated with the intake of pickled vegetables, and perhaps stronger associations in the Republic of Korea and China (156). Within the context of *H. pylori* infection, high dietary salt intake and low iron levels are most highly associated with an increased risk for developing gastric cancer (137,161,162).

Alternatively, adherence to a Mediterranean diet has been shown to be associated with a 33 percent reduction in gastric cancer (163). This diet is characterized by high consumption of fruit, vegetables, cereals, legumes, nuts and seeds, and seafood, with olive oil as the main fat source, moderate alcohol consumption (particularly red wine), low to moderate consumption of dairy products, and low consumption of red and processed meat (164–166).

Smoking. An association has been shown between smoking and stomach cancer that could not be explained by bias or confounding factors (167,168). Smoking also potentiates the carcinogenic effect of infection with CagA-positive *H. pylori* (169–171).

Genetic Predisposition and Hereditary Syndromes

First-degree relatives of patients with gastric cancer are almost three times as likely as the general population to develop gastric cancer (172). This may be partly attributable to *H. pylori* infection being common in families and to the potential role of *IL-1* gene polymorphisms (146,173). However, susceptibility to carcinogens may play a role as well. For example, polymorphisms of genes encoding for glutathione S-transferase enzymes, known to metabolize tobacco-related carcinogens and N-acetyltransferase 1, increase the risk of gastric cancer development (174,175). There also is evidence of familial clustering: about 10 percent of stomach cancers show evidence of a familial component and approximately 1 to 3 percent of gastric cancers are a result of an inherited predisposition (176–178).

CLINICAL FEATURES

Gastric cancer can develop without symptoms, with nonspecific symptoms such as dyspepsia or, in some patients, with so-called "alarm" symptoms, which consist of weight loss, signs and symptoms of upper gastrointestinal hemorrhage, anemia, and vomiting. The clinical presentation is related to topography, growth pattern, and stage of the disease. Apart from Japan and Korea, where screening programs have resulted in early diagnosis in asymptomatic patients, in most Western countries the diagnosis of gastric cancer is made because of dyspeptic and alarm symptoms, which may also be of prognostic significance when reported by the patient at diagnosis (179,180).

Symptoms of early stage cancer may be indistinguishable from those of benign dyspepsia, while the presence of alarm symptoms may imply advanced and often inoperable disease. Most guidelines recommend immediate endoscopy in all patients presenting with alarm symptoms. However, their use as selection criteria for endoscopy seems to be inconsistent since alarm symptoms are not sufficiently sensitive to detect malignancies. When caused by gastric cancer, alarm symptoms are independently related to survival and an increased number, as well as specific alarm symptoms, are closely correlated to the risk of death (179). Dysphagia, weight loss, and a palpable abdominal mass appear to be major independent prognostic factors in gastric cancer, while gastrointestinal bleeding, vomiting and duration of symptoms do not seem to have a significant prognostic impact on survival in gastric cancer (179).

Endoscopy is a sensitive and specific diagnostic test for gastric cancer. Modern video-endoscopy allows the recognition of subtle changes in color, relief, and architecture of the mucosal surface. Although detection of lesions associated with early gastric cancer can be improved using chromoendoscopy and narrow-band imaging, a substantial number of such lesions still escape detection. Tumor staging before treatment decision involves endoscopic ultrasound for characterization of the primary tumor, but is less useful for nodal (N) staging, whereas computerized tomography (CT) is used to detect lymph node and liver metastases. Positron emission tomography (PET) in combination with CT imaging may be superior to either alone for preoperative staging. Laparoscopic staging may be the only way to exclude peritoneal seeding in the absence of ascites. Despite improvements in endoscopic, surgical, and systemic treatments, and an increasing emphasis on multidisciplinary evaluation and treatment of patients, the global 5-year survival rates remain unsatisfactory (25 to 30 percent), with the exception of patients in Japan and South Korea (over 50 percent) (181).

GROSS FINDINGS

Gastric adenocarcinoma can present at an early or advanced disease stage. Early gastric carcinoma is defined as a carcinoma that has infiltrated the mucosa or submucosa regardless of the presence or absence of lymph node metastases (182,183). Gastric carcinoma infiltrating into the muscularis propria and beyond is defined as advanced.

Early Gastric Cancer

Most EGCs measure 2 to 5 cm and are localized on the lesser curvature around the angulus (184–187). Some remain confined to the superficial layers for several years, although potentially expanding laterally to a considerable degree; others penetrate the gastric wall rapidly and can then invade into the submucosa when they are only about 3 to 5 mm in size (188,189). Minute EGCs that measure less than 5 mm in diameter and superficial spreading EGCs with neoplastic cells spreading over large areas are observed (183).

Endoscopists divide EGCs into three types based on the endoscopic appearance: type 0-I (protruded), polypoid growth (subcategorized into Ip [pedunculated] and Is [sessile]); type 0-II (superficial), nonpolypoid growth (subcategorized into type 0-IIa [slightly elevated], type 0-IIb [flat], and type 0-IIc [slightly depressed]); and type 0-III, excavated growth (190) (figs. 9-2–9-4).

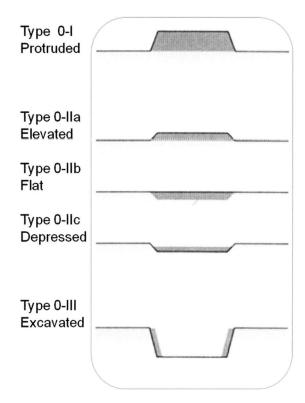

Figure 9-2

ENDOSCOPIC CLASSIFICATION OF EARLY GASTRIC CARCINOMA GROWTH PATTERNS

Growth patterns of early gastric carcinoma (EGC) according to the Paris classification.

Advanced Gastric Cancer

Advanced gastric carcinomas can display various gross appearances. The Borrmann classification remains the most widely used. It divides gastric carcinomas into four types: polypoid carcinoma (type 1), fungating carcinoma (type 2), ulcerated carcinoma (type 3), and diffusely infiltrative carcinoma (type 4) (191) (fig. 9-5).

Polypoid and fungating tumors typically consist of friable masses that bleed easily and project from a broad base in the gastric lumen. They tend to develop in the body of the stomach, in the region of the greater curvature, posterior wall, or fundus. Ulcerated tumors occur frequently in the EGJ, antrum, or lesser curvature. They differ from benign ulcers by an irregular margin with raised borders and thickened, uneven and indurated surrounding mucosa. The ulcer base is necrotic, shaggy, and often nodular. Mucosal folds radiating from

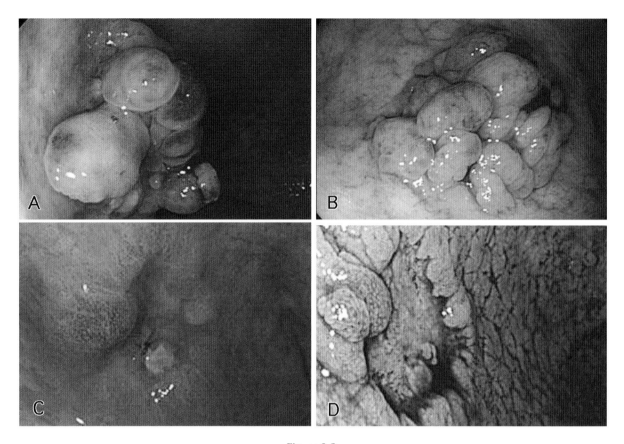

Figure 9-3

EARLY GASTRIC CARCINOMA: ENDOSCOPY

A: Type 0-I: well-demarcated multinodular polypoid lesion by white conventional endoscopy.
B: Same as A, by chromoendoscopy.
C: Type 0-IIc: deep mucosal depression with irregular margin by white conventional endoscopy.
D: Same as C, by chromoendoscopy. (Courtesy of Dr. Tadakazu Shimoda, Japan.)

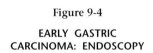

Figure 9-4

EARLY GASTRIC CARCINOMA: ENDOSCOPY

Type 0-IIa, seen by narrow band imaging (NBI), displays an irregular mucosal pattern compared to surrounding mucosa. (Courtesy of Dr. Tadakazu Shimoda, Japan.)

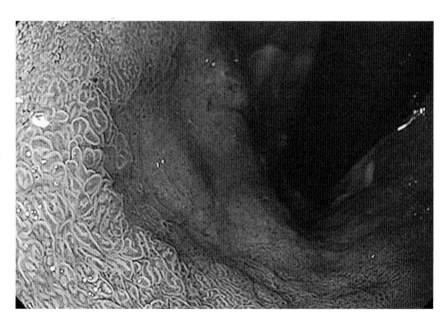

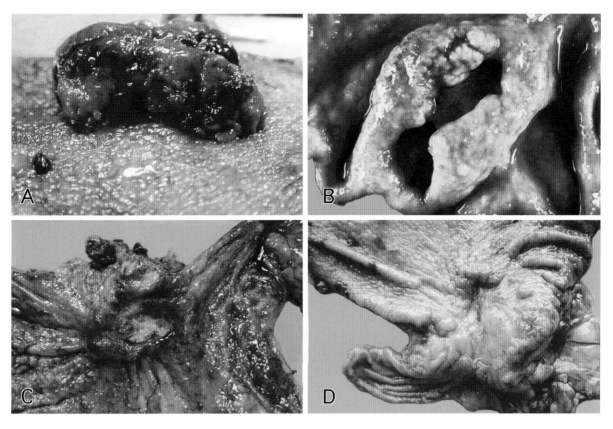

Figure 9-5

GASTRIC ADENOCARCINOMA: BORRMANN CLASSIFICATION

A: Type 1 (polypoid): well-defined polypoid tumor with inflamed nodular surface. (Courtesy of Prof. Pinto de Sousa, Portugal.)

B: Type 2 (fungating): elevated tumor mass with central ulceration, crater formation, and raised irregular margin. (Courtesy of Dr. Tadakazu Shimoda, Japan.)

C: Type 3 (ulcerated): central crater with necrotic base, surrounded by a raised rolled margin. (Courtesy of Prof. Pinto de Sousa, Portugal.)

D: Type 4 (infiltrative): plaque-like lesion with flattening of the rugal folds, with an irregular surface and focal ulceration. (Courtesy of Prof. Pinto de Sousa, Portugal.)

the crater are irregular and frequently show club-like thickening and fusion. Malignant ulcers tend to be larger than their benign counterparts. However, many malignant ulcers lack these typical features and, therefore, endoscopic appearance is not a sufficiently reliable guide to diagnosis (192) and should be complemented by numerous systematic biopsies.

Invasive adenocarcinoma, particularly when composed of poorly cohesive neoplastic cells, may spread superficially in the mucosa and submucosa, giving rise to plaque-like lesions with flattening of the rugal folds. In some cases, superficial ulceration supervenes. Frequently, the infiltration involves the entire thickness of the wall, usually over a limited area but sometimes extensively, to produce the so-called linitis plastica or "leather bottle" stomach. In these cases, the wall assumes a stiff consistency due to an extensive desmoplastic response to tumor cells. There is usually no visible localized growth. A characteristic feature, at endoscopy, is that, because of the diffuse involvement of the stomach, it fails to inflate, in marked contrast to the normal stomach. Other gastric carcinomas, irrespective of histologic type, may secrete considerable amounts of mucin, which gives the tumor a gelatinous appearance to the naked eye. These are referred to as mucinous or colloid carcinomas.

Table 9-1

WORLD HEALTH ORGANIZATION (WHO) CLASSIFICATION OF EPITHELIAL TUMORS OF THE STOMACH: MALIGNANCY-ASSOCIATED AND PREMALIGNANT LESIONS[a]

Glandular intraepithelial neoplasia (dysplasia), low grade

Glandular intraepithelial neoplasia (dysplasia), high grade

Adenoma

Adenocarcinoma

Papillary adenocarcinoma

Tubular adenocarcinoma

Mucinous adenocarcinoma

Poorly cohesive carcinoma (including signet ring cell carcinoma and other variants)

Mixed carcinoma

Adenosquamous carcinoma

Squamous cell carcinoma

Hepatoid adenocarcinoma

Carcinoma with lymphoid stroma (medullary carcinoma)

Undifferentiated carcinoma

Hereditary diffuse gastric cancer

[a]Data reference 193.

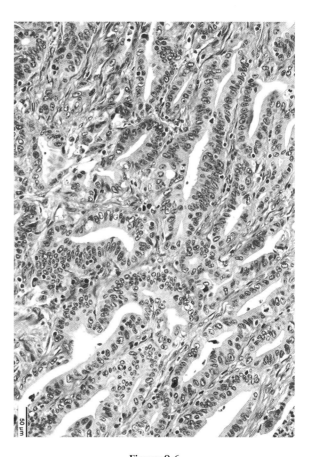

Figure 9-6

TUBULAR CARCINOMA

Well-differentiated tubular adenocarcinoma shows well-defined, closely packed tubules lined by columnar neoplastic cells, with minimal intervening stroma.

MICROSCOPIC FINDINGS AND HISTOLOGIC CLASSIFICATION

Despite epidemiologic differences, adenocarcinomas of the proximal and distal stomach show similar microscopic features. The histologic classification of gastric adenocarcinoma is challenging because of intratumoral variations in architecture or differentiation, and several histologic classifications have been proposed over the years.

World Health Organization (WHO) Classification

The WHO classification, which does not take into account histogenesis and differentiation, recognizes five main types of gastric adenocarcinoma (tubular, papillary, mucinous, poorly cohesive, and mixed), as well as rare variants (Table 9-1) (193).

Tubular Adenocarcinoma. This type consists of tubular structures, branching glands, or acinar structures surrounded by various degrees of desmoplasia. Individual neoplastic cells can be columnar, cuboidal or flattened by intraluminal mucin (figs. 9-6–9-8). A clear cell variant also has been recognized. Nuclear atypia ranging from low to high grade can be seen (194,195). A poorly differentiated component may coexist, composed of compact sheets of tumor cells (fig. 9-9). At the other end of the spectrum, (extremely) well-differentiated gastric adenocarcinoma has been described (195), either with gastric or intestinal differentiation (196–198), some mimicking complete-type intestinal metaplasia in the stomach (fig. 9-10) (194). Tubular adenocarcinomas develop mainly in the antrum and body of the stomach and are strongly linked to chronic *H. pylori* infection, atrophic gastritis, and intestinal metaplasia.

Papillary Adenocarcinoma. Typically, this tumor grows as an exophytic polypoid mass with a sharply demarcated invading edge. It is composed of pointed or blunted papillary epithelial processes

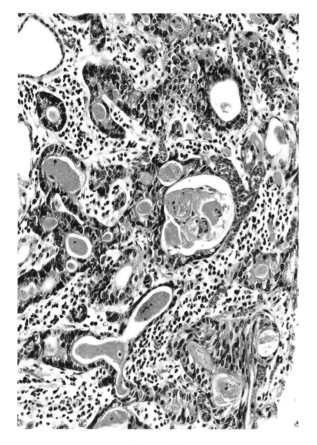

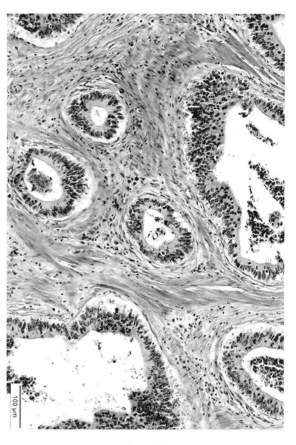

Figure 9-7

TUBULAR CARCINOMA

Moderately differentiated tubular adenocarcinoma composed of irregular tubular structures lined by cuboidal cells. Some glands are dilated and filled with colloid-like material or necrotic debris.

Figure 9-8

TUBULAR CARCINOMA

The tumor invades the muscle layer.

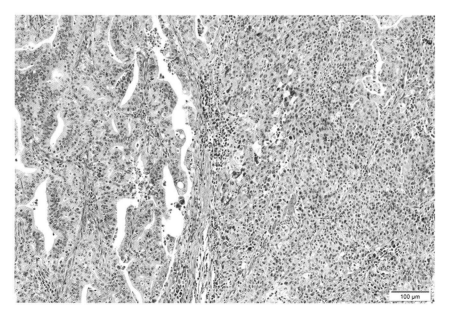

Figure 9-9

TUBULOPAPILLARY ADENOCARCINOMA WITH A POORLY DIFFERENTIATED COMPONENT

A moderately differentiated component is seen on the left and a poorly differentiated component on the right.

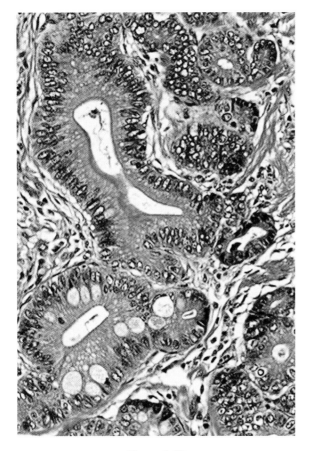

Figure 9-10

WELL-DIFFERENTIATED TUBULAR ADENOCARCINOMA: INTESTINAL DIFFERENTIATION

The neoplasm is composed of irregularly shaped tubules lined by columnar and goblet cells (mimicking intestinal metaplasia).

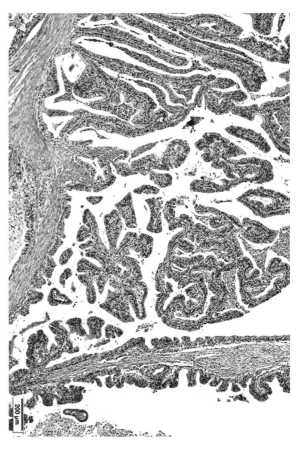

Figure 9-11

PAPILLARY CARCINOMA

Finger-like fibrovascular cores lined by neoplastic cells are characteristic of this tumor type.

with fibrovascular cores (fig. 9-11). Tubulocystic formation may be observed but the papillary pattern predominates. The neoplastic cells tend to maintain their polarity, and the degree of cellular atypia and mitotic index can vary significantly. A dense acute and chronic inflammatory infiltrate may be noted. Papillary adenocarcinomas occur mainly in the proximal stomach, and are frequently associated with liver metastases.

Mucinous Adenocarcinoma. Mucinous adenocarcinomas (also described as *mucoid* or *colloid carcinomas*) are composed of malignant epithelium mixed with extracellular mucin pools. By convention, the tumor shows more than 50 percent extracellular mucin. Marked heterogeneity is seen in some tumors, with the epithelial component forming glands or disag-

gregated ribbons or clusters of cells floating in lakes of mucin (fig. 9-12).

Poorly Cohesive Carcinomas, Including Signet Ring Cell Carcinoma. Poorly cohesive tumors were previously inaccurately included in a general category of signet ring cell carcinoma even in cases in which signet ring cells were not identified. The current WHO classification recognizes that a general category of poorly cohesive tumors better reflects the wide diversity of tumors composed of neoplastic cells that are isolated or arranged in small aggregates and may display various morphologies. One such tumor is the *signet ring cell type*, a tumor composed predominantly or exclusively of signet ring cells characterized by a central, optically clear or eosinophilic, globoid droplet of cytoplasmic mucin with an eccentrically placed nucleus (fig. 9-13).

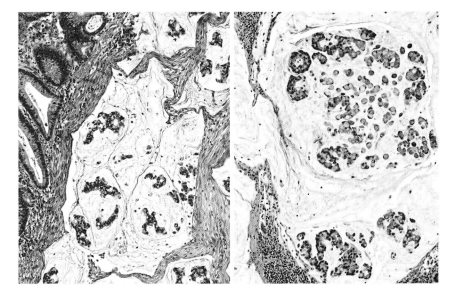

Figure 9-12

MUCINOUS CARCINOMA

The tumor is characterized by a large amount of extracellular mucin in which the neoplastic epithelium is floating within pools of mucin.

Left: The malignant epithelium consists of irregular glands.

Right: The neoplastic epithelium consists mainly of signet ring cells.

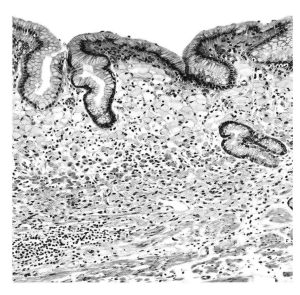

Figure 9-13

POORLY COHESIVE CARCINOMA: SIGNET RING CELL TYPE

The tumor is composed of signet ring cells, characterized by an eccentrically placed nucleus and eosinophilic cytoplasm. The neoplastic cells are small in the deep region of the mucosa and much larger in the superficial part of the lamina propria. (Courtesy of Dr. Tadakazu Shimoda, Japan.)

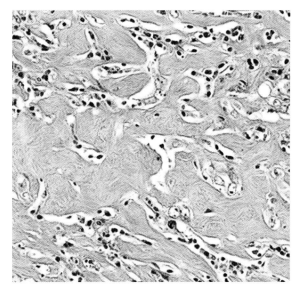

Figure 9-14

POORLY COHESIVE CARCINOMA

This tumor deeply invades the gastric wall, and is associated with marked desmoplasia.

The cells may form a lace-like or delicate microtrabecular pattern (usually when intramucosal) or are accompanied by marked desmoplasia in deeper levels of the gastric wall, losing the morphologic features of signet ring cells (fig. 9-14). In some cases, signet ring cells may be restricted to the superficial aspect of the mucosa with a transition toward other variants of discohesive cells within the deeper levels of the gastric wall. Tumors composed predominantly of signet ring cells are more common in younger patients and in the distal stomach (199).

Other poorly cohesive variants include tumors composed of neoplastic cells resembling histiocytes or lymphocytes; others have deeply

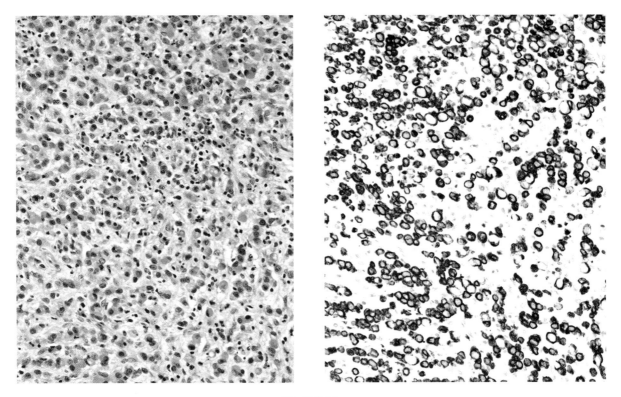

Figure 9-15

POORLY COHESIVE CARCINOMA: NON-SIGNET RING CELL TYPE

Left: The neoplastic cells display a plasmacytoid phenotype.
Right: The neoplastic cells are immunoreactive for cytokeratin.

eosinophilic cytoplasm sometimes mimicking plasma cells (fig. 9-15) (200). Some poorly cohesive cells may show significant nuclear irregularity, including particularly bizarre nuclei (fig. 9-16). A mixture of the different cell types can be seen, including signet ring cells.

Mixed Carcinoma. Mixed adenocarcinomas show a mixture of morphologically identifiable glandular (tubular/papillary) and poorly cohesive cellular histologic components (figs. 9-17, 9-18). Mixed carcinomas have been shown to be clonal (201,202) and the phenotypic divergence has been attributed to somatic mutation in the E-cadherin gene (*CDH1*), restricted to the poorly cohesive component (fig. 9-19) (203). Enhanced promoter CpG island hypermethylation also has been implicated in the histogenesis of mixed carcinoma (204).

Laurén Classification

The Laurén classification (205) maintains historic value, since it has proven useful in evalu-

ating the natural history of gastric carcinoma, especially with regard to its association with environmental factors, incidence trends, and precursors. The tumors are classified into one of two major types, intestinal or diffuse. Tumors that contain approximately equal quantities of intestinal and diffuse components are called mixed carcinomas. Carcinomas too undifferentiated to fit neatly into either category are placed in the indeterminate category.

Intestinal Carcinomas. The intestinal type is more common in males and older age groups. It usually has a polypoid or fungating gross appearance and often an expansile growth pattern. These neoplasms form glands with various degrees of differentiation, sometimes with poorly differentiated tumor areas mixed in. The glandular epithelium consists of large pleomorphic cells with hyperchromatic nuclei, often with numerous mitoses. Mucin secretion is variable and occurs either focally in the cytoplasm of scattered cells or extracellularly

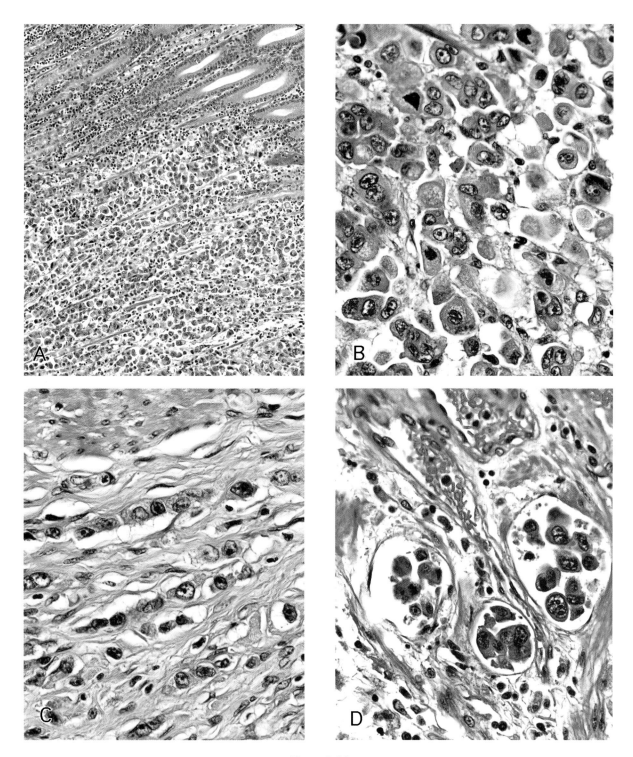

Figure 9-16

POORLY COHESIVE CARCINOMA: NON-SIGNET RING CELL TYPE, COMPOSED OF BIZARRE, ATYPICAL CELLS

A: The gastric mucosa is extensively infiltrated by poorly cohesive carcinoma, non-signet ring cell type.
B: At higher magnification, the neoplastic cells are highly atypical, and show bizarre nuclei.
C: The muscle layer is invaded by tumor.
D: Lymphatic permeation by bizarre-shaped tumor cells.

Tumors of the Esophagus and Stomach

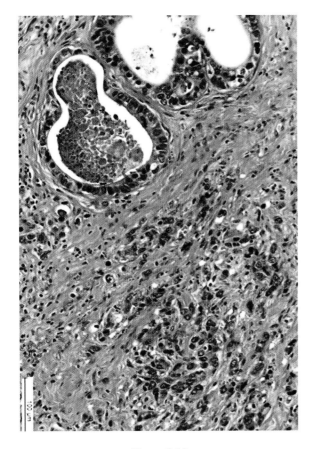

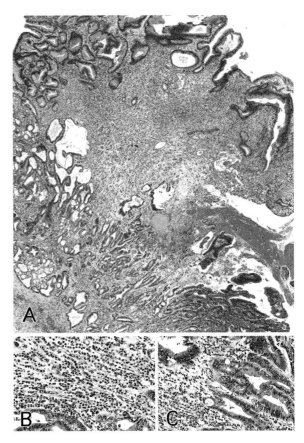

Figure 9-17

MIXED CARCINOMA

The tumor displays two morphologically identifiable components: a tubular component (top) and a poorly cohesive component (bottom).

Figure 9-18

MIXED CARCINOMA

A: This mixed carcinoma is composed of a tubular component (bottom and left side) and a poorly cohesive, non-signet ring cell component (central part). (Courtesy of Prof. Jean-François Fléjou, France.)

B: Poorly cohesive, non-signet ring cell component at higher magnification.

C: Tubular component at higher magnification.

Figure 9-19

MIXED CARCINOMA

Left: The tubular component (left) transforms into a poorly cohesive component with signet ring cells (right).

Right: Loss or decreased expression of E-cadherin in the poorly cohesive component (right), but present at the cell membrane in the tubular component (left).

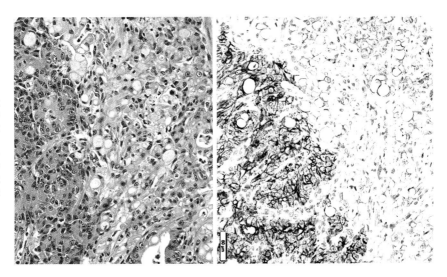

214

in the lumens of neoplastic glands. Intestinal carcinomas typically arise on a background of intestinal metaplasia. At the cellular level, despite being classified as intestinal, the neoplastic cells may show morphologic or immunophenotypic evidence not only of intestinal differentiation but also of gastric, gastrointestinal, unclassifiable, or null differentiation, underscoring the inadequacies of this classification.

Diffuse Carcinomas. The diffuse type shows a more equal male to female ratio and is more frequent in younger individuals. It has an ulcerative or infiltrative gross appearance and a diffuse, infiltrative growth pattern. These tumors are classified as "poorly cohesive carcinomas, including signet ring cell carcinoma" in the current WHO classification (193). In this type, poorly cohesive cells diffusely infiltrate the gastric wall, with little or no gland formation. Mucin secretion is common, and can be widespread throughout the tumor. Desmoplastic connective tissue proliferation is usually more marked than in intestinal cancers and inflammatory cell infiltration less prominent.

Of the 1,344 tumors originally described by Laurén (205), 53 percent were intestinal and 33 percent diffuse, and the remainder included tumors that contained equal proportions of intestinal and diffuse types (mixed) or were undifferentiated with a solid growth pattern. The decreasing incidence of gastric cancer appears to result from a reduction in intestinal-type tumors, while diffuse tumors remain constant.

Other Classifications

The Laurén and WHO classifications are the ones most commonly used outside of Japan. In Japan, the Japanese Gastric Cancer Association, updated in 2017, recommends a histologic typing system that is similar but not 100 percent identical to the WHO classification (Table 9-2) (182).

The Nakamura classification (206) extensively used in Japan divides gastric cancer in two groups: differentiated and undifferentiated. The former encompasses tubular and papillary adenocarcinomas, the latter includes poorly differentiated adenocarcinoma and signet ring cell carcinoma (Table 9-2).

The classification of Mulligan and Rember (207) is based on cell differentiation and recognizes a third subtype, pyloro-cardiac gland type,

characterized by glands of various sizes lined by stratified or singly oriented cylindrical cells that often show striking vacuolization or clear cell changes. Notably, it occurs predominantly in the "cardia" or pylorus.

The classification proposed by Ming (208) is based on the pattern of growth and invasion at the advancing edge, dividing tumors into an expansile type (about 67 percent), for those composed of discrete tumor nodules with a pushing edge, and an infiltrative type (about 33 percent), for those formed of widely infiltrative tumor cells with a poor inflammatory cell response and desmoplasia. In general, Ming's expansile and infiltrative tumors correspond to Laurén's intestinal and diffuse tumor types, with a similar number of cases showing overlap in patterns.

The Goseki classification (209) is a four-grade scheme based on tubular differentiation and intracellular mucin production: group I consists of well-differentiated tubules with poor intracellular mucin production; group II consists of well-differentiated tubules and plentiful intracellular mucin; group III has poorly differentiated tubules and poor intracellular mucin; and group IV tumors are made up of poorly differentiated tubules and plentiful intracellular mucin. Prognostic value has been attributed to this classification system (209,210).

A three-tiered prognostic classification based on histologic, clinico-pathologic, and molecular parameters was proposed by Italian authors (211,212).

Phenotypic Classification

In 1997, Carneiro et al. (213) proposed a classification based on four histotypes: glandular and isolated cell carcinomas (roughly equivalent to the intestinal and diffuse carcinomas of the Laurén classification); a solid type (composed of sheets, trabeculae, or islands of undifferentiated cells with no gland formation); and a mixed type (consisting of a mixture of glandular and isolated cell types). This classification suggests that intestinal carcinoma is a misnomer, since a large proportion of these tumors displays a gastric phenotype, as demonstrated by mucin and trefoil factor peptide expression (discussed below). This classification was shown to have prognostic significance (214). Some studies also have shown that "mixed" carcinomas have

Table 9-2

COMPARISON OF DIFFERENT CLASSIFICATION SYSTEMS FOR GASTRIC CANCER[a]

Laurén (1965)	Nakamura (1968)	Word Health Organization (WHO) (2010)	Japanese Classification (2017)
Intestinal	Differentiated	Papillary Tubular, well-differentiated Tubular, moderately-differentiated	Papillary: pap Tubular 1 (well-differentiated): tub1 Tubular 2 (moderately-differentiated): tub2
Intermediate	Undifferentiated	Tubular, poorly-differentiated	Poorly 1 (solid type)
Intestinal/diffuse	Differentiated/ Undifferentiated	Mucinous	Mucinous
Diffuse	Undifferentiated	Poorly cohesive, SRC[b] phenotype Poorly cohesive, other cell types	SRC carcinoma: sig Poorly 2 (non-solid type): por2
Mixed	Undifferentiated	Mixed	Description according to the proportion (e.g., por2>sig>tub2)
		Histologic variants[c]: Adenosquamous carcinoma Squamous cell carcinoma Undifferentiated carcinoma Carcinoma with lymphoid stroma Hepatoid adenocarcinoma Adenocarcinoma of fundic gland type Micropapillary adenocarcinoma Miscellaneous carcinomas[d]	**Special types[d]:** Adenosquamous carcinoma Squamous cell carcinoma Undifferentiated carcinoma Carcinoma with lymphoid stroma Hepatoid adenocarcinoma Adenocarcinoma with enteroblastic differentiation Miscellaneous carcinomas[e]

[a]Table prepared in collaboration with Prof. Ryoji Kushima, Japan.
[b]SRC = signet ring cell.
[c]Neuroendocrine neoplasms are not included.
[d]Miscellaneous carcinomas (WHO): carcinosarcoma, choriocarcinoma, malignant rhabdoid tumor, mucoepidermoid carcinoma, parietal carcinoma, Paneth cell carcinoma, pure gastric yolk-sac tumor.
[e]Miscellaneous carcinomas (JGCA): carcinosarcoma, choriocarcinoma, invasive micropapillary carcinoma, yolk sac tumor-like carcinoma.

distinct patterns of invasion, and are more aggressive than pure types (202,215). The mixed histotype was shown to be an independent risk factor for nodal metastases in submucosal gastric cancers (216).

An increasing interest in cell differentiation has allowed for a better understanding of tumor histogenesis. The data emerged from ultrastructural (217) and immunohistochemical studies using markers of cell differentiation, such as 1) markers of surface epithelium (foveolar cells): MUC5AC and trefoil peptide TFF1; 2) markers of mucous neck cell, pyloric gland, and Brunner gland cells: mucin MUC6 and trefoil peptide TFF2; and 3) markers of intestinal (columnar) and goblet cells: MUC2, CDX-2, and CD10.

According to their immunohistochemical expression, four gastric cancer immunophenotypes have been described: intestinal (expressing MUC2, CD10, CDX2) (fig. 9-20), gastric (expressing MUC5AC/TTF1 and/or MUC6/TTF2) (fig. 9-21), hybrid (expressing intestinal and gastric markers), and null phenotype (Table 9-3) (218–221). The expression of p53 is frequently observed in tumors with intestinal-type differentiation. These phenotypes have been recognized also in gastric cancer precursor lesions (42,222). The mixed phenotype may be further subdivided into gastric predominant type and intestinal predominant type. In addition, pepsinogen-1 staining has been used to distinguish mucous neck/pseudopyloric type from the true pyloric type (220). These findings challenge the classic proposed histogenetic pathway from chronic atrophic gastritis through intestinal metaplasia to intestinal-type carcinoma (213,223–225) and also show that the phenotype may impact prognosis, although the proportion of each variant differs in various studies and the findings are not universal (226–231).

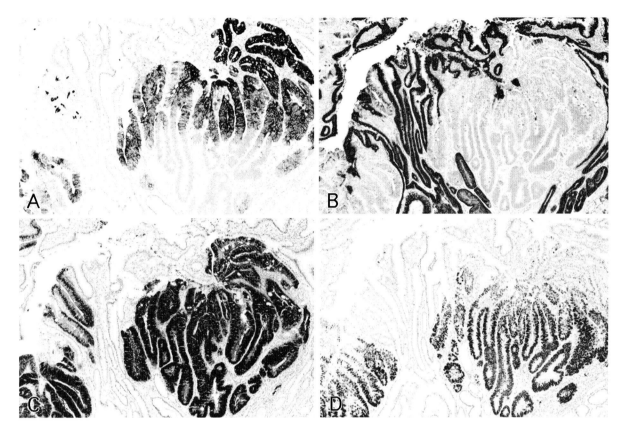

Figure 9-20

INTRAMUCOSAL TUBULAR ADENOCARCINOMA WITH INTESTINAL PHENOTYPE

A: Expression of MUC2.
B: Lack of expression of MUC5AC.
C: Diffuse and intense expression of CDX2.
D: Expression of p53.

Table 9-3

PHENOTYPIC DIFFERENTIATION OF GASTRIC CARCINOMA

Histologic Type	Cell Differentiation	Markers
Tubular and papillary adenocarcinomas	Intestinal type	MUC2 CD10 CDX2 (high)
Signet ring cell carcinoma	Gastric type	MUC5AC MUC6 CDX2 (low/absent)
Mucinous adenocarcinoma	Gastric and/or intestinal type	MUC5Ac MUC6 MUC2 CD10 CDX2 (variable)
Undifferentiated carcinoma	Null	

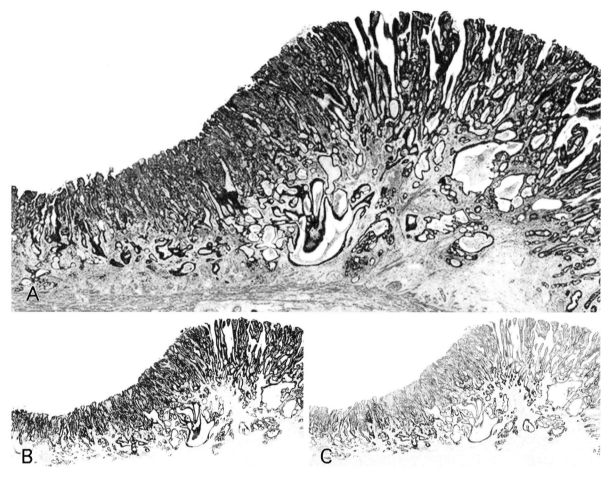

Figure 9-21

TUBULOPAPILLARY ADENOCARCINOMA WITH GASTRIC PHENOTYPE

A: Panoramic view of the lesion.
B: Diffuse and intense expression MUC5AC.
C: Mild expression of MUC6 in the deep part of the tumor. (Courtesy of Dr. Tadakazu Shimoda, Japan.)

Merits of the Various Classifications of Gastric Cancer

None of the current schemes are fully satisfactory. None offers ease of use and reproducibility, combined with prognostic relevance and histogenesis. The WHO and Laurén classifications are widely used, but are of little prognostic value. One drawback of the various classifications is that many gastric carcinomas are heterogenous.

Early Gastric Cancer

Most early gastric cancers (EGCs) are well-differentiated glandular carcinomas. This is particularly true for small (less than 2 cm) lesions.

However, when the size increases and submucosal invasion develops, histologic diversity also develops, with mixed or poorly differentiated components commonly detected as well. Tubular and papillary variants represent over 50 and 30 percent of EGCs, respectively, and are usually polypoid or elevated (type 0-I and 0-IIa) (fig. 9-22). Signet ring cell carcinoma and poorly differentiated carcinoma represent 25 and 15 percent of the cases, respectively, and are usually depressed or ulcerated types (types 0-IIc and 0-III) (fig. 9-23) (184,232,233).

A biopsy diagnosis of EGC may be challenging. A small number of signet ring cells infiltrating the lamina propria can be overlooked easily but their

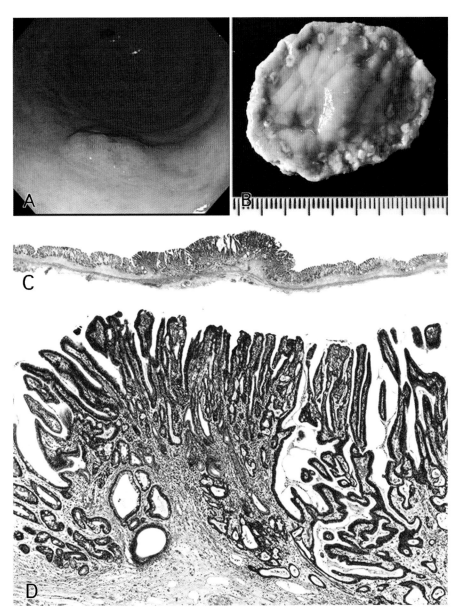

Figure 9-22

EARLY GASTRIC CANCER: TYPE 0-IIA, INTESTINAL TYPE

A: Conventional (white light) endoscopic appearance of a slightly elevated lesion.

B: A well-demarcated elevated lesion is identified in the endoscopic submucosal dissection (ESD) specimen.

C,D: Histologic features at low (C) and high (D) magnification. A tubulopapillary adenocarcinoma (papillary component at the surface; tubular component in the deep region) is seen in D. (Courtesy of Dr. Tadakazu Shimoda, Japan.)

detection can be facilitated by special stains (234). Conversely, muciphages and the finely vacuolated cells of a gastric xanthoma/xanthelasma may be mistaken for signet ring cell carcinoma as well. In such cases, careful attention to the nuclear morphology and the use of immunohistochemical (epithelial and macrophage) markers are helpful. Other histologic mimics of poorly cohesive gastric carcinoma include artifactual extrusion of highly proliferative benign mucous neck cells with prominent mitoses that form sheets of discohesive cells; these represent detachment of the highly proliferative neck zone from the surrounding mucosa (235). Similar lesions have been described by Wu et al. (236).

For gland-forming neoplasms, distinction between high-grade intraepithelial neoplasia/dysplasia and well-differentiated tubular carcinoma, especially of type 0-I and 0-IIa EGCs, can be difficult to make on biopsy material. Furthermore, there is good evidence that a proportion of type 0-I and 0-IIa EGCs result from malignant transformation of an adenoma (234,237). Fortunately, distinction between high-grade intraepithelial neoplasia/dysplasia and well-differentiated tubular carcinoma is of

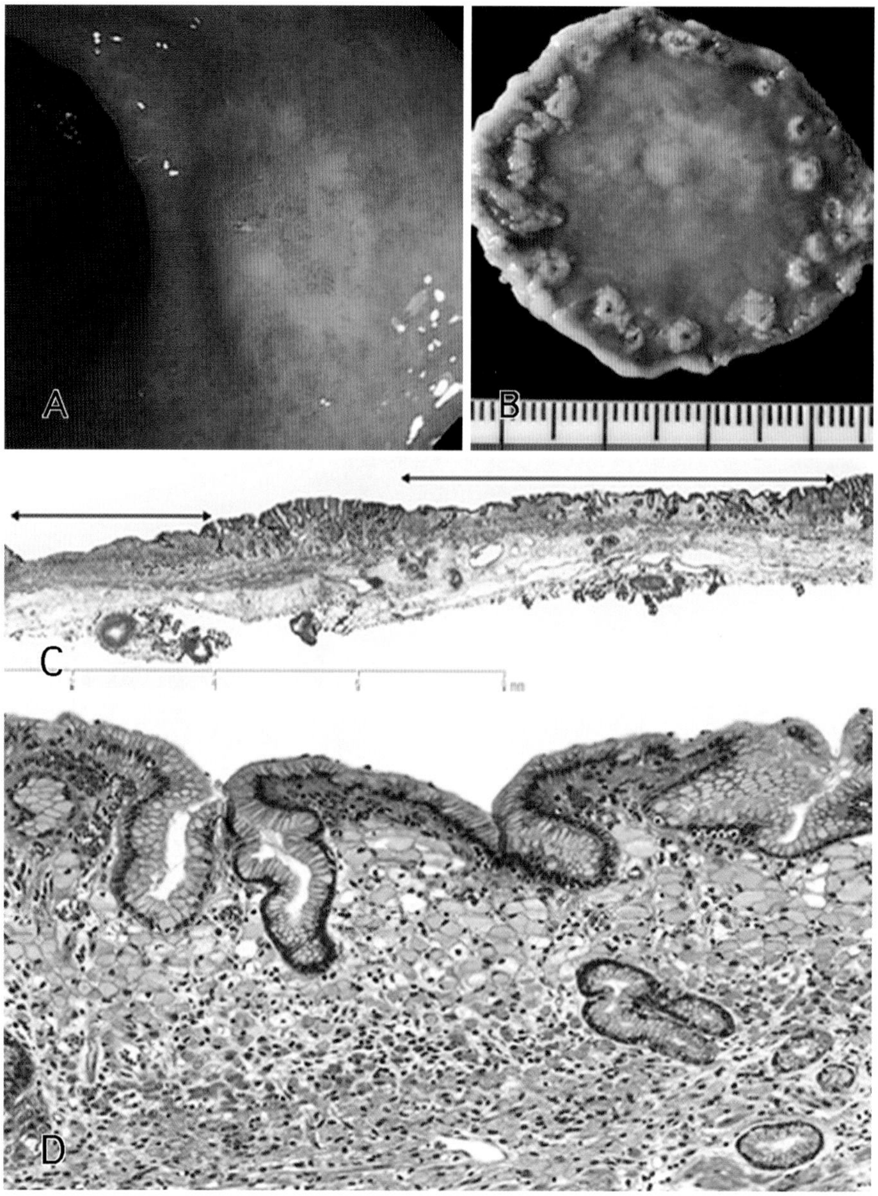

Figure 9-23

EARLY GASTRIC CANCER: TYPE 0-IIC, DIFFUSE TYPE

A: Conventional (white light) endoscopic appearance of a slightly depressed lesion.

B: A well-demarcated shallow mucosal depression with discoloration is seen.

C: Panoramic view of lesion (black line).

D: High magnification displays a signet ring cell carcinoma. (Courtesy of Dr. Tadakazu Shimoda, Japan.)

limited clinical value, since these two conditions are both managed endoscopically. The location, size, and configuration of the lesion and the patient's physical condition are important features that help guide therapeutic decisions.

Careful histologic assessment of submucosal invasion, particularly depth of invasion, is important in evaluating resected EGCs because it correlates with the likelihood of lymph node metastasis (238). Submucosal invasion occurs in about 50 percent of cases, a figure that varies remarkably little between series (232), and is less common in flat (type 0-IIb)

lesions (239). Lymph node metastasis occurs in 3 to 20 percent of all EGCs (35,232,238,240) and correlates with the depth of submucosal invasion and increasing tumor diameter (232,238,241,242).

Endoscopic resection has become the reference standard in the treatment of superficial gastric cancers. The following data are recommended to assess the curability of endoscopic resection: 1) status of resection margins, particularly the deep margin, 2) tumor size, 3) depth of invasion, 4) presence of ulcer scar, 5) lymphovascular invasion, and 6) histologic type (243).

When a tumor involves the submucosal layer, the depth of submucosal invasion must be recorded. To facilitate objective and reproducible evaluation, immunohistochemistry for desmin may be useful to measure the absolute distance between the lower aspect of the muscularis mucosae and the deepest portion of the tumor (243). Special stains, such as antipodoplanin (D2-40) antibody (244) and elastic stains in lesions with submucosal invasion, significantly improve the detection sensitivity of lymphovascular invasion, even when the submucosal invasion is limited.

HISTOLOGIC GRADING

Grading applies primarily to tubular and papillary carcinomas. Other types of gastric carcinoma are not normally graded (193). Well-differentiated adenocarcinomas are composed of preserved glands, sometimes resembling metaplastic intestinal epithelium (194). Poorly differentiated adenocarcinomas are composed of irregular glandular structures. Moderately differentiated adenocarcinomas display features intermediate between well and poorly differentiated ones. Given the interobserver variability in grading lesions, we favor gastric cancers being reported as either low grade (well and moderately differentiated) or high grade (poorly differentiated).

CYTOLOGIC FINDINGS

Well-/Moderately Differentiated Gastric Adenocarcinomas

A well-differentiated intestinal-type adenocarcinoma needs to be distinguished from an adenoma on the basis of cellularity and dyshesion. Adenocarcinomas are much more cellular and show more obvious dyshesion and architectural atypia, depending on the degree of differentiation. Well-differentiated adenocarcinomas may show minimal dyshesion, with cells arranged in a discernible glandular configuration showing polarization of nuclei and lumen formation (fig. 9-24). Stratification of nuclei is easily appreciated, especially when strips of cells are viewed from the side. The N/C ratio is moderately increased, with a fair amount of granular or vacuolated cytoplasm. Nuclei are oval to elongated with either fine, open chromatin and prominent single nucle-

oli or hyperchromatic, coarse chromatin and multiple small nucleoli.

Well-differentiated adenocarcinomas also need to be distinguished from reactive/reparative changes. While reactive/reparative cells are usually arranged in orderly, cohesive, two-dimensional sheets with a streaming pattern (fig. 9-25), adenocarcinomas are disorderly arranged in dyshesive or loosely cohesive three-dimensional clusters. At least a few atypical epithelial cells should be present before a definitive diagnosis of adenocarcinoma can be made. Significant cytologic atypia, including macronucleoli, chromatin aberration, or sharp nuclear membrane irregularity should also be present for a definitive diagnosis of carcinoma. Dyshesion and cytologic atypia become more pronounced and gland formation becomes less apparent for less well-differentiated/moderately differentiated adenocarcinomas (fig. 9-26).

Poorly Cohesive Gastric Adenocarcinomas

Poorly cohesive gastric adenocarcinomas (signet ring cell carcinoma and other subtypes) represent a diagnostic challenge. Since the tumor cells in the mucosa primarily involve the lamina propria, they may not be sampled on cytologic specimens unless the epithelium is eroded or ulcerated. Endoscopic fine-needle aspirations are more likely than endoscopic brushings to yield tumor cells in this situation. Erosion/ulceration of surface epithelium is associated with an inflammatory response and reactive epithelial changes that may detract from the main lesion. In addition, signet ring carcinoma cells may show a range of cytologic atypia. Signet ring carcinoma cells typically present as single cells in a background of mixed inflammatory cells. Small cohesive clusters of a few tumor cells may be present and help confirm the epithelial nature of the cells. The more anaplastic type of tumor cells can be recognized as malignant by their high N/C ratio, irregular nuclear membranes with notches and sharp indentations, and aberrant chromatin pattern (fig. 9-27). Nucleoli may or may not be present. The most banal signet ring carcinoma cells are easily mistaken as histiocytes. This more banal type of tumor cell shows a moderately increased N/C ratio, subtle nuclear membrane irregularities, and homogeneous chromatin (fig.

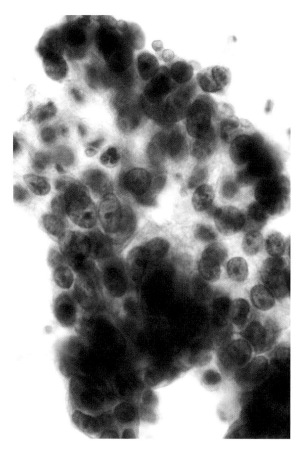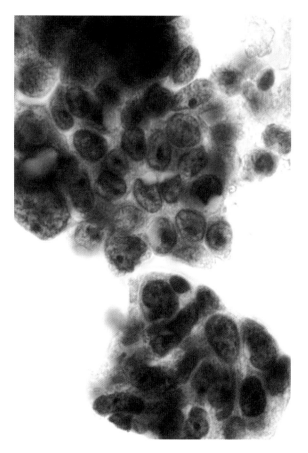

Figure 9-24

WELL-DIFFERENTIATED ADENOCARCINOMA

Left: Partly cohesive and partly dyshesive three-dimensional groups of epithelial cells are present. The nuclei show mild variation in size and shape, with polarization and lumen formation (Papanicolaou stain).

Right: Two three-dimensional cohesive groups of glandular epithelial cells with moderate nuclear variation and shape are present. Vacuolated cytoplasm is appreciated in the cells at the periphery. Although lumen formation is not seen, focal nuclear polarization is present (Papanicolaou stain).

9-28). They are distinguished from histiocytes by the higher N/C ratio, a single large distinct cytoplasmic vacuole that indents the nucleus, and the lack of phagocytized intracytoplasmic material. The awareness of this diagnostic pitfall is probably the best safeguard against a false-negative diagnosis.

Poorly Differentiated Gastric Adenocarcinomas

Poorly differentiated gastric adenocarcinomas need to be differentiated from large cell lymphoma. These tumor cells share some features with large lymphoma cells, such as isolated tumor cells and very high N/C ratio with scant cytoplasm. Carcinoma cells, however, tend to be more pleomorphic than lymphoma cells,

and they also show a tendency to cluster (fig. 9-29). The finding of small cohesive clusters of even two or three tumor cells helps determine the epithelial nature of the tumor (fig. 9-30). Intracytoplasmic vacuoles are also useful for a diagnosis of adenocarcinoma. Poorly differentiated carcinoma cells show more chromatin aberration than lymphoma cells, whereas the latter are more likely to show large prominent nucleoli.

MOLECULAR GENETIC FINDINGS

Gastric carcinoma is the result of accumulated genomic damage affecting cellular functions, including self-sufficiency in growth signals, escape from antigrowth signals, apoptosis resistance, sustained replicative potential, angiogenesis

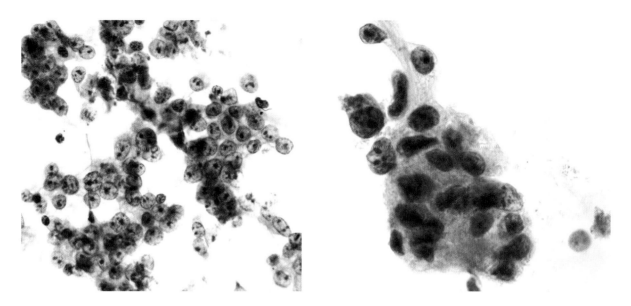

Figure 9-25

REACTIVE CHANGES

Left: Irregular branching of loose sheets of uniformly enlarged, stripped nuclei is present. Although the nuclei appear enlarged and alarming, they have similar shape and size as well as uniform prominent nucleoli. The loss of cytoplasm in most of the cells makes them appear dyshesive. Two subsequent endoscopies with biopsies were both benign (Papanicolaou stain).

Right: A cohesive, vaguely streaming sheet of glandular epithelial cells is present. A few nuclei overlap; however, abundant cytoplasm and normal nuclear/cytoplasmic (N/C) ratio are apparent. Prominent nucleoli are noted in some of the cells (Papanicolaou stain).

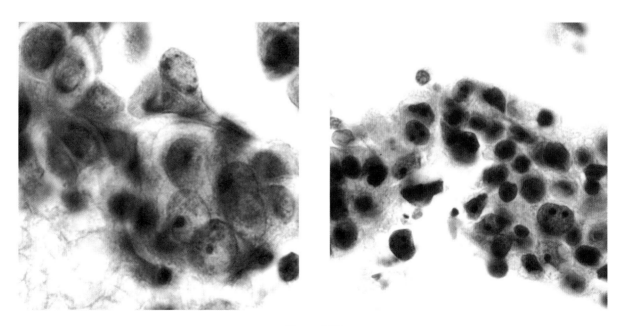

Figure 9-26

MODERATELY DIFFERENTIATED ADENOCARCINOMA

Left: A three-dimensional group of atypical glandular epithelial cells is seen. Cytoplasmic vacuolization is apparent. Nuclear polarization can be appreciated, although no lumen formation is present (Papanicolaou stain).

Right: There is a loose group of atypical glandular epithelial cells with crowding and overlapping. Cytoplasmic vacuolization is obvious without nuclear polarization or lumen formation (Papanicolaou stain).

Figure 9-27

SIGNET RING CELL CARCINOMA

Left: Signet ring cells with a single cytoplasmic vacuole indenting the nucleus are present singly and in files of single cells. The nuclei show hyperchromasia and irregular nuclear membranes (Papanicolaou stain).

Right: A loose group of signet ring cells shows a variable amount of vacuolated cytoplasm. Nuclei show hyperchromasia and irregular indentations (Papanicolaou stain).

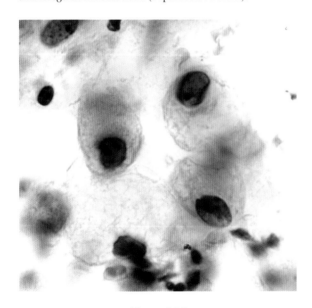

Figure 9-28

SIGNET RING CELL CARCINOMA

A few isolated signet ring cells show abundant vacuolated cytoplasm without any phagocytized material. The N/C ratio resembles that of histiocytes. The nuclei show subtle nuclear membrane irregularities and small prominent nucleoli. It may be difficult to appreciate the malignant nature of these cells; however, the lesion proved to be a signet ring cell carcinoma on biopsy (Papanicolaou stain).

induction, and invasive or metastatic potential, but also deregulation of cell energy, escape from immune destruction, tumor-promoting inflammation, genomic instability, deregulation of cell energy, and escape from immune destruction (245,246).

Molecular Subtypes

Several groups (247–250) have analyzed molecular alterations of gastric cancer at high resolution. These studies attempted to achieve an integrated molecular classification scheme, clustering the comprehensive molecular data obtained into subgroups with different molecular signatures and clinical phenotypes (Table 9-4). Key challenges for the future will involve translation of molecular findings to clinical utility, thus enabling novel strategies for early gastric carcinoma detection and precision therapies for individual patients (251).

The Cancer Genome Atlas (TCGA) Research Network. The landmark study of gastric carcinoma molecular-based stratification was carried out by The Cancer Genome Atlas (TCGA) research network (249). They combined data from different platforms such as array-based somatic

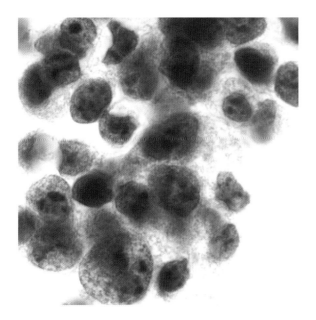

Figure 9-29

POORLY DIFFERENTIATED ADENOCARCINOMA

There is a loose group of pleomorphic nuclei. The vaguely vacuolated cytoplasm seems to be falling apart. The marked variation in nuclear size and shape and the clumpy chromatin separate the cells from those of a lymphoma (Papanicolaou stain).

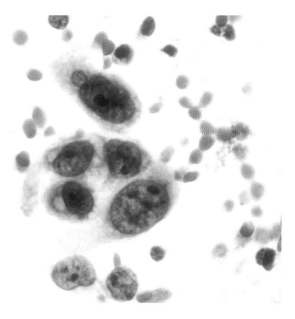

Figure 9-30

POORLY DIFFERENTIATED ADENOCARCINOMA

A cluster and a few single apparently glandular epithelial cells are present. Glandular differentiation is only seen in the cytoplasmic vacuolization (Papanicolaou stain).

copy number analysis, whole exome and genome sequencing, messenger RNA-sequencing, microRNA sequencing, and reverse-phase protein array profiling. TGCA proposed a four-tiered molecular classification of gastric cancer that includes: 1) Epstein-Barr virus positive (EBV+) gastric carcinoma, characterized by a stable genome, lack of *TP53* mutation, prevalent *ARID1A* mutation, recurrent *PIK3CA* mutations, frequent *JAK2* and *PD-L1* amplifications, and an extensive degree of genome-wide hypermethylation; 2) gastric carcinoma with microsatellite instability (MSI-high), characterized by chromosome stability, hypermethylation and demethylation of the genome, *MLH1* silencing, lack of *TP53* mutation, and mutation in druggable target genes such as *RNF43* and *ERBB2*; 3) genomically stable (GS) gastric carcinoma, associated with diffuse morphology and recurrent *CDH1* and *RHOA* events, as confirmed by previous studies (252,253); and 4) gastric carcinoma with chromosomal instability (CIN), exhibiting intestinal morphology, high number of *TP53* mutations, and amplifications of tyrosine kinase receptors (TKR).

The Asian Cancer Research Group (ACRG). ACRG described four molecular subtypes with distinct prognostic impact (250): 1) MSI-high tumors, with intestinal morphology and the best prognosis; 2) microsatellite stable/epithelial to mesenchymal transition (MSS/EMT) gastric carcinoma, with diffuse morphology and the worst prognosis; and 3,4) microsatellite-stable adenocarcinomas (MSS), with no EMT signature, either TP53 active (MSS/TP53+) or inactive (MSS/TP53-), and with an intermediate prognosis. The MSS/TP53- subtype (roughly corresponds to the proliferative and CIN subtypes) is frequent (36 to 50 percent of gastric carcinomas) and harbors genomic amplification of *TKR* and/or *RAS*, which are in-use or potential therapeutic targets. In keeping with a previous study by Deng et al. (254), the ACRG found that *TKR* and *RAS* amplifications tend to be mutually exclusive, emphasizing intertumor heterogeneity and the importance of investigating molecular alterations for targeted therapy.

In-depth studies combining molecular features with histopathologic and immunohistochemical profiles have revealed interesting associations and are currently feasible, thanks to new molecular profiling technologies

Table 9-4

MOLECULAR CLASSIFICATIONS OF GASTRIC CANCER[a]

Lei et al., 2013 (248) (n = 248)			**Mesenchymal** High *TP53* mutations Low E-cadherin mRNA MSS/EMT[b] properties mTOR inhibitors Diffuse GC	**Proliferative** *TP53* mutations Genomic instability Oncogene amplification DNA hypomethylation Intestinal GC (intestinal phenotype)	**Metabolic** Low *TP53* mutations Normal gastric mucosa gene expression 5-FU sensitive Intestinal GC (gastric phenotype)
Bass et al., 2014 (249) The Cancer Genome Atlas (TCGA) (n=295)	**EBV** (9%) *EBV-CIMP* *CDKN2A* silencing *PIK3CA* mutations *ARID1A* mutations *PD-L1/2* amplification *JAK2* amplification	**MSI** (22%) Gastric-CIMP *MLH1* silencing *PIK3CA* mutations *ARID1A* mutations *ERBB2/3* mutations *EGFR* mutations	**GS** (20%) *CDH1* mutations *RHOA* mutations *CLDN18-ARHGAP* fusion (RhoA-GTPase) Diffuse GC	**CIN** (50%) High *TP53* mutations *TKR-RAS* amplification Amplification of cell-cycle mediators Intestinal GC	
Cristescu et al., (250) Asian Cancer Research Group (ACRG) (n = 251)	EBV+ cases included in MSS/TP53+	**MSI** (23%) *MLH1* loss Hypermutation (*KRAS, ARID1A, PIK3A*) Best prognosis Intestinal GC	**MSS/EMT** (15%) *CDH1* loss Worst prognosis Diffuse GC	**MSS/TP53- (inactive)** (36%) High *TP53* mutations Genomic instability Oncogene amplification Intermediate prognosis Intestinal GC	**MSS/TP3+ (active)** (26%) Intermediate prognosis Intestinal GC

[a]Adapted from reference 251.

[b]MSS/EMT = microsatellite stable/epithelial to mesenchymal transition; GC = gastric cancer; EBV = Epstein-Barr virus; MSI = microsatellite instability; GS = genomically stable; CIN = chromosomal instability; MSS = microsatellite stable; CIMP = CpG island methylator phenotype.

generating accurate molecular information from formalin-fixed paraffin-embedded (FFPE) tissues (255,256). Setia et al. (257) proposed a practical algorithm based on immunohistochemical and in situ hybridization techniques available in routine diagnostic practice. The authors translated molecular subgroups into specific immunophenotypes with prognostic and predictive significance in 149 gastric cancer cases in a Western population. More recently, a validation study was performed in a large-scale Asian cohort (n=349), providing similar results (258).

Tumor Suppressor Genes

Many tumor suppressor genes have been implicated in gastric carcinoma development, including *APC* (259–262) and *DCC* (263,264) in intestinal-type carcinomas, as well as *CDH1* (265–270) and *RB1* (271) in diffuse carcinomas. Other tumor suppressor genes are altered in both types of gastric carcinoma, such as *PTEN* (272) and *TP53* (261,273–275), although the latter are more common in intestinal-type carcinoma.

Oncogenes

Some oncogenes are altered preferentially in diffuse-type carcinoma, such as *BCL2* (276,277) and *FGFR2* (formerly *K-SAM*) (278,279). Other oncogenes are altered both in intestinal and diffuse carcinomas, including *CTNNB1* (encoding beta-catenin) (280), *MET* (281), and *MYC* (282,283). The expression of genes involved in the regulation of the cell cycle, such as *CDKN1B* (284–286) and cyclin E (287), is deregulated as well in gastric cancer.

Some oncogenes are preferentially altered in intestinal-type carcinoma, such as *KRAS* (288–291), and *ERBB2/HER2* (292–294). *HER2* overexpression or amplification is present in about 20 percent of gastric cancers (295). There is current interest in the immunohistochemical and in situ hybridization detection of HER2 expression in gastric cancer since these tumors may respond well to therapy with the humanized monoclonal antibody trastuzumab (Herceptin®), as shown in the trastuzumab in gastric adenocarcinoma (ToGA) trial (296). Compared to breast carcinoma, HER2 positivity in gastric cancer is frequently heterogenous and there is less stringent correlation between *ERBB2* amplification and protein overexpression (295).

The European Medicines Agency (EMEA) recommends HER2 testing by immunohistochemistry as a first evaluation assay, followed by fluorescence in situ hybridization (FISH) in IHC 2+ cases (297). The presence of five intensely positive neoplastic cells in a biopsy, or at least 10 percent in a surgical specimen, is the criteria for an IHC 3+ score. Notably, U-shaped or lateral staining is more common than complete membrane staining in gastric cancer (295,298,299). EMEA recommends that trastuzumab should only be used in patients whose tumors have IHC 2+ HER2 overexpression and a confirmed FISH result, or IHC 3+ (fig. 9-31), as determined by an accurate and validated assay (297). Recently, a guideline was published from the College of American Pathologists, American Society for Clinical Pathology, and American Society of Clinical Oncology (299) that establishes an evidence-based guideline for HER2 testing in patients with gastric or EGJ cancer. It formalizes the algorithms for methods to improve the accuracy of HER2 testing (fig. 9-32), and provides several recommendations (Table 9-5).

Given the issue of intratumoral heterogeneity in gastroesophageal adenocarcinoma specimens (fig. 9-33), testing of multiple biopsy fragments (from a primary or metastatic site) or from the resected primary tumor is preferred. For biopsy specimens, current recommendations state that when possible, a minimum of 5 biopsy specimens (300) and optimally, 6 to 8, should be obtained to account for intratumoral heterogeneity and to provide sufficient tumor specimens for diagnosis and biomarker testing (300,301).

The gastric cancer epigenome has been recently analyzed in depth through targeted and genome-wide technologies, focusing on DNA

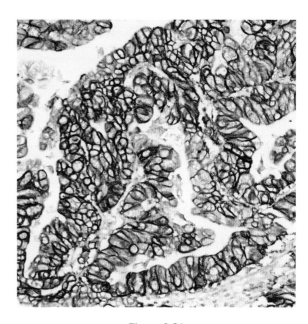

Figure 9-31

HER2 EXPRESSION

Strong and complete, basolateral membranous expression of HER2 (IHC 3+).

methylation and histone modifications, as well as epigenomic promoter alterations, linking these findings to potential therapeutic opportunities (302,303). Special interest has been dedicated to the tumor microenvironment, which is a complex mixture of tumor cells, cancer-associated fibroblasts (CAFs), tumor-associated macrophages (TAMs), and other infiltrating immune cells, endothelial cells, extracellular matrix proteins, and signalling molecules, such as cytokines; it is now known that the microenvironment has a role in gastric carcinoma progression and metastasis (181).

SPREAD AND METASTASES

Gastric carcinomas spread via direct extension to adjacent organs, by lymphatic and/or hematogenous spread, or by peritoneal dissemination.

Direct Extension of Tumor. According to the primary site, penetration of the serosa may result in direct spread to the pancreas, liver, spleen, transverse colon, and greater omentum, and this often leads to early transperitoneal dissemination. Tumors at the EGJ infiltrate the lower end of the esophagus, while distal tumors, particularly poorly cohesive neoplasms,

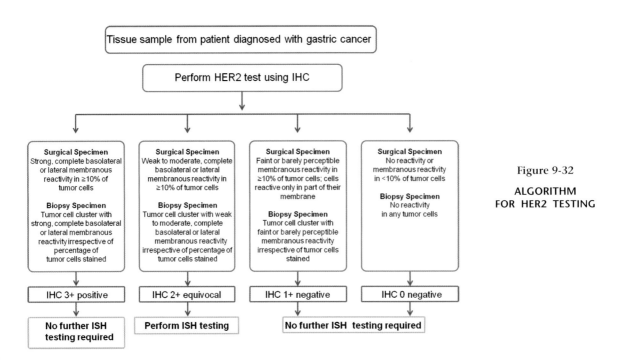

Figure 9-32

ALGORITHM FOR HER2 TESTING

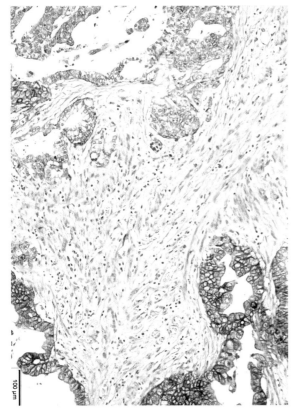

Figure 9-33

IMMUNOEXPRESSION OF HER2 IN GASTRIC CANCER

Heterogeneous expression is present, from IHC 1+ (top, left) to IHC 3+ (bottom, right).

commonly extend into the duodenum (304). Widespread tumor extension is particularly common in poorly cohesive carcinomas, which frequently show extensive spread on the serosal surface, well beyond the macroscopically visible tumor. Intramural permeation of small lympho-vascular vessels is marked in these neoplasms. There is a high propensity to invade the duodenum via submucosal or subserosal routes or via the submucosal lymphatics (305). Consequently, frozen section examination of margins is desirable, particularly when the clearance is less than 4 cm, to ensure completeness of resection.

Lymphatic Spread. The incidence of lymph node metastasis increases with the depth of tumor invasion (306) and occurs with equal frequency regardless of histologic type. The distribution varies according to the location of the tumor. Involvement of nodes along the lesser and greater curvatures is common, and extension to the next zone often occurs as well (for example along the left gastric, common hepatic, and celiac arteries). Distant spread may involve para-aortic and mesenteric nodes. Tumors of the mid-portion of the stomach give rise to metastases in pancreatic and splenic nodes and lesions of the proximal stomach metastasize to mediastinal lymph nodes. It is important for the surgeon to perform an exhaustive lymphadenectomy, and

Table 9-5

HER2 TESTING AND CLINICAL DECISION MAKING IN GASTROESOPHAGEAL ADENOCARCINOMA[a]

Guideline Statement	Strength of Recommendation
1. In patients with GEA[b] who are potential candidates for HER2-targeted therapy, the treating clinician should request HER2 testing on tumor tissue.	strong recommendation
2. Treating clinicians or pathologist should request HER2 testing on tumor tissue in the biopsy or resection specimens (primary or metastasis) preferably before the initiation of trastuzumab therapy if such specimens are available and adequate. HER2 testing on FNA specimens (cell blocks) is an acceptable alternative.	recommendation
3. Treating clinicians should offer combination chemotherapy and HER2-targeted therapy as the initial treatment for appropriate patients with HER2-positive tumors who have metastatic or recurrent GEA.	recommendation
4. Laboratories/pathologists must specify the antibodies and probes used for the test and ensure that assays are appropriately validated for HER2 IHC and ISH on GEA specimens.	strong recommendation
5. When GEA HER2 status is being evaluated, laboratories/pathologists should perform/order IHC testing first followed by ISH when IHC result is 2+ (equivocal). Positive (3+) or negative (0 or 1+) HER2 IHC results do not require further ISH testing.	strong recommendation
6. Pathologists should use the Ruschoff/Hofmann method in scoring HER2 IHC and ISH results for GEA.	strong recommendation
7. Pathologists should select the tissue block with the areas of lowest grade tumor morphology in biopsy and resection specimens. More than 1 tissue block may be selected if different morphologic patterns are present.	recommendation
8. Laboratories should report HER2 testing results in GEA specimens in accordance with the CAP "Template for Reporting Results of HER2 (ERBB2) Biomarker Testing of Specimens from Patients with Adenocarcinoma of the Stomach or Esophagogastric Junction."	strong recommendation
9. Pathologists should identify areas of invasive adenocarcinoma and also mark areas with strongest intensity of HER2 expression by IHC in GEA specimens for subsequent ISH scoring when required.	strong recommendation
10. Laboratories must incorporate GEA HER2 testing methods into their overall laboratory quality improvement program, establishing appropriate quality improvement monitors as needed to ensure consistent performance in all steps of the testing and reporting process. In particular, laboratories performing GEA HER2 testing must participate in a formal proficiency testing program, if available, or an alternative proficiency assurance activity.	strong recommendation
11. There is insufficient evidence to recommend for or against genomic testing in patients with GEA at this time.	no recommendation

[a]Guidelines from the College of American Pathologists, American Society for Clinical Pathology, and American Society of Clinical Oncology (299).
[b]GEA = gastric and esophagogastric junction adenocarcinoma; FNA = fine-needle aspirate; IHC = immunohistochemistry; ISH = in situ hybridization.

for the pathologist to examine all lymph nodes, since there is good evidence that prognosis depends on the number of nodes involved (307). Further, the ratio of metastatic to examined nodes (node ratio) has been suggested as an independent prognostic factor (308).

Hematogenous Spread. Spread via the bloodstream occurs from invasion of tributaries of the portal venous system and may develop in the absence of lymph node involvement. Any organ can be affected, but metastases are most common in the liver, followed by the lung, peritoneum, adrenal gland, skin, and ovary; the latter can also be involved by transperitoneal spread. The distribution of metastases is also dictated, to some extent, by the histologic tumor type. Gland-forming carcinomas are more likely to give rise to liver metastases by hematogenous spread while poorly cohesive carcinomas are more likely to involve the peritoneum and disseminate widely, infiltrating lungs more extensively than nodular metastases

Table 9-6

MAIN CHANGES IN TNM CLASSIFICATION (8TH EDITION) OF GASTRIC CANCER

Change	Details of Change	Levels of Evidence
Anatomy - Primary Site(s)	Anatomic boundary between esophagus and stomach: tumors involving the esophagogastric junction (EGJ) with the tumor epicenter no more than 2 cm into the proximal stomach are staged as esophageal cancers; EGJ tumors with their epicenter located greater than 2 cm into the proximal stomach are staged as stomach cancers. Cardia cancer not involving the EGJ is staged as stomach cancer	III
AJCC Prognostic Stage Groups	cTNM: stage groupings of cTNM differ from those of pTNM	III
AJCC Prognostic Stage Groups	ypTNM: stage groupings are the same as those for pTNM; however prognostic information is presented using only the four broad stage categories (stage I-IV)	III
AJCC Prognostic Stage Groups	In pathologic classification (pTNM), T4aN2 and T4bN0 are now classified as stage IIIA	II

associated with gland-forming tumors and more often involving unusual sites such as the kidney, spleen, uterus, and meninges (309,310). Peritoneal involvement is also more common in younger patients. In adenocarcinomas with unusual metastasis (for instance, gland-forming carcinomas involving the peritoneum or poorly cohesive carcinomas involving the liver), the primary tumor often shows a mixed histologic pattern (311).

Transperitoneal Spread. Secondary tumor deposits are common in the omentum, peritoneum, and mesentery but are rare in the spleen. Secondary ovarian deposits are one form of Krukenberg tumor for which bloodstream spread is as likely as transperitoneal spread. Krukenberg tumors are more frequently associated with diffuse primary carcinomas than gland-forming tumors. The presence of signet ring cells within an ovarian mucinous tumor, however, should not necessarily exclude a primary ovarian tumor (312).

STAGING

Staging for carcinoma of the stomach was modified in 2017 (313). A comparison with the previous TNM classification (7th edition) (186,187) is shown in Table 9-6. Major changes include staging according to the anatomic boundary between the esophagus and stomach: tumors involving the EGJ with the tumor epicenter no more than 2 cm into the proximal stomach are staged as esophageal cancers; EGJ

tumors with their epicenter located greater than 2 cm into the proximal stomach are staged as stomach cancers. Cardia cancer not involving the EGJ is staged as a stomach cancer.

Table 9-7 shows the definitions of T (primary tumor) and N (regional lymph node) stages (313). American Joint Committee on Cancer (AJCC) prognostic stage groups are available for cTNM, pTNM, and ypTNM (postneoadjuvant therapy) (313). The pTNM categories are almost identical to those for esophagus and EGJ tumors, except that N3 (metastasis in 7 or more regional lymph nodes) is divided into N3a (7 to 15 nodes) and N3b (16 or more nodes) for gastric carcinomas but not for esophageal carcinomas (313).

TREATMENT

Therapeutic approaches vary according to the location of the tumor, stage of the disease, and expression of predictive biomarkers for target therapy.

Early Gastric Cancer

Endoscopic resection is generally indicated when the probability of lymph node metastasis is low. Since the estimated incidences of lymph node metastasis in mucosal and submucosal gastric cancers are approximately 3 and 20 percent, respectively (221,314), the indication for endoscopic resection in these patients is based on careful evaluation of clinicopathologic, endoscopic, and imaging features indicating a negligible

Table 9-7

TNM CLASSIFICATION OF GASTRIC CANCER

T – Primary Tumor

TX	Primary tumor cannot be assessed
T0	No evidence of primary tumor
Tis	Carcinoma *in situ*: intraepithelial tumor without invasion of the lamina propria, high-grade dysplasia
T1	Tumor invades the lamina propria, muscularis mucosae, or submucosa
T1a	Tumor invades the lamina propria or muscularis mucosae
T1b	Tumor invades the submucosa
T2	Tumor invades the muscularis propria
T3	Tumor penetrates the subserosal connective tissue without invasion of the visceral peritoneum or adjacent structures
T4	Tumor invades the serosa (visceral peritoneum) or adjacent structures
T4a	Tumor invades the serosa (visceral peritoneum)
T4b	Tumor invades adjacent structures/organs

N – Regional Lymph Node

NX	Regional lymph node(s) cannot be assessed
N0	No regional lymph node metastasis
N1	Metastasis in one or two regional lymph nodes
N2	Metastasis in three to six regional lymph nodes
N3	Metastasis in seven or more regional lymph nodes
N3a	Metastasis in seven to 15 regional lymph nodes
N3b	Metastasis in 16 or more regional lymph nodes

M – Distant Metastasis

M0	No distant metastasis
M1	Distant metastasis

pTNM – Pathologic Stage Grouping

Stage 0	Tis	N0	M0
Stage IA	T1	N0	M0
Stage IB	T1	N1	M0
Stage IB	T2	N0	M0
Stage IIA	T1	N2	M0
Stage IIA	T2	N1	M0
Stage IIA	T3	N0	M0
Stage IIB	T1	N3a	M0
Stage IIB	T2	N2	M0
Stage IIB	T3	N1	M0
Stage IIB	T4a	N0	M0
Stage IIIA	T2	N3a	M0
Stage IIIA	T3	N2	M0
Stage IIIA	T4a	N1	M0
Stage IIIA	T4a	N2	M0
Stage IIIA	T4b	N0	M0
Stage IIIB	T1	N3b	M0
Stage IIIB	T2	N3b	M0
Stage IIIB	T3	N3a	M0
Stage IIIB	T4a	N3a	M0
Stage IIIB	T4b	N1	M0
Stage IIIB	T4b	N2	M0
Stage IIIC	T3	N3b	M0
Stage IIIC	T4a	N3b	M0
Stage IIIC	T4b	N3a	M0
Stage IIIC	T4b	N3b	M0
Stage IV	Any T	Any N	M1

Table 9-8

INDICATIONS FOR ENDOSCOPIC SUBMUCOSAL DISSECTION

Well- to moderately differentiated histopathologic type, intramucosal cancer (size ≤2 cm — absolute indication, >2cm — expanded indication), without ulceration.

Well- to moderately differentiated histopathologic type, intramucosal cancer, ≤3 cm in diameter, with ulceration (expanded indication).

Well- to moderately differentiated histopathologic type, ≤3 cm in diameter, minute submucosal (SM1 ≤500 µm) cancer (expanded indication).

Poorly differentiated histopathologic type, intramucosal cancer, ≤2 cm in diameter, without ulceration (expanded indication).

risk of nodal metastasis. Endoscopic resection encompasses endoscopic mucosal resection (EMR) and endoscopic submucosal dissection (ESD), the latter allowing en bloc resection of the lesions.

EMR alone was considered in the past for well- or moderately differentiated tumors that were not ulcerated, smaller than 30 mm in diameter, without submucosal or lymphovascular invasion and complete local excision (315). However, evidence accumulated in recent years (221, 314) led to the publication of the European and Japanese guidelines for the endoscopic resection of gastric carcinoma (316,317). The indications for ESD are shown in Table 9-8. The expanded indications now include larger lesions and lesions with ulceration that can be removed en bloc by ESD. Such lesions were previously resected surgically because of the difficulty in effectively using EMR techniques for resection in this context. Lymphovascular infiltration, both ly(+) and v(+), should always be excluded as this finding correlates with a greatly increased risk of lymph node metastases.

Advanced Gastric Cancer

Treatment of potentially resectable advanced gastric cancer is based on surgery and chemotherapy/chemoradiotherapy. For patients with inoperable cancer or metastatic disease, systemic therapy is indicated, encompassing conventional chemotherapy and targeted therapy with monoclonal antibodies directed to HER2 and VEGFR2 (180,181,318). Immune checkpoint therapies based on antibodies that block the three key components of immune checkpoints, CTLA4, PD1, and PD-L1, are promising tools for gastric cancer therapy (319,320); FDA approval was granted to pembrolizumab for patients with advanced gastric or EGJ adenocarcinoma whose

tumors express PD-L1, and numerous studies are ongoing (181).

PROGNOSIS

In Japan, the 5-year survival rate for patients with T2 adenocarcinoma is 60 to 80 percent. This decreases to 50 percent for T3 tumors (321,322). Lower survival rates have been observed in the West (323). Female sex and Japanese ethnicity are associated with a survival advantage (324). Higher frequency of early-stage carcinomas, accurate staging, and surgical expertise are also associated with improved survival in Japan compared to Western nations (325,326).

At the time of diagnosis, most patients with advanced carcinoma present with lymph node metastases (327). Lymphatic and vascular invasion, often seen in advanced cases, are associated with a poor prognosis. In patients with involvement of 1 to 6 lymph nodes, the 5-year survival rate is 46 percent, compared with 30 percent in patients with 7 to 15 involved lymph nodes (328). The extent of the regional lymphadenectomy performed, and the quality of lymph node evaluation are salient. Patients undergoing a "curative" gastrectomy but limited lymph node dissection (D1/D0) have an overall 5-year survival rate of only 23 percent versus more than 50 percent for those undergoing more aggressive lymphadenectomy (D2) (329). Adequate N staging requires that at least 15 lymph nodes be examined.

In resectable cases, complete tumor removal with negative margins is important (330). The depth of invasion, the number of positive lymph nodes, and the postoperative complications are important independent prognostic factors (331). After curative resection, recurrence is locoregional (resection margins, surgical bed, or regional lymph nodes) in 40 percent of cases and systemic (liver and peritoneum) in 60 percent (332–334). Whether patients with distal adenocarcinomas have a better prognosis than those with proximal carcinomas is debated (326,335). Saito et al. (336) reported a 5-year survival rate of 62 percent in patients with carcinoma of the cardia versus 83 percent for those with carcinoma of the lower third of the stomach. Others found the prognoses to be equally grim, with 28 and 29 percent survival rates, respectively (335).

Preoperative/neoadjuvant treatment, namely, neoadjuvant chemotherapy, is associated with a survival benefit compared to surgery alone in locally advanced gastric cancer. Accordingly, the TNM classification encompasses a postneoadjuvant therapy pathology classification (ypTNM stage) (313). The tumor regression grade (TRG) has been shown to provide highly valuable prognostic information. As in most cases, complete or subtotal tumor regression after neoadjuvant treatment is associated with better patient outcome (337,338). In cases of complete tumor regression, malignant cells are destroyed and the tumor is replaced by fibrous or fibroinflammatory granulation tissue. Residual tumor, in contrast, may be abundant or only consist of small single cells or tumor cell groups/clusters. The residual tumor cells show characteristic abundant cytoplasm, with vacuolization or oncocytic differentiation (337). Nuclear atypia, including hyperchromasia and large, bizarre nuclei, is frequent, but mitoses are rare; giant cells may be present (fig. 9-34) (337). These changes may be localized, regardless of the tumor regression grade. Several systems are available for evaluation of tumor regression in gastric cancer (339–341).

Histologic Features and Prognosis

The value of histologic typing in predicting prognosis is controversial. Whether the prognosis for diffuse carcinoma (Laurén classification) is equal to or worse than intestinal carcinoma is still debated (210,342). It has been suggested that diffuse carcinomas encompass lesions with different prognoses, such as a low-grade desmoplastic subtype (with no or scarce angiolympho-neuroinvasion) and a high-grade subtype (with anaplastic cells) (343). In a large study performed in a single high-volume cen-

ter in Asia (344), it was shown that early-stage signet ring cell/diffuse carcinomas can be indolent. More than half present as localized gastric carcinoma. On the other hand, signet ring cell/diffuse carcinomas in advanced stages bestow a worse prognosis than well/moderately differentiated carcinomas. Therefore, the context-dependent nature of signet ring cell/diffuse carcinoma must be considered when predicting prognosis (344). The prognosis is particularly grim for children and young adults with poorly cohesive carcinomas, for whom the diagnosis is often delayed (345,346).

Mixed gastric carcinoma (193,205), defined by a dual pattern of differentiation (tubulo-papillary/intestinal and poorly cohesive [signet ring cell]/diffuse) carried, in one multivariate analysis, a significantly worse prognosis than the two main types in the Laurén classification (226). Several authors demonstrated that mixed gastric carcinoma displays more aggressive features than "pure" intestinal and diffuse gastric cancer, including larger tumor size, deeper invasion, lymphatic invasion, and lymph node metastases (202,226,229,347–350). Interestingly, the mixed type shows a dual metastatic pattern (hematogenous metastases and peritoneal dissemination with lymph node metastases), suggesting a cumulative effect of the adverse behaviors of both intestinal and diffuse-type gastric carcinoma (311).

VARIANTS OF GASTRIC CARCINOMA

Morphologic variants of gastric carcinoma encompass EGJ gastric adenocarcinoma (discussed in chapter 4) and unusual histologic variants (about 5 percent of gastric cancers).

Gastric Carcinoma with Lymphoid Stroma and Other Epstein-Barr Virus-Associated (EBVaGC) Variants

Gastric carcinoma with lymphoid stroma (351) is also termed *medullary carcinoma with lymphocytic infiltration* (352), *undifferentiated gastric carcinoma with intense lymphocytic infiltrate* (353), and *lymphoepithelioma-like carcinoma* (354). Over 80 percent of these tumors are associated with EBV infection; designated as EBVaGCs (355,356). A similar morphology can be observed in gastric cancers with microsatellite instability (357–359).

233

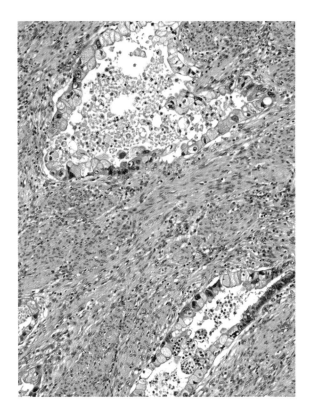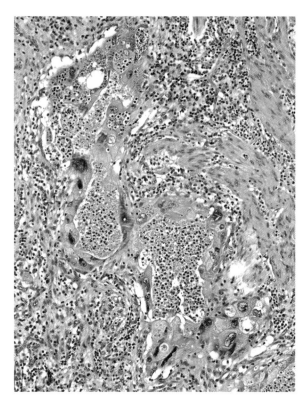

Figure 9-34

CYTOLOGIC EFFECTS INDUCED BY NEOADJUVANT CHEMOTHERAPY

Left: Neoplastic glands are dilated, filled with necrotic debris, and lined by vacuolated epithelium with hyperchromatic nuclei.
Right: Neoplastic cells display abundant cytoplasm, hyperchromatic bizarre nuclei, and multinucleated cells. There is an abundant inflammatory reaction and necrotic debris in the lumen of glands.

The frequency of EBV infection in gastric carcinoma ranges from 2 to 20 percent, with a worldwide average of nearly 10 percent (360–363). Differences in reported frequencies may be due to geographic and environmental factors, although this remains controversial (362,364). In a meta-analysis by Murphy et al. (355), the pooled estimates of EBVaGC frequency in America, Europe, and Asia were 9.9, 9.2, and 8.3 percent, respectively, with an overall frequency of 8.7 percent. Camargo et al. (365) found a similar overall frequency (8.2 percent), although the frequencies they found were slightly higher in American (12.5 percent) and European (13.9 percent) cases and lower in Asian (7.5 percent) cases.

EBVaGCs display certain distinctive macroscopic and histologic characteristics (351,352, 366). Gastric carcinoma with lymphoid stroma, the main histologic variant, occurs predominantly in the proximal stomach, including the cardia, fundus, and body (367,368) and in the

gastric stump of patients with previous subtotal gastrectomy (369). The age at presentation is slightly younger than for conventional carcinoma and males are affected more often than females (351,352,356,367).

On gross examination, the tumors commonly involve the proximal stomach and are usually ulcerated, with well-circumscribed borders. Necrosis or hemorrhage is notably absent. Histologically, the tumors usually have a well-demarcated pushing, rather than infiltrating, margin. They are typically composed of irregular sheets, trabeculae, ill-defined tubules or syncytia of polygonal-shaped cells embedded within a prominent lymphocytic infiltrate, with occasional lymphoid follicles (fig. 9-35, left). In its early stage, EBVaGCs show a characteristic "lace-like pattern" (362,368), with anastomosing or branching glandular structures (fig. 9-35, right). In some cases, the lymphocytic infiltrate may be so intense that a diagnosis of gastric

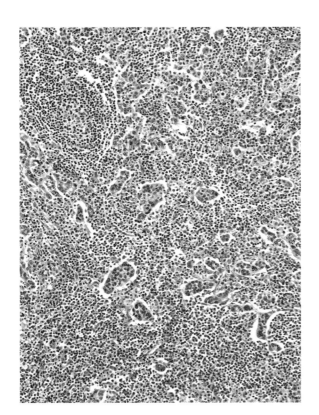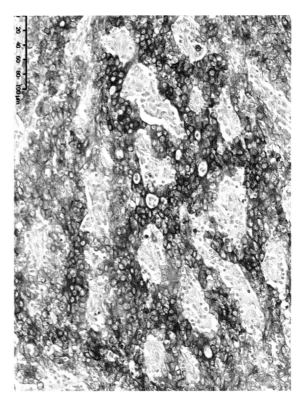

Figure 9-35

GASTRIC CARCINOMA WITH LYMPHOID STROMA

Left: The tumor is composed of solid sheets of polygonal-shaped epithelial cells intermixed with a prominent lymphocytic infiltrate.
Right: Intramucosal tumor-forming, irregularly anastomosing tubules and cords result in a lace-like or a reticular pattern, which is highlighted by immunostaining for cytokeratin.

lymphoma is considered until the tumor cells are confirmed by immunostaining for epithelial markers. Rarely, giant cells are observed (370).

Two other histologic variants of EBVaGCs have been reported. Tubular carcinomas with limited desmoplasia, a smaller number of lymphocytes than tumor cells, and prominent lymphoid follicles with active germinal centers, are termed *carcinoma with Crohn disease-like lymphoid reaction* (368). The other is *conventional-type adenocarcinomas with scant lymphocytic infiltrate* (368). Immunophenotypic analysis reveals that CD8-positive cytotoxic T lymphocytes form the predominant inflammatory component, which also contains B lymphocytes, plasma cells, neutrophils, and eosinophils.

The prognosis of patients with these tumors is better than typical gastric cancers (352,354,356, 365,366,369,371,372), possibly as a result of the immunologic factors at play in the associated lymphocytic infiltrate. Patients with gastric carcino-ma with lymphoid stroma have the best overall and disease-free survival rates, followed by those with Crohn disease-like reactions, and finally, conventional-type adenocarcinoma (373).

There is some debate about the role that EBV plays in carcinogenesis; either a direct role or simply a secondary effect (374). Infection likely occurs early in the process since EBV can be found in adjacent dysplasia (375), although it has not been observed in normal gastric mucosa or intestinal metaplasia (376). In EBVaGC there is a monoclonal proliferation of carcinoma cells with latent EBV infection, as demonstrated by polymerase chain reaction (PCR) and EBV-encoded small RNA (EBER) in situ hybridization (fig. 9-36) (377). EBVaGC is characterized by a stable genome, without p53 expression or *TP53* mutations, and generally is not associated with *H. pylori* infection (240). In rare instances of co-infection (*H. pylori* and EBV) EBV potentiates the oncogenic effects of *H. pylori* in the stomach (378,379).

Previous studies have shown that some EBV latent genes have oncogenic properties. Recent advances in genome-wide and comprehensive molecular analyses (249) have demonstrated that both genetic and epigenetic changes contribute to EBVaGC carcinogenesis. Genetic changes characteristic of EBVaGC include frequent mutations in *PIK3CA* and *ARID1A* and amplification of *JAK2* and *PD-L1/L2* (249). Global CpG island hypermethylation, which induces epigenetic silencing of tumor suppressor genes, is also a unique feature of EBVaGC and is considered to be crucial for carcinogenesis. Furthermore, post-transcriptional gene expression regulation by cellular and/or EBV-derived microRNAs has attracted considerable attention (380). These abnormalities result in significant alterations in gene expression related to cell proliferation, apoptosis, migration, and immune signaling pathways (362).

Due to the overexpression/amplification of *PD-L1/L2* (fig. 9-37), EBVaGCs are good candidates for therapy with immune checkpoint inhibitors (381,382).

Adenosquamous and Squamous Cell Carcinomas

Adenosquamous carcinoma accounts for 0.5 percent of all gastric cancers. It is defined as a tumor in which the neoplastic squamous component comprises at least 25 percent of the tumor volume; the diagnosis requires the presence of a neoplastic squamous component characterized by keratin pearl formation and intercellular bridges, in addition to a glandular element (fig. 9-38) (383). The transition between the elements may be abrupt or there may be intermingling of squamous foci within neoplastic glands (383–385). Ultrastructural evaluation shows evidence of both squamous and adenosquamous differentiation, supporting the view that this neoplastic type arises from a multipotential stem cell (386).

These tumors occur most often in the antrum, and most present as advanced carcinomas, although rare cases of EGC have been reported (387). Lymphovascular permeation is common and the prognosis poor (383,385,387–389), although some exhibit a favorable response to chemotherapy (390). Metastases usually contain both glandular and squamous components but, in some instances, only one component is present (385). Tumors

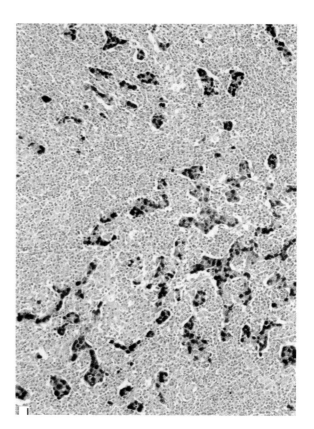

Figure 9-36

GASTRIC CARCINOMA WITH LYMPHOID STROMA

The presence of Epstein-Barr virus (EBV) infection is demonstrated by EBV-encoded small RNA (EBER) in situ hybridization.

with a distinct boundary between components may represent a rare collision tumor. Rare tumors containing discrete foci of benign-appearing squamous metaplasia have been observed, and have been termed *adenocarcinoma with squamous differentiation*, or *adenoacanthoma*.

Pure *squamous cell carcinomas* develop rarely in the stomach, representing from 0.04 to 0.09 percent of all gastric carcinomas (388,391,392). Men are affected four times as often as women (392,393). The tumors are usually diagnosed at a late stage and confer a poor prognosis (392). A glandular component is often present when such tumors are extensively sampled (383). At the EGJ and in the proximal stomach, caudal extension of an esophageal squamous cell carcinoma should be excluded.

Squamous cell carcinomas possibly arise from squamous metaplasia of an adenocarcinoma,

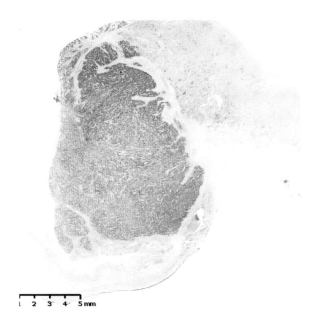
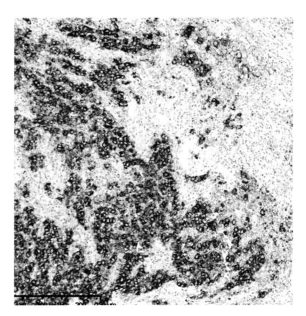

Figure 9-37

OVEREXPRESSION OF PD-L1 IN GASTRIC CARCINOMA WITH LYMPHOID STROMA

Left: Panoramic view highlighting the heterogeneous expression of PD-L1.
Right: Strong, membranous expression of PD-L1 in epithelial neoplastic cells (left); granular expression of PD-L1 in stromal cells (right).

from heterotopic squamous epithelium, or from multipotential stem cells with bidirectional differentiation (387,392). Gastric squamous cell carcinomas have also been described as a complication of gastric involvement in tertiary syphilis (394), after ingestion of corrosive acids (395), and following long-term cyclophosphamide therapy (396).

Micropapillary Carcinoma

Micropapillary carcinoma (MPC) is a rare, distinctive tumor characterized by irregular small mole-like clusters of tumor cells lying within clear lacunar spaces that simulate lymphatic or vascular channels (fig. 9-39). Most gastric MPCs arise from tubular or papillary adenocarcinomas, with an incidence of about 6 percent. The proportion of the micropapillary component ranges from 5 to 80 percent (397). Epithelial membrane antigen shows a characteristic inside-out staining pattern (398).

MPC carcinoma is an aggressive neoplasm, with a high incidence of lymphovascular invasion and nodal metastasis and high TNM stage (398–400). One case confined to the mucosa has been reported (401). In one study (402), the follow-up data showed that the prognosis of patients with

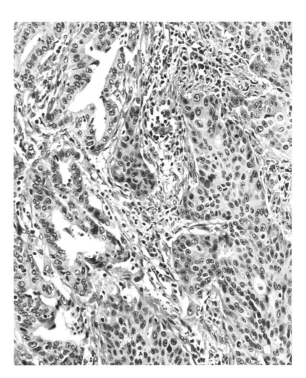

Figure 9-38

ADENOSQUAMOUS GASTRIC CARCINOMA

The tumor is composed of neoplastic squamous and glandular components.

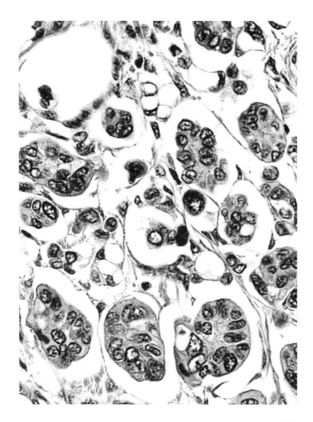 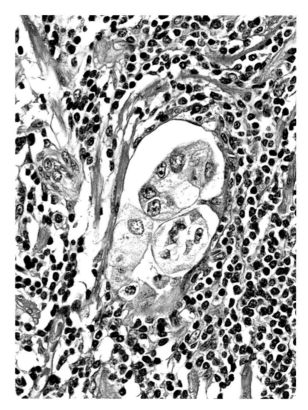

Figure 9-39

MICROPAPILLARY CARCINOMA

Left: This variant of adenocarcinoma has neoplastic cells that are surrounded by clear spaces, resembling lymphatic tumor emboli. Right: Invasive front.

MPC was not significantly different from conventional tubular or papillary adenocarcinoma. More recent studies, however, show that overall 5-year survival rates for patients with MPC are significantly worse than for those with non-MPC carcinomas (397,398).

Hepatoid Adenocarcinoma and Other Alpha-Fetoprotein-Producing Gastric Carcinomas

A small number of gastric adenocarcinomas contain variable amounts of tumor cells resembling hepatocellular carcinoma (fig. 9-40), usually interspersed with areas of more typical adenocarcinoma. *Hepatoid adenocarcinomas* may produce large amounts of alpha-fetoprotein (AFP), which is detectable in the serum and demonstrated by immunohistochemistry (403). Molecular evidence supports the clonal origin of hepatoid adenocarcinoma and coexistent adenocarcinoma (404). This subtype is commonly diagnosed in patients over the age of 50 years and, although occa-

sional early cases have been detected (405,406), most are advanced bulky polypoid tumors with ulceration and areas of necrosis and hemorrhage (407). The antrum appears to be the most common location, followed by the fundus, and occasionally, the cardia (405).

These tumors are commonly heterogeneous, with hepatoid foci intermingled with adenocarcinoma, often showing a papillary pattern, and less-differentiated areas containing bizarre giant cells (fig. 9-41) and spindle cells (403,408). Large, polygonal-shaped cells with prominent eosinophilic cytoplasm, resembling those of hepatocellular carcinoma (403,409), arranged in trabeculae, wide sheets, or acinar structures, are characteristic. These cells may contain periodic acid–Schiff (PAS)-diastase-resistant hyaline globules (fig. 9-42) (405,408). Based on the immunohistochemical expression of CD10, MUC2, MUC5AC, MUC6, and CDX-2, Kumashiro et al. (410) suggested that these

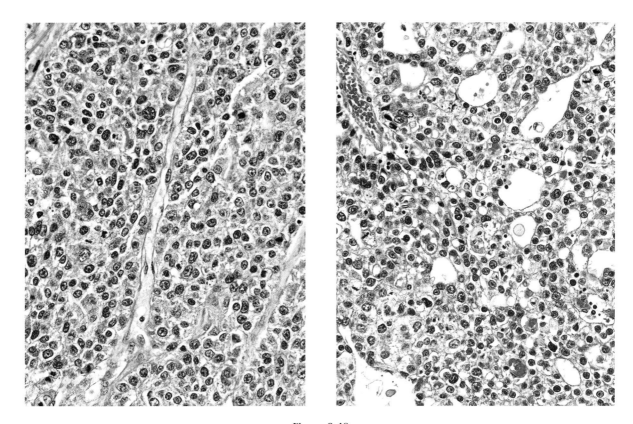

Figure 9-40

HEPATOID ADENOCARCINOMA

The tumor consists of polygonal-shaped neoplastic cells with eosinophilic cytoplasm.
Left: A solid/trabecular growth pattern, resembling hepatocellular carcinoma, is present.
Right: Rare gland-like spaces are present.

tumors arise from carcinomas with an intestinal phenotype. Clinically, one characteristic of these neoplasms is the extensive vascular infiltration, reflected in the high incidence of hepatic and nodal metastases and a poorer prognosis compared to conventional adenocarcinoma (403,406,407,411–413).

Immunohistochemical and in situ hybridization studies have documented albumin, AFP, α_1-antichymotrypsin, and bile production within the tumor cells (409,414,415). Positivity for AFP on immunohistochemistry is usually, but not invariably present, and overexpression of p53 has been described (408). Gene expression profiling has identified PLUNC [palate, lung, and nasal epithelium carcinoma-associated protein) as a marker for gastric hepatoid adenocarcinoma (416).

Other types of gastric neoplasms also produce AFP, including well-differentiated papillary/

tubular adenocarcinoma with clear cytoplasm, yolk sac tumor-like carcinoma, and fetal-type adenocarcinoma (409,414). Gastric adenocarcinomas with enteroblastic differentiation (GAED) have been recognized as a variant of AFP-producing gastric carcinomas (417). GAED may be a representative example of "primitive enterocyte phenotype" cancer because of its morphologic resemblance to early fetal gut epithelium as well as frequent upregulation of oncofetal proteins such as AFP and glypican 3 (GPC3) (fig. 9-43) as well several embryonic stem cell marker genes, including spalt-like transcription factor 4 (SALL4), LIN28, and claudin-6 (CLDN6) (418). GAED/primitive enterocyte phenotype are associated with highly aggressive biological behavior (417,418). Molecular characteristics include frequent *TP53* mutations and weak association with EBV and MSI. In terms of TCGA molecular subclassification, this group comprises a distinct subset of CIN tumors (418).

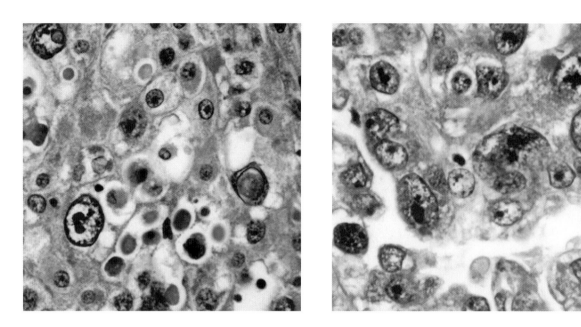

Figure 9-41

HEPATOID ADENOCARCINOMA

Left: Some nuclei display intranuclear cytoplasmic inclusions.
Right: Nuclei are large and bizarre and several mitoses are present.

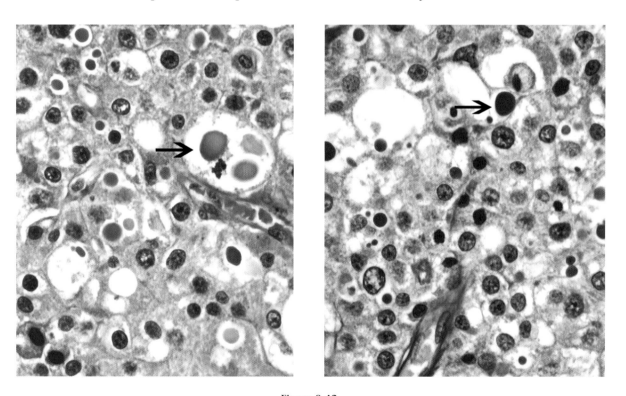

Figure 9-42

HEPATOID ADENOCARCINOMA

Left: Hyaline globules (arrow) are seen in the cytoplasm of neoplastic cells.
Right: Hyaline bodies are highlighted by periodic acid–Schiff (PAS) staining after diastase digestion (arrow).

It may be difficult to distinguish a liver metastasis from a gastric hepatoid adenocarcinoma from a primary hepatocellular carcinoma (HCC). Immunostaining for HepPar1, CK19, or CK20 is useful: most HCCs show extensive staining with HepPar1, whereas only focal staining is observed in gastric hepatoid adenocarcinoma (419). SALL4 is a sensitive marker for AFP-producing gastric carcinoma and may be useful in differentiation from primary hepatocellular carcinoma (420). In one study, however, SALL4 immunoreactivity (defined as greater than 5 percent of tumor cells) was seen in 3 of 236 cases of hepatocellular carcinoma (1.3 percent) (421). Accordingly, SALL4 expression should be interpreted with caution. Arginase-1, a sensitive and specific marker for hepatocellular carcinoma, is commonly expressed (62.5 percent) in hepatoid adenocarcinoma and hence is not useful (422).

Choriocarcinoma

A small number of gastric tumors, affecting both sexes, have been reported in which areas of *choriocarcinoma,* containing syncytiotrophoblast and cytotrophoblast, occur in association with poorly differentiated adenocarcinoma with no evidence of primary choriocarcinoma elsewhere (423,424). The tumor often contains widespread areas of hemorrhagic necrosis that can be detected macroscopically (425,426). The commonly accepted pathogenetic explanation is that these tumors represent choriocarcinomatous differentiation or transformation of conventional adenocarcinoma (427).

Immunohistochemical evidence of human chorionic gonadotrophin (HCG) expression within trophoblastic areas has been shown (426–429) and markedly elevated levels of circulating HCG are often present (427,428,430). Placental lactogen and pregnancy-specific glycoprotein have also been demonstrated by immunohistochemistry within the trophoblastic elements of the tumor. In occasional cases, other germ cell tumor-like elements coexist, such as embryonal carcinoma and yolk sac tumor (430,431). Metastases to the liver and lung are common and the prognosis is typically poor, with survival a matter of months following diagnosis (424,426,432).

Only a few cases of pure gastric yolk sac tumor have been reported (433,434). Recent publications have described a case of choriocarcinoma admixed with an AFP-producing adenocarcinoma and "separated" adenocarcinoma (435), as well as a case of combined choriocarcinoma, neuroendocrine cell carcinoma, and tubular adenocarcinoma (436).

Gastric Adenocarcinoma of Fundic Gland Type

Gastric adenocarcinoma of fundic gland type (chief cell-predominant type) (437), a rare variant of gastric cancer, is associated with both activation of the Wnt/β-catenin signaling pathway and mutations in guanine nucleotide binding protein, alpha-stimulating complex (*GNAS*) (438,439). Gastric adenocarcinoma of fundic gland type shares common genetic and phenotypic features with pyloric gland adenoma (440).

Even when submucosal invasion occurs, this subtype is a low-grade malignancy when it is the chief cell-predominant type (441). Gastric adenocarcinomas of fundic gland type typically display irregularly anastomosing glands with mildly enlarged and hyperchromatic nuclei (fig. 9-44, left). The tumors arise within the deeper zone of the gastric mucosa and are covered with a non-neoplastic epithelium. Accordingly, the neoplastic cells express MUC6 (fig. 9-44, right) and pepsinogen-I (gastric phenotype) and are negative for MUC2 and CD10.

Despite the presence of minimal invasion into the submucosal layer, lymphatic or venous invasion is rare (442). Because of the lack of tumor recurrence or metastasis, some authors question whether the term oxyntic gland polyp/ adenoma is more appropriate for this type of lesion (443,444). Other authors claim that chief cell-predominant gastric polyps, encompassing oxyntic gland polyp/adenoma and gastric adenocarcinoma of fundic gland type, appear to show a morphologic continuum (445).

Parietal Cell Carcinoma

These exceedingly rare tumors present as bulky lesions involving both the gastric body and antrum (446). Histologically, they have an expansile rather than infiltrating growth pattern and are composed of sheets of cells that may contain small gland-like clefts. The tumor cells resemble acid-secreting parietal cells in that they have eosinophilic granular cytoplasm and stain with phosphotungstic acid hematoxylin (PTAH)

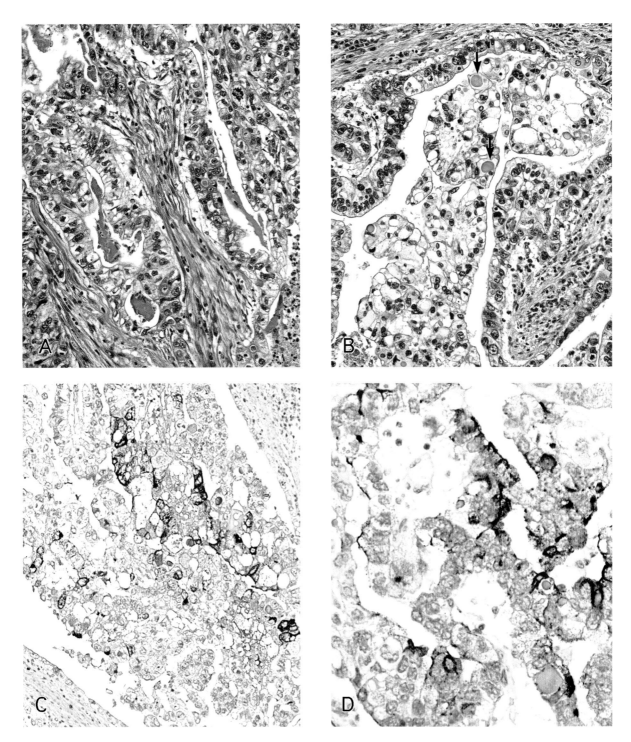

Figure 9-43

GASTRIC ADENOCARCINOMA WITH ENTEROBLASTIC DIFFERENTIATION

A: The neoplastic glands are lined by columnar cells with clear cytoplasm (fetal gut-like). In some areas the neoplastic cells display high-grade nuclear atypia and mitoses (upper, right).

B: Hyaline globules (arrows) are observed in the cytoplasm of some neoplastic cells.

C: Immunoexpression of alpha-fetoprotein (AFP).

D: Immunoexpression of glypican-3 (GPC3).

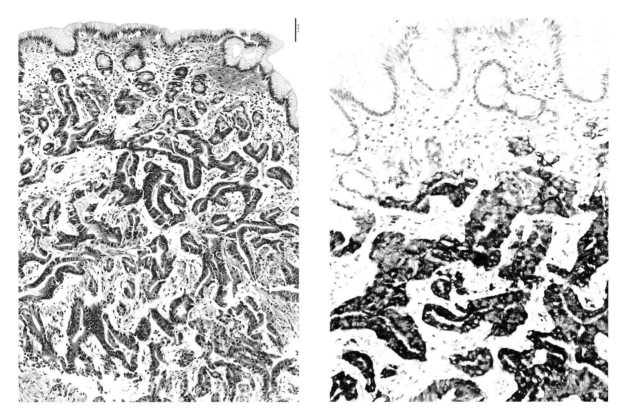

Figure 9-44

GASTRIC ADENOCARCINOMA OF FUNDIC GLAND TYPE

Left: Irregularly anastomosing glands are characteristic.
Right: The neoplastic cells express MUC6.

and Luxol fast blue. They also are positive for parietal cell-specific antibodies and human milk fat globule-2. Ultrastructural evaluation reveals numerous mitochondria and intracellular canaliculi (446–448). Focal parietal cell differentiation has been reported in a well-differentiated (gland-forming) EGC (449). Lymph node metastases occur but are not extensive. It has been suggested that the prognosis of patients with parietal cell carcinoma is better than that for those with usual gastric carcinomas (447). Some cases of oncocytic gastric carcinomas negative for antiparietal cell antibodies have been reported (450).

Paneth Cell Carcinoma

Paneth cell carcinoma is characterized by a predominance of Paneth cells characteristically showing eosinophilic cytoplasmic granules that are positive for lysozyme and defensin-5 by immunohistochemistry (451–453). These tu-

mors are exceedingly rare and have no distinctive clinicopathologic features (451,454). Neoplastic Paneth cells can be identified dispersed among typical gastric adenocarcinomas (455,456).

Mucoepidermoid Carcinoma

These neoplasms are exceedingly rare. Morphologically, the characteristic admixture of mucus-producing and squamous epithelia is present (457).

Carcinosarcoma (Sarcomatoid Carcinoma)

Gastric carcinosarcoma (sarcomatoid carcinoma) is composed of admixed carcinomatous and sarcomatous elements (fig. 9-45), both displaying epithelial markers (fig. 9-46). The sarcomatous component may include elements of chondrosarcomatous, osteosarcomatous, rhabdomyosarcomatous, or leiomyosarcomatous differentiation (458–462). Cases have been reported in the EGJ and gastric stump

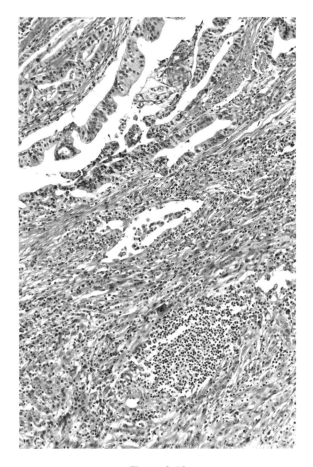

Figure 9-45

**GASTRIC CARCINOSARCOMA
(SARCOMATOID CARCINOMA)**

The tumor is composed of admixed carcinomatous and sarcomatous elements.

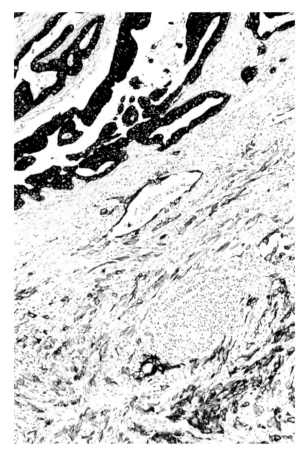

Figure 9-46

**GASTRIC CARCINOSARCOMA
(SARCOMATOID CARCINOMA)**

Both components of the tumor express an epithelial marker (cytokeratin).

(463–465). Neoplasms combining adenosquamous and neuroendocrine components have also been reported (462,466–469). Most cases present as large polypoid tumors and are associated with a poor outcome (470). A case has been reported of gastric adenosarcoma composed of benign tubular and cystic glands embedded in a leiomyosarcomatous stroma (471).

Gastroblastoma

A distinctive well-differentiated epithelial and predominantly mesenchymal biphasic tumor (*gastroblastoma*) has been described in young adults (fig. 9-47) (see also chapter 12) (472–476). The epithelial component is arranged in nests, cords, and tubules that contain luminal eosinophilic secretory material (fig. 9-48, left).

The mesenchymal component is composed of short bundles of spindle cells and variable myxoid or collagenous stroma (fig. 9-48, right). Neither component displays sufficient atypia to be diagnosed as a carcinosarcoma or other malignancy (473). Foci of multinucleated cells are observed in some cases (476).

Malignant Rhabdoid Tumor

Gastric malignant rhabdoid tumors are composed of poorly cohesive, round to polygonal-shaped cells characterized by eosinophilic or clear cytoplasm and large nuclei with predominant nucleoli. The neoplastic cells show strong cellular immunoreactivity for vimentin as well as positivity for cytokeratin, epithelial membrane antigen (EMA), and focal neuron-specific

esterase (NSE) but are negative for carcinoembryonic antigen (CEA) (477–479). The prognosis
of patients with these tumors is dismal, with
early metastases (480).

Undifferentiated Carcinoma

Undifferentiated carcinoma is a term used to
categorize carcinomas lacking any differentiated
features (fig. 9-49) but showing an epithelial
phenotype, at least in part (for example by
cytokeratin expression). They fall into the indeterminate category of the Laurén classification.

Small Cell Carcinoma

This tumor is considered in the chapter on
endocrine cell tumors.

HEREDITARY GASTRIC CANCER SYNDROMES AND INHERITED CANCER PREDISPOSITION SYNDROMES

Although most gastric carcinomas are sporadic, familial aggregation is known to occur in
around 10 to 20 percent of patients. Incidences
range from 2.8 percent in Sweden to 36.6 percent
in Japan and differ between low- and high-risk
gastric carcinoma areas (172,481–483). Familial

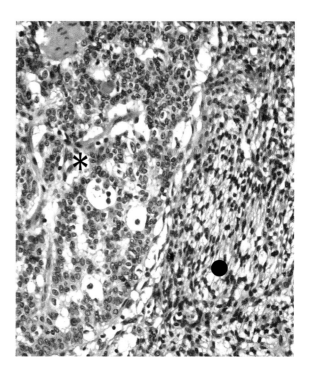

Figure 9-47

GASTROBLASTOMA

The tumor is biphasic, with a sharply defined demarcation
between the epithelial (asterisk) and mesenchymal (dot)
components.

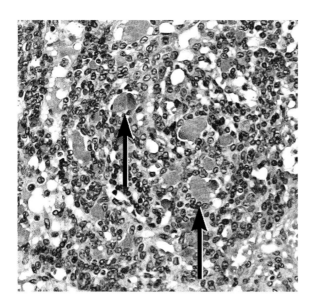
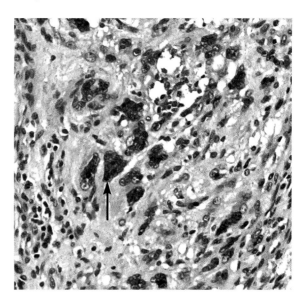

Figure 9-48

GASTROBLASTOMA

Left: The epithelial component is arranged in nests, cords, and tubules that contain luminal eosinophilic secretory
material (arrows).

Right: The mesenchymal component is composed of short bundles of spindle cells and variable myxoid or collagenous stroma.
Note the multinucleated giant cells (arrow).

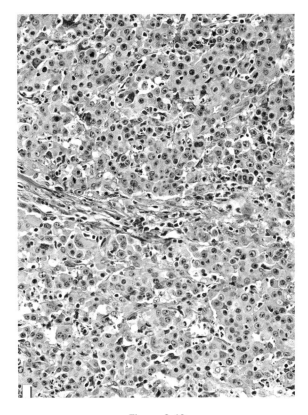

Figure 9-49

UNDIFFERENTIATED CARCINOMA

Malignant cells show minimal differentiation and immunolabeling is required to exclude lymphoma, melanoma, and other malignant neoplasms.

gastric cancer is classified as *hereditary diffuse gastric cancer* (HDGC), *familial intestinal gastric cancer* (FIGC), and, when the histopathology of the tumor is unknown, as *familial gastric cancer* (FGC) (484). Among these groups, only 1 to 3 percent are related to known specific genetic causes, with the most important susceptibility gene for HDGC being *CDH1*. In 2012, a new hereditary cancer syndrome was identified, and was coined GAPPS (*gastric adenocarcinoma and proximal polyposis of the stomach*), which is an autosomal dominant condition characterized by fundic gland polyposis with increased risk of developing gastric carcinoma (485,486), and currently considered a variant of familial adenomatous polyposis (FAP).

Inherited Cancer Predisposition Syndromes

Several inherited cancer predisposition syndromes are associated with an increased risk of gastric cancer. These include familial adenomatous polyposis (FAP), Lynch syndrome (LS), Li-Fraumeni syndrome (LFS), Peutz-Jeghers syndrome (PJS), *MUTYH*-associated polyposis, and juvenile polyposis syndrome (JPS) (486,487).

Familial Adenomatous Polyposis. The presence of gastric polyps is a known manifestation of FAP, with a reported incidence varying from 51 percent (488) to 88 percent (489). The incidence of gastric polyps in attenuated FAP has been reported to be even higher (93 percent) (490). Stomach polyps include predominantly fundic gland polyps; sometimes gastric foveolar adenomas and pyloric gland adenomas also occur (491,492). The risk of gastric carcinoma in FAP varies geographically. A high risk has been reported in Japan and Korea (4.5 to 13.6 percent) (493,494) but has not been confirmed in the West, where the risk is low (0.6 to 4.2 percent) (495,496). In Western countries, the risk of gastric adenocarcinoma does not seem appreciably higher in patients with FAP compared to those with sporadic fundic gland polyps (497,498). Patients with FAP usually undergo esophagogastroduodenoscopy primarily for surveillance of duodenal and ampullary adenomas and cancer (499). Prophylactic gastrectomy has been discussed for patients with FAP (including those with attenuated disease) displaying diffuse fundic gland polyps and high-grade dysplasia or large polyps (500).

Lynch Syndrome. There is also an increased frequency of gastric cancers in patients with LS. The tumors arise at an earlier age than sporadic neoplasms and most are of intestinal type, even though coincidental *H. pylori* infection is uncommon (501). In LS, the cumulative risk of developing gastric cancer by the age of 70 years is approximately 5 percent (502). Recent studies have shown that there is no evidence for the clustering of gastric cancer in specific LS families (503). In parts of the world with a high background incidence of gastric cancer in the population (Korea, Japan), the risk of developing gastric cancer in LS families is also higher, suggesting the role of environmental factors. There is the impression that the incidence of gastric cancer in LS in the Western world is decreasing in parallel to the declining incidence of gastric cancer in the general population (503).

According to the guidelines by the American College of Gastroenterology, screening for gastric and duodenal cancer should be considered in individuals at risk for or affected with LS by baseline esophagogastroduodenoscopy, with gastric biopsy at age 30 to 35 years and treatment of *H. pylori* infection when found (504). These guidelines recommend ongoing surveillance every 3 to 5 years if there is a family history of gastric or duodenal cancer (504). In view of the low risk of gastric cancer and the lack of established benefit, however, the Mallorca group (502) does not advise regular surveillance for gastric cancer, although they recommend screening mutation carriers for the presence of an *H. pylori* infection and subsequent eradication if detected, and indicate that surveillance might be performed in a research setting in countries with a high incidence of gastric cancer.

Li-Fraumeni Syndrome. LFS is caused by germline mutations in the tumor suppressor gene *TP53* (505). Gastrointestinal cancers are rare, representing less than 10 percent of malignancies associated with the syndrome, but gastric cancer represents 50 percent of these. Gastric cancers are detected in 1.8 to 4.9 percent of carriers (506,507). The adenocarcinomas can be detected as early as 12 years of age and most are detected before the patient is 50. Most cases are diagnosed in the proximal stomach (508). Although no specific surveillance guidelines exist, it has been suggested that screening upper endoscopy be considered in patient with a family member affected by gastric cancer (508).

Peutz-Jeghers Syndrome. PJS is caused by mutations in the tumor suppressor gene *STK11* (serine-threonine kinase 1, also known as liver kinase B1 [*LKB1*]). It is characterized by the association of hamartomatous gastrointestinal polyps with mucocutaneous pigmentation and increased cancer risk, particularly for gastrointestinal and breast cancers, which develop at younger ages than in the general population (509–512).

A meta-analysis suggested a cumulative risk of gastric cancer of 29 percent by age 65 years (511). Based on the increased cancer risk, surveillance recommendations for patients with PJS include esophagogastroduodenoscopy (repeated every 2 to 5 years depending on endoscopic and histologic findings) (511). It has been suggested that the site and type of *STK11* gene mutations are predictors of the development of gastric polyps

and malignancies; individuals with truncating mutations develop an earlier onset of gastric polyps in comparison with those with missense mutations (487). Germline mutations have been identified in patients with PJS and gastric cancer (513,514).

Juvenile Polyposis Syndrome. JPS is a rare syndrome characterized by multiple juvenile polyps in the colorectum, small intestine, and stomach. It is caused by a germline mutation in *SMAD4* or *BMPR1A*. JPS is subdivided into four major groups: juvenile polyposis of infancy, juvenile polyposis coli, generalized juvenile polyposis, and juvenile polyposis of the stomach, the latter corresponding to polyps limited to the stomach at the time of the initial diagnosis. *SMAD4* mutations are associated with a higher incidence of gastric polyposis (515).

Clinical criteria to evaluate JPS include individuals with five or more juvenile polyps in the colorectum, any juvenile polyp in other parts of the gastrointestinal tract, or any number of juvenile polyps and a family history of juvenile polyps (504). The cancer risk is believed to arise from dysplasia (foveolar type) in juvenile polyps, which was seen in 32 percent of cases in the study by Gonzalez et al. (516). In another study, it was observed that dysplasia in gastric juvenile polyps may be associated with foveolar, intestinal, and pyloric differentiation (517). The gastric cancer risk is 10 to 30 percent in those with *SMAD4* mutations (504,516). A case of JPS of the stomach with multiple early gastric cancers has been reported (518). Complete or partial gastrectomy may be needed for patients with massive gastric polyposis, high-grade dysplasia, and cancer (516).

Gastric Hyperplastic Polyposis. Gastric cancer has also been described in the rare case of gastric hyperplastic polyposis, an inherited autosomal dominant syndrome characterized by the presence of hyperplastic gastric polyposis, severe psoriasis, and a high incidence of gastric cancer of the diffuse type (519,520).

Hereditary Breast and Ovarian Cancer (HBOC) Syndrome Caused by *BRCA1* and *BRCA2* Mutations. The incidence of gastric cancer before the age of 70 years is twice as common in these patients compared to the general population (521,522). In one study all gastric carcinomas were diagnosed at a young age (under the age of 55 years) (523).

Hereditary Diffuse Gastric Cancer

Definition. *Hereditary diffuse gastric cancer* (HDGC) is an autosomal dominant cancer susceptibility syndrome characterized by signet ring cell (diffuse) gastric cancer and lobular breast cancer.

General Features. The genetic basis of HDGC was discovered in 1998 by Guilford et al. (524), who studied three Maori kindreds in New Zealand with multigenerational diffuse gastric cancer, in which germline mutations of the E-cadherin (*CDH1*) gene (OMIM# 192090) were identified by linkage analysis and mutation screening. Other susceptibility genes have been identified, as described below.

Genetic Susceptibility. Germline *CDH1* mutations can affect the whole gene coding sequence. So far, more than 150 *CDH1* germline mutations have been described (486,525–527), including by frequency, small frameshift insertions and deletions, splice-site, missense and nonsense mutations, large rearrangements and, rarely, germline promoter methylation (487,528,529). About 80 percent of mutations are pathogenic (e.g., truncating mutations), leading to protein dysfunction. The remaining 20 percent are of uncertain significance (e.g., missense mutations) and require additional functional studies to address their pathogenicity (530–534).

According to the two-hit hypothesis, a second somatic event, leading to biallelic inactivation, is necessary for E-cadherin disruption and the development of HDGC. *CDH1* second-hit mechanisms include promoter hypermethylation and, less frequently, loss of heterozygosity or intragenic deletions (535–538).

Another gene involved in intercellular cell adhesion (*CTNNA1*, encoding α–E-catenin) has also been implicated in HDGC (529,539). Recently, exome and multiplexed targeted sequencing has led to the identification of new candidate HDGC susceptibility genes, some of which are associated with other hereditary cancer predisposition syndromes, namely, *BRCA2, STK11, SDHB, PRSS1, ATM, MSR1, PALB2, INSR, FBXO24,* and *DOT1L (529, 540)*.

Clinical Features. The age of onset of clinically significant HGDC is extremely variable (range, 14 to 85 years), even within families. On the basis of clinical criteria, the International Gastric Cancer Linkage Consortium (IGCLC) defined families with HDGC syndrome as meeting one of two criteria: 1) two or more documented cases of diffuse gastric cancer in first- or second-degree relatives with at least one being diagnosed before the age of 50 years or 2) three or more cases of documented diffuse gastric cancer in first- or second-degree relatives, independent of age of diagnosis (484). Women in these families have an elevated risk of lobular breast cancer (526,541–544). The IGCLC criteria for genetic testing were updated in 2010 (545). An alternative genetically based nomenclature has been proposed, in which the term "HDGC" is restricted to families with germline mutations in the *CDH1* gene (524,546).

In clinically defined HDGC, *CDH1* mutations are detected in 30 to 40 percent of cases (178,527,543). The cumulative risk of HDGC for *CDH1* mutation carriers by age 80 years is reported to be 70 percent for men (95 percent CI, 59 to 80 percent) and 56 percent for women (95 percent CI, 44 to 69 percent) (530). The cumulative risk of lobular breast cancer for women with a *CDH1* mutation is estimated to be 42 percent (95 percent CI, 23 to 68 percent) by 80 years (530). There is currently no evidence that the risk of other cancer types in individuals with a *CDH1* mutation is significantly increased.

Endoscopic Findings. It is recommended that individuals with HDGC having endoscopy who do not know their mutation status or those who do not have a proven pathogenic *CDH1* mutation undergo screening whereas mutation-positive individuals undergo surveillance. In asymptomatic *CDH1* mutation carriers, no lesions are observed at endoscopy in the majority of the cases. In some apparently normal stomachs, subtle pale areas are visible on standard white-light endoscopy (530,547) and narrow-band imaging may make them easier to visualize (530). Chromoendoscopy with Congo red and methylene blue is no longer recommended due to concerns over toxicity (530).

It is recommended that individuals with HDGC should be offered annual endoscopy. A minimum of 30 biopsies is recommended, as described in the Cambridge protocol (530). Any malignant lesions detected endoscopically should prompt a referral for gastrectomy. All patients undergoing endoscopy for HDGC should be informed that, given the very focal and often

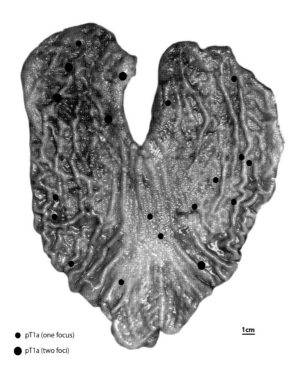

● pT1a (one focus)

● pT1a (two foci)

1cm

Figure 9-50

HEREDITARY DIFFUSE GASTRIC CANCER (HDGC) CARRIER: GROSS APPEARANCE

Resection specimen from a prophylactic/risk reducing gastrectomy performed in one carrier of a germline *CDH1* mutation. The stomach appears normal to the naked eye, without mass lesions. Black dots indicate the sites where microscopic lesions were identified.

endoscopically invisible nature of these lesions, it is possible that lesions will not be detected by random biopsies (530).

Gross Findings. Macroscopic features differ in stomachs from asymptomatic *CDH1* mutation carriers submitted to prophylactic/risk reducing gastrectomy and index cases with HDGC. In the former, stomachs nearly always appear normal to the naked eye, there is no mass lesion (fig. 9-50), and slicing shows normal mucosal thickness (548–551). In some apparently normal stomachs, subtle pale areas are visible on standard white-light endoscopy (547), and close inspection may show white patches that after formalin fixation correspond to intramucosal signet ring cell (diffuse) carcinoma. Most index cases with HDGC present with cancers that are indistinguishable from sporadic diffuse gastric cancer, often with linitis plastica, which can involve all topographic regions within the stomach.

Microscopic Features. Early-stage HDGC in *CDH1* mutation carriers is characterized by multiple foci of invasive (T1a) signet-ring cell (diffuse) carcinoma in the superficial gastric mucosa (fig. 9-51, left), without nodal metastases. Some of the foci are tiny and contain few signet ring cells (fig. 9-51, right); in some cases the population of neoplastic cells is heterogeneous (fig. 9-52) (549,552–554). Mapping of the entire gastric mucosa performed in many stomachs from kindred with different *CDH1* mutations (548–550,552,553,555–557) has shown that there is wide variation in the number of T1a foci observed in these stomachs, both within and between kindreds, ranging from one focus (548) to hundreds of tiny foci (549,553). Histologic examination of the entire gastric mucosa is required before the absence of neoplasia can be claimed. The cause of this variation in number of foci currently is unknown. Early invasive carcinoma is not restricted to any topographic region in the stomach (548,550,552,555). As all regions of the gastric mucosa can be affected, pathologic examination of the resected specimen should include confirmation of the presence of a complete cuff of proximal squamous esophageal mucosa and distal duodenal mucosa.

Two precursors (Tis) to T1a signet ring cell carcinoma are recognized in HDGC: 1) pagetoid spread of signet ring cells situated underneath the normal epithelium of glands and foveolae, but within the confines of the basement membrane (fig. 9-53) and 2) in situ signet ring cell carcinoma, corresponding to the presence of signet ring cells within the basement membrane, replacing the normal epithelial cells (fig. 9-54), generally with hyperchromatic and depolarized nuclei (548). In these lesions, E-cadherin immunoexpression is reduced or absent (178,548). Confirmation of in situ carcinoma by an independent histopathologist with experience in this area is strongly recommended. A case seen in consultation, with a tiny focus of intramucosal carcinoma and focal transformation of the glandular epithelium (isthmus/neck zone) into in situ carcinoma is seen in figure 9-55.

Advanced HDGC presents as a poorly differentiated diffuse carcinoma, sometimes with a few signet ring cells, that invades widely the whole thickness of the gastric wall, which becomes rigid (linitis plastica). It also presents

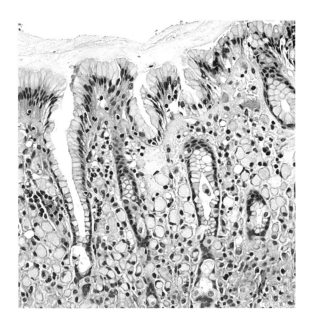 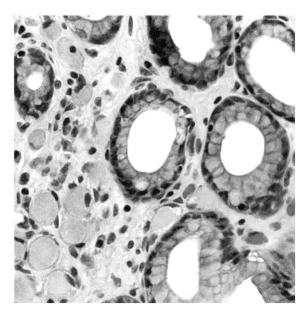

Figure 9-51

HEREDITARY DIFFUSE GASTRIC CANCER

Left: Panoramic view of signet ring cell/diffuse carcinoma restricted to the mucosa. The neoplastic cells display the typical features of signet ring cells.

Right: Tiny focus of T1a signet ring cell carcinoma constituted by few signet ring cells.

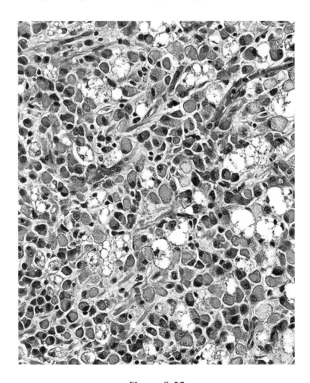

Figure 9-52

HEREDITARY DIFFUSE GASTRIC CANCER

In this case, the population of neoplastic cells is heterogeneous.

as undifferentiated or mixed subtypes with mucinous and occasionally tubular components. These advanced gastric carcinomas of *CDH1* mutation carriers do not have any characteristics that can be used to differentiate them from sporadic gastric cancers.

Background changes in the gastric mucosa of prophylactic gastrectomy specimens encompass mild chronic gastritis, foveolar hyperplasia, and tufting of surface epithelium (551). Occasionally, an inflammatory granulomatous reaction is observed. In almost all prophylactic gastrectomies studied so far, intestinal metaplasia and *H. pylori* infection are absent, namely, in families from North America and Europe.

Immunohistochemical Findings. Consistent with the biallelic *CDH1* inactivation and consequent E-cadherin loss of function, E-cadherin protein expression by immunohistochemistry is almost always abnormal in HDGC, in contrast to the normal complete membranous expression in adjacent normal (nontumoral) epithelium (30,548,554–556). Aberrant E-cadherin staining patterns include absence of immunoreactivity as well as reduced membranous, dotted, and

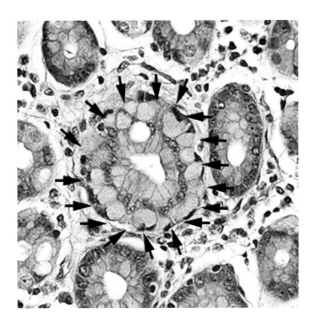
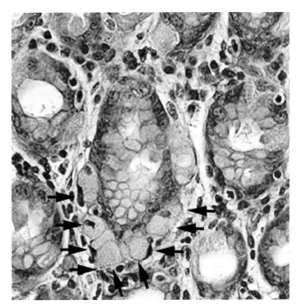

Figure 9-53

HEREDITARY DIFFUSE GASTRIC CANCER

Pagetoid spread of signet ring cells (arrows). The cells spread underneath the epithelium of glands and foveolae, within the basement membrane.

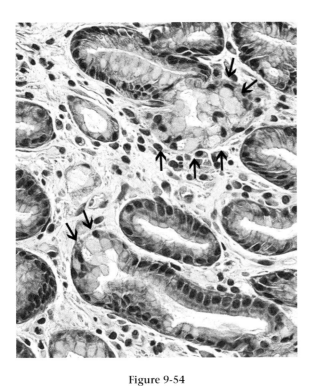

Figure 9-54

HEREDITARY DIFFUSE GASTRIC CANCER

In situ signet ring cell carcinoma is characterized by the presence of signet ring cells (arrows) within the basement membrane, replacing the normal epithelial cells.

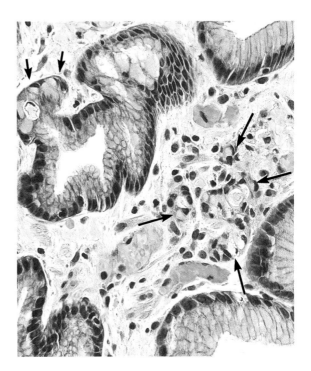

Figure 9-55

HEREDITARY DIFFUSE GASTRIC CANCER

Intramucosal carcinoma (tiny focus [arrows]) and focal in situ carcinoma in an adjacent gland.

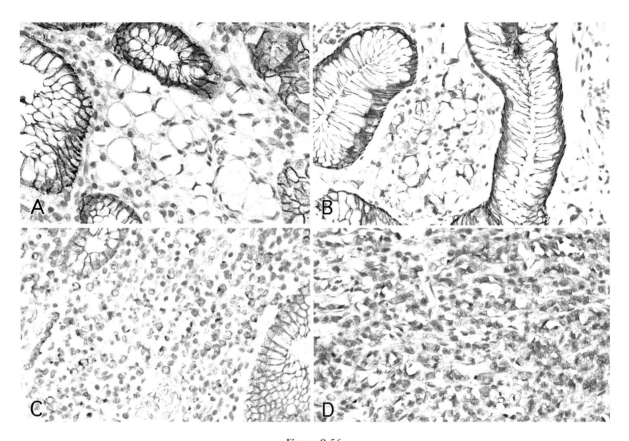

Figure 9-56

HEREDITARY DIFFUSE GASTRIC CANCER

Patterns of E-cadherin immunoexpression. (Adapted from figure in reference 558.)
A: Absence of immunoreactivity.
B: Reduced E-cadherin membranous expression.
C: "Dotted" pattern of expression.
D: Cytoplasmic staining.

cytoplasmic staining (fig. 9-56) (558). The dotted staining pattern is probably due to persistence of E-cadherin nonfunctional domains in the Golgi apparatus (536). Abnormal immunoreactivity of E-cadherin has been described in precursor lesions (in situ signet ring cell carcinoma and pagetoid spread of signet ring cells) as well as in early or advanced carcinomas, suggesting that the inactivation of E-cadherin is probably a key initiating event in HDGC tumorigenesis (548). Moreover, normal immunoreactivity of the gastric mucosa between lesions suggests a clonal origin of the individual cancer foci.

One report described abnormal patterns of expression of both α- and β-catenin in early HDGCs (536), suggesting that the absence of a normal E-cadherin protein may lead to the disruption of the cell-cell adhesion complex. Furthermore, β-actin, p120 catenin, and Lin7 were shown to be reduced or absent in HDGC in another study (559).

Early HDGCs present with an indolent phenotype, with typical signet ring cells, without proliferation, and normal immunohistochemical staining of p53. Advanced HDGCs display an aggressive phenotype, with a mixture of pleomorphic cells and a high proliferative index with increased staining of Ki-67 and p53 (558). Figure 9-57 shows two cases in the same family, with the same germline *CDH1* mutation: one case with an indolent phenotype and the other with an aggressive phenotype. The latter corresponded to an 18-year-old patient who died shortly after the diagnosis with widely invasive HDGC. Based

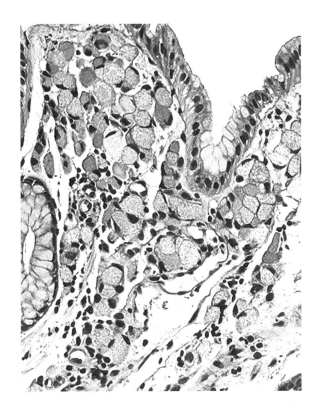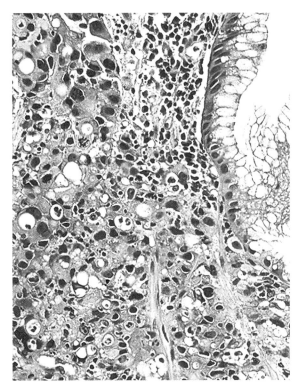

Figure 9-57

HEREDITARY DIFFUSE GASTRIC CANCER: INDOLENT AND AGGRESSIVE PHENOTYPES

Left: The neoplastic cells are localized below the preserved superficial epithelium and display the typical features of signet ring cells.

Right: The neoplastic cels are bizarre and pleomorphic, with hyperchromatic nuclei.

on available evidence, the finding of gastric carcinoma with an aggressive phenotype in a screening biopsy performed in a *CDH1* germline mutation carrier should be taken as a predictive sign of widely invasive carcinoma, and prompt staging and surgical treatment.

Molecular Genetic Findings. In HDGC, most *CDH1* mutations (75 to 80 percent) are truncating and the remainder are missense (530,553,560). Large germline deletions have been found in 6.5 percent of HDGC families who tested negatively for point mutations (527). Unlike the somatic mutations in *CDH1* that occur in sporadic gastric cancers and cluster around exons 7 and 8, the germline mutations in *CDH1* in HDGC families span the whole length of the gene and no hot spots have been identified.

In HDGC, the *CDH1* gene can be inactivated by a number of mechanisms. Most frequently, this occurs via promoter hypermethylation (epigenetic modification) and less frequently by loss

of heterozygosity (LOH) and *CDH1* mutations (535,537,538). An intragenic deletion in the wild-type allele is also reported (536). Humar et al. (559) have suggested that the initiation of diffuse gastric cancer seems to occur at the proliferative zone of the gastric epithelium and correlates with absent or reduced expression of junctional proteins, activation of the c-SRC system and epithelial-mesenchymal transition. In about two thirds of HDGC patients, *CDH1* germline mutations are not identified. Germline mutations in *TP53* were detected in two studies of families with gastric cancer and no mutation in *CDH1* (561,562).

Differential Diagnosis. Confirmation of carcinoma in situ and pagetoid spread of signet ring cells by an independent pathologist with experience in this area is strongly recommended, and will help pathologists to distinguish legitimate precursor lesions and tiny foci of early intramucosal carcinoma from mimics of signet ring cells (e.g., telescoped normal glands, globoid cells in hyperplastic lesions [fig. 9-58A], clear or glassy cell change of mucous glands [fig. 9-58B], xanthomatous cells [fig. 9-58C], and neuroendocrine cell nests [fig. 9-58D]) (530).

In patients with both lobular breast cancer and diffuse gastric cancer, either synchronously or metachronously, a metastasis should be considered. Two primary tumors may be indicative of a hereditary background, but this is not always the underlying reason. Metastases from these tumors are often morphologically indistinguishable (563). Breast-associated immunomarkers are ER, BRST-2, and mammaglobin; CK20 and HNF4A are suggestive of gastric cancer (564).

Staging. At the time of prophylactic gastrectomy, most carriers of *CDH1* germline mutations are found to have T1 N0 stage tumors (556). It has been suggested that there is a dormant period in which the signet ring cell adenocarcinoma does not spread or progress due to the low proliferative index of the neoplastic cells. In symptomatic patients, the gastric cancer stage is usually advanced.

Treatment. The age at which to offer genetic testing to at-risk relatives should take into consideration the earliest age of cancer onset in that family. Testing from the late teens or early 20s is favored in families with early-onset gastric cancer (543). Current guidelines recommend that asymptomatic carriers of *CDH1* mutations be offered prophylactic gastrectomy, or for selected groups, annual endoscopic surveillance, as risk-reduction strategies. Surveillance is recommended for individuals aged less than 20 years; for those aged more than 20 years who elect to delay surgery; for those for whom prophylactic gastrectomy (biopsy negative) is unacceptable but gastrectomy with curative intent (biopsy positive) is acceptable; and for those with mutations of undetermined significance (e.g., missense) (543,547). Total gastrectomy is recommended in at-risk family members who have a *CDH1* germline mutation, in early adulthood, between the ages of 20 and 30 years (530,553). In biopsy-positive individuals, a curative total gastrectomy is advised, regardless of age.

The diagnosis of HDGC offers the opportunity for presymptomatic genetic screening for at-risk family members and life-saving cancer risk-reduction surgery for carriers of *CDH1* mutations. Prophylactic gastrectomy after age 75 should be carefully considered (530). Family phenotype, especially age of onset of clinical cancer in probands, should be taken into account.

Prognosis. If foci of carcinoma are limited to the gastric mucosa, the prognosis is likely to be excellent after total gastrectomy, although long-term survival with HDGC after gastrectomy remains unknown. It is possible that curative gastrectomies for gastric disease will unmask an additional risk for carcinoma at other sites in HDGC patients. Patients who develop symptomatic, widely invasive HDGC have a poor prognosis, with as few as 10 percent having potentially curable disease (17). Even if potentially curable, the 5-year survival rate of widely invasive HDGC does not exceed 30 percent (565).

Procedure for Pathologic Examination. The analysis of the pathologic changes in HDGC prophylactic gastrectomy specimens includes a thorough microscopic assessment of the complete stomach with a hematoxylin and eosin (H&E) stain. A mucin stain, such as periodic acid–Schiff (PAS) (530,545), may increase the detection rate of small invasive cancers and reduce screening time. The Swiss roll technique, consisting of rolling up the gastrectomy specimen lengthwise, can be used to include the complete mucosa. The pathology report should mention all gastric abnormalities and localization. Histologic confirmation of resection margins consisting of proximal esophageal and distal duodenal mucosa is essential because new gastric cancer can develop in remaining gastric mucosa (545,548).

GASTRIC ADENOCARCINOMA AND PROXIMAL POLYPOSIS OF THE STOMACH

Definition. *Gastric adenocarcinoma and proximal polyposis of the stomach* (GAPPS) is an autosomal-dominant cancer-predisposition syndrome with a significant risk of gastric, but not colorectal, adenocarcinoma (485). In 2012, after the initial description of three GAPPS families from Australia, the United States, and Canada (485), two Japanese families with similar clinicopathologic features were reported (566). In 2016, the first European GAPPS family was described (567). To date, more than ten families with GAPPS are reported worldwide; the youngest patient presented with generalized gastric adenocarcinoma at the age of 26 years (485,566–570).

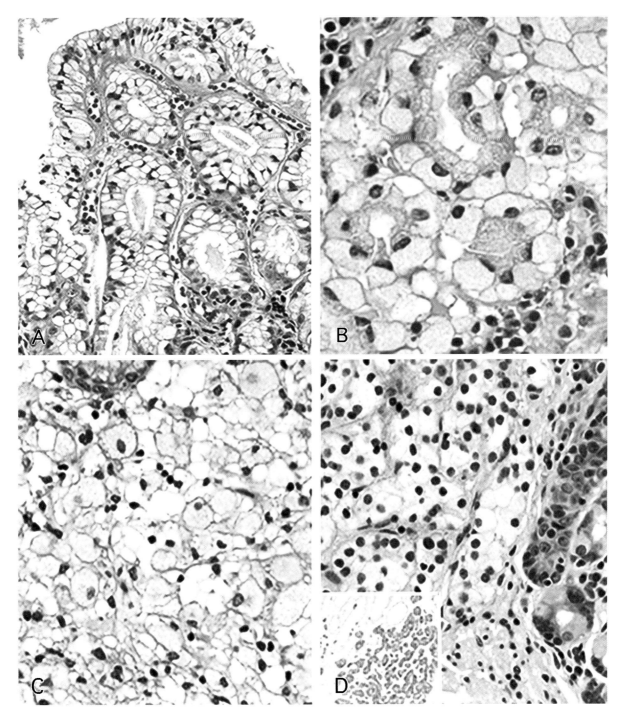

Figure 9-58

HEREDITARY DIFFUSE GASTRIC CANCER MIMICS

A: Globoid change of foveolar epithelium.

B: Clear cell change of pyloric glands, characterized by a cytoplasmic vacuole occupying the basal portion of the cells; a preserved rim of cytoplasm is seen at the apical pole.

C: Xanthoma consists of macrophages with clear, microvacuolated cytoplasm and centrally located nuclei.

D: Neuroendocrine tumor. The neoplastic cells are polyhedral with small nuclei and express neuroendocrine markers (Inset: immunoexpression of synaptophysin).

Clinical Features. GAPPS presents as an incomplete penetrance, as proven by the evidence of normal endoscopies in elderly obligate carriers (485). The age of onset of gastric carcinoma is variable, ranging from 23 to 75 years (median, 50 years) and the typical fundic gland polyposis with multifocal dysplasia is detected as early as 10 years of age (485,567).

Gross Findings. Florid gastric polyposis, mainly with polyps less than 10 mm in size, is the main gross feature (fig. 9-59). More than 100 polyps usually carpet the gastric body and fundus, with relative sparing along the lesser curve of the stomach (485,566). The esophagus, gastric antrum, pylorus, and duodenum are usually unaffected.

Microscopic Findings. Microscopy shows mainly fundic gland polyposis (fig. 9-60) and regions of dysplasia (fig. 9-61). Occasional hyperplastic and pure adenomatous polyps and some mixed polyps containing discrete areas of fundic gland polyp-like, adenomatous, and hyperplastic features are detected among the fundic gland polyps (485,571). Gastric cancers that develop in patients with GAPPS display features of both intestinal-type or mixed gastric cancer (485,567).

The following diagnostic criteria have been proposed: 1) gastric polyps restricted to the body and fundus without colorectal or duodenal polyposis; 2) more than 100 polyps in the proximal stomach of the index or more than 30 polyps in a first-degree relative; 3) mainly fundic gland polyps with or without dysplasia or adenocarcinoma; 4) autosomal dominant pattern of inheritance; and 5) exclusion of another gastric polyposis syndrome and use of proton-pump inhibitors (485).

Immunohistochemical Findings. Fundic gland polyps and gastric cancers display increased expression of nuclear β-catenin, Ki-67, and p53 (569). These features are shared by the few colonic polyps identified in GAPPS syndrome. Both gastric and colonic lesions harbor activating somatic variants of β-catenin signaling (569).

Molecular Genetic Findings. Recently, the genetic defect in GAPPS was identified as point mutations in promoter 1B of the *APC* gene that co-segregated with disease in six GAPPS families (568). Similar mutations in *APC* promoter 1B occur in rare families (0.9 percent) with FAP and gastric fundic gland polyposis; further, gastric cancer has been previously described in some FAP-affected individuals with large deletions around promoter 1B. These findings suggest that families with mutations affecting the promoter 1B are at risk of gastric adenocarcinoma, regardless of whether or not colorectal polyps are present. Based on this evidence, GAPPS has been considered a FAP variant (568).

Differential Diagnosis. The major entity in the differential diagnosis is fundic gland polyposis in the setting of FAP. The unique noninvolvement of the antrum in patients with GAPPS, coupled with the absence of a colonic polyposis phenotype, is an important clinical feature that distinguishes GAPPS and FAP. The prolonged use of proton-pump inhibitors may be the cause of fundic gland polyps/polyposis without dysplasia and should be considered in the differential diagnosis.

Treatment and Prognosis. Clinically accepted approaches to the management of GAPPS families include endoscopic surveillance with random biopsies or preferably polypectomies directed to large/irregular polyps and, eventually, prophylactic gastrectomy. The limitations of endoscopic surveillance, the patient-specific risk of morbidity associated with prophylactic surgery and the risk of gastric cancer within the specific family need to be balanced. Patients with biopsy-proven gastric adenocarcinoma are candidates for standard therapy.

All first-degree relatives of affected patients should be advised to undergo esophagogastroduodenoscopy and colonoscopy (568,572). The prognosis is dismal in patients with gastric adenocarcinoma.

Procedure for Pathologic Examination. Surgical specimens should be carefully examined and polyps generously sampled and submitted for histology. No specific protocol for the study of these specimens is available for the moment.

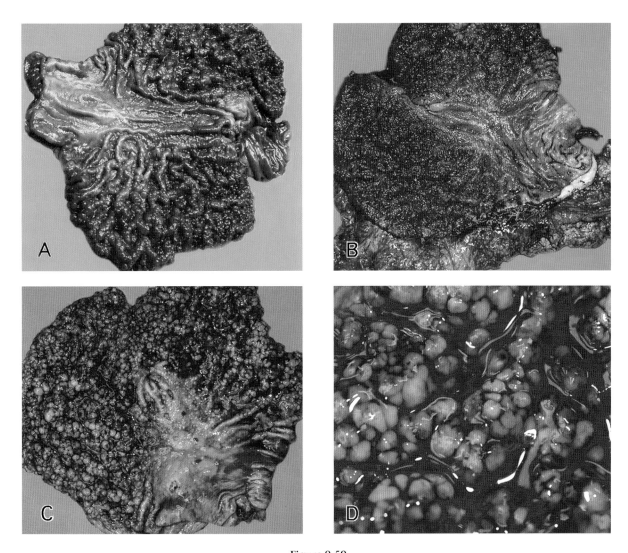

Figure 9-59

GASTRIC ADENOCARCINOMA AND PROXIMAL POLYPOSIS OF THE STOMACH (GAPPS)

A–C: Resection specimens (total gastrectomies) displaying florid gastric polyposis. More than 100 small polyps carpet the gastric body and fundus, with relative sparing of the lesser curve of the stomach.

D: At higher magnification, the polyps are roundish with a smooth glistering surface. (Courtesy of Dr. Priyanthi Kumarasinghe and Dr. Bastiaan de Boer, Australia.)

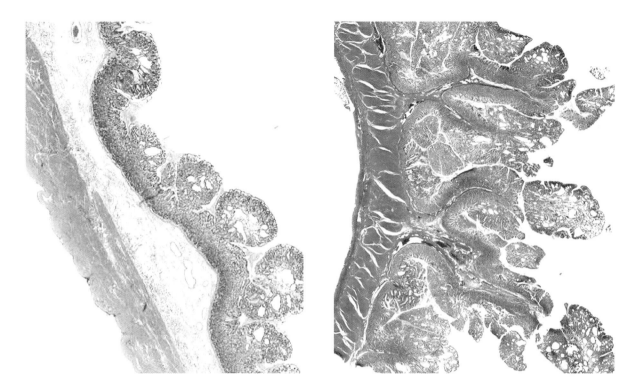

Figure 9-60

GASTRIC ADENOCARCINOMA AND PROXIMAL POLYPOSIS OF THE STOMACH

Panoramic views of polyposis in the body mucosa. The polyps display the features of fundic gland polyps, with cystic dilatation of the glands. (Courtesy of Dr. Priyanthi Kumarasinghe and Dr. Bastiaan de Boer, Australia.)

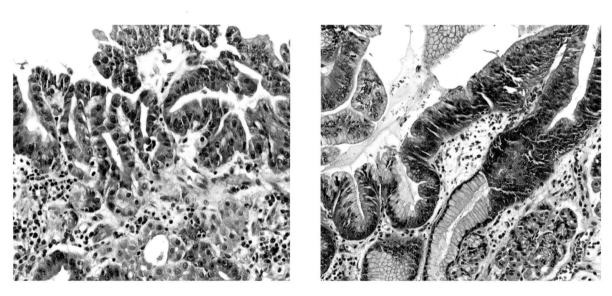

Figure 9-61

GASTRIC ADENOCARCINOMA AND PROXIMAL POLYPOSIS OF THE STOMACH

Left: High-grade dysplasia is observed in the surface of a fundic gland polyp (the dysplastic glands are tortuous, lined by cuboidal cells with hyperchromatic nuclei).

Right: High-grade dysplasia is observed at the surface of the mucosa. It shows an abrupt transition from normal-appearing foveolar epithelium.

REFERENCES

1. Ferlay J, Soerjomataram I, Dikshit R, et al. Cancer incidence and mortality worldwide: sources, methods and major patterns in GLOBOCAN 2012. Int J Cancer 2015;136:E359-86.
2. Bray F, Jemal A, Grey N, Ferlay J, Forman D. Global cancer transitions according to the Human Development Index (2008-2030): a population-based study. Lancet Oncol 2012;13:790-801.
3. Sonnenberg A. Time trends of mortality from gastric cancer in Europe. Digestive diseases and sciences. 2011;56(4):1112-8.
4. Carneiro F. Stomach cancer. In: Steward BW, Wild CP, eds. World Cancer Report 2014. Lyon: IARC Press; 2014:382-91.
5. Torre LA, Siegel RL, Ward EM, Jemal A. Global cancer incidence and mortality rates and trends—an update. Cancer Epidemiol Biomarkers Prev 2016;25:16-27.
6. Parkin DM. The global health burden of infection-associated cancers in the year 2002. Int J Cancer 2006;118:3030-44.
7. Keeney S, Bauer TL. Epidemiology of adenocarcinoma of the esophagogastric junction. Surg Oncol Clin N Am 2006;15:687-96.
8. Zheng T, Mayne ST, Holford TR, et al. The time trend and age-period-cohort effects on incidence of adenocarcinoma of the stomach in Connecticut from 1955-1989. Cancer 1993;72:330-40.
9. Deans C, Yeo MS, Soe MY, Shabbir A, Ti TK, So JB. Cancer of the gastric cardia is rising in incidence in an Asian population and is associated with adverse outcome. World J Surg 2011;35:617-24.
10. Blot WJ, Devesa SS, Kneller RW, Fraumeni JF Jr. Rising incidence of adenocarcinoma of the esophagus and gastric cardia. JAMA 1991;265: 1287-9.
11. Pohl H, Welch HG. The role of overdiagnosis and reclassification in the marked increase of esophageal adenocarcinoma incidence. J Natl Cancer Inst 2005;97:142-6.
12. Botterweck AA, Schouten LJ, Volovics A, Dorant E, van Den Brandt PA. Trends in incidence of adenocarcinoma of the oesophagus and gastric cardia in ten European countries. Int J Epidemiol 2000;29:645-54.
13. Pera M, Manterola C, Vidal O, Grande L. Epidemiology of esophageal adenocarcinoma. J Surg Oncol 2005;92:151-9.
14. Brown LM, Devesa SS, Chow WH. Incidence of adenocarcinoma of the esophagus among white Americans by sex, stage, and age. J Natl Cancer Inst 2008;100:1184-7.
15. Kokkola A, Sipponen P. Gastric carcinoma in young adults. Hepatogastroenterology 2001;48:1552-5.
16. Milne AN, Sitarz R, Carvalho R, Carneiro F, Offerhaus GJ. Early onset gastric cancer: on the road to unraveling gastric carcinogenesis. Curr Mol Med 2007;7:15-28.
17. Koea JB, Karpeh MS, Brennan MF. Gastric cancer in young patients: demographic, clinicopathological, and prognostic factors in 92 patients. Ann Surg Oncol 2000;7:346-51.
18. Moreira H, Pinto-de-Sousa J, Carneiro F, Cardoso de Oliveira M, Pimenta A. Early onset gastric cancer no longer presents as an advanced disease with ominous prognosis. Dig Surg 2009;26:215-21.
19. Park JC, Lee YC, Kim JH, et al. Clinicopathological aspects and prognostic value with respect to age: an analysis of 3,362 consecutive gastric cancer patients. J Surg Oncol 2009;99:395-401.
20. Theuer CP, de Virgilio C, Keese G, et al. Gastric adenocarcinoma in patients 40 years of age or younger. Am J Surg 1996;172:473-6; discussion 6-7.
21. Seruca R, Sobrinho-Simoes M. Assessment of microsatellite alterations in young patients with gastric adenocarcinoma. Cancer 1997;80:1358-60.
22. Hayden JD, Cawkwell L, Dixon MF, et al. A comparison of microsatellite instability in early onset gastric carcinomas from relatively low and high incidence European populations. Int J Cancer 2000;85:189-91.
23. Lim S, Lee HS, Kim HS, Kim YI, Kim WH. Alteration of E-cadherin-mediated adhesion protein is common, but microsatellite instability is uncommon in young age gastric cancers. Histopathology 2003;42:128-36.
24. Milne AN, Carvalho R, Morsink FM, et al. Early-onset gastric cancers have a different molecular expression profile than conventional gastric cancers. Mod Pathol 2006;19:564-72.
25. Carvalho R, Milne AN, Polak M, Offerhaus GJ, Weterman MA. A novel region of amplification at 11p12-13 in gastric cancer, revealed by representational difference analysis, is associated with overexpression of CD44v6, especially in early-onset gastric carcinomas. Genes Chromosomes Cancer 2006;45:967-75.
26. Buffart TE, Carvalho B, Hopmans E, et al. Gastric cancers in young and elderly patients show different genomic profiles. J Pathol 2007;211:45-51.
27. Silva EM, Begnami MD, Fregnani JH, et al. Cadherin-catenin adhesion system and mucin expression: a comparison between young and older patients with gastric carcinoma. Gastric Cancer 2008;11:149-59.

28. Rugge M, Busatto G, Cassaro M, et al. Patients younger than 40 years with gastric carcinoma: Helicobacter pylori genotype and associated gastritis phenotype. Cancer 1999;85:2506-11.

29. Koshida Y, Koizumi W, Sasabe M, Katoh Y, Okayasu I. Association of Helicobacter pylori-dependent gastritis with gastric carcinomas in young Japanese patients: histopathological comparison of diffuse and intestinal type cancer cases. Histopathology 2000;37:124-30.

30. Huntsman DG, Carneiro F, Lewis FR, et al. Early gastric cancer in young, asymptomatic carriers of germ-line E-cadherin mutations. N Engl J Med 2001;344:1904-9.

31. Skierucha M, Milne AN, Offerhaus GJ, Polkowski WP, Maciejewski R, Sitarz R. Molecular alterations in gastric cancer with special reference to the early-onset subtype. World J Gastroenterol 2016;22:2460-74.

32. Murakami T. Pathomorphological diagnosis. Definition and growth classification of early gastric cancer. In: Murakami T, ed. Early gastric cancer. Gann monograph on cancer research 11. Tokyo: University of Tokyo Press; 1971:55-66.

33. Crew KD, Neugut AI. Epidemiology of gastric cancer. World J Gastroenterol 2006;12:354-62.

34. Tsukuma H, Mishima T, Oshima A. Prospective study of "early" gastric cancer. Int J Cancer 1983; 31:421-6.

35. Ohta H, Noguchi Y, Takagi K, Nishi M, Kajitani T, Kato Y. Early gastric carcinoma with special reference to macroscopic classification. Cancer 1987;60:1099-106.

36. Hisamichi S, Sugawara N. Mass screening for gastric cancer by X-ray examination. Jpn J Clin Oncol 1984;14:211-23.

37. Green PH, O'Toole KM, Weinberg LM, Goldfarb JP. Early gastric cancer. Gastroenterology 1981;81:247-56.

38. Carter KJ, Schaffer HA, Ritchie WP Jr. Early gastric cancer. Ann Surg 1984;199:604-9.

39. Grigioni WF, D'Errico A, Milani M, et al. Early gastric cancer. Clinico-pathological analysis of 125 cases of early gastric cancer (EGC). Acta Pathol Jpn 1984;34:979-89.

40. Correa P. A human model of gastric carcinogenesis. Cancer Res 1988;48:3554-60.

41. Correa P. Human gastric carcinogenesis: a multistep and multifactorial process—First American Cancer Society Award Lecture on Cancer Epidemiology and Prevention. Cancer Res 1992;52: 6735-40.

42. Valente P, Garrido M, Gullo I, et al. Epithelial dysplasia of the stomach with gastric immunophenotype shows features of biological aggressiveness. Gastric Cancer 2015;18:720-8.

43. Imai T, Kubo T, Watanabe H. Chronic gastritis in Japanese with reference to high incidence of gastric carcinoma. J Natl Cancer Inst 1971;47:179-95.

44. Correa P, Cuello C, Duque E. Carcinoma and intestinal metaplasia of the stomach in Colombian migrants. J Natl Cancer Inst 1970;44:297-306.

45. Siurala M, Varis K, Wiljasalo M. Studies of patients with atrophic gastritis: a 10-15-year follow-up. Scand J Gastroenterol 1966;1:40-8.

46. Walker IR, Strickland RG, Ungar B, Mackay IR. Simple atrophic gastritis and gastric carcinoma. Gut 1971;12:906-11.

47. Goldenring JR, Nam KT. Oxyntic atrophy, metaplasia, and gastric cancer. Prog Mol Biol Transl Sci 2010;96:117-31.

48. Price AB. The Sydney System: histological division. J Gastroenterol Hepatol 1991;6:209-22.

49. Dixon MF, Genta RM, Yardley JH, Correa P. Classification and grading of gastritis. The updated Sydney System. International Workshop on the Histopathology of Gastritis, Houston 1994. Am J Surg Pathol 1996;20:1161-81.

50. El-Zimaity HM, Graham DY, al-Assi MT, et al. Interobserver variation in the histopathological assessment of Helicobacter pylori gastritis. Hum Pathol 1996;27:35-41.

51. Offerhaus GJ, Price AB, Haot J, et al. Observer agreement on the grading of gastric atrophy. Histopathology 1999;34:320-5.

52. Chen XY, van der Hulst RW, Bruno MJ, et al. Interobserver variation in the histopathological scoring of Helicobacter pylori related gastritis. J Clin Pathol 1999;52:612-5.

53. Rugge M, Correa P, Dixon MF, et al. Gastric mucosal atrophy: interobserver consistency using new criteria for classification and grading. Alimentary Pharmacol Ther 2002;16:1249-59.

54. Meining A, Bayerdorffer E, Muller P, et al. Gastric carcinoma risk index in patients infected with Helicobacter pylori. Virchows Arch 1998;432:311-4.

55. Rugge M, Meggio A, Pennelli G, et al. Gastritis staging in clinical practice: the OLGA staging system. Gut 2007;56:631-6.

56. Rugge M, Genta RM. Staging gastritis: an international proposal. Gastroenterology 2005;129: 1807-8.

57. Graham DY, Nurgalieva ZZ, El-Zimaity HM, et al. Noninvasive versus histologic detection of gastric atrophy in a Hispanic population in North America. Clin Gastroenterol Hepatol 2006;4:306-14.

58. Capelle LG, de Vries AC, Haringsma J, et al. The staging of gastritis with the OLGA system by using intestinal metaplasia as an accurate alternative for atrophic gastritis. Gastrointest Endosc 2010;71:1150-8.

59. Rugge M, de Boni M, Pennelli G, et al. Gastritis OLGA-staging and gastric cancer risk: a twelve-year clinico-pathological follow-up study. Alimentary Pharmacol Ther 2010;31:1104-11.

60. Isajevs S, Liepniece-Karele I, Janciauskas D, et al. Gastritis staging: interobserver agreement by applying OLGA and OLGIM systems. Virchows Arch 2014;464:403-7.

61. Rugge M, Genta RM, Graham DY, et al. Chronicles of a cancer foretold: 35 years of gastric cancer risk assessment. Gut 2016;65:721-5.

62. Dinis-Ribeiro M, Areia M, de Vries AC, et al. Management of precancerous conditions and lesions in the stomach (MAPS): guideline from the European Society of Gastrointestinal Endoscopy (ESGE), European Helicobacter Study Group (EHSG), European Society of Pathology (ESP), and the Sociedade Portuguesa de Endoscopia Digestiva (SPED). Endoscopy 2012;44(1):74-94.

63. Filipe MI, Potet F, Bogomoletz WV, et al. Incomplete sulphomucin-secreting intestinal metaplasia for gastric cancer. Preliminary data from a prospective study from three centres. Gut 1985;26:1319-26.

64. Filipe MI, Jass JR. Intestinal metaplasia subtypes and cancer risk. In: Filipe MI, Jass JR, eds. Gastric carcinoma. Edinburgh: Churchill Livingstone; 1986:87-115.

65. Jass JR. Role of intestinal metaplasia in the histogenesis of gastric carcinoma. J Clin Pathol 1980;33:801-10.

66. Filipe MI, Munoz N, Matko I, et al. Intestinal metaplasia types and the risk of gastric cancer: a cohort study in Slovenia. Int J Cancer 1994;57:324-9.

67. Reis CA, David L, Correa P, et al. Intestinal metaplasia of human stomach displays distinct patterns of mucin (MUC1, MUC2, MUC5AC, and MUC6) expression. Cancer Res 1999;59:1003-7.

68. Rokkas T, Filipe MI, Sladen GE. Detection of an increased incidence of early gastric cancer in patients with intestinal metaplasia type III who are closely followed up. Gut 1991;32:1110-3.

69. Rubio CA, Jonasson J, Nesi G, et al. Extensive intestinal metaplasia in gastric carcinoma and in other lesions requiring surgery: a study of 3,421 gastrectomy specimens from dwellers of the Atlantic and Pacific basins. J Clin Pathol 2005;58:1271-7.

70. de Vries AC, Haringsma J, de Vries RA, et al. The use of clinical, histologic, and serologic parameters to predict the intragastric extent of intestinal metaplasia: a recommendation for routine practice. Gastrointest Endosc 2009;70:18-25.

71. El-Zimaity HM, Ramchatesingh J, Saeed MA, Graham DY. Gastric intestinal metaplasia: subtypes and natural history. J Clin Pathol 2001;54:679-83.

72. Smith JL, Dixon MF. Is subtyping of intestinal metaplasia in the upper gastrointestinal tract a worthwhile exercise? An evaluation of current mucin histochemical stains. Br J Biomed Sci 2003;60:180-6.

73. Kang KP, Lee HS, Kim N, et al. Role of intestinal metaplasia subtyping in the risk of gastric cancer in Korea. J Gastroenterol Hepatol 2009;24:140-8.

74. Kakinoki R, Kushima R, Matsubara A, et al. Re-evaluation of histogenesis of gastric carcinomas: a comparative histopathological study between Helicobacter pylori-negative and H. pylori-positive cases. Dig Dis Sci 2009;54:614-20.

75. Gutierrez-Gonzalez L, Wright NA. Biology of intestinal metaplasia in 2008: more than a simple phenotypic alteration. Dig Liver Dis 2008;40:510-22.

76. Goldenring JR, Nam KT, Wang TC, Mills JC, Wright NA. Spasmolytic polypeptide-expressing metaplasia and intestinal metaplasia: time for reevaluation of metaplasias and the origins of gastric cancer. Gastroenterology 2010;138:2207-10.

77. Armbrecht U, Stockbrugger RW, Rode J, Menon GG, Cotton PB. Development of gastric dysplasia in pernicious anaemia: a clinical and endoscopic follow up study of 80 patients. Gut 1990; 31:1105-9.

78. Mosbech J, Videbaek A. Mortality from and risk of gastric carcinoma among patients with pernicious anaemia. Br Med J 1950;2:390-4.

79. Magnus HA. A re-assessment of the gastric lesion in pernicious anaemia. J Clin Pathol 1958;11:289-95.

80. Coati I, Fassan M, Farinati F, Graham DY, Genta RM, Rugge M. Autoimmune gastritis: pathologist's viewpoint. World J Gastroenterol 2015;21:12179-89.

81. Brinton LA, Gridley G, Hrubec Z, Hoover R, Fraumeni JF Jr. Cancer risk following pernicious anaemia. Br J Cancer 1989;59:810-3.

82. Hsing AW, Hansson LE, McLaughlin JK, et al. Pernicious anemia and subsequent cancer. A population-based cohort study. Cancer 1993;71:745-50.

83. Mellemkjaer L, Gridley G, Moller H, et al. Pernicious anaemia and cancer risk in Denmark. Br J Cancer 1996;73:998-1000.

84. Karlson BM, Ekbom A, Wacholder S, McLaughlin JK, Hsing AW. Cancer of the upper gastrointestinal tract among patients with pernicious anemia: a case-cohort study. Scand J Gastroenterol 2000;35:847-51.

85. Ye W, Nyren O. Risk of cancers of the oesophagus and stomach by histology or subsite in patients hospitalised for pernicious anaemia. Gut 2003;52:938-41.

86. Schafer LW, Larson DE, Melton LJ, 3rd, Higgins JA, Zinsmeister AR. Risk of development of gastric carcinoma in patients with pernicious anemia: a population-based study in Rochester, Minnesota. Mayo Clin Proc 1985;60:444-8.

87. Rugge M, Fassan M, Pizzi M, et al. Autoimmune gastritis: histology phenotype and OLGA staging. Aliment Pharmacol Ther 2012;35(12):1460-6.

88. Stockbrugger RW, Menon GG, Beilby JO, Mason RR, Cotton PB. Gastroscopic screening in 80 patients with pernicious anaemia. Gut 1983;24:1141-7.

89. Park JY, Cornish TC, Lam-Himlin D, Shi C, Montgomery E. Gastric lesions in patients with autoimmune metaplastic atrophic gastritis (AMAG) in a tertiary care setting. Am J Surg Pathol 2010;34:1591-8.

90. Solcia E, Rindi G, Fiocca R, et al. Distinct patterns of chronic gastritis associated with carcinoid and cancer and their role in tumorigenesis. Yale J Biol Med 1992;65(6):793-804; discussion 27-9.

91. Kokkola A, Sjoblom SM, Haapiainen R, Sipponen P, Puolakkainen P, Jarvinen H. The risk of gastric carcinoma and carcinoid tumours in patients with pernicious anaemia. A prospective follow-up study. Scand J Gastroenterol 1998;33:88-92.

92. Bordi C, D'Adda T, Azzoni C, Pilato FP, Caruana P. Hypergastrinemia and gastric enterochromaffin-like cells. Am J Surg Pathol 1995;19(Suppl 1):S8-19.

93. Viste A, Bjornestad E, Opheim P, et al. Risk of carcinoma following gastric operations for benign disease. A historical cohort study of 3,470 patients. Lancet 1986;2:502-5.

94. Offerhaus GJ, Tersmette AC, Huibregtse K, et al. Mortality caused by stomach cancer after remote partial gastrectomy for benign conditions: 40 years of follow up of an Amsterdam cohort of 2,633 postgastrectomy patients. Gut 1988;29:1588-90.

95. Sitarz R, Maciejewski R, Polkowski WP, Offerhaus GJ. Gastroenterostoma after Billroth antrectomy as a premalignant condition. World J Gastroenterol 2012;18:3201-6.

96. Caygill CP, Hill MJ, Hall CN, Kirkham JS, Northfield TC. Increased risk of cancer at multiple sites after gastric surgery for peptic ulcer. Gut 1987;28:924-8.

97. Toftgaard C. Gastric cancer after peptic ulcer surgery. A historic prospective cohort investigation. Ann Surg 1989;210:159-64.

98. Safatle-Ribeiro AV, Ribeiro U Jr, Reynolds JC. Gastric stump cancer: what is the risk? Dig Dis 1998;16:159-68.

99. La Vecchia C, Negri E, D'Avanzo B, Moller H, Franceschi S. Partial gastrectomy and subsequent gastric cancer risk. J Epidemiol Community Health 1992;46:12-4.

100. Tersmette AC, Offerhaus GJ, Tersmette KW, et al. Meta-analysis of the risk of gastric stump cancer: detection of high risk patient subsets for stomach cancer after remote partial gastrectomy for benign conditions. Cancer Res 1990;50:6486-9.

101. Ohira M, Toyokawa T, Sakurai K, et al. Current status in remnant gastric cancer after distal gastrectomy. World J Gastroenterol 2016;22:2424-33.

102. Tanigawa N, Nomura E, Lee SW, et al. Current state of gastric stump carcinoma in Japan: based on the results of a nationwide survey. World J Surg 2010;34:1540-7.

103. Hole DJ, Quigley EM, Gillis CR, Watkinson G. Peptic ulcer and cancer: an examination of the relationship between chronic peptic ulcer and gastric carcinoma. Scand J Gastroenterol 1987;22:17-23.

104. Hansson LE, Nyren O, Hsing AW, et al. The risk of stomach cancer in patients with gastric or duodenal ulcer disease. N Engl J Med 1996;335:242-9.

105. Wu CY, Kuo KN, Wu MS, Chen YJ, Wang CB, Lin JT. Early Helicobacter pylori eradication decreases risk of gastric cancer in patients with peptic ulcer disease. Gastroenterology 2009;137:1641-8.

106. Asaka M, Kimura T, Kato M, et al. Possible role of Helicobacter pylori infection in early gastric cancer development. Cancer 1994;73:2691-4.

107. Plummer M, Franceschi S, Vignat J, Forman D, de Martel C. Global burden of gastric cancer attributable to Helicobacter pylori. Int J Cancer 2015;136:487-90.

108. Møller H, Heseltine E, Vainio H. Working group report on schistosomes, liver flukes and Helicobacter pylori. Int J Cancer 1995;60:587-9.

109. Forman D, Newell DG, Fullerton F, et al. Association between infection with Helicobacter pylori and risk of gastric cancer: evidence from a prospective investigation. BMJ 1991;302:1302-5.

110. Nomura A, Stemmermann GN, Chyou PH, Kato I, Perez-Perez GI, Blaser MJ. Helicobacter pylori infection and gastric carcinoma among Japanese Americans in Hawaii. N Engl J Med 1991;325:1132-6.

111. Parsonnet J, Friedman GD, Vandersteen DP, et al. Helicobacter pylori infection and the risk of gastric carcinoma. N Engl J Med 1991;325:1127-31.

112. Hooi JK, Lai WY, Ng WK, et al. Global prevalence of Helicobacter pylori infection: Systematic review and meta-analysis. Gastroenterology 2017;153:420-9.

113. Helicobacter and Cancer Collaborative Group. Gastric cancer and Helicobacter pylori: a combined analysis of 12 case control studies nested within prospective cohorts. Gut 2001;49:347-53.

114. Gonzalez CA, Megraud F, Buissonniere A, et al. Helicobacter pylori infection assessed by ELISA and by immunoblot and noncardia gastric cancer risk in a prospective study: the Eurgast-EPIC project. Ann Oncol 2012;23:1320-4.

115. Ekstrom AM, Held M, Hansson LE, Engstrand L, Nyren O. Helicobacter pylori in gastric cancer established by CagA immunoblot as a marker of past infection. Gastroenterology 2001;121:784-91.

116. Gonzalez CA, Jakszyn P, Pera G, et al. Meat intake and risk of stomach and esophageal adenocarcinoma within the European Prospective Investigation Into Cancer and Nutrition (EPIC). J Natl Cancer Inst 2006;98:345-54.

117. Watanabe T, Tada M, Nagai H, Sasaki S, Nakao M. Helicobacter pylori infection induces gastric cancer in mongolian gerbils. Gastroenterology 1998;115:642-8.

118. Honda S, Fujioka T, Tokieda M, Satoh R, Nishizono A, Nasu M. Development of Helicobacter pylori-induced gastric carcinoma in Mongolian gerbils. Cancer Res 1998;58:4255-9.

119. Sugiyama A, Maruta F, Ikeno T, et al. Helicobacter pylori infection enhances N-methyl-N-nitrosourea-induced stomach carcinogenesis in the Mongolian gerbil. Cancer Res 1998; 58:2067-9.

120. Shimizu N, Inada K, Nakanishi H, et al. Helicobacter pylori infection enhances glandular stomach carcinogenesis in Mongolian gerbils treated with chemical carcinogens. Carcinogenesis 1999;20:669-76.

121. Ford AC, Forman D, Hunt R, Yuan Y, Moayyedi P. Helicobacter pylori eradication for the prevention of gastric neoplasia. Cochrane Database Syst Re 2015:Cd005583.

122. Uemura N, Okamoto S, Yamamoto S, et al. Helicobacter pylori infection and the development of gastric cancer. N Engl J Med 2001;345:784-9.

123. Figueiredo C, Machado JC, Pharoah P, et al. Helicobacter pylori and interleukin 1 genotyping: an opportunity to identify high-risk individuals for gastric carcinoma. J Natl Cancer Inst 2002;94:1680-7.

124. Ferreira RM, Machado JC, Figueiredo C. Clinical relevance of Helicobacter pylori vacA and cagA genotypes in gastric carcinoma. Best Pract Res Clin Gastroenterol 2014;28:1003-15.

125. Plummer M, van Doorn LJ, Franceschi S, et al. Helicobacter pylori cytotoxin-associated genotype and gastric precancerous lesions. J Natl Cancer Inst 2007;99:1328-34.

126. Gonzalez CA, Figueiredo C, Lic CB, et al. Helicobacter pylori cagA and vacA genotypes as predictors of progression of gastric preneoplastic lesions: a long-term follow-up in a high-risk area in Spain. The Am J Gastroenterol 2011;106:867-74.

127. Basso D, Zambon CF, Letley DP, et al. Clinical relevance of Helicobacter pylori cagA and vacA gene polymorphisms. Gastroenterology 2008;135:91-9.

128. Batista SA, Rocha GA, Rocha AM, et al. Higher number of Helicobacter pylori CagA EPIYA C phosphorylation sites increases the risk of gastric cancer, but not duodenal ulcer. BMC Microbiol 2011;11:61.

129. Ferreira RM, Machado JC, Leite M, Carneiro F, Figueiredo C. The number of Helicobacter pylori CagA EPIYA C tyrosine phosphorylation motifs influences the pattern of gastritis and the development of gastric carcinoma. Histopathology 2012;60:992-8.

130. Ferreira RM, Pinto-Ribeiro I, Wen X, et al. Helicobacter pylori cagA promoter region sequences influence cagA expression and interleukin 8 secretion. The J Infect Dis 2016;213:669-73.

131. Loh JT, Shaffer CL, Piazuelo MB, et al. Analysis of cagA in Helicobacter pylori strains from Colombian populations with contrasting gastric cancer risk reveals a biomarker for disease severity. Cancer Epidemiol Biomarkers Prev 2011;20:2237-49.

132. Atherton JC, Cao P, Peek RM Jr, Tummuru MK, Blaser MJ, Cover TL. Mosaicism in vacuolating cytotoxin alleles of Helicobacter pylori. Association of specific vacA types with cytotoxin production and peptic ulceration. J Biol Chem 1995;270:17771-7.

133. Rhead JL, Letley DP, Mohammadi M, et al. A new Helicobacter pylori vacuolating cytotoxin determinant, the intermediate region, is associated with gastric cancer. Gastroenterology 2007;133:926-36.

134. Ferreira RM, Machado JC, Letley D, et al. A novel method for genotyping the Helicobacter pylori vacA intermediate region directly in gastric biopsy specimens. J Clin Microbiol 2012;50:3983-9.

135. Nogueira C, Figueiredo C, Carneiro F, et al. Helicobacter pylori genotypes may determine gastric histopathology. Am J Pathol 2001;158:647-54.

136. Pinto-Ribeiro I, Ferreira RM, Batalha S, et al. Helicobacter pylori vacA genotypes in chronic gastritis and gastric carcinoma patients from Macau, China. Toxins (Basel) 2016;8:pii.

137. Amieva M, Peek RM Jr. Pathobiology of Helicobacter pylori-induced gastric cancer. Gastroenterology 2016;150:64-78.

138. Wroblewski LE, Peek RM Jr. Helicobacter pylori, cancer, and the gastric microbiota. Adv Exp Med Biol 2016;908:393-408.

139. Wroblewski LE, Peek RM Jr, Coburn LA. The role of the microbiome in gastrointestinal cancer. Gastroenterol Clin North Am 2016;45:543-56.

140. Plottel CS, Blaser MJ. Microbiome and malignancy. Cell Host Microbe 2011;10:324-35.

141. Graham DY. Helicobacter pylori update: gastric cancer, reliable therapy, and possible benefits. Gastroenterology 2015;148:719-31.e3.

142. El-Omar EM, Carrington M, Chow WH, et al. The role of interleukin-1 polymorphisms in the pathogenesis of gastric cancer. Nature 2001;412:99.

143. El-Omar EM, Rabkin CS, Gammon MD, et al. Increased risk of noncardia gastric cancer associated with proinflammatory cytokine gene polymorphisms. Gastroenterology 2003;124:1193-201.

144. Machado JC, Pharoah P, Sousa S, et al. Interleukin 1B and interleukin 1RN polymorphisms are associated with increased risk of gastric carcinoma. Gastroenterology 2001;121:823-9.

145. Machado JC, Figueiredo C, Canedo P, et al. A proinflammatory genetic profile increases the risk for chronic atrophic gastritis and gastric carcinoma. Gastroenterology 2003;125:364-71.

146. El-Omar EM, Carrington M, Chow WH, et al. Interleukin-1 polymorphisms associated with increased risk of gastric cancer. Nature 2000;404:398-402.

147. Bessede E, Dubus P, Megraud F, Varon C. Helicobacter pylori infection and stem cells at the origin of gastric cancer. Oncogene. 2015; 34:2547-55.

148. Houghton J, Stoicov C, Nomura S, et al. Gastric cancer originating from bone marrow-derived cells. Science 2004;306:1568-71.

149. Correa P, Houghton J. Carcinogenesis of Helicobacter pylori. Gastroenterology 2007;133:659-72.

150. Eguchi H, Herschenhous N, Kuzushita N, Moss SF. Helicobacter pylori increases proteasome-mediated degradation of p27(kip1) in gastric epithelial cells. Cancer Res 2003;63:4739-46.

151. Franco AT, Israel DA, Washington MK, et al. Activation of beta-catenin by carcinogenic Helicobacter pylori. Proc Natl Acad Sci U S A 2005;102:10646-51.

152. Wei J, O'Brien D, Vilgelm A, et al. Interaction of Helicobacter pylori with gastric epithelial cells is mediated by the p53 protein family. Gastroenterology 2008;134:1412-23.

153. Tsugane S, Sasazuki S. Diet and the risk of gastric cancer: review of epidemiological evidence. Gastric Cancer 2007;10:75-83.

154. Epplein M, Nomura AM, Hankin JH, et al. Association of Helicobacter pylori infection and diet on the risk of gastric cancer: a case-control study in Hawaii. Cancer Causes Control 2008;19:869-77.

155. Kim HJ, Lim SY, Lee JS, et al. Fresh and pickled vegetable consumption and gastric cancer in Japanese and Korean populations: a meta-analysis of observational studies. Cancer Sci 2010;101:508-16.

156. Ren JS, Kamangar F, Forman D, Islami F. Pickled food and risk of gastric cancer—a systematic review and meta-analysis of English and Chinese literature. Cancer Epidemiol Biomarkers Prev 2012;21:905-15.

157. Lee SA, Kang D, Shim KN, Choe JW, Hong WS, Choi H. Effect of diet and Helicobacter pylori infection to the risk of early gastric cancer. J Epidemiol 2003;13:162-8.

158. Wang T, Cai H, Sasazuki S, et al. Fruit and vegetable consumption, Helicobacter pylori antibodies, and gastric cancer risk: a pooled analysis of prospective studies in China, Japan, and Korea. Int J Cancer 2017;140:591-9.

159. Raei N, Behrouz B, Zahri S, Latifi-Navid S. Helicobacter pylori infection and dietary factors act synergistically to promote gastric cancer. Asian Pac J Cancer Prev 2016;17:917-21.

160. Fang X, Wei J, He X, et al. Landscape of dietary factors associated with risk of gastric cancer: a systematic review and dose-response meta-analysis of prospective cohort studies. Eur J Cancer 2015;51:2820-32.

161. Noto JM, Gaddy JA, Lee JY, et al. Iron deficiency accelerates Helicobacter pylori-induced carcinogenesis in rodents and humans. J Clin Invest 2013;123:479-92.

162. Shikata K, Kiyohara Y, Kubo M, et al. A prospective study of dietary salt intake and gastric cancer incidence in a defined Japanese population: the Hisayama study. Int J Cancer 2006; 119:196-201.

163. Buckland G, Agudo A, Lujan L, et al. Adherence to a Mediterranean diet and risk of gastric adenocarcinoma within the European prospective investigation into cancer and nutrition cohort study. Am J Clin Nutr 2010;91:381-90.

164. Gonzalez CA, Lujan-Barroso L, Bueno-de-Mesquita HB, et al. Fruit and vegetable intake and the risk of gastric adenocarcinoma: a reanalysis of the European Prospective Investigation into Cancer and Nutrition (EPIC-EURGAST) study after a longer follow-up. Int J Cancer 2012;131:2910-9.

165. Gonzalez CA, Pera G, Agudo A, et al. Fruit and vegetable intake and the risk of stomach and oesophagus adenocarcinoma in the European Prospective Investigation into Cancer and Nutrition (EPIC-EURGAST). Int J Cancer 2006;118per:2559-66.

166. M A M, Pera G, Agudo A, et al. Cereal fiber intake may reduce risk of gastric adenocarcinomas: the EPIC-EURGAST study. Int J Cancer 2007;121:1618-23.

167. Gonzalez CA, Pera G, Agudo A, et al. Smoking and the risk of gastric cancer in the European Prospective Investigation Into Cancer and Nutrition (EPIC). Int J Cancer 2003;107:629-34.

168. IARC Working Group on the Evaluation of the Carcinogenic Risks to Humans, World Health Organization, IARC. Tobacco Smoke and Involuntary Smoking IARC monographs on the evaluation of carcinogenic risks to humans, vol. 83. Lyon: IARC Press; 2004.

169. Brenner H, Arndt V, Bode G, Stegmaier C, Ziegler H, Stumer T. Risk of gastric cancer among smokers infected with Helicobacter pylori. Int J Cancer 2002;98:446-9.

170. Siman JH, Forsgren A, Berglund G, Floren CH. Tobacco smoking increases the risk for gastric adenocarcinoma among Helicobacter pylori-infected individuals. Scand J Gastroenterol 2001;36:208-13.

171. Zaridze D, Borisova E, Maximovitch D, Chkhikvadze V. Alcohol consumption, smoking and risk of gastric cancer: case-control study from Moscow, Russia. Cancer Causes Control 2000;11:363-71.

172. La Vecchia C, Negri E, Franceschi S, Gentile A. Family history and the risk of stomach and colorectal cancer. Cancer 1992;70:50-5.

173. El-Omar EM. The importance of interleukin 1beta in Helicobacter pylori associated disease. Gut 2001;48:743-7.

174. Saadat M. Genetic polymorphisms of glutathione S-transferase T1 (GSTT1) and susceptibility to gastric cancer: a meta-analysis. Cancer Sci 2006;97:505-9.

175. Wideroff L, Vaughan TL, Farin FM, et al. GST, NAT1, CYP1A1 polymorphisms and risk of esophageal and gastric adenocarcinomas. Cancer Detect Prev 2007;31:233-6.

176. Palli D, Galli M, Caporaso NE, et al. Family history and risk of stomach cancer in Italy. Cancer Epidemiol Biomarkers Prev 1994;3:15-8.

177. Fitzgerald RC, Caldas C. Familial gastric cancer—clinical management. Best Pract Res Clin Gastroenterol 2006;20:735-43.

178. Oliveira C, Seruca R, Carneiro F. Hereditary gastric cancer. Best Pract Res Clin Gastroenterol 2009;23:147-57.

179. Maconi G, Manes G, Porro GB. Role of symptoms in diagnosis and outcome of gastric cancer. World J Gastroenterol 2008;14:1149-55.

180. Lordick F, Allum W, Carneiro F, et al. Unmet needs and challenges in gastric cancer: the way forward. Cancer Treat Rev 2014;40:692-700.

181. Ajani JA, Lee J, Sano T, Janjigian YY, Fan D, Song S. Gastric adenocarcinoma. Nat Rev Dis Primers 2017;3:17036.

182. Japanese Gastric Cancer Assocociation. Japanese classification of gastric carcinoma: 3rd English edition. Gastric Cancer 2011;14:101-12.

183. Lewin KJ, Appelman HD. Carcinoma of the stomach. In: Lewin KJ, Appelman HD, eds. Tumors of the esophagus and stomach. AFIP Atlas of Tumor Pathology, 3rd Series, Fascicle 18. Washington, D.C.: American Registry of Pathology; 1996:245-330.

184. Gotoda T. Endoscopic resection of early gastric cancer. Gastric Cancer 2007;10:1-11.

185. Ming SC, Hirota T. Malignant epithelial tumors of the stomach. In: Ming SC, Goldman H, eds. Pathology of the gastrointestinal tract, 2nd ed. Baltimore: Williams & Wilkins; 1998.

186. Sobin LH, Gospodarowicz MK, Wittekind C, eds. TNM classification of malignant tumours. West Sussex: Wiley-Blackwell, 2010.

187. Edge SB, Byrd DR, Compton CC, Fritz AG, Greene FL, Trotti A, eds. AJCC cancer staging manual. New York: Springer, 2010.

188. Oohara T, Tohma H, Takezoe K, et al. Minute gastric cancers less than 5 mm in diameter. Cancer 1982;50:801-10.

189. Kodama Y, Inokuchi K, Soejima K, Matsusaka T, Okamura T. Growth patterns and prognosis in early gastric carcinoma. Superficially spreading and penetrating growth types. Cancer 1983;51:320-6.

190. The Paris endoscopic classification of superficial neoplastic lesions: esophagus, stomach, and colon: November 30 to December 1, 2002. Gastrointest Endosc 2003;58(6 Suppl):S3-43.

191. Borrmann R. Geshwulste des Magens und Duodenums. In: Henke F, Lubarsch O, eds. Handbuch der speziellen pathologischen Anatomie und Histologie. Berlin: Springer-Verlag; 1926:865.

192. Dekker W, Tytgat GN. Diagnostic accuracy of fiberendoscopy in the detection of upper intestinal malignancy. A follow-up analysis. Gastroenterology 1977;73(Pt 1):710-4.

193. Lauwers GY, Carneiro F, Graham DY, et al. Gastric carcinoma. In: Bosman FT, Carneiro F, Hruban RH, Theise ND, eds. WHO classification of tumours of the digestive system, 4th ed. Lyon: IARC Press; 2010:48-58.

194. Endoh Y, Tamura G, Motoyama T, Ajioka Y, Watanabe H. Well-differentiated adenocarcinoma mimicking complete-type intestinal metaplasia in the stomach. Hum Pathol 1999;30:826-32.

195. Yao T, Utsunomiya T, Oya M, Nishiyama K, Tsuneyoshi M. Extremely well-differentiated adenocarcinoma of the stomach: clinicopathological and immunohistochemical features. World J Gastroenterol 2006;12:2510-6.

196. Lee WA. Gastric extremely well differentiated adenocarcinoma of gastric phenotype: as a gastric counterpart of adenoma malignum of the uterine cervix. World J Surg Oncol 2005;3:28.

197. Joo M, Han SH. Gastric-type extremely well-differentiated adenocarcinoma of the stomach: a challenge for preoperative diagnosis. J Pathol Transl Med 2016;50:71-4.

198. Ushiku T, Arnason T, Ban S, et al. Very well-differentiated gastric carcinoma of intestinal type: analysis of diagnostic criteria. Mod Pathol 2013;26:1620-31.

199. Wang HH, Antonioli DA, Goldman H. Comparative features of esophageal and gastric adenocarcinomas: recent changes in type and frequency. Hum Pathol 1986;17:482-7.

200. Gupta R, Arora R, Das P, Singh MK. Deeply eosinophilic cell variant of signet-ring type of gastric carcinoma: a diagnostic dilemma. Int J Clin Oncol 2008;13:181-4.

201. Carvalho B, Buffart TE, Reis RM, et al. Mixed gastric carcinomas show similar chromosomal aberrations in both their diffuse and glandular components. Cell Oncol 2006;28:283-94.

202. Zheng HC, Li XH, Hara T, et al. Mixed-type gastric carcinomas exhibit more aggressive features and indicate the histogenesis of carcinomas. Virchows Arch 2008;452:525-34.

203. Machado JC, Soares P, Carneiro F, et al. E-cadherin gene mutations provide a genetic basis for the phenotypic divergence of mixed gastric carcinomas. Lab Invest 1999;79:459-65.

204. Park SY, Kook MC, Kim YW, Cho NY, Kim TY, Kang GH. Mixed-type gastric cancer and its association with high-frequency CpG island hypermethylation. Virchows Arch 2010;456:625-33.

205. Lauren P. The two histological main types of gastric carcinoma: diffuse and so-called intestinal-type carcinoma. An attempt at a histo-clinical classification. Acta Pathol Microbiol Scand 1965;64:31-49.

206. Nakamura K, Sugano H, Takagi K. Carcinoma of the stomach in incipient phase: its histogenesis and histological appearances. Gan 1968;59:251-8.

207. Mulligan RM. Histogenesis and biologic behavior of gastric carcinoma. Pathol Annu 1972;7:349-415.

208. Ming SC. Gastric carcinoma. A pathobiological classification. Cancer 1977;39:2475-85.

209. Goseki N, Takizawa T, Koike M. Differences in the mode of the extension of gastric cancer classified by histological type: new histological classification of gastric carcinoma. Gut 1992;33:606-12.

210. Martin IG, Dixon MF, Sue-Ling H, Axon AT, Johnston D. Goseki histological grading of gastric cancer is an important predictor of outcome. Gut 1994;35:758-63.

211. Chiaravalli AM, Klersy C, Vanoli A, Ferretti A, Capella C, Solcia E. Histotype-based prognostic classification of gastric cancer. World J Gastroenterol 2012;18:896-904.

212. Solcia E, Klersy C, Mastracci L, et al. A combined histologic and molecular approach identifies three groups of gastric cancer with different prognosis. Virchows Arch 2009;455:197-211.

213. Carneiro F. Classification of gastric carcinoma. Curr Diag Pathol. 1997;4:5.

214. Carneiro F, Seixas M, Sobrinho-Simoes M. New elements for an updated classification of the carcinomas of the stomach. Pathol Res Practice 1995;191:571-84.

215. Stelzner S, Emmrich P. The mixed type in Lauren's classification of gastric carcinoma. Histologic description and biologic behavior. Gen Diagn Pathol 1997;143:39-48.

216. Miyamae M, Komatsu S, Ichikawa D, et al. Histological mixed-type as an independent risk factor for nodal metastasis in submucosal gastric cancer. Tumour Biol 2016;37:709-14.

217. Fiocca R, Villani L, Tenti P, et al. Characterization of four main cell types in gastric cancer: foveolar, mucopeptic, intestinal columnar and goblet cells. An histopathologic, histochemical and ultrastructural study of "early" and "advanced" tumours. Pathol Res Pract 1987;182:308-25.

218. Machado JC, Carneiro F, Ribeiro P, Blin N, Sobrinho-Simoes M. pS2 protein expression in gastric carcinoma. An immunohistochemical and immunoradiometric study. Eur J Cancer 1996;32A:1585-90.

219. Machado JC, Nogueira AM, Carneiro F, Reis CA, Sobrinho-Simoes M. Gastric carcinoma exhibits distinct types of cell differentiation: an immunohistochemical study of trefoil peptides (TFF1 and TFF2) and mucins (MUC1, MUC2, MUC5AC, and MUC6). J Pathol 2000;190:437-43.

220. Kushima R, Vieth M, Borchard F, Stolte M, Mukaisho K, Hattori T. Gastric-type well-differentiated adenocarcinoma and pyloric gland adenoma of the stomach. Gastric Cancer 2006;9:177-84.

221. Kim DH, Shin N, Kim GH, et al. Mucin expression in gastric cancer: reappraisal of its clinicopathologic and prognostic significance. Arch Pathol Lab Med 2013;137:1047-53.

222. Park DY, Srivastava A, Kim GH, et al. Adenomatous and foveolar gastric dysplasia: distinct patterns of mucin expression and background intestinal metaplasia. Am J Surg Pathol 2008;32:524-33.

223. Kushima R, Hattori T. Histogenesis and characteristics of gastric-type adenocarcinomas in the stomach. J Cancer Res Clin Oncol 1993;120:103-11.

224. Tsukashita S, Kushima R, Bamba M, Sugihara H, Hattori T. MUC gene expression and histogenesis of adenocarcinoma of the stomach. Int J Cancer 2001;94:166-70.

225. Shiroshita H, Watanabe H, Ajioka Y, Watanabe G, Nishikura K, Kitano S. Re-evaluation of mucin phenotypes of gastric minute well-differentiated-type adenocarcinomas using a series of HGM, MUC5AC, MUC6, M-GGMC, MUC2 and CD10 stains. Pathol Int 2004;54:311-21.

226. Wakatsuki K, Yamada Y, Narikiyo M, et al. Clinicopathological and prognostic significance of mucin phenotype in gastric cancer. J Surg Oncol 2008;98:124-9.

227. Lee OJ, Kim HJ, Kim JR, Watanabe H. The prognostic significance of the mucin phenotype of gastric adenocarcinoma and its relationship with histologic classifications. Oncol Rep 2009;21:387-93.

228. Han HS, Lee SY, Lee KY, et al. Unclassified mucin phenotype of gastric adenocarcinoma exhibits the highest invasiveness. J Gastroenterol Hepatol 2009;24:658-66.

229. Zhang CT, He KC, Pan F, Li Y, Wu J. Prognostic value of Muc5AC in gastric cancer: A meta-analysis. World J Gastroenterol 2015;21:10453-60.

230. Kim SM, Kwon CH, Shin N, et al. Decreased Muc5AC expression is associated with poor prognosis in gastric cancer. Int J Cancer 2014;134:114-24.

231. Oue N, Sentani K, Sakamoto N, Yasui W. Clinicopathologic and molecular characteristics of gastric cancer showing gastric and intestinal mucin phenotype. Cancer Sci 2015;106:951-8.

232. Everett SM, Axon AT. Early gastric cancer in Europe. Gut 1997;41:142-50.

233. Xuan ZX, Ueyama T, Yao T, Tsuneyoshi M. Time trends of early gastric carcinoma. A clinicopathologic analysis of 2846 cases. Cancer 1993;72:2889-94.

234. Yamashina M. A variant of early gastric carcinoma. Histologic and histochemical studies of early signet ring cell carcinomas discovered beneath preserved surface epithelium. Cancer 1986;58:1333-9.

235. Arnason T, Lauwers GY. Extruded highly proliferative benign mucous neck cells: a peculiar histologic mimic of poorly cohesive gastric carcinoma. Int J Surg Pathol 2014;22:623-8.

236. Wu ML, Natarajan S, Lewin KJ. Peculiar artifacts mimicking carcinoma. Arch Pathol Lab Med 2001;125:1173 6.

237. Johansen A. Elevated early gastric carcinoma. Differential diagnosis as regards adenomatous polyps. Pathol Res Pract 1979;164:316-30.

238. Yasuda K, Shiraishi N, Suematsu T, Yamaguchi K, Adachi Y, Kitano S. Rate of detection of lymph node metastasis is correlated with the depth of submucosal invasion in early stage gastric carcinoma. Cancer 1999;85:2119-23.

239. Fukutomi H, Sakita T. Analysis of early gastric cancer cases collected from major hospitals and institutes in Japan. Jpn J Clin Oncol 1984;14:169-79.

240. Gotoda T, Yanagisawa A, Sasako M, et al. Incidence of lymph node metastasis from early gastric cancer: estimation with a large number of cases at two large centers. Gastric Cancer 2000;3:219-25.

241. Kurihara N, Kubota T, Otani Y, et al. Lymph node metastasis of early gastric cancer with submucosal invasion. Br J Surg 1998;85:835-9.

242. Ishigami S, Hokita S, Natsugoe S, et al. Carcinomatous infiltration into the submucosa as a predictor of lymph node involvement in early gastric cancer. World J Surg 1998;22:1056-9; discussion 1059-60.

243. Sekine S, Yoshida H, Jansen M, Kushima R. The Japanese viewpoint on the histopathology of early gastric cancer. Adv Exp Med Biol 2016;908:331-46.

244. Arigami T, Natsugoe S, Uenosono Y, et al. Lymphatic invasion using D2-40 monoclonal antibody and its relationship to lymph node micrometastasis in pN0 gastric cancer. Br J Cancer 2005;93:688-93.

245. Hanahan D, Weinberg RA. The hallmarks of cancer. Cell 2000;100:57-70.

246. Hanahan D, Weinberg RA. Hallmarks of cancer: the next generation. Cell 2011;144:646-74.

247. Tan IB, Ivanova T, Lim KH, et al. Intrinsic subtypes of gastric cancer, based on gene expression pattern, predict survival and respond differently to chemotherapy. Gastroenterology 2011;141:476-85, 85.e1-11.

248. Lei Z, Tan IB, Das K, et al. Identification of molecular subtypes of gastric cancer with different responses to PI3-kinase inhibitors and 5-fluorouracil. Gastroenterology 2013;145:554-65.

249. Cancer Genome Atlas Research Network. Comprehensive molecular characterization of gastric adenocarcinoma. Nature 2014;513:202-9.

250. Cristescu R, Lee J, Nebozhyn M, et al. Molecular analysis of gastric cancer identifies subtypes associated with distinct clinical outcomes. Nat Med 2015;21:449-56.

251. Gullo I, Carneiro F, Oliveira C, Almeida GM. Heterogeneity in gastric cancer: from pure morphology to molecular classifications. Pathobiology 2017. [Epub ahead of print]

252. Lee YS, Cho YS, Lee GK, et al. Genomic profile analysis of diffuse-type gastric cancers. Genome Biol 2014;15:R55.

253. Kakiuchi M, Nishizawa T, Ueda H, et al. Recurrent gain-of-function mutations of RHOA in diffuse-type gastric carcinoma. Nat Genet 2014;46:583-7.

254. Deng N, Goh LK, Wang H, et al. A comprehensive survey of genomic alterations in gastric cancer reveals systematic patterns of molecular exclusivity and co-occurrence among distinct therapeutic targets. Gut 2012;61:673-84.

255. Mafficini A, Amato E, Fassan M, et al. Reporting tumor molecular heterogeneity in histopathological diagnosis. PloS One 2014;9:e104979.

256. Das K, Chan XB, Epstein D, et al. NanoString expression profiling identifies candidate biomarkers of RAD001 response in metastatic gastric cancer. ESMO Open. 2016;1:e000009.

257. Setia N, Agoston AT, Han HS, et al. A protein and mRNA expression-based classification of gastric cancer. Mod Pathol 2016;29:772-84.

258. Ahn S, Lee SJ, Kim Y, et al. High-throughput protein and mRNA expression-based classification of gastric cancers can identify clinically distinct subtypes, concordant with recent molecular classifications. Am J Surg Pathol 2017;41:106-15.

259. Nakatsuru S, Yanagisawa A, Ichii S, et al. Somatic mutation of the APC gene in gastric cancer: frequent mutations in very well differentiated adenocarcinoma and signet-ring cell carcinoma. Hum Mol Genet 1992;1:559-63.

260. Tamura G, Maesawa C, Suzuki Y, et al. Mutations of the APC gene occur during early stages of gastric adenoma development. Cancer Res 1994;54:1149-51.

261. Seruca R, David L, Castedo S, Veiga I, Borresen AL, Sobrinho-Simoes M. p53 alterations in gastric carcinoma: a study of 56 primary tumors and 204 nodal metastases. Cancer Genet Cytogenet 1994;75:45-50.

262. Lee JH, Abraham SC, Kim HS, et al. Inverse relationship between APC gene mutation in gastric adenomas and development of adenocarcinoma. Am J Pathol 2002;161:611-8.

263. Nishizuka S, Tamura G, Terashima M, Satodate R. Loss of heterozygosity during the development and progression of differentiated adenocarcinoma of the stomach. J Pathol 1998;185:38-43.

264. Uchino S, Tsuda H, Noguchi M, et al. Frequent loss of heterozygosity at the DCC locus in gastric cancer. Cancer Res 1992;52:3099-102.

265. Becker KF, Atkinson MJ, Reich U, et al. E-cadherin gene mutations provide clues to diffuse type gastric carcinomas. Cancer Res 1994;54:3845-52.

266. Jawhari A, Jordan S, Poole S, Browne P, Pignatelli M, Farthing MJ. Abnormal immunoreactivity of the E-cadherin-catenin complex in gastric carcinoma: relationship with patient survival. Gastroenterology 1997;112:46-54.

267. Machado JC, Carneiro F, Beck S, et al. E-cadherin expression is correlated with the isolated cell diffuse histotype and with features of biological aggressiveness of gastric carcinoma. Int J Surg Pathol 1998;6:135-44.

268. Ascano JJ, Frierson H Jr, Moskaluk CA, et al. Inactivation of the E-cadherin gene in sporadic diffuse-type gastric cancer. Mod Pathol 2001;14:942-9.

269. Machado JC, Oliveira C, Carvalho R, et al. E-cadherin gene (CDH1) promoter methylation as the second hit in sporadic diffuse gastric carcinoma. Oncogene 2001;20:1525-8.

270. Chan AO. E-cadherin in gastric cancer. World J Gastroenterol 2006;12:199-203.

271. Feakins RM, Nickols CD, Bidd H, Walton SJ. Abnormal expression of pRb, p16, and cyclin D1 in gastric adenocarcinoma and its lymph node metastases: relationship with pathological features and survival. Hum Pathol 2003;34:1276-82.

272. Li YL, Tian Z, Wu DY, Fu BY, Xin Y. Loss of heterozygosity on 10q23.3 and mutation of tumor suppressor gene PTEN in gastric cancer and precancerous lesions. World J Gastroenterol 2005;11:285-8.

273. Kakeji Y, Korenaga D, Tsujitani S, et al. Gastric cancer with p53 overexpression has high potential for metastasising to lymph nodes. Br J Cancer 1993;67:589-93.

274. Yonemura Y, Fushida S, Tsugawa K. Correlation of p53 expression and proliferative activity in gastric cancer. Anal Cell Pathol 1993;5:277-88.

275. Ikeguchi M, Saito H, Kondo A, Tsujitani S, Maeta M, Kaibara N. Mutated p53 protein expression and proliferative activity in advanced gastric cancer. Hepatogastroenterology 1999;46:2648-53.

276. Ayhan A, Yasui W, Yokozaki H, Seto M, Ueda R, Tahara E. Loss of heterozygosity at the bcl-2 gene locus and expression of bcl-2 in human gastric and colorectal carcinomas. Jpn J Cancer Res 1994;85:584-91.

277. Lee HK, Lee HS, Yang HK, et al. Prognostic significance of Bcl-2 and p53 expression in gastric cancer. Int J Colorectal Dis 2003;18:518-25.

278. Hattori Y, Odagiri H, Nakatani H, et al. K sam, an amplified gene in stomach cancer, is a member of the heparin-binding growth factor receptor genes. Proc Natl Acad Sci U S A 1990;87:5983-7.

279. Smith MG, Hold GL, Tahara E, El-Omar EM. Cellular and molecular aspects of gastric cancer. World J Gastroenterol 2006;12:2979-90.

280. Wang L, Zhang F, Wu PP, Jiang XC, Zheng L, Yu YY. Disordered beta-catenin expression and E-cadherin/CDH1 promoter methylation in gastric carcinoma. World J Gastroenterol 2006; 12:4228-31.

281. Kuniyasu H, Yasui W, Kitadai Y, Yokozaki H, Ito H, Tahara E. Frequent amplification of the c-met gene in scirrhous type stomach cancer. Biochem Biophys Res Commun 1992;189:227-32.

282. Kozma L, Kiss I, Hajdu J, Szentkereszty Z, Szakall S, Ember I. C-myc amplification and cluster analysis in human gastric carcinoma. Anticancer Res 2001;21:707-10.

283. Calcagno DQ, Leal MF, Seabra AD, et al. Interrelationship between chromosome 8 aneuploidy, C-MYC amplification and increased expression in individuals from northern Brazil with gastric adenocarcinoma. World J Gastroenterol 2006;12:6207-11.

284. Yasui W, Kudo Y, Semba S, Yokozaki H, Tahara E. Reduced expression of cyclin-dependent kinase inhibitor p27Kip1 is associated with advanced stage and invasiveness of gastric carcinomas. Jpn J Cancer Res 1997;88:625-9.

285. Xiangming C, Natsugoe S, Takao S, et al. The cooperative role of p27 with cyclin E in the prognosis of advanced gastric carcinoma. Cancer 2000;89:1214-9.

286. Kim DH, Lee HI, Nam ES, et al. Reduced expression of the cell-cycle inhibitor p27Kip1 is associated with progression and lymph node metastasis of gastric carcinoma. Histopathology 2000;36:245-51.

287. Akama Y, Yasui W, Yokozaki H, et al. Frequent amplification of the cyclin E gene in human gastric carcinomas. Jpn J Cancer Res 1995;86:617-21.

288. Brennetot C, Duval A, Hamelin R, et al. Frequent Ki-ras mutations in gastric tumors of the MSI phenotype. Gastroenterology 2003;125:1282.

289. Kim IJ, Park JH, Kang HC, et al. Mutational analysis of BRAF and K-ras in gastric cancers: absence of BRAF mutations in gastric cancers. Hum Genet 2003;114:118-20.

290. Oliveira C, Pinto M, Duval A, et al. BRAF mutations characterize colon but not gastric cancer with mismatch repair deficiency. Oncogene 2003;22:9192-6.

291. Wu M, Semba S, Oue N, Ikehara N, Yasui W, Yokozaki H. BRAF/K-ras mutation, microsatellite instability, and promoter hypermethylation of hMLH1/MGMT in human gastric carcinomas. Gastric Cancer 2004;7:246-53.

292. Oda N, Tsujino T, Tsuda T, et al. DNA ploidy pattern and amplification of ERBB and ERBB2 genes in human gastric carcinomas. Virchows Arch B Cell Pathol Incl Mol Pathol 1990;58:273-7.

293. Varis A, Zaika A, Puolakkainen P, et al. Coamplified and overexpressed genes at ERBB2 locus in gastric cancer. Int J Cancer 2004;109:548-53.

294. Barros-Silva JD, Leitao D, Afonso L, et al. Association of ERBB2 gene status with histopathological parameters and disease-specific survival in gastric carcinoma patients. Br J Cancer 2009;100:487-93.

295. Ruschoff J, Dietel M, Baretton G, et al. HER2 diagnostics in gastric cancer-guideline validation and development of standardized immunohistochemical testing. Virchows Arch 2010;457:299-307.

296. Bang YJ, Van Cutsem E, Feyereislova A, et al. Trastuzumab in combination with chemotherapy versus chemotherapy alone for treatment of HER2-positive advanced gastric or gastro-oesophageal junction cancer (ToGA): a phase 3, open-label, randomised controlled trial. Lancet 2010;376:687-97.

297. EMEA, European Medicines Agency (2009): Opinion. http://www.emea.europa.eu/pdfs/human/opinion/Herceptin_82246709en.pdf.

298. Albarello L, Pecciarini L, Doglioni C. HER2 testing in gastric cancer. Adv Anat Pathol 2011;18:53-9.

299. Bartley AN, Washington MK, Ventura CB, et al. HER2 testing and clinical decision making in gastroesophageal adenocarcinoma: guideline from the College of American Pathologists, American Society for Clinical Pathology, and American Society of Clinical Oncology. Arch Pathol Lab Med 2016;140:1345-63.

300. Gullo I, Grillo F, Molinaro L, et al. Minimum biopsy set for HER2 evaluation in gastric and gastro-esophageal junction cancer. Endosc Int Open 2015;3:E165-70.

301. Grillo F, Fassan M, Sarocchi F, Fiocca R, Mastracci L. HER2 heterogeneity in gastric/gastro-esophageal cancers: from benchside to practice. World J Gastroenterol 2016;22:5879-87.
302. Padmanabhan N, Ushijima T, Tan P. How to stomach an epigenetic insult: the gastric cancer epigenome. Nat Rev Gastroenterol Hepatol 2017;14:467-78.
303. Qamra A, Xing M, Padmanabhan N, et al. Epigenomic promoter alterations amplify gene isoform and immunogenic diversity in gastric adenocarcinoma. Cancer Discov 2017;7:630-51.
304. Zinninger MM, Collins WT. Extension of carcinoma of the stomach into the duodenum and esophagus. Ann Surg 1949;130:557-66.
305. Fernet P, Azar HA, Stout AP. Intramural (tubal) spread of linitis plastica along the alimentary tract. Gastroenterology 1965;48:419-24.
306. Maruyama K, Gunven P, Okabayashi K, Sasako M, Kinoshita T. Lymph node metastases of gastric cancer. General pattern in 1931 patients. Ann Surg 1989;210:596-602.
307. Ahn HS, Lee HJ, Hahn S, et al. Evaluation of the Seventh American Joint Committee on Cancer/International Union Against Cancer Classification of gastric adenocarcinoma in comparison with the sixth classification. Cancer 2010;116:5592-8.
308. Maduekwe UN, Lauwers GY, Fernandez-Del-Castillo C, et al. New metastatic lymph node ratio system reduces stage migration in patients undergoing D1 lymphadenectomy for gastric adenocarcinoma. Ann Surg Oncol 2010;17:1267-77.
309. Duarte I, Llanos O. Patterns of metastases in intestinal and diffuse types of carcinoma of the stomach. Hum Pathol 1981;12:237-42.
310. Esaki Y, Hirayama R, Hirokawa K. A comparison of patterns of metastasis in gastric cancer by histologic type and age. Cancer 1990;65:2086-90.
311. Mori M, Sakaguchi H, Akazawa K, Tsuneyoshi M, Sueishi K, Sugimachi K. Correlation between metastatic site, histological type, and serum tumor markers of gastric carcinoma. Hum Pathol 1995;26:504-8.
312. McCluggage WG, Young RH. Primary ovarian mucinous tumors with signet ring cells: report of 3 cases with discussion of so-called primary Krukenberg tumor. Am J Surg Pathol 2008;32:1373-9.
313. Ajani JA, In H, Sano T, et al. Stomach. In: Amin MB, Edge S, Greene F, Byrd DR, Brookland RK, Washington MK, et al., eds. AJCC Cancer Staging Manual, 8th ed 2017.
314. Hirasawa T, Gotoda T, Miyata S, et al. Incidence of lymph node metastasis and the feasibility of endoscopic resection for undifferentiated-type early gastric cancer. Gastric Cancer 2009;12:148-52.
315. Ono H, Kondo H, Gotoda T, et al. Endoscopic mucosal resection for treatment of early gastric cancer. Gut 2001;48:225-9.
316. Ono H, Yao K, Fujishiro M, et al. Guidelines for endoscopic submucosal dissection and endoscopic mucosal resection for early gastric cancer. Dig Endosc 2016;28:3-15.
317. Pimentel-Nunes P, Dinis-Ribeiro M, Ponchon T, et al. Endoscopic submucosal dissection: European Society of Gastrointestinal Endoscopy (ESGE) Guideline. Endoscopy 2015;47:829-54.
318. Smyth EC, Verheij M, Allum W, Cunningham D, Cervantes A, Arnold D. Gastric cancer: ESMO Clinical Practice Guidelines for diagnosis, treatment and follow-up. Ann Oncol 2016;27(suppl 5):v38-v49.
319. Fridman WH, Zitvogel L, Sautes-Fridman C, Kroemer G. The immune contexture in cancer prognosis and treatment. Nat Rev Clin Oncol 2017;14:717-34.
320. Dai C, Geng R, Wang C, et al. Concordance of immune checkpoints within tumor immune contexture and their prognostic significance in gastric cancer. Mol Oncol 2016;10:1551-8.
321. Ishigami S, Natsugoe S, Miyazono F, et al. Clinical merit of subdividing gastric cancer according to invasion of the muscularis propria. Hepatogastroenterology 2004;51:869-71.
322. Yoshikawa K, Maruyama K. Characteristics of gastric cancer invading to the proper muscle layer—with special reference to mortality and cause of death. Jpn J Clin Oncol 1985;15:499-503.
323. Harrison JC, Dean PJ, Vander Zwaag R, el-Zeky F, Wruble LD. Adenocarcinoma of the stomach with invasion limited to the muscularis propria. Hum Pathol 1991;22:111-7.
324. Hundahl SA, Phillips JL, Menck HR. The National Cancer Data Base Report on poor survival of U.S. gastric carcinoma patients treated with gastrectomy: Fifth Edition American Joint Committee on Cancer staging, proximal disease, and the "different disease" hypothesis. Cancer 2000;88:921-32.
325. Reid-Lombardo KM, Gay G, Patel-Parekh L, Ajani JA, Donohue JH. Treatment of gastric adenocarcinoma may differ among hospital types in the United States, a report from the National Cancer Data Base. J Gastrointest Surg 2007;11:410-9; discussion 9-20.
326. Noguchi Y, Yoshikawa T, Tsuburaya A, Motohashi H, Karpeh MS, Brennan MF. Is gastric carcinoma different between Japan and the United States? Cancer 2000;89:2237-46.
327. Fielding JW, Roginski C, Ellis DJ, et al. Clinicopathological staging of gastric cancer. Br J Surg 1984;71:677-80.

328. Roder JD, Bottcher K, Busch R, Wittekind C, Hermanek P, Siewert JR. Classification of regional lymph node metastasis from gastric carcinoma. German Gastric Cancer Study Group. Cancer 1998;82:621-31.

329. Kappas AM, Fatouros M, Roukos DH. Is it time to change surgical strategy for gastric cancer in the United States? Ann Surg Oncol 2004;11:727-30.

330. Bizer LS. Adenocarcinoma of the stomach: current results of treatment. Cancer 1983;51:743-5.

331. Siewert JR, Bottcher K, Stein HJ, Roder JD. Relevant prognostic factors in gastric cancer: ten-year results of the German Gastric Cancer Study. Ann Surg 1998;228:449-61.

332. Wanebo HJ, Kennedy BJ, Chmiel J, Steele G Jr, Winchester D, Osteen R. Cancer of the stomach. A patient care study by the American College of Surgeons. Ann Surg 1993;218:583-92.

333. Karpeh MS, Leon L, Klimstra D, Brennan MF. Lymph node staging in gastric cancer: is location more important than Number? An analysis of 1,038 patients. Ann Surg 2000;232:362-71.

334. Landry J, Tepper JE, Wood WC, Moulton EO, Koerner F, Sullinger J. Patterns of failure following curative resection of gastric carcinoma. Int J Radiat Oncol Biol Phys 1990;19:1357-62.

335. Cunningham SC, Kamangar F, Kim MP, et al. Survival after gastric adenocarcinoma resection: eighteen-year experience at a single institution. J Gastrointest Surg 2005;9:718-25.

336. Saito H, Fukumoto Y, Osaki T, et al. Distinct recurrence pattern and outcome of adenocarcinoma of the gastric cardia in comparison with carcinoma of other regions of the stomach. World J Surg 2006;30:1864-9.

337. Thies S, Langer R. Tumor regression grading of gastrointestinal carcinomas after neoadjuvant treatment. Front Oncol 2013;3:262.

338. Becker K, Langer R, Reim D, et al. Significance of histopathological tumor regression after neoadjuvant chemotherapy in gastric adenocarcinomas: a summary of 480 cases. Ann Surg 2011;253:934-9.

339. Mandard AM, Dalibard F, Mandard JC, et al. Pathologic assessment of tumor regression after preoperative chemoradiotherapy of esophageal carcinoma. Clinicopathologic correlations. Cancer 1994;73:2680-6.

340. Becker K, Mueller JD, Schulmacher C, et al. Histomorphology and grading of regression in gastric carcinoma treated with neoadjuvant chemotherapy. Cancer 2003;98:1521-30.

341. Sano T, Aiko T. New Japanese classifications and treatment guidelines for gastric cancer: revision concepts and major revised points. Gastric Cancer 2011;14:97-100.

342. Songun I, van de Velde CJ, Arends JW, et al. Classification of gastric carcinoma using the Goseki system provides prognostic information additional to TNM staging. Cancer 1999;85:2114-8.

343. Chiaravalli AM, Klersy C, Tava F, et al. Lower- and higher-grade subtypes of diffuse gastric cancer. Hum Pathol 2009;40:1591-9.

344. Chon HJ, Hyung WJ, Kim C, et al. Differential prognostic implications of gastric signet ring cell carcinoma: stage adjusted analysis from a single high-volume center in Asia. Ann Surg 2017;265:946-53.

345. Radi MJ, Fenoglio-Preiser CM, Bartow SA, Key CR, Pathak DR. Gastric carcinoma in the young: a clinicopathological and immunohistochemical study. Am J Gastroenterol 1986;81:747-56.

346. Umeyama K, Sowa M, Kamino K, Kato Y, Satake K. Gastric carcinoma in young adults in Japan. Anticancer Res 1982;2:283-6.

347. Shimizu H, Ichikawa D, Komatsu S, et al. The decision criterion of histological mixed type in "T1/T2" gastric carcinoma—comparison between TNM classification and Japanese classification of gastric cancer. J Surg Oncol 2012;105:800-4.

348. Min BH, Kim KM, Park CK, et al. Outcomes of endoscopic submucosal dissection for differentiated-type early gastric cancer with histological heterogeneity. Gastric Cancer 2015;18:618-26.

349. Hanaoka N, Tanabe S, Mikami T, Okayasu I, Saigenji K. Mixed-histologic-type submucosal invasive gastric cancer as a risk factor for lymph node metastasis: feasibility of endoscopic submucosal dissection. Endoscopy 2009;41:427-32.

350. Park HK, Lee KY, Yoo MW, Hwang TS, Han HS. Mixed carcinoma as an independent prognostic factor in submucosal invasive gastric carcinoma. J Korean Med Sci 2016;31:866-72.

351. Watanabe H, Enjoji M, Imai T. Gastric carcinoma with lymphoid stroma. Its morphologic characteristics and prognostic correlations. Cancer 1976;38:232-43.

352. Minamoto T, Mai M, Watanabe K, et al. Medullary carcinoma with lymphocytic infiltration of the stomach. Clinicopathologic study of 27 cases and immunohistochemical analysis of the subpopulations of infiltrating lymphocytes in the tumor. Cancer 1990;66:945-52.

353. Shibata D, Tokunaga M, Uemura Y, Sato E, Tanaka S, Weiss LM. Association of Epstein-Barr virus with undifferentiated gastric carcinomas with intense lymphoid infiltration. Lymphoepithelioma-like carcinoma. Am J Pathol 1991;139:469-74.

354. Wang HH, Wu MS, Shun CT, Wang HP, Lin CC, Lin JT. Lymphoepithelioma-like carcinoma of the stomach: a subset of gastric carcinoma with distinct clinicopathological features and high prevalence of Epstein-Barr virus infection. Hepatogastroenterology 1999;46:1214-9.

355. Murphy G, Pfeiffer R, Camargo MC, Rabkin CS. Meta-analysis shows that prevalence of Epstein-Barr virus-positive gastric cancer differs based on sex and anatomic location. Gastroenterology 2009;137:824-33.

356. Lim H, Park YS, Lee JH, et al. Features of gastric carcinoma with lymphoid stroma associated with Epstein-Barr virus. Clin Gastroenterol Hepatol 2015;13:1738-44.e2.

357. Grogg KL, Lohse CM, Pankratz VS, Halling KC, Smyrk TC. Lymphocyte-rich gastric cancer: associations with Epstein-Barr virus, microsatellite instability, histology, and survival. Mod Pathol 2003;16:641-51.

358. Cheng N, Hui DY, Liu Y, et al. Is gastric lymphoepithelioma-like carcinoma a special subtype of EBV-associated gastric carcinoma? New insight based on clinicopathological features and EBV genome polymorphisms. Gastric Cancer 2015;18:246-55.

359. Chiaravalli AM, Cornaggia M, Furlan D, et al. The role of histological investigation in prognostic evaluation of advanced gastric cancer. Analysis of histological structure and molecular changes compared with invasive pattern and stage. Virchows Arch 2001;439:158-69.

360. Young LS, Rickinson AB. Epstein-Barr virus: 40 years on. Nat Rev Cancer 2004;4:757-68.

361. Fukayama M, Ushiku T. Epstein-Barr virus-associated gastric carcinoma. Pathol Res Pract 2011;207:529-37.

362. Shinozaki-Ushiku A, Kunita A, Fukayama M. Update on Epstein-Barr virus and gastric cancer (review). Int J Oncol 2015;46:1421-34.

363. Chen JN, He D, Tang F, Shao CK. Epstein-Barr virus-associated gastric carcinoma: a newly defined entity. J Clin Gastroenterol 2012;46:262-71.

364. Fukayama M, Hino R, Uozaki H. Epstein-Barr virus and gastric carcinoma: virus-host interactions leading to carcinoma. Cancer Sci 2008;99:1726-33.

365. Camargo MC, Kim WH, Chiaravalli AM, et al. Improved survival of gastric cancer with tumour Epstein-Barr virus positivity: an international pooled analysis. Gut 2014;63:236-43.

366. Park S, Choi MG, Kim KM, et al. Lymphoepithelioma-like carcinoma: a distinct type of gastric cancer. J Surg Res 2015;194:458-63.

367. Lee JH, Kim SH, Han SH, An JS, Lee ES, Kim YS. Clinicopathological and molecular characteristics of Epstein-Barr virus-associated gastric carcinoma: a meta-analysis. J Gastroenterol Hepatol 2009;24:354-65.

368. Song HJ, Kim KM. Pathology of Epstein-Barr virus-associated gastric carcinoma and its relationship to prognosis. Gut Liver 2011;5:143-8.

369. Yamamoto N, Tokunaga M, Uemura Y, et al. Epstein-Barr virus and gastric remnant cancer. Cancer 1994;74:805-9.

370. Willems S, Carneiro F, Geboes K. Gastric carcinoma with osteoclast-like giant cells and lymphoepithelioma-like carcinoma of the stomach: two of a kind? Histopathology 2005;47:331-3.

371. Matsunou H, Konishi F, Hori H, et al. Characteristics of Epstein-Barr virus-associated gastric carcinoma with lymphoid stroma in Japan. Cancer 1996;77:1998-2004.

372. Tak DH, Jeong HY, Seong JK, Moon HS, Kang SH. [Comparison of clinical characteristics and prognostic factors between gastric lymphoepithelioma-like carcinoma and gastric adenocarcinoma.] Korean J Gastroenterol 2013;62:272-7. [Korean]

373. Song HJ, Srivastava A, Lee J, et al. Host inflammatory response predicts survival of patients with Epstein-Barr virus-associated gastric carcinoma. Gastroenterology 2010;139:84-92 e2.

374. Fukayama M, Chong JM, Kaizaki Y. Epstein-Barr virus and gastric carcinoma. Gastric Cancer 1998;1:104-14.

375. Gulley ML, Pulitzer DR, Eagan PA, Schneider BG. Epstein-Barr virus infection is an early event in gastric carcinogenesis and is independent of bcl-2 expression and p53 accumulation. Hum Pathol 1996;27:20-7.

376. Truong CD, Feng W, Li W, et al. Characteristics of Epstein-Barr virus-associated gastric cancer: a study of 235 cases at a comprehensive cancer center in U.S.A. J Exp Clin Cancer Res 2009;28:14.

377. Chang MS, Kim WH, Kim CW, Kim YI. Epstein-Barr virus in gastric carcinomas with lymphoid stroma. Histopathology 2000;37:309-15.

378. Saju P, Murata-Kamiya N, Hayashi T, et al. Host SHP1 phosphatase antagonizes Helicobacter pylori CagA and can be downregulated by Epstein-Barr virus. Nat Microbiol 2016;1:16026.

379. Wroblewski LE, Peek RM Jr. Helicobacter pylori: pathogenic enablers—toxic relationships in the stomach. Nat Rev Gastroenterol Hepatol 2016;13:317-8.

380. Shinozaki-Ushiku A, Kunita A, Isogai M, et al. Profiling of virus-encoded microRNAs in Epstein-Barr Virus-associated gastric carcinoma and their roles in gastric carcinogenesis. J Virol 2015;89:5581-91.

381. Saito R, Abe H, Kunita A, Yamashita H, Seto Y, Fukayama M. Overexpression and gene amplification of PD-L1 in cancer cells and PD-L1+ immune cells in Epstein-Barr virus-associated gastric cancer: the prognostic implications. Mod Pathol 2017;30:427-39.

382. Ma C, Patel K, Singhi AD, et al. Programmed death-ligand 1 expression is common in gastric cancer associated with Epstein-Barr virus or Microsatellite instability. Am J Surg Pathol 2016;40:1496-506.

383. Mori M, Iwashita A, Enjoji M. Adenosquamous carcinoma of the stomach. A clinicopathologic analysis of 28 cases. Cancer 1986;57:333-9.

384. Donald KJ. Adenocarcinoma of the pyloric antrum with extensive squamous differentiation. J Clin Pathol 1967;20:136-8.

385. Chen H, Shen C, Yin R, et al. Clinicopathological characteristics, diagnosis, treatment, and outcomes of primary gastric adenosquamous carcinoma. World J Surg Oncol 2015;13:136.

386. Mori M, Fukuda T, Enjoji M. Adenosquamous carcinoma of the stomach. Histogenetic and ultrastructural studies. Gastroenterology 1987;92:1078-82.

387. Yoshida K, Manabe T, Tsunoda T, Kimoto M, Tadaoka Y, Shimizu M. Early gastric cancer of adenosquamous carcinoma type: report of a case and review of literature. Jpn J Clin Oncol 1996;26:252-7.

388. Boswell JT, Helwig EB. Squamous cell carcinoma and adenoacanthoma of the stomach. A clinicopathologic study. Cancer 1965;18:181-92.

389. Namatame K, Ookubo M, Suzuki K, et al. [A clinicopathological study of five cases of adenosquamous carcinoma of the stomach.] Gan No Rinsho 1986;32:170-5. [Japanese]

390. Ikeda E, Shigematsu T, Hidaka K, et al. [A case of adenosquamous gastric carcinoma successfully treated with TS-1, low-dose CDDP and docetaxel as neoadjuvant chemotherapy.] Gan To Kagaku Ryoho 2007;34:423-6. [Japanese]

391. Bonnheim DC, Sarac OK, Fett W. Primary squamous cell carcinoma of the stomach. Am J Gastroenterol 1985;80:91-4.

392. Marubashi S, Yano H, Monden T, et al. Primary squamous cell carcinoma of the stomach. Gastric Cancer 1999;2:136-41.

393. Won OH, Farman J, Krishnan MN, Iyer SK, Vuletin JC. Squamous cell carcinoma of the stomach. Am J Gastroenterol 1978;69:594-8.

394. Vaughan WP, Straus FH 2nd, Paloyan D. Squamous carcinoma of the stomach after luetic linitis plastica. Gastroenterology 1977;72(Pt 1):945-8.

395. Eaton H, Tennekoon GE. Squamous carcinoma of the stomach following corrosive acid burns. Br J Surg 1972;59:382-7.

396. McLoughlin GA, Cave-Bigley DJ, Tagore V, Kirkham N. Cyclophosphamide and pure squamous-cell carcinoma of the stomach. Br Med J 1980;280:524-5.

397. Eom DW, Kang GH, Han SH, et al. Gastric micropapillary carcinoma: a distinct subtype with a significantly worse prognosis in TNM stages I and II. Am J Surg Pathol 2011;35:84-91.

398. Zhang Q, Ming J, Zhang S, Li B, Yin L, Qiu X. Micropapillary component in gastric adenocarcinoma: an aggressive variant associated with poor prognosis. Gastric Cancer 2015;18:93-9.

399. Fujita T, Gotohda N, Kato Y, et al. Clinicopathological features of stomach cancer with invasive micropapillary component. Gastric Cancer 2012;15:179-87.

400. Ushiku T, Matsusaka K, Iwasaki Y, et al. Gastric carcinoma with invasive micropapillary pattern and its association with lymph node metastasis. Histopathology 2011;59:1081-9.

401. Tanaka H, Baba Y, Sase T, et al. Gastric intramucosal adenocarcinoma with an invasive micropapillary carcinoma component. Clin J Gastroenterology 2015;8:14-7.

402. Roh JH, Srivastava A, Lauwers GY, et al. Micropapillary carcinoma of stomach: a clinicopathologic and immunohistochemical study of 11 cases. Am J Surg Pathol 2010;34:1139-46.

403. Ishikura H, Kirimoto K, Shamoto M, et al. Hepatoid adenocarcinomas of the stomach. An analysis of seven cases. Cancer 1986;58:119-26.

404. Akiyama S, Tamura G, Endoh Y, et al. Histogenesis of hepatoid adenocarcinoma of the stomach: molecular evidence of identical origin with coexistent tubular adenocarcinoma. Int J Cancer 2003;106:510-5.

405. Nagai E, Ueyama T, Yao T, Tsuneyoshi M. Hepatoid adenocarcinoma of the stomach. A clinicopathologic and immunohistochemical analysis. Cancer 1993;72:1827-35.

406. Chang YC, Nagasue N, Kohno H, et al. Clinicopathologic features and long-term results of alpha-fetoprotein-producing gastric cancer. Am J Gastroenterol 1990;85:1480-5.

407. Lin CY, Yeh HC, Hsu CM, Lin WR, Chiu CT. Clinicopathologial features of gastric hepatoid adenocarcinoma. Biomed J 2015;38:65-9.

408. Petrella T, Montagnon J, Roignot P, et al. Alphafetoprotein-producing gastric adenocarcinoma. Histopathology 1995;26:171-5.

409. Motoyama T, Aizawa K, Watanabe H, Fukase M, Saito K. Alpha-fetoprotein producing gastric carcinomas: a comparative study of three different subtypes. Acta Pathol Jpn 1993;43:654-61.

410. Kumashiro Y, Yao T, Aishima S, et al. Hepatoid adenocarcinoma of the stomach: histogenesis and progression in association with intestinal phenotype. Hum Pathol 2007;38:857-63.

411. Ishikura H, Kishimoto T, Andachi H, Kakuta Y, Yoshiki T. Gastrointestinal hepatoid adeno-carcinoma: venous permeation and mimicry of hepatocellular carcinoma, a report of four cases. Histopathology 1997;31:47-54.

412. Liu X, Cheng Y, Sheng W, et al. Analysis of clin-icopathologic features and prognostic factors in hepatoid adenocarcinoma of the stomach. Am J Surg Pathol 2010;34:1465-71.

413. Su JS, Chen YT, Wang RC, Wu CY, Lee SW, Lee TY. Clinicopathological characteristics in the differential diagnosis of hepatoid adenocarci-noma: a literature review. World J Gastroenterol 2013;19:321-7.

414. Inagawa S, Shimazaki J, Hori M, et al. Hepatoid adenocarcinoma of the stomach. Gastric Can-cer 2001;4:43-52.

415. Supriatna Y, Kishimoto T, Uno T, Nagai Y, Ishikura H. Evidence for hepatocellular differ-entiation in alpha-fetoprotein-negative gastric adenocarcinoma with hepatoid morphology: a study with in situ hybridisation for albumin mRNA. Pathology 2005;37:211-5.

416. Sentani K, Oue N, Sakamoto N, et al. Gene expression profiling with microarray and SAGE identifies PLUNC as a marker for hepatoid adenocarcinoma of the stomach. Mod Pathol 2008;21:464-75.

417. Murakami T, Yao T, Mitomi H, et al. Clin-icopathologic and immunohistochemical characteristics of gastric adenocarcinoma with enteroblastic differentiation: a study of 29 cases. Gastric Cancer 2016;19:498-507.

418. Yamazawa S, Ushiku T, Shinozaki-Ushiku A, et al. Gastric cancer with primitive enterocyte phenotype: an aggressive subgroup of intesti-nal-type adenocarcinoma. Am J Surg Pathol 2017;41:989-97.

419. Terracciano LM, Glatz K, Mhawech P, et al. Hepatoid adenocarcinoma with liver metas-tasis mimicking hepatocellular carcinoma: an immunohistochemical and molecular study of eight cases. Am J Surg Pathol 2003;27:1302-12.

420. Ushiku T, Shinozaki A, Shibahara J, et al. SALL4 represents fetal gut differentiation of gastric cancer, and is diagnostically useful in distinguishing hepatoid gastric carcinoma from hepatocellular carcinoma. Am J Surg Pathol 2010;34:533-40.

421. Liu TC, Vachharajani N, Chapman WC, Brunt EM. SALL4 immunoreactivity predicts prog-nosis in Western hepatocellular carcinoma

patients but is a rare event: a study of 236 cases. Am J Surg Pathol 2014;38:966-72.

422. Chandan VS, Shah SS, Torbenson MS, Wu TT. Arginase-1 is frequently positive in hepatoid adenocarcinomas. Human Pathol 2016;55:11-6.

423. Wurzel J, Brooks JJ. Primary gastric choriocar-cinoma: immunohistochemistry, postmortem documentation, and hormonal effects in a post-menopausal female. Cancer 1981;48:2756-61.

424. Kobayashi A, Hasebe T, Endo Y, et al. Primary gastric choriocarcinoma: two case reports and a pooled analysis of 53 cases. Gastric Cancer 2005;8:178-85.

425. Imai Y, Kawabe T, Takahashi M, et al. A case of primary gastric choriocarcinoma and a review of the Japanese literature. J Gastroenterol 1994;29:642-6.

426. Saigo PE, Brigati DJ, Sternberg SS, Rosen PP, Turnbull AD. Primary gastric choriocarcinoma. An immunohistological study. Am J Surg Pathol 1981;5:333-42.

427. Liu AY, Chan WY, Ng EK, et al. Gastric cho-riocarcinoma shows characteristics of adeno-carcinoma and gestational choriocarcinoma: a comparative genomic hybridization and fluorescence in situ hybridization study. Diagn Mol Pathol 2001;10:161-5.

428. Smith FR, Barkin JS, Hensley G. Choriocar-cinoma of the stomach. Am J Gastroenterol 1980;73:45-8.

429. Yonezawa S, Maruyama I, Tanaka S, Nakamura T, Sato E. Immunohistochemical localization of thrombomodulin in chorionic diseases of the uterus and choriocarcinoma of the stomach. A comparative study with the distribution of human chorionic gonadotropin. Cancer 1988;62:569-76.

430. Krulewski T, Cohen LB. Choriocarcinoma of the stomach: pathogenesis and clinical char-acteristics. Am J Gastroenterol 1988;83:1172-5.

431. Garcia RL, Ghali VS. Gastric choriocarcino-ma and yolk sac tumor in a man: observa-tions about its possible origin. Hum Pathol 1985;16:955-8.

432. Jindrak K, Bochetto JF, Alpert LI. Primary gastric choriocarcinoma: case report with review of world literature. Hum Pathol 1976;7:595-604.

433. Kanai M, Torii A, Hamada A, et al. Pure gastric yolk sac tumor that was diagnosed after cura-tive resection: case report and review of litera-ture. Int J Gastrointest Cancer 2005;35:77-81.

434. Satake N, Chikakiyo M, Yagi T, Suzuki Y, Hirose T. Gastric cancer with choriocarcinoma and yolk sac tumor components: case report. Pathol Int 2011;61:156-60.

435. Eom BW, Jung SY, Yoon H, et al. Gastric choriocarcinoma admixed with an alpha-fetoprotein-producing adenocarcinoma and separated adenocarcinoma. World J Gastroenterol 2009;15:5106-8.

436. Hirano Y, Hara T, Nozawa H, et al. Combined choriocarcinoma, neuroendocrine cell carcinoma and tubular adenocarcinoma in the stomach. World J Gastroenterol 2008;14.3269-72.

437. Ueyama H, Yao T, Nakashima Y, et al. Gastric adenocarcinoma of fundic gland type (chief cell predominant type): proposal for a new entity of gastric adenocarcinoma. Am J Surg Pathol 2010;34:609-19.

438. Hidaka Y, Mitomi H, Saito T, et al. Alteration in the Wnt/beta-catenin signaling pathway in gastric neoplasias of fundic gland (chief cell predominant) type. Hum Pathol 2013;44:2438-48.

439. Nomura R, Saito T, Mitomi H, et al. GNAS mutation as an alternative mechanism of activation of the Wnt/beta-catenin signaling pathway in gastric adenocarcinoma of the fundic gland type. Hum Pathol 2014;45:2488-96.

440. Kushima R, Sekine S, Matsubara A, Taniguchi H, Ikegami M, Tsuda H. Gastric adenocarcinoma of the fundic gland type shares common genetic and phenotypic features with pyloric gland adenoma. Pathol Int 2013;63:318-25.

441. Chiba T, Kato K, Masuda T, et al. Clinicopathological features of gastric adenocarcinoma of the fundic gland (chief cell predominant type) by retrospective and prospective analyses of endoscopic findings. Dig Endosc 2016;28:722-30.

442. Tohda G, Osawa T, Asada Y, Dochin M, Terahata S. Gastric adenocarcinoma of fundic gland type: endoscopic and clinicopathological features. World J Gastrointest Endosc 2016;8:244-51.

443. Parikh ND, Gibson J, Aslanian H. Gastric fundic gland adenocarcinoma with chief cell differentiation. Clin Gastroenterol Hepatol 2015;13:A17-8.

444. Singhi AD, Lazenby AJ, Montgomery EA. Gastric adenocarcinoma with chief cell differentiation: a proposal for reclassification as oxyntic gland polyp/adenoma. Am J Surg Pathol 2012;36:1030-5.

445. Chan K, Brown IS, Kyle T, Lauwers GY, Kumarasinghe MP. Chief cell-predominant gastric polyps: a series of 12 cases with literature review. Histopathology 2016;68:825-33.

446. Capella C, Frigerio B, Cornaggia M, Solcia E, Pinzon-Trujillo Y, Chejfec G. Gastric parietal cell carcinoma—a newly recognized entity: light microscopic and ultrastructural features. Histopathology 1984;8:813-24.

447. Byrne D, Holley MP, Cuschieri A. Parietal cell carcinoma of the stomach: association with long-term survival after curative resection. Br J Cancer 1988;58:85-7.

448. Yang GY, Liao J, Cassai ND, Smolka AJ, Sidhu GS. Parietal cell carcinoma of gastric cardia: immunophenotype and ultrastructure. Ultrastruct Pathol 2003;27:87-94.

449. Caruso RA, Fabiano V, Rigoli L, Inferrera A. Focal parietal cell differentiation in a well-differentiated (intestinal-type) early gastric cancer. Ultrastruct Pathol 2000;24:417-22.

450. Takubo K, Honma N, Sawabe M, et al. Oncocytic adenocarcinoma of the stomach: parietal cell carcinoma. Am J Surg Pathol 2002;26:458-65.

451. Kazzaz BA, Eulderink F. Paneth cell-rich carcinoma of the stomach. Histopathology 1989;15:303-5.

452. Ooi A, Nakanishi I, Itoh T, Ueda H, Mai M. Predominant Paneth cell differentiation in an intestinal type gastric cancer. Pathol Res Pract 1991;187:220-5.

453. Inada KI, Mizoshita T, Tsukamoto T, Porter EM, Tatematsu M. Paneth type gastric cancer cells exhibit expression of human defensin-5. Histopathology 2005;47:330-1.

454. Ooi A, Ota M, Katsuda S, Nakanishi I, Sugawara H, Takahashi I. An unusual case of multiple gastric carcinoids associated with diffuse endocrine cell hyperplasia and parietal cell hypertrophy. Endocr Pathol 1995;6:229-37.

455. Lev R, DeNucci TD. Neoplastic Paneth cells in the stomach. Report of two cases and review of the literature. Arch Pathol Lab Med 1989;113:129-33.

456. Caruso RA, Famulari C. Neoplastic Paneth cells in adenocarcinoma of the stomach: a case report. Hepatogastroenterology 1992;39:264-6.

457. Hayashi I, Muto Y, Fujii Y, Morimatsu M. Mucoepidermoid carcinoma of the stomach. J Surg Oncol 1987;34:94-9.

458. Cho KJ, Myong NH, Choi DW, Jang JJ. Carcinosarcoma of the stomach. A case report with light microscopic, immunohistochemical, and electron microscopic study. APMIS 1990;98:991-5.

459. Nakayama Y, Murayama H, Iwasaki H, et al. Gastric carcinosarcoma (sarcomatoid carcinoma) with rhabdomyoblastic and osteoblastic differentiation. Pathol Int 1997;47:557-63.

460. Sato Y, Shimozono T, Kawano S, et al. Gastric carcinosarcoma, coexistence of adenosquamous carcinoma and rhabdomyosarcoma: a case report. Histopathology 2001;39:543-4.

461. Randjelovic T, Filipovic B, Babic D, Cemerikic V. Carcinosarcoma of the stomach: a case report and review of the literature. World J Gastroenterol 2007;13:5533-6.

462. Fujiie M, Yamamoto M, Taguchi K, et al. Gastric carcinosarcoma with rhabdomyosarcomatous differentiation: a case report and review. Surg Case Rep 2016;2:52.

463. Solerio D, Ruffini E, Camandona M, Raggio E, Castellano I, Dei Poli M. Carcinosarcoma of the esophagogastric junction. Tumori 2008;94:416-8.

464. Matsukuma S, Wada R, Hase K, Sakai Y, Ogata S, Kuwabara N. Gastric stump carcinosarcoma with rhabdomyosarcomatous differentiation. Pathol Int 1997;47:73-7.

465. Sato A, Oki E, Kohso H, et al. Sarcomatoid carcinoma of the remnant stomach: report of a case. Surg Today 2013;43:308-12.

466. Tsuneyama K, Sasaki M, Sabit A, et al. A case report of gastric carcinosarcoma with rhabdomyosarcomatous and neuroendocrinal differentiation. Pathol Res Pract 1999;195:93-7; discussion 8.

467. Yamazaki K. A gastric carcinosarcoma with neuroendocrine cell differentiation and undifferentiated spindle-shaped sarcoma component possibly progressing from the conventional tubular adenocarcinoma; an immunohistochemical and ultrastructural study. Virchows Arch 2003;442:77-81.

468. Teramachi K, Kanomata N, Hasebe T, Ishii G, Sugito M, Ochiai A. Carcinosarcoma (pure endocrine cell carcinoma with sarcoma components) of the stomach. Pathol Int 2003;53:552-6.

469. Kuroda N, Oonishi K, Iwamura S, et al. Gastric carcinosarcoma with neuroendocrine differentiation as the carcinoma component and leiomyosarcomatous and myofibroblastic differentiation as the sarcomatous component. APMIS 2006;114:234-8.

470. Ikeda Y, Kosugi S, Nishikura K, et al. Gastric carcinosarcoma presenting as a huge epigastric mass. Gastric Cancer 2007;10:63-8.

471. Kallakury BV, Bui HX, delRosario A, Wallace J, Solis OG, Ross JS. Primary gastric adenosarcoma. Arch Pathol Lab Med 1993;117:299-301.

472. Miettinen M, Dow N, Lasota J, Sobin LH. A distinctive novel epitheliomesenchymal biphasic tumor of the stomach in young adults ("gastroblastoma"): a series of 3 cases. Am J Surg Pathol 2009;33:1370-7.

473. Shin DH, Lee JH, Kang HJ, et al. Novel epitheliomesenchymal biphasic stomach tumour (gastroblastoma) in a 9-year-old: morphological, usltrastructural and immunohistochemical findings. J Clin Pathol 2010;63:270-4.

474. Ma Y, Zheng J, Zhu H, et al. Gastroblastoma in a 12-year-old Chinese boy. Int J Clin Exp Pathol 2014;7:3380-4.

475. Wey EA, Britton AJ, Sferra JJ, Kasunic T, Pepe LR, Appelman HD. Gastroblastoma in a 28-year-

476. Fernandes T, Silva R, Devesa V, Lopes JM, Carneiro F, Viamonte B. AIRP best cases in radiologic-pathologic correlation: gastroblastoma: a rare biphasic gastric tumor. Radiographics 2014;34:1929-33.

477. Ueyama T, Nagai E, Yao T, Tsuneyoshi M. Vimentin-positive gastric carcinomas with rhabdoid features. A clinicopathologic and immunohistochemical study. Am J Surg Pathol 1993;17:813-9.

478. Pinto JA, Gonzalez Alfonso JE, Gonzalez L, Stevenson N. Well differentiated gastric adenocarcinoma with rhabdoid areas: a case report with immunohistochemical analysis. Pathol Res Pract 1997;193:801-5; discussion 6-8.

479. Rivera-Hueto F, Rios-Martin JJ, Dominguez-Triano R, Herrerias-Gutierrez JM. Early gastric stump carcinoma with rhabdoid features. Case report. Pathol Res Pract 1999;195:841-6.

480. Ofkeli O, Bulut A, Yuksek YN, Yildiz HI. Malignant rhabdoid tumour in the stomach. Ulus Cerrahi Derg 2015;31:55-7.

481. Kawasaki K, Kanemitsu K, Yasuda T, Kamigaki T, Kuroda D, Kuroda Y. Family history of cancer in Japanese gastric cancer patients. Gastric Cancer 2007;10:173-5.

482. Hemminki K, Sundquist J, Ji J. Familial risk for gastric carcinoma: an updated study from Sweden. Br J Cancer 2007;96:1272-7.

483. Carneiro F. Pathology of hereditary gastric cancer. Spotlight on Familial and hereditary gastric cancer. Corso G, Roviello F, eds. Dordrecht: Springer; 2013:141-56.

484. Caldas C, Carneiro F, Lynch HT, et al. Familial gastric cancer: overview and guidelines for management. J Med Genet 1999;36:873-80.

485. Worthley DL, Phillips KD, Wayte N, et al. Gastric adenocarcinoma and proximal polyposis of the stomach (GAPPS): a new autosomal dominant syndrome. Gut 2012;61:774-9.

486. Oliveira C, Pinheiro H, Figueiredo J, Seruca R, Carneiro F. Familial gastric cancer: genetic susceptibility, pathology, and implications for management. Lancet Oncol 2015;16:e60-70.

487. Setia N, Clark JW, Duda DG, et al. Familial gastric cancers. Oncologist 2015;20:1365-77.

488. Attard TM, Cuffari C, Tajouri T, et al. Multicenter experience with upper gastrointestinal polyps in pediatric patients with familial adenomatous polyposis. Am J Gastroenterol 2004;99:681-6.

489. Bianchi LK, Burke CA, Bennett AE, Lopez R, Hasson H, Church JM. Fundic gland polyp dysplasia is common in familial adenomatous polyposis. Clin Gastroenterol Hepatol 2008;6:180-5.

490. Lynch HT, Smyrk T, McGinn T, et al. Attenuated familial adenomatous polyposis (AFAP). A phenotypically and genotypically distinctive variant of FAP. Cancer 1995;76.2427-33.

491. Wood LD, Salaria SN, Cruise MW, Giardiello FM, Montgomery EA. Upper GI tract lesions in familial adenomatous polyposis (FAP): enrichment of pyloric gland adenomas and other gastric and duodenal neoplasms. Am J Surg Pathol 2014;38:389-93.

492. Brosens LA, Giardiello FM, Offerhaus GJ, Montgomery EA. Syndromic gastric polyps: at the crossroads of genetic and environmental cancer predisposition. Adv Exp Med Biol 2016;908:347-69.

493. Iwama T, Mishima Y, Utsunomiya J. The impact of familial adenomatous polyposis on the tumorigenesis and mortality at the several organs. Its rational treatment. Ann Surg 1993;217:101-8.

494. Park JG, Park KJ, Ahn YO, et al. Risk of gastric cancer among Korean familial adenomatous polyposis patients. Report of three cases. Dis Colon Rectum 1992;35:996-8.

495. Offerhaus GJ, Giardiello FM, Krush AJ, et al. The risk of upper gastrointestinal cancer in familial adenomatous polyposis. Gastroenterology 1992;102:1980-2.

496. Jagelman DG, DeCosse JJ, Bussey HJ. Upper gastrointestinal cancer in familial adenomatous polyposis. Lancet 1988;1:1149-51.

497. Lynch HT, Grady W, Suriano G, Huntsman D. Gastric cancer: new genetic developments. J Surg Oncol 2005;90:114-33; discussion 33.

498. Arnason T, Liang WY, Alfaro E, et al. Morphology and natural history of familial adenomatous polyposis-associated dysplastic fundic gland polyps. Histopathology 2014;65:353-62.

499. Offerhaus GJ, Entius MM, Giardiello FM. Upper gastrointestinal polyps in familial adenomatous polyposis. Hepatogastroenterology 1999;46:667-9.

500. Ong ES, Alassas MA, Bogner PN, Bullard Dunn K, Chey WY, Gibbs JF. Total gastrectomy for gastric dysplasia in a patient with attenuated familial adenomatous polyposis syndrome. J Clin Oncol 2008;26:3641-2.

501. Aarnio M, Salovaara R, Aaltonen LA, Mecklin JP, Jarvinen HJ. Features of gastric cancer in hereditary non-polyposis colorectal cancer syndrome. Int J Cancer 1997;74:551-5.

502. Vasen HF, Blanco I, Aktan-Collan K, et al. Revised guidelines for the clinical management of Lynch syndrome (HNPCC): recommendations by a group of European experts. Gut 2013;62:812-23.

503. Capelle LG, Van Grieken NC, Lingsma HF, et al. Risk and epidemiological time trends of gastric cancer in Lynch syndrome carriers in the Netherlands. Gastroenterology 2010;138:487-92.

504. Syngal S, Brand RE, Church JM, et al. ACG clinical guideline: genetic testing and management of hereditary gastrointestinal cancer syndromes. Am J Gastroenterol 2015;110:223-62.

505. Varley JM, McGown G, Thorncroft M, et al. An extended Li-Fraumeni kindred with gastric carcinoma and a codon 175 mutation in TP53. J Med Genet 1995;32:942-5.

506. Li FP, Fraumeni JF Jr. Soft-tissue sarcomas, breast cancer, and other neoplasms. A familial syndrome? Ann Intern Med 1969;71:747-52.

507. Bouaoun L, Sonkin D, Ardin M, et al. TP53 Variations in human cancers: new lessons from the IARC TP53 database and genomics data. Hum Mutat 2016;37:865-76.

508. Masciari S, Dewanwala A, Stoffel EM, et al. Gastric cancer in individuals with Li-Fraumeni syndrome. Genet Med 2011;13:651-7.

509. Giardiello FM, Brensinger JD, Tersmette AC, et al. Very high risk of cancer in familial Peutz-Jeghers syndrome. Gastroenterology 2000;119:1447-53.

510. van Lier MG, Westerman AM, Wagner A, et al. High cancer risk and increased mortality in patients with Peutz-Jeghers syndrome. Gut 2011;60:141-7.

511. van Lier MG, Wagner A, Mathus-Vliegen EM, Kuipers EJ, Steyerberg EW, van Leerdam ME. High cancer risk in Peutz-Jeghers syndrome: a systematic review and surveillance recommendations. The Am J Gastroenterol 2010; 105:1258-64; author reply 65.

512. Utsunomiya J, Gocho H, Miyanaga T, Hamaguchi E, Kashimure A. Peutz-Jeghers syndrome: its natural course and management. Johns Hopkins Med J 1975;136:71-82.

513. Shinmura K, Goto M, Tao H, et al. A novel STK11 germline mutation in two siblings with Peutz-Jeghers syndrome complicated by primary gastric cancer. Clin Genet 2005;67:81-6.

514. Takahashi M, Sakayori M, Takahashi S, et al. A novel germline mutation of the LKB1 gene in a patient with Peutz-Jeghers syndrome with early-onset gastric cancer. J Gastroenterol 2004;39:1210-4.

515. Soer E, de Vos Tot Nederveen Cappel WH, Ligtenberg MJ, et al. Massive gastric polyposis associated with a germline SMAD4 gene mutation. Fam Cancer 2015;14:569-73.

516. Gonzalez RS, Adsay V, Graham RP, et al. Massive Gastric juvenile-type polyposis: a clinicopathologic analysis of 22 cases. Histopathology 2017;70:918-28.

517. Ma C, Giardiello FM, Montgomery EA. Upper tract juvenile polyps in juvenile polyposis patients: dysplasia and malignancy are associated with foveolar, intestinal, and pyloric differentiation. Am J Surg Pathol 2014;38:1618-26.

518. Saito R, Fukuda T, Fujikuni N, et al. A case of juvenile polyposis of the stomach with multiple early gastric cancers. Mol Clin Oncol 2016;4:851-4.

519. Seruca R, Carneiro F, Castedo S, David L, Lopes C, Sobrinho-Simoes M. Familial gastric polyposis revisited. Autosomal dominant inheritance confirmed. Cancer Genet Cytogenet 1991;53:97-100.

520. Carneiro F, David L, Seruca R, Castedo S, Nesland JM, Sobrinho-Simoes M. Hyperplastic polyposis and diffuse carcinoma of the stomach. A study of a family. Cancer 1993;72:323-9.

521. Lorenzo Bermejo J, Hemminki K. Risk of cancer at sites other than the breast in Swedish families eligible for BRCA1 or BRCA2 mutation testing. Ann Oncol 2004;15:1834-41.

522. Gallardo M, Silva A, Rubio L, et al. Incidence of BRCA1 and BRCA2 mutations in 54 Chilean families with breast/ovarian cancer, genotype-phenotype correlations. Breast Cancer Res Treat 2006;95:81-7.

523. Jakubowska A, Nej K, Huzarski T, Scott RJ, Lubinski J. BRCA2 gene mutations in families with aggregations of breast and stomach cancers. Br J Cancer 2002;87:888-91.

524. Guilford P, Hopkins J, Harraway J, et al. E-cadherin germline mutations in familial gastric cancer. Nature 1998;392:402-5.

525. Seevaratnam R, Coburn N, Cardoso R, Dixon M, Bocicariu A, Helyer L. A systematic review of the indications for genetic testing and prophylactic gastrectomy among patients with hereditary diffuse gastric cancer. Gastric Cancer 2012;15(Suppl 1):S153-63.

526. Brooks-Wilson AR, Kaurah P, Suriano G, et al. Germline E-cadherin mutations in hereditary diffuse gastric cancer: assessment of 42 new families and review of genetic screening criteria. J Med Genet 2004;41:508-17.

527. Oliveira C, Senz J, Kaurah P, et al. Germline CDH1 deletions in hereditary diffuse gastric cancer families. Hum Mol Genet 2009;18:1545-55.

528. Oliveira C, Seruca R, Hoogerbrugge N, Ligtenberg M, Carneiro F. Clinical utility gene card for: Hereditary diffuse gastric cancer (HDGC). Eur J Hum Genet 2013;21(8).

529. Hansford S, Kaurah P, Li-Chang H, et al. Hereditary Diffuse Gastric Cancer Syndrome: CDH1 Mutations and Beyond. JAMA oncology. 2015;1(1):23-32.

530. van der Post RS, Vogelaar IP, Carneiro F, et al. Hereditary diffuse gastric cancer: updated clinical guidelines with an emphasis on germline CDH1 mutation carriers. J Med Genet 2015;52:361-74.

531. Suriano G, Seixas S, Rocha J, Seruca R. A model to infer the pathogenic significance of CDH1 germline missense variants. J Mol Med (Berl) 2006;84:1023-31.

532. Figueiredo J, Soderberg O, Simoes-Correia J, Grannas K, Suriano G, Seruca R. The importance of E-cadherin binding partners to evaluate the pathogenicity of E-cadherin missense mutations associated to HDGC. Eur J Hum Genet 2013;21:301-9.

533. Sanches JM, Figueiredo J, Fonseca M, et al. Quantification of mutant E-cadherin using bioimaging analysis of in situ fluorescence microscopy. A new approach to CDH1 missense variants. Eur J Hum Genet 2015;23:1072-9.

534. Simoes-Correia J, Figueiredo J, Lopes R, et al. E-cadherin destabilization accounts for the pathogenicity of missense mutations in hereditary diffuse gastric cancer. PloS One 2012;7:e33783.

535. Grady WM, Willis J, Guilford PJ, et al. Methylation of the CDH1 promoter as the second genetic hit in hereditary diffuse gastric cancer. Nat Genet 2000;26:16-7.

536. Oliveira C, de Bruin J, Nabais S, et al. Intragenic deletion of CDH1 as the inactivating mechanism of the wild-type allele in an HDGC tumour. Oncogene 2004;23:2236-40.

537. Oliveira C, Sousa S, Pinheiro H, et al. Quantification of epigenetic and genetic 2nd hits in CDH1 during hereditary diffuse gastric cancer syndrome progression. Gastroenterology 2009;136:2137-48.

538. Barber M, Murrell A, Ito Y, et al. Mechanisms and sequelae of E-cadherin silencing in hereditary diffuse gastric cancer. J Pathol 2008;216:295-306.

539. Majewski IJ, Kluijt I, Cats A, et al. An alpha-E-catenin (CTNNA1) mutation in hereditary diffuse gastric cancer. J Pathol 2013;229:621-9.

540. Donner I, Kiviluoto T, Ristimaki A, Aaltonen LA, Vahteristo P. Exome sequencing reveals three novel candidate predisposition genes for diffuse gastric cancer. Fam Cancer 2015;14:241-6.

541. Keller G, Vogelsang H, Becker I, et al. Diffuse type gastric and lobular breast carcinoma in a familial gastric cancer patient with an E-cadherin germline mutation. Am J Pathol 1999;155:337-42.

542. Suriano G, Yew S, Ferreira P, et al. Characterization of a recurrent germ line mutation of the E-cadherin gene: implications for genetic testing and clinical management. Clin Cancer Res 2005;11:5401-9.

543. Kaurah P, MacMillan A, Boyd N, et al. Founder and recurrent CDH1 mutations in families with hereditary diffuse gastric cancer. JAMA 2007;297:2360-72.

544. Schrader KA, Masciari S, Boyd N, et al. Hereditary diffuse gastric cancer: association with lobular breast cancer. Fam Cancer 2008;7:73-82.

545. Fitzgerald RC, Hardwick R, Huntsman D, et al. Hereditary diffuse gastric cancer: updated consensus guidelines for clinical management and directions for future research. J Med Genet 2010;47:436-44.

546. Guilford PJ, Hopkins JB, Grady WM, et al. E-cadherin germline mutations define an inherited cancer syndrome dominated by diffuse gastric cancer. Hum Mutat 1999;14:249-55.

547. Shaw D, Blair V, Framp A, et al. Chromoendoscopic surveillance in hereditary diffuse gastric cancer: an alternative to prophylactic gastrectomy? Gut 2005;54:461-8.

548. Carneiro F, Huntsman DG, Smyrk TC, et al. Model of the early development of diffuse gastric cancer in E-cadherin mutation carriers and its implications for patient screening. J Pathol 2004;203:681-7.

549. Charlton A, Blair V, Shaw D, Parry S, Guilford P, Martin IG. Hereditary diffuse gastric cancer: predominance of multiple foci of signet ring cell carcinoma in distal stomach and transitional zone. Gut 2004;53:814-20.

550. Rogers WM, Dobo E, Norton JA, et al. Risk-reducing total gastrectomy for germline mutations in E-cadherin (CDH1): pathologic findings with clinical implications. Am J Surg Pathol 2008;32:799-809.

551. Carneiro F, Charlton A, Huntsman DG. Hereditary diffuse gastric cancer. In: Bosman FT, Carneiro F, Hruban RH, Theise ND, editors. WHO Classification of Tumours of the Digestive System, Fouth Edition. Lyon: IARC Press; 2010:59-63.

552. Richards FM, McKee SA, Rajpar MH, et al. Germline E-cadherin gene (CDH1) mutations predispose to familial gastric cancer and colorectal cancer. Hum Mol Genet 1999;8:607-10.

553. Blair V, Martin I, Shaw D, et al. Hereditary diffuse gastric cancer: diagnosis and management. Clin Gastroenterol Hepatol 2006;4:262-75.

554. Chun YS, Lindor NM, Smyrk TC, et al. Germline E-cadherin gene mutations: is prophylactic total gastrectomy indicated? Cancer 2001;92:181-7.

555. Barber ME, Save V, Carneiro F, et al. Histopathological and molecular analysis of gastrectomy specimens from hereditary diffuse gastric cancer patients has implications for endoscopic surveillance of individuals at risk. J Pathol 2008;216:286-94.

556. Norton JA, Ham CM, Van Dam J, et al. CDH1 truncating mutations in the E-cadherin gene: an indication for total gastrectomy to treat hereditary diffuse gastric cancer. Ann Surg 2007;245:873-9.

557. Hebbard PC, Macmillan A, Huntsman D, et al. Prophylactic total gastrectomy (PTG) for hereditary diffuse gastric cancer (HDGC): the Newfoundland experience with 23 patients. Ann Surg Oncol 2009;16:1890-5.

558. van der Post RS, Gullo I, Oliveira C, et al. Histopathological, molecular, and genetic profile of hereditary diffuse gastric cancer: current knowledge and challenges for the future. Adv Exp Med Biol 2016;908:371-91.

559. Humar B, Fukuzawa R, Blair V, et al. Destabilized adhesion in the gastric proliferative zone and c-Src kinase activation mark the development of early diffuse gastric cancer. Cancer Res 2007;67:2480-9.

560. Carneiro F, Oliveira C, Suriano G, Seruca R. Molecular pathology of familial gastric cancer, with an emphasis on hereditary diffuse gastric cancer. J Clin Pathol 2008;61:25-30.

561. Oliveira C, Ferreira P, Nabais S, et al. E-cadherin (CDH1) and p53 rather than SMAD4 and caspase-10 germline mutations contribute to genetic predisposition in Portuguese gastric cancer patients. Eur J Cancer 2004;40:1897-903.

562. Keller G, Vogelsang H, Becker I, et al. Germline mutations of the E-cadherin(CDH1) and TP53 genes, rather than of RUNX3 and HPP1, contribute to genetic predisposition in German gastric cancer patients. J Med Genet 2004;41:e89.

563. Mahmud N, Ford JM, Longacre TA, Parent R, Norton JA. Metastatic lobular breast carcinoma mimicking primary signet ring adenocarcinoma in a patient with a suspected CDH1 mutation. J Clin Oncol 2015;33:e19-21.

564. van der Post RS, Bult P, Vogelaar IP, Ligtenberg MJ, Hoogerbrugge N, van Krieken JH. HNF4A immunohistochemistry facilitates distinction between primary and metastatic breast and gastric carcinoma. Virchows Arch 2014;464:673-9.

565. Stiekema J, Cats A, Kuijpers A, et al. Surgical treatment results of intestinal and diffuse type gastric cancer. Implications for a differentiated therapeutic approach? Eur J Surg Oncol 2013;39:686-93.

566. Yanaru-Fujisawa R, Nakamura S, Moriyama T, et al. Familial fundic gland polyposis with gastric cancer. Gut 2012;61:1103-4.

567. Repak R, Kohoutova D, Podhola M, et al. The first European family with gastric adenocarcinoma and proximal polyposis of the stomach: case report and review of the literature. Gastrointest Endosc 2016;84:718-25.

568. Li J, Woods SL, Healey S, et al. Point mutations in exon 1B of APC reveal gastric adenocarcinoma and proximal polyposis of the stomach as a familial adenomatous polyposis variant. Am J Hum Genet 2016;98:830-42.

569. Beer A, Streubel B, Asari R, Dejaco C Oberhuber G. Gastric adenocarcinoma and proximal polyposis of the stomach (GAPPS)—a rare recently described gastric polyposis syndrome—report of a case. Gastroenterol 2017;55:1131-4.

570. Mitsui Y, Yokoyama R, Fujimoto S, et al. First report of an Asian family with gastric adenocarcinoma and proximal polyposis of the stomach (GAPPS) revealed with the germline mutation of the APC exon 1B promoter region. Gastric Cancer 2018;21:1058-63.

571. de Boer WB, Ee H, Kumarasinghe MP. Neoplastic lesions of gastric adenocarcinoma and proximal polyposis syndrome (GAPPS) are gastric phenotype. Am J Surg Pathol 2018;42:1-8.

572. McDuffie LA, Sabesan A, Allgaeuer M, et al. beta-Catenin activation in fundic gland polyps, gastric cancer and colonic polyps in families afflicted by 'gastric adenocarcinoma and proximal polyposis of the stomach' (GAPPS). J Clin Pathol 2016;69:826-33.

10 GASTRIC NEUROENDOCRINE NEOPLASMS

Gastric neuroendocrine neoplasms are a group of tumors composed of neoplastic cells with neuroendocrine differentiation. The majority are low-grade well-differentiated and nonfunctioning neoplasms. Most develop from histamine-secreting enterochromaffin-like cells, many in the setting of hypergastrinemia (see below). Biologically more aggressive and poorly differentiated tumors, i.e., neuroendocrine carcinomas, are also recognized. These tumors are rare, and not associated with hypergastrinemia.

In this chapter, a modified classification scheme is used in which six types of gastric neuroendocrine neoplasms are described. These neoplasms are separated by different clinical, pathologic, and pathophysiologic characteristics (Table 10-1). The six categories include neuroendocrine tumors, type I to IV, neuroendocrine carcinoma, and mixed adenoneuroendocrine carcinoma (1–3).

NEUROENDOCRINE TUMORS

Neuroendocrine tumors (NETs) of the stomach are composed of well-differentiated cells with neuroendocrine differentiation. They are a heterogenous group of low- and intermediate-grade neoplasms usually associated with a good to intermediate prognosis (3).

General Features

Gastric NETs are an uncommon group of neoplasms. In an analysis of the Surveillance, Epidemiology and End Results (SEER) database, the incidence of well-differentiated NET was 0.4/100,000. Recent epidemiologic surveys, however, have indicated that these lesions have been diagnosed with increased frequency in recent years. The annual increase in incidence is 9 percent per year. From 1950 to 1999, the relative prevalence rate of gastric NET, compared to all other types of gastric malignancies, increased from 0.5 to 1.77 percent. During that same time period, gastric NETs represented 2.4 to 8.7 percent of all gastrointestinal NETs (4–10).

The reasons for the increasing rates of NET are multifactorial. These factors include the increasing use of upper endoscopy, increasing awareness by clinicians, further development of immunohistochemical techniques that help in establishing a more accurate diagnosis, and possibly, the increasing use of proton pump inhibitors by clinicians.

Gastric Neuroendocrine Cells

Normal gastric mucosa has five types of endocrine cells: histamine-secreting enterochromaffin-like cells (ECL cells); serotonin-secreting

Table 10-1

CLASSIFICATION OF GASTRIC NEUROENDOCRINE NEOPLASMS

Tumor	Frequency	Multiplicity	Biologic Behavior
NET[a] type I	65-80% of NET	Common	Benign/low-grade
NET type II	6% of NET	Common	Benign/low-grade
NET type III	10-15% of NET	Uncommon	Moderate
NET type IV	Extremely rare	No	Benign/low-grade
NEC	Rare	No	Malignant
MANEC	Rare	No	Malignant

[a]NET = neuroendocrine tumor; NEC = neuroendocrine carcinoma; MANEC = mixed adenocarcinoma and neuroendocrine carcinoma.

Table 10-2

GASTRIC NEUROENDOCRINE CELL CHARACTERISTICS

Cell Type	Fundus	Antrum	Relative Frequency	Main Secretory Product
ECL	yes	no	40-60%	Histamine
P/D1	yes	yes	10-15%	Ghrelin
D	yes	yes	15-25%	Somatostatin
EC	yes	yes	10-20%	Serotonin
G	no	yes	40-60%	Gastrin

enterochromaffin cells (EC cells); gastrin cells (G cells), somatostatin cells (D cells), and ghrelin-producing cells (P cells) (11,12). These cells are distributed throughout the columnar epithelium. Less commonly, they are scattered in the lamina propria near the base of the gastric glands, in a site-dependent distribution (Table 10-2) (11). The neuroendocrine products secreted by these cells are important regulators of gastrointestinal physiology.

Neuroendocrine cells are most often wedged between the basement membrane and other cells in the epithelium. G cells are preferentially located in the neck and upper gland regions, and are limited to the gastric antrum. They have round nuclei with clear or pale cytoplasm. The other neuroendocrine cells are pyramidal-shaped and contain eosinophilic cytoplasm. Their cytoplasm contains granules that are smaller than Paneth cells. The granules are either dispersed in the cytoplasm diffusely, in a supranuclear location, or concentrated solely beneath the nucleus.

Most endocrine cells of the body and fundus are ECL cells. The second most common are ghrelin-producing cells. In combination these represent more than 50 percent of the neuroendocrine cells of the oxyntic mucosa (11,13,14).

ECL cells are predominantly located in the basal third of the gastric glands and are usually difficult to detect on routine hematoxylin and eosin (H&E)-stained sections. They are located exclusively in the oxyntic mucosa of the stomach.

Gastric neuroendocrine cells are recognized using immunohistochemical stains against general endocrine markers (e.g., chromogranin and synaptophysin). Antibodies against amines or polypeptide products specific to each endocrine cell type, such as somatostatin and ghrelin,

identify particular neuroendocrine cells of the gastric mucosa (13–15).

Ultrastructurally, endocrine cells in antral mucosa have a narrow apex in which the neuroendocrine vesicles open into the gland lumen of the stomach (open type). Neuroendocrine cells in fundic mucosa are of the closed type: they do not secrete their protein into the gastric lumen directly. Each type of endocrine cell contains spherical granules of various size. They have a variably electron-dense core and an average diameter of 150 to 350 nm (11,13,14).

Pathogenesis

Despite the diversity of gastric endocrine cells, most NETs are composed of gastric ECL cells. Prolonged hypergastrinemia is the most important factor contributing to the proliferation of ECL cells and their neoplastic progression.

Common causes of hypergastrinemia include: 1) achlorhydria as a result of autoimmune chronic atrophic gastritis; 2) gastrin-producing NETs (gastrinoma) in the setting of Zollinger-Ellison syndrome (ZES), with or without multiple endocrine neoplasia syndrome type 1 (MEN1); and 3) long-term proton-pump inhibitor (PPI) therapy (16,17). Hypergastrinemia alone is insufficient for the development of NET, since it occurs in the setting of long-term PPI use with no established relationship with the development of NET. The roles of other regulatory factors such as TGFalpha, betaFGF, CCN2, and Reg in the development of gastric NETs is not fully understood (2,18).

Rare cases of gastric NET are composed of cells other than histamine-producing ECL cells. Gastric NETs with G cells are associated with gastrin production and gastrinoma syndrome (19,20). EC cell NETs are associated with serotonin production. P/D1 cell NETs have been noted as well. These rarer cases of NET present as sporadic (type III) lesions (Table 10-3) (3,18,21,22).

Clinical Features

Regardless of the specific type, most patients with gastric NETs are asymptomatic. Nevertheless, nonspecific symptoms such as dyspepsia, vomiting, and abdominal pain (69 percent) are common. Patients may also have heme-positive stools and anemia (72 percent), the most common clinical signs at presentation. Affected individuals may present with symptoms related to the specific underlying pathogenetic condition. For instance, patients who develop type I NET may present with endocrine diseases like pernicious anemia (58 percent), hypothyroidism (39 percent), diabetes (19 percent), Addison disease (6 percent), and hypoparathyroidism (6 percent) (21,23). Some patients, particularly with large NETs, have signs and symptoms of gastric adenocarcinoma, such as loss of appetite, weight loss, and anemia (2,7).

In less than 10 percent of cases, patients with gastric NETs present with a hormone hyperfunction syndrome (flushing, itching, and bronchospasm) related to the release of histamine or bradykinin-related peptides by the tumor. These symptoms are more commonly attributed to the sporadic (type III) NETs, compared to type I or II tumors (24). More specific syndromes, such as Zollinger-Ellison syndrome and adrenocorticotropic hormone (ACTH) production with Cushing syndrome from ectopic corticotropin secretion, have also been reported in some type II and III NETs (20,25,26). The etiopathogenesis and clinical features of the four subtypes of NET are shown in Table 10-4.

Subtypes of NET

Type I ECL Tumor. Type I tumors are the most common type of gastric NET. They represent 46 to 80 percent of all gastric NETs. Type I NETs are much more common in middle-aged females (70 to 80 percent of all patients). Most patients are in the 5th to 7th decades of life at initial presentation (1,7,22,27–29).

These tumors develop exclusively within atrophic body/fundic mucosa, as a consequence of hypochlorhydria and secondary compensatory hypergastrinemia due to autoimmune gastritis (28,29). The frequency of developing gastric NET in patients with autoimmune gastritis ranges from 1.6 to 10.0 percent. In these patients, there is uncontrolled proliferation of ECL cells in the fundus which leads to ECL hyperplasia. Thus, most patients with type I NET show evidence of neuroendocrine cell hyperplasia and dysplasia (see below). Associated clinicopathologic characteristics include antral gastrin cell hyperplasia and increased serum gastrin levels. Corpus mucosal atrophy related to longstanding *H. pylori* infection may be, in rare cases, causative of type I gastric NET (30).

Table 10-3

NEUROENDOCRINE TUMOR (NET): PATHOGENESIS AND CELL TYPE

	Type I	Type II	Type III	Type IV
Pathogenesis	Hypergastrinemia	MEN 1	Sporadic	Sporadic
Cell	ECL	ECL	ECL/others	ECL

ECL = enterochromaffin-like; MEN = multiple endocrine neoplasia.

Table 10-4

CLINICOPATHOLOGIC CHARACTERISTICS OF NEUROENDOCRINE TUMORS

	Type I	Type II	Type III	Type IV
Frequency	70-80%	5%	15-20%	Rare
Demographics	F: 70-80%	Male = Female	Male>Female	?
	50-60 years	Mean age 50	Mean age 55	
Location	Corpus/body	Corpus/body	Anywhere	Corpus/body
Number of NET	Multifocal	Multifocal	Solitary	Multifocal
Size	0.5-1.0 cm	1.5 cm or less	variable	small
Behavior	Low-grade	30% metastasis	71% metastasis over 2 cm	Low-grade

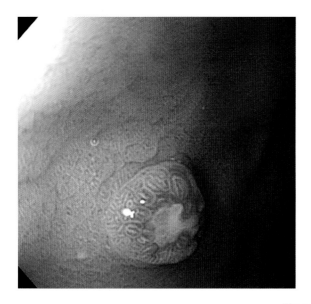 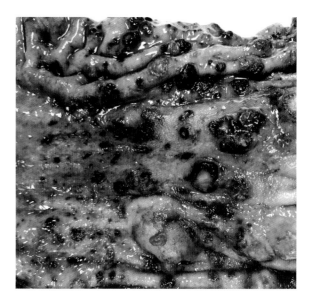

Figure 10-1

NEUROENDOCRINE TUMOR (NET): ENDOSCOPIC AND MACROSCOPIC APPEARANCE

This is a broad-based and well-circumscribed yellowish nodule. The surrounding mucosa is unremarkable, but ulceration of the mucosa is common (left). Types I (right) and II NETs are often multicentric.

Type II NET. Type II NETs are rare. They account for about 6 percent of all gastric NETs. No sex predominance is recognized for patients with this type of NET. Most patients are in the 4th to 7th decades of life at initial presentation (22,29,31).

Type II NETs develop in less than 1 percent of patients with Zollinger-Ellison syndrome, unless associated with MEN1. In one recent large series of MEN1 patients, the incidence of ECL tumors was 23 percent (32). Type II NETs are usually accompanied by hyperchlorhydria, as well as hypergastrinemia. Thus, like type I NET, most patients (53 percent) with type II NET show evidence of advance neuroendocrine cell hyperplasia and dysplasia. Cases of multiple gastric NETs in the setting of MEN1 without hypergastrinemia have been observed (33). Like type I NETs, type II NETs develop almost exclusively in the body fundic mucosa. However, cases of antral tumors have been reported (32,34,35).

Type III NET. Type III gastric NETs are the second most common group. They represent 6 to 21 percent of all gastric NETs and are more common in men (68 percent). Most patients are in the 5th to 7th decades of life at initial presentation (7,27,29,31).

These NETs develop sporadically, and are not associated with hypergastrinemia or any other spe-

cific pathogenetic association or genetic condition. Type III NETs are typically solitary large tumors, with a mean size of 3.2 cm (31). Giant examples measuring up to 10 cm have been reported. Patients present with hematochezia and melena (36).

Type IV NET. Type IV NETs are also gastrin-dependent tumors and extremely rare: only two cases of multiple low-grade gastric NET have been reported. The surrounding oxyntic mucosa is hypertrophic and shows prominent rugae. The oxyntic glands are distended and lined by hyperplastic and vacuolated parietal cells. The suspected pathogenetic mechanism is a failure of the parietal cells to produce HCl, with subsequent achlorhydria and hypergastrinemia. Thus, like type I and type II NET, ECL cell hyperplasia and dysplasia is detected (37,38).

Gross Findings

Endoscopically, most NETs, regardless of the type, appear as broad-based and well-circumscribed yellowish nodules covered by unremarkable normal-appearing mucosa. Most NETs are small, particularly types I and II. Of the former, 77 percent measure less than 1 cm, and 97 percent are less than 1.5 cm (7,22). Multicentricity of tumors is also common for types I, II, and IV NETs (fig. 10-1) (29,35).

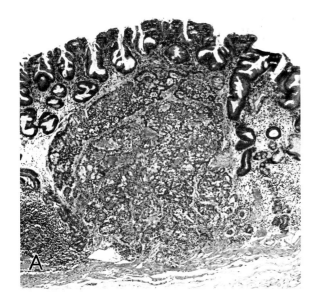

Figure 10-2

NEUROENDOCRINE TUMOR

A: This type I NET is well circumscribed and limited to the mucosa. The adjoining oxyntic mucosa shows features of autoimmune gastritis (parietal cell loss and intestinal metaplasia).

B: A large NET invades the submucosa, with a pushing interface.

C: Type III NET reveals an expansive submucosal invasion pattern with vascular invasion. The adjoining oxyntic mucosa is normal.

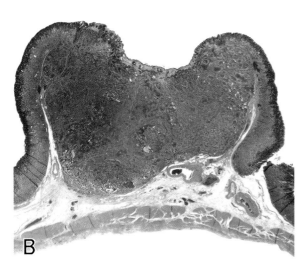

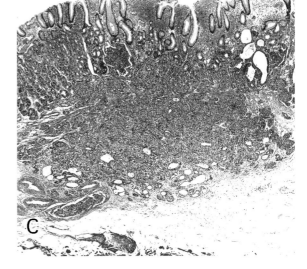

Most NETs, particularly types I and II, involve only the mucosa. Larger tumors may invade the submucosa and even extend into the muscularis propria. Deeply invasive tumors are more commonly observed in type III NETs (fig. 10-2) (21,22,28,39,40).

The features of the background mucosa vary substantially according to the pathogenesis, and thus, the type, of NET. For instance, atrophic gastritis secondary to autoimmune gastritis is associated with type I NETs. Type II NETs arise against a backdrop of hypertrophic mucosa, with grossly apparent prominent rugae which reflect parietal cell hyperplasia secondary to MEN1 or ZES (35). The rare type IV NETs are also associated with hypertrophic corpus mucosa (37,38).

Microscopic Findings

Gastric NETs have a variety of architectural growth patterns, including cellular nests and ribbons, tubules, pseudoglandular rosettes, solid islands, and acinar or trabecular growth, either alone or in combination. Some types, such as type III, often have a more uniform pattern of growth, being formed of broad trabeculae and solid nests of cells (fig. 10-3) (41). Regardless of the growth pattern, the tumor cells are usually found within a loose connective tissue stroma. Desmoplasia is uncommon.

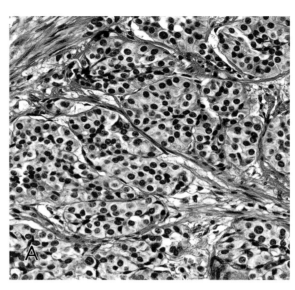

Figure 10-3

GASTRIC NET: GROWTH PATTERNS

Cellular nests (A), broad trabeculae (B), and tubules (C) are evident.

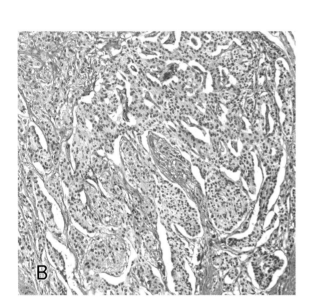

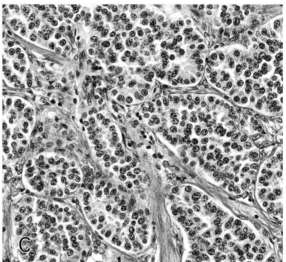

Typical gastric NETs display uniform small polygonal- or cuboidal-shaped cells with pale eosinophilic, finely granular cytoplasm. Focal mucin production is occasionally detected in cases with a typical histologic appearance (fig. 10-4) (42). The nuclei of typical gastric NETs are usually inconspicuous, with regular contours, round or oval shape, and stippled chromatin. Most gastric NETs show only mild cellular atypia. Nuclear polymorphism is rare (fig. 10-5). In some cases, small nucleoli are present, particularly types II and III NETs. In type III NET, round to spindle-shaped cells with large nuclei and prominent nucleoli are more common (41).

There have been several histologic variants described. These include NETs that show plas-macytoid, spindle cell, clear cell, rhabdoid, or anaplastic cellular features (fig. 10-6) (43). Most types of NETs show either no, or only few, mitoses, particularly in type I. Types II and III NETs can show increased mitotic rates (fig. 10-7) (see grading) (41).

Neuroendocrine Hyperplasia and Dysplasia

As discussed above, gastrin-dependent NET types I, II, and IV are typically associated with a background of endocrine cell proliferation in the gastric mucosa. These changes are believed to predispose patients to the development of NET. Neuroendocrine hyperplasia has been separated into four categories (Table 10-5) based on the extent, location, pattern of growth, and size of the

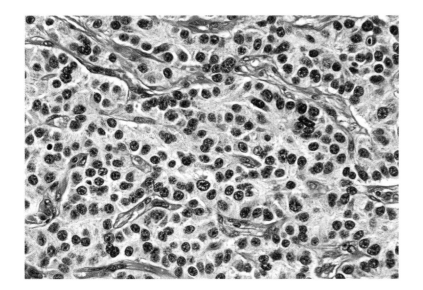

Figure 10-4

GASTRIC NET: HISTOLOGIC FEATURES

This tumor characteristically displays a uniform population of small cuboidal-shaped cells with pale eosinophilic cytoplasm. The nuclei are typically round and show regular contours with stippled chromatin.

Figure 10-5

GASTRIC NET: CELLULAR ATYPIA

A,B: Although uncommon, cellular pleomorphism occurs in a small subset of gastric NETs (A). However, the lesion is a well-differentiated NET since it has a low Ki-67 proliferative index (B).

C: This case also showed focal mucin production.

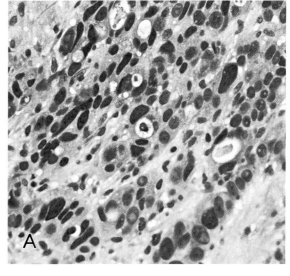

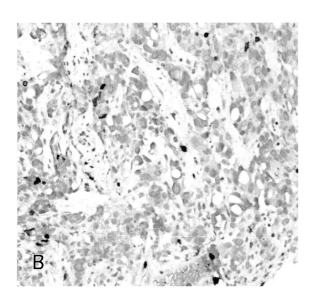

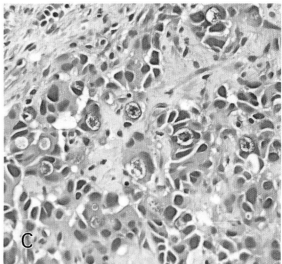

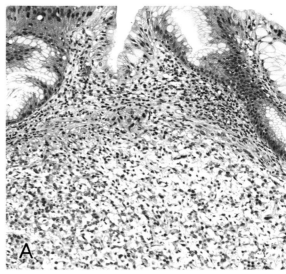

Figure 10-6

GASTRIC NET: CLEAR CELL VARIANT

Synaptophysin is positive in C.

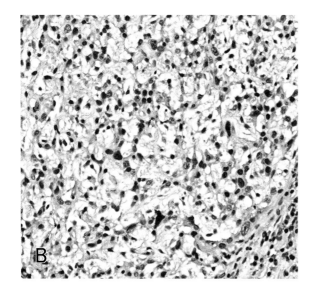

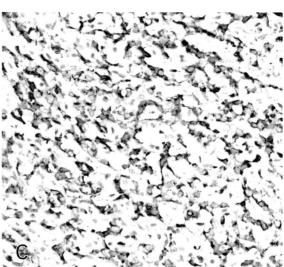

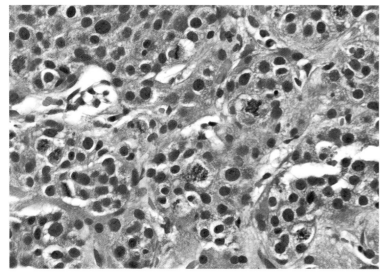

Figure 10-7

GASTRIC NET: HIGH MITOTIC INDEX

This tumor showed a high mitotic rate and would be classified as NEC per the 2010 World Health Organization (WHO) classification. Some data, however, suggest that well-differentiated NETs with a high mitotic rate confer a better prognosis than NEC and thus, should be classified as a grade 3 NET.

Table 10-5

CLASSIFICATION OF PROLIFERATION OF ECL NEUROENDOCRINE CELLS

Terminology	Definition	Distribution	Size
Simple ECL[a]-cell hyperplasia	Generalized increase of scattered cells	Epithelium	–
Linear ECL-cell hyperplasia	≤5 cells in single-file pattern	Epithelium	–
Micronodular ECL-cell hyperplasia	Cluster of 5 or more cells	Epithelium or lamina propria	30-150 μm
Adenomatoid hyperplasia	Expansion and fusion of 5 or more micronodular hyperplastic nodules	Lamina propria	
Dysplasia	Expansile nodules of variable growth pattern	Lamina propria	>150 μm but ≤500 μm
Intramucosal NET	Expansile nodules	Lamina propria	>500 μm

[a]ECL = enterochromaffin-like; NET = neuroendocrine tumor.

lesions (6). The true risk of neoplastic transformation for each category of proliferation has not been fully determined; thus, to date, it remains a system of limited clinical utility. However, one large series of patients with autoimmune gastritis (n=100) reported a rate of neoplastic transformation of 25 percent in patients with ECL cell dysplasia but a rate of 2.5 percent in patients with ECL cell hyperplasia during a median follow-up of 90 months (44). The risk was highest in patients with ECL cell microinvasive dysplastic lesions of the glandular proliferative type.

A six-biopsy protocol, with sampling of the antrum (x2 biopsies) and oxyntic mucosa (x4 biopsies from corpus and fundus), has been recommended to fully assess the precursor changes in patients with corpus-predominant atrophic gastritis and elevated gastrin levels. Although the risk of developing NETs in patient with ECL cell dysplasia is recognized, the amplitude of the risk has not been fully evaluated and there are no generally accepted surveillance guidelines for this category of precursor lesion.

The four categories of hyperplasia include: *simple ECL cell hyperplasia, linear ECL cell hyperplasia, micronodular ECL cell hyperplasia*, and *adenomatoid hyperplasia* (Table 10-5). ECL cell hyperplasia represents groups of cells, which can either be limited by the basement membrane or present within the lamina propria. Simple (diffuse) hyperplasia is characterized by a generalized increased of neuroendocrine cells scattered within the epithelium. Linear (or chain-forming) hyperplasia is defined as the presence of a minimum of five neuroendocrine

cells in a single-file pattern, within the epithelium and limited by the basement membrane. Micronodular hyperplasia is defined as a cluster of five or more cells, measuring 30 to 150 μm, either limited by the basement membrane or present within the lamina propria.

Adenomatoid hyperplasia is the expansion and fusion of five or more micronodular hyperplastic nodules. *Neuroendocrine dysplasia* is arbitrarily defined as nodules of neuroendocrine cells that measure over 150 μm but less than 500 μm. The growth patterns of dysplastic foci are variable. Intramucosal lesions greater than 0.5 mm in diameter are considered intramucosal NET, by convention. Regardless of the size or pattern of growth, the presence of submucosal extension defines an invasive NET (fig. 10-8) (27,45,46).

The surrounding gastric oxyntic mucosa can offer additional diagnostic clues with regard to the pathogenesis of NET. Type I NETs are associated with features of autoimmune atrophic gastritis, i.e., pyloric and intestinal metaplasia. These changes are not observed at the periphery of type II NETs, which instead, are surrounded by elongated foveolae with hypertrophic oxyntic glands and parietal cell hyperplasia characteristic of Zollinger-Ellison syndrome. Notably, the mucosa surrounding type III NETs is devoid of gastrin-dependent ECL cell hyperplasia. Parietal cell hyperplasia and hypertrophy are noted in the vicinity of type IV NETs (37,38). In those cases, however, the parietal cells are vacuolated, and show protrusion of their cytoplasm into oxyntic glands containing inspissated eosinophilic material.

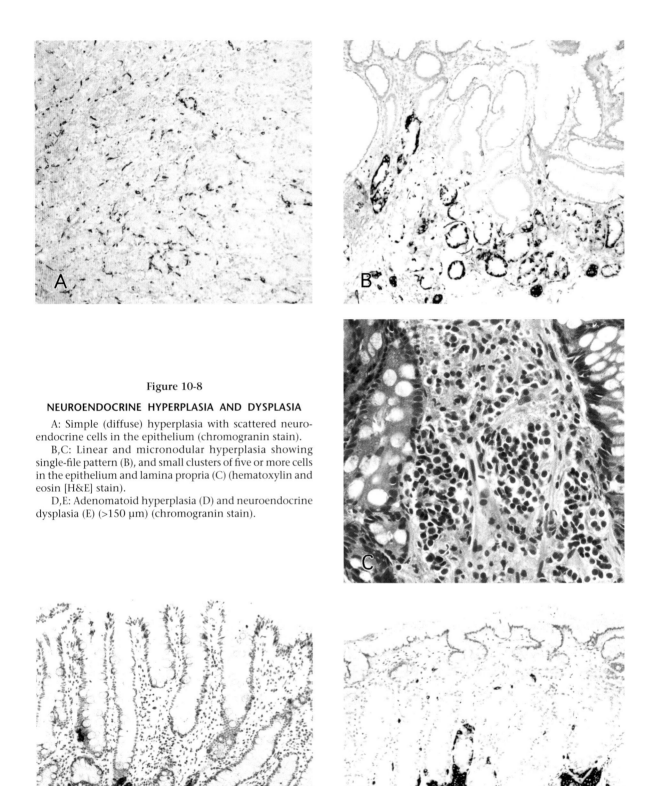

Figure 10-8

NEUROENDOCRINE HYPERPLASIA AND DYSPLASIA

A: Simple (diffuse) hyperplasia with scattered neuroendocrine cells in the epithelium (chromogranin stain).

B,C: Linear and micronodular hyperplasia showing single-file pattern (B), and small clusters of five or more cells in the epithelium and lamina propria (C) (hematoxylin and eosin [H&E] stain).

D,E: Adenomatoid hyperplasia (D) and neuroendocrine dysplasia (E) (>150 μm) (chromogranin stain).

Grading

The histologic grading of gastric NETs is based on the mitotic activity and Ki-67 proliferative index, both of which have shown correlation with prognosis (9). More specifically, the mitotic count should be evaluated per area of mucosa measuring 2 mm^2 (10 high-power fields) in the region of highest mitotic activity. The Ki-67 index should be established after counting 500 to 2000 tumor cells in the areas of highest nuclear labeling (Table 10-6). When discrepancies exist between the mitotic rate and the Ki-67 index, the highest grade of the two should be used to grade the NET.

Most gastric NETs are grade 1, or at most, grade 2. Rare cases show well-differentiated morphology but with a high mitotic activity or Ki-67 index. These tumors should be classified as well-differentiated (G3) NETs, since several studies have revealed a better prognosis than for neuroendocrine carcinoma (NEC) (9).

Immunohistochemical Findings

Gastric neuroendocrine tumors are most frequently positive for chromogranin A, but not necessarily for chromogranin B. Synaptophysin is positive in about 50 percent of cases. Leu-7, PGP 9.5, and carcinoembryonic antigen (CEA) are positive in most cases as well. Vesicular monoamine transporter type 2 (VMAT-2) is a specific marker of ECL cells (47). Although these tumors may also contain histamine and histidine decarboxylase, these are difficult to demonstrate in routinely fixed tissue sections.

Other peptide hormones, such as serotonin, histamine, gastrin, somatostatin, pancreatic polypeptide, glucagon, calcitonin, alpha-human chorionic gonadotropin (HCG), and ACTH, can be detected in NET, but are usually only present as a minor component of the tumor (fig. 10-9) (48,49).

Molecular Genetic Findings

Frequent loss of heterozygosity (LOH) of the *MEN1* locus is recognized in type I and type II gastric NETs. The much lower rate in type III is suggestive of different genetic mechanisms (50). When evaluating a panel of three genes including *CgA, MAGE-D2,* and *MTA1* some investigators were able to segregate the different subtypes of gastric neuroendocrine neoplasms

Table 10-6

HISTOLOGIC GRADING OF GASTRIC NEUROENDOCRINE TUMORS

Grade	Definition
Grade 1	Mitotic count/10 HPF[a]: <2; Ki-67: <3%
Grade 2	Mitotic count/10 HPF: 2 – 20; Ki-67: 3-20%
Grade 3	Mitotic count/10 HPF: >20; Ki-67: >20%

[a]HPF = high-power fields.

(51). Type III NETs and NECs were differentiated from less aggressive type I/II tumors by higher levels of *CgA*, and the expression of *MAGE-D2* and *MTA1*. Furthermore, protein expression of MTA1 was associated with tumor invasion. Mutation of *REG1A*, a gene implicated in the cell cycle regulation of ECL cells, has also been reported in type I NET (52). Several miRNAs, including miR-202-3p, have been reported to be upregulated in type I NET and may target *DUSP1* (53).

Differential Diagnosis

In most instances, gastric NETs do not represent a diagnostic problem. There are few neoplasms that show a proliferation of round to oval neoplastic cells with scant cytoplasm, round nuclei, and inconspicuous nucleoli that can mimic gastric NET. These include melanoma, glomus tumor, epithelioid gastrointestinal stromal tumor, lymphoma, and metastatic carcinoma, particularly of breast origin. In each, attention to specific microscopic details, evaluation of clinical history, review of endoscopic images, and appropriate use of immunohistochemistry help yield a correct diagnosis (Table 10-7).

Spread and Metastasis

Most gastric NETs are slow-growing, locally infiltrative, low-grade neoplasms. Size and invasiveness correlate best with the probability of metastases. For instance, NETs less than 1 cm in diameter, and limited to the mucosa or submucosa, usually remain stable over the course of many years. They only rarely show lymphovascular invasion, and even more rarely distant metastases (22,29).

Lymph node metastases are observed in up to 6 percent of cases of type I NET. Distant metastases are uncommon, unless associated with large lesions with deep invasion. As a result, type

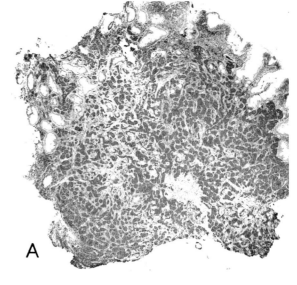

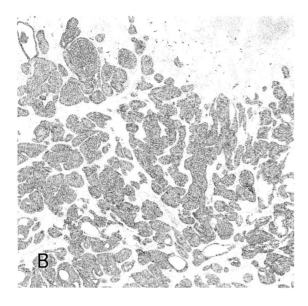

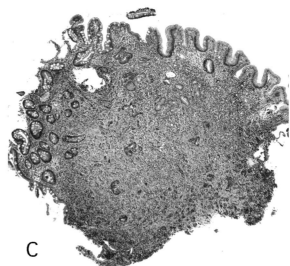

Figure 10-9

GASTRIC NET: IMMUNOHISTOCHEMISTRY

A: The use of neuroendocrine markers like synaptophysin facilitates diagnosis at low-power examination.

B: Synaptophysin is the most sensitive immunohistochemical stain for gastric NET.

C: This type 1 NET is associated with loss of parietal cells and intestinal metaplasia in the overlying gastric mucosa.

I NETs are usually associated with excellent long-term survival (fig. 10-10) (22,29).

Type II NETs more frequently present with submucosal invasion, and as a result, metastases are more common. Metastases occur in 12 to 15 percent of cases (21,22).

Type III NETs are usually deeply invasive neoplasms, and are more likely to spread, usually to regional lymph nodes and liver. The risk of metastasis correlates best with the size of the NET, but small tumors can metastasize as well. At diagnosis, 15 percent of patients with type III NETs present with local spread. Metastases have been recorded in 24 to 61 percent of cases (51). The 5-year survival rate is higher for those with localized disease (64.3 percent) and those with local metastases (regional lymph nodes) (29.9 percent) than those with distant metastases (10 percent). The degree of cellular atypia, high mitotic rate, angioinvasion, and deep invasion correlate with aggressive behavior (2,4,22,29,54).

TNM Staging

The 2017 American Joint Commission on Cancer (AJCC) developed a specific system to be used uniquely for NETs of grade 1 and grade 2, and the rare well-differentiated grade 3. NEC and mixed adenocarcinoma-neuroendocrine carcinoma (MANEC) are staged according to the gastric cancer protocol (see chapter 9).

Table 10-7

DIFFERENTIAL DIAGNOSIS OF GASTRIC NEUROENDOCRINE TUMORS

	SYN[a] CHR, CD56	CK, CAM5.2	LCA CD20, CD3	HMB-45 SOX10	GATA3 Mammoglobin	CD117 DOG1
Melanoma	(-) (rare CD56 positivity)	(-)	(-)	(+)	(-)	(-)
Glomus tumor	(+)/(-)	(-)	(-)	(-)	(-)	(-)
Epithelioid GIST	(-)	(-)	(-)	( )	(-)	(+)
Large cell lymphoma	(-)	(-)	(+)	(-)	(-)	(-)
Metastatic breast ca	(-)	(+)	(-)	(-)	(+)	(-)

[a]SYN = synaptophysin; CHR = chromogranin; CK = cytokeratin; LCA = leukocyte common antigen; GIST = gastrointestinal stromal tumor; Ca = carcinoma.

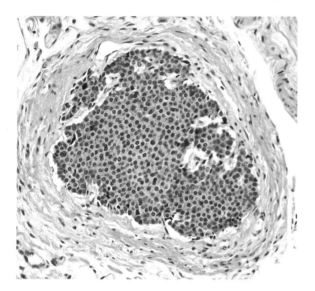
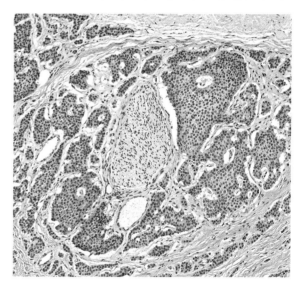

Figure 10-10

AGGRESSIVE NET

This NET measured over 1 cm and involved the deeper layers of the gastric wall. It shows lymphovascular (left) and perineural (right) invasion.

Table 10-8 presents the definition of T (primary tumor) and N (regional lymph node) classification (9). The m prefix is used when multiple tumors are identified and the pT assessed on the most advanced. The r prefix is used for recurrent tumor after a post-treatment disease-free interval (rTNM).

Although not yet universally endorsed, the 2017 AJCC suggests the evaluation of serologic markers, i.e., gastrin and chromogranin A, in addition to the traditional pathologic prognostic markers. Normal serum gastrin level is associated with a worse prognosis (22). Elevated chromogranin A serum level is an indicator of poor prognosis (55).

Treatment

Given the heterogeneity of gastric NETs, it is not surprising that the treatment of patients is highly dependent on the specific subtype. In patients with type I NET, the major goal is to assure removal of the lesion(s). Patients are then followed by endoscopic surveillance and extirpation of new lesions as they arise (1). Conservative endoscopic management (i.e., endoscopic polypectomy, endoscopic mucosal resection, endoscopic submucosal/mucosal dissection) is advocated over surgical resection whenever possible.

The typical proposed size cutoff for recommending surgical resection over endoscopic resection is 2 cm, since the risk of metastasis is limited (56). When surgery is performed, two types of procedures are usually considered. Antrectomy is the treatment of choice to remove the antral G cells that provide the hypergastrinemic drive. This is done when the lesions are too large or too numerous to be effectively managed by endoscopy. Reduction of hypergastrinemia induces a dramatic decrease in ECL proliferation, sometimes with complete disappearance of hyperplastic changes, as well as in one report, of the NET tumors (57).

In rare cases of type II NET, management is based on excising the gastrin-producing tumor (duodenal or pancreatic) in the context of MEN1 syndrome. Local or limited resection of gastric lesions is usually recommended (1).

Type III NETs represent a different therapeutic challenge. Several authorities have proposed endoscopic resection of small lesions. Nevertheless, surgical resection remains the treatment of choice, including partial or total gastrectomy with lymph node dissection. Adjuvant therapy is used for patients with metastatic disease. The various options include somatostatin analogs, radiolabeled somatostatin analogs, mTOR inhibitors, and the tyrosine kinase inhibitor sunitinib (58).

Prognosis

Patients with type I NET have an excellent prognosis, with reports of recurrence-free survival rates of 100 percent about 2 years postresection. The 5- and 10-year survival rates are reported at 96 and 74 percent, respectively (1,29), figures identical to those for the general population. Metastases, however, are reported (in up to 2 percent of the cases), as is tumor-related death (29).

The outcome of patients with type II NET is more difficult to assess since it is linked to the outcome of gastrinemia. Recurrence-free survival 71 months post diagnosis of type II is recorded (29).

The prognosis of patients with type III NET is more guarded, with 25 percent dead within 26 months. At diagnosis, 15 percent of patients with type III NET have local spread and close to half have hepatic metastases. The 5-year survival rate is higher for those with localized disease (64.3 percent) and those with regional metastases (29.9 percent) than those with distant metastases (10 percent). The 5-year and 10-year

Table 10-8

AMERICAN JOINT COMMISSION ON CANCER TNM STAGING OF GASTRIC NEUROENDOCRINE TUMORS

T0	No evidence of tumor
T1	Tumor limited to lamina propria or submucosa and <1 cm in size
T2	Tumor invades the muscularis propria or >1 cm in size
T3	Tumor invades into subserosal tissue without penetration of overlying serosa
T4	Tumor invades the serosa or other organs
N0	Negative regional lymph nodes
N1	Positive regional lymph nodes
M0	No distant metastasis
M1a	Hepatic metastasis
M1b	Metastasis to extrahepatic organ(s)
M1c	Hepatic and extrahepatic metastasis

survival rates after diagnosis are reported at 33 and 22 percent, respectively (2,4,29,54).

NEUROENDOCRINE CARCINOMA

Neuroendocrine carcinoma (NEC) of the stomach is a malignant tumor composed of cells with neuroendocrine differentiation exclusively. NECs are rare and represent a group of heterogeneous high-grade neoplasms associated with a dismal prognosis. There are two main morphologic variants: small cell and large cell types. In addition, a substantial number of NECs is associated with a traditional adenocarcinoma component, which suggests a genetic link. These tumors are termed mixed adenocarcinoma-neuroendocrine carcinoma (MANEC) when either component exceeds 30 percent of the tumor volume (3).

General Features

NECs are rare sporadic neoplasms. They account for up to 1.5 percent of all gastric cancers, and represent 6 to 16 percent of all gastric endocrine neoplasms (31,59–61). The clinical and demographic characteristics of MANECs are similar to those of NECs (31,59,61–65).

Pathogenesis

The overwhelming majority of gastric NECs develops in the absence of hypergastrinemia. Compared to type I and II gastrin-dependent

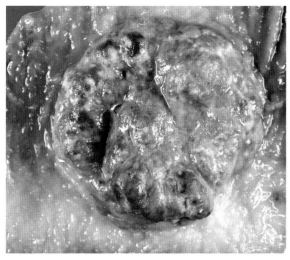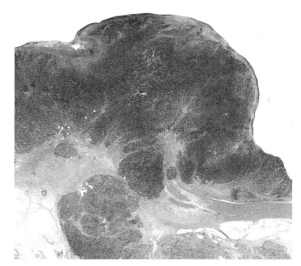

Figure 10-11

NEUROENDOCRINE CARCINOMA (NEC)

Left: A fungating mass projects into the gastric lumen.
Right: Low-power view displays transmural infiltration.

NETs, the overexpression of p53, the diverse genetic background, and the frequent detection of foci of adenocarcinoma suggest a different pathogenesis from NET related to hypergastrinemia, but possibly one that is closer to that of type III NETs and even adenocarcinoma (59). Some cases are associated with well-differentiated NETs associated with autoimmune gastritis or MEN1/ZES, suggesting a potential for progression from these neoplasms in some cases (6,66,67).

An immunohistochemical evaluation of exocrine markers, including MUC5AC, human gastric mucin, MUC6, MUC2, and CDX2 concluded that gastric NETs (G1 and G2) and NECs have different carcinogenesis, and that the latter may develop from a preexisting adenocarcinoma (68). The conclusion was based on the lack of expression of exocrine markers except CDX2 in NET cases and their presence in NEC cases (86.5 percent). Double immunohistochemistry revealed dual expression of CDX2 and chromogranin A in 50 percent of the NEC cases.

Clinical Features

NECs usually present as large and symptomatic neoplasm. The patients may complain of epigastric pain or present with gastrointestinal bleeding or weight loss. In practice, NECs cannot normally be differentiated from gastric adenocarcinoma prior to microscopic analysis. However, rare cases of hyperfunctioning gastric NEC, including one with heterotopic Cushing syndrome, have been reported (29).

Gastric NECs occur in both sexes, but are more common in males (72 to 80 percent) compared to females (20 to 28 percent) (61,62,65,69). Most affected patients are in the 6th to 7th decades of life, with a range from 35 to 86 years.

Gross Findings

NECs and MANECs develop in any portion of the stomach, but are more frequent in the upper third, where over 40 percent of cases occur (61,63). Other series have reported NECs in the body and antrum in 42.6 and 38.3 percent of cases, respectively (64).

Gastric NECs have a mean size of 5.0 to 6.4 cm, but some are much larger (over 13 cm) (61,64). In most cases, NECs present as solitary tumors; however, two concurrent lesions have been reported in up to 12.5 percent of patients in a series of 16 cases (59).

NECs display various gross characteristics. Most develop as fungating masses that project into the gastric lumen (Borrmann type 2) and represent 46 to 64 percent of cases. Ulcerated tumors (Borrmann type 3) are also common (16 to 20 percent of the cases) (fig. 10-11) (61).

Figure 10-12

NEC: GROWTH PATTERN

These tumors are commonly composed of either sheets (A) or nests (B) of cells. A trabecular pattern (C) is common.

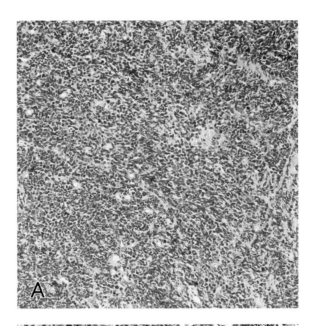

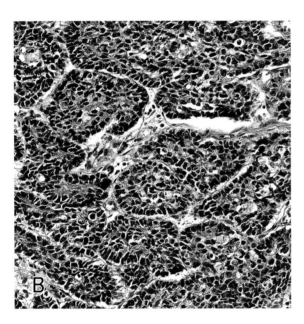

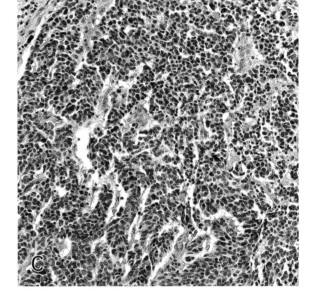

Microscopic Findings

The majority of NECs show a solid growth pattern (94 percent) composed of either nests or sheets of cells with a homogeneous appearance. A trabecular pattern occurs in 18 percent of cases. Scirrhous and tubular growth patterns are less common, seen in less than 10 percent of NECs. Up to one third of cases show more than one growth pattern (fig. 10-12) (62).

NECs are composed of anaplastic cellular elements that range in shape from round to polyhedral and spindled with scant cytoplasm.

Mitoses and apoptosis are normally conspicuous. One study reported a median mitotic count of 42 per 10 high-power fields (range, 11 to 198 per 10 high-power fields) (62). Necrosis, particularly multifocal, is common and is observed in nearly all cases at least focally. In some cases, abundant geographic necrosis is observed (fig. 10-13) (62).

Depending on the size of the cell types and the amount of cytoplasm, small and large cells may be present. This morphologic diversity occasionally makes a diagnosis difficult to establish. To date, the clinical significance of this histologic subclassification has not been validated (70).

296

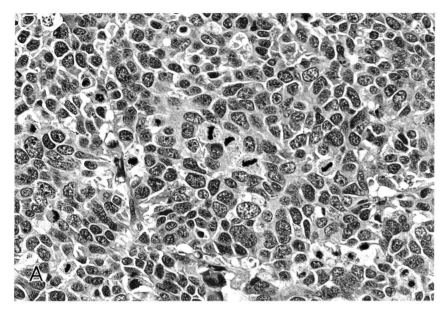

Figure 10-13

NEC: HISTOLOGIC FEATURES

A: These tumors are char-acteristically composed of anaplastic cells with scant cytoplasm and high nuclear/cytoplasmic (N/C) ratio. Mitoses and apoptosis are normally conspicuous.

B,C: Necrosis is also common (B) and can be marked (C).

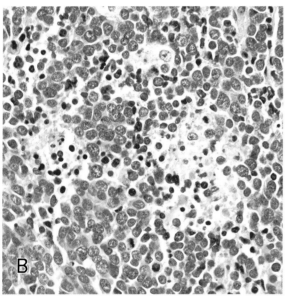

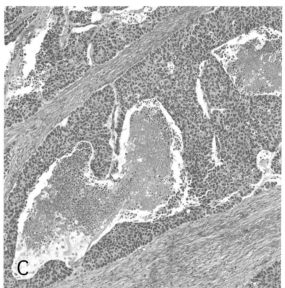

Large Cell NECs. Large cell NEC is the most common type of gastric NEC. Up to 85 percent of NECs are of the large cell type. The tumors are defined by the presence large polygonal-shaped cells with enlarged vesicular nuclei and prominent nucleoli. The cytoplasm is usually abundant. They are prone to form organoid structures, a feature that suggests neuroendocrine differentiation. Rosettes and pseudorosettes are common (45 percent of cases), but are rare in small cell NECs (62–64). Mucin droplets are detected in 57 percent of cases, which reinforces the possibility of a histogenetic link with gastric adenocarcinoma (fig. 10-14) (61).

Small Cells NECs. Small cell NECs are characterized by cells with high nuclear/cytoplasmic (N/C) ratios and scant cytoplasm. They represent 15 to 39 percent of NECs. Nuclear molding is common, observed in over 90 percent of cases, but in less than 20 percent of the large cell variant (62–64). Both histologic variants are usually mixed: in one study, 63 percent of small cell NECs contained a large cell component (fig. 10-15) (62).

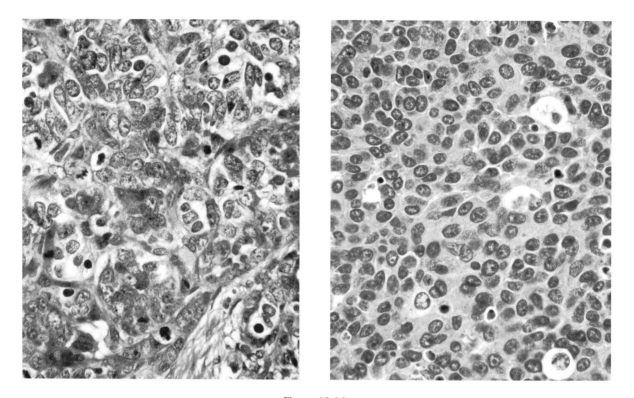

Figure 10-14

LARGE CELL NEC

Left: Large cell NECs are composed of large polygonal-shaped cells with abundant cytoplasm. Enlarged vesicular nuclei and prominent nucleoli are common.

Right: Pseudorosettes are also common.

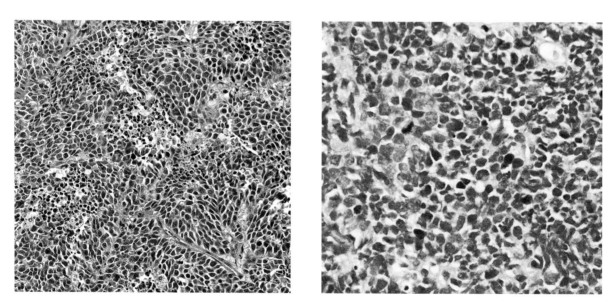

Figure 10-15

SMALL CELL NEC

Left: Small cell NECs are characterized by cells with a high N/C ratio.

Right: Scant cytoplasm and nuclear molding are common.

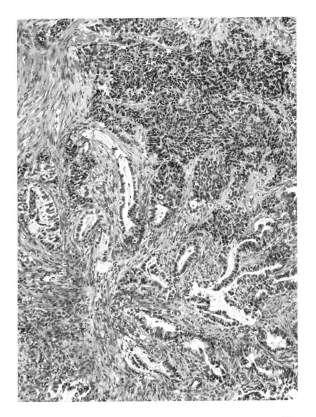 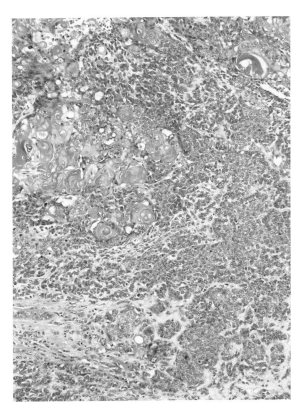

Figure 10-16

MIXED ADENOCARCINOMA AND NEUROENDOCRINE CARCINOMA (MANEC)

Left: This case is a combination of a large cell NEC and adenocarcinoma.
Right: Some cases of gastric NEC show squamous differentiation (top of image).

Similar to gastric adenocarcinoma, the background mucosa surrounding NECs may be unremarkable, or show chronic atrophic gastritis and intestinal metaplasia. In most cases, ECL cell hyperplasia is not detected at the periphery of NEC.

Composite Tumors

Composite tumors, which are defined as tumors composed of both neuroendocrine and non-neuroendocrine epithelial elements, are common: 71 percent of NECs are associated with adenocarcinoma or epithelial dysplasia. MANECs (mixed adenocarcinoma and neuroendocrine carcinomas) contain at least 30 percent of one of the components. They are rare in the stomach. The neuroendocrine component is usually composed of large cells, but rarely, of NET. MANEC expresses neuroendocrine markers in the NEC component, similar to pure NEC. The exocrine component of MANEC is usually composed of an adenocarcinoma, which may be well, moderately, or poorly differentiated. In a recent series of MANECs, the adenocarcinoma component was poorly differentiated in most cases (80 percent). Moderately differentiated adenocarcinomas or a signet ring cell component are less common (10 percent) (fig. 10-16) (61–64,71).

Histologic Grading

NECs are poorly differentiated by definition.

Immunohistochemical Findings

NECs are typically reactive for general neuroendocrine markers, such as chromogranin A, synaptophysin, CD56, neural cell adhesion molecule (N-CAM), protein gene product 9.5 (PGP9.5), and neuron-specific enolase (NSE). Other peptide hormones, such as serotonin, ghrelin, peptide YY, somatostatin, and gastrin may be demonstrated (3,70,71).

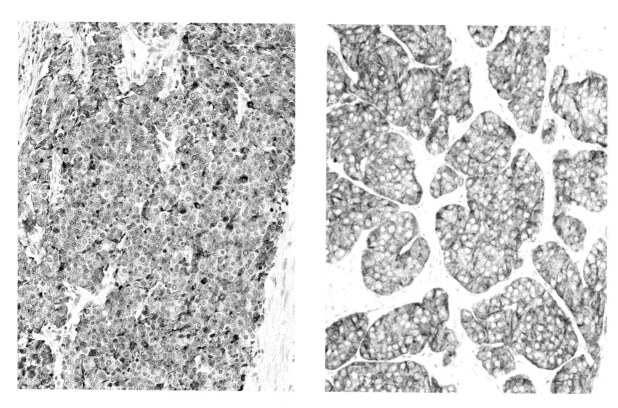

Figure 10-17

NEC: IMMUNOHISTOCHEMISTRY

Chromogranin A (left) is the most specific marker, whereas synaptophysin is the most sensitive (right).

Chromogranin A and synaptophysin are sensitive markers of neuroendocrine differentiation. Synaptophysin, the most reliable marker, is positive in 94 to 98 percent of the cases. Chromogranin A (64 to 86 percent) and CD56 (47 to 60 percent) are less sensitive, although 96 percent of cases express either or both in a diffuse fashion. Some authors advocate the use of these two markers for first-line screening of neuroendocrine differentiation, and CD56 as an additional marker, since few NECs are positive for CD56 only. There is no immunohistochemical difference between the large cell and the small cell types of NECs. TTF-1, used for the identification of metastatic carcinomas of pulmonary and thyroid gland origin, is aberrantly expressed in up to 37 percent of gastric NECs as well as other gastrointestinal NECs (fig. 10-17) (62,65).

Novel neuroendocrine markers, such as ASH1 and NKX2.2, have been recently investigated in NECs. ASH1 is a transcription factor. It plays a role in neuronal/neuroendocrine cell differentiation during development. It has been suggested to be more sensitive than conventional neuroendocrine markers, although it was expressed in only 40 percent of all gastric NECs in one study. NKX2.2 is another transcription factor important for differentiation of pancreatic islet cells. It was reported in 83 percent of neuroendocrine tumors of gastrointestinal origin (62,72,73), although one study reported expression in less than half of all gastric NECs.

Molecular Genetic Findings

Genome-wide molecular studies have shown differences between low-grade and high-grade NETs. Somatic mutations of *BRAF*, *PIK3CA*, *PTEN*, and *WNT*, among others, have been reported in NEC, but not in well-differentiated NET (74). Gastric NECs show a high rate of loss of heterozygosity (LOH) of chromosomes 8p, 15q, 17p, 11p, 12p (50 percent), and 13q (50 percent) and chromosomal abnormalities involving *TP53* (the most frequent), *SMAD4* (18q), and *MEN1*, with a higher frequency of allelic imbalances than in NETs (75,76).

Table 10-9

DIFFERENTIAL DIAGNOSIS OF NEUROENDOCRINE CARCINOMA

	SYN [a] CHR, CD56	CK7/CK20 CAM5.2	CK5/6 P40/P63	LCA CD20, CD3	S-100 Protein SOX10	GATA3 Mammoglobin
Melanoma	(-)	(+)/(-)	(-)	(-)	(+)	(-)
Undiff ca	(-)	(+) (variable)	(-)	(-)	(-)	(-)
Poorly diff SCC	(-)	(-)	(+)	(-)	(-)	(-)
Large cell lymphoma	(-)	(-)	(-)	(+) (variable)	(-)	(-)
Metastatic breast ca	(-)	(+)	(-)	(-)	(-)	(+)

[a]SYN = synaptophysin; CHR = chromogranin; CK = cytokeratin; LCA = leukocyte common antigen; SCC = squamous cell carcinoma; Undiff = undifferentiated; ca = carcinoma.

Data on gastric MANEC indicate a relatively higher frequency of chromosomal abnormalities in the NEC component than the adenocarcinoma component. Shared LOH at chromosomes 5q, 11q, 17p, and 18q, however, suggests a close genetic relationship (77).

Some studies have shown that SV40 TAg is capable of inducing a neuroendocrine gene signature in gastric carcinomas of some transgenic mice, an oncogenic effect that seems to be related to inactivation of the tumor suppressor proteins p53 and RB1. Interestingly, alterations of these proteins is a common event in human NECs, suggesting again similarity with gastric adenocarcinoma (78).

Microsatellite instability (MSI) is noted in 36 percent of gastric NEC/MANECs with methylation-mediated silencing of the *MLH1* gene. Loss of MLH1 and PMS2 occurs in tumor development. MSI status imparts a more favorable prognosis than microsatellite stability in NEC/MANECs. MSI status is an independent prognostic factor at multivariable analysis together with vascular invasion (79).

Differential Diagnosis

The limited awareness of gastric NECs, their undifferentiated high-grade morphology, and the frequent admixture with adenocarcinoma, may lead to their misdiagnosis as poorly differentiated adenocarcinoma. Lymphoma, metastatic malignant melanoma, and even poorly differentiated squamous cell carcinoma should be considered when the morphology is atypical. In these cases, judicious use of immunohistochemistry usually leads to the proper diagnosis of these neoplasms (Table 10-9).

Spread and Metastases

In a series of 47 patients with NEC, pT1 and pT2 tumors represented 14.9 and 23.4 percent, respectively, whereas pT3 and pT4 tumors constituted 44.7 and 17.0 percent at the time of initial presentation (64). In another series of 51 NECs, early cancers represented 9.75 percent of the cases (61).

Lymphatic and vascular involvement are common in NEC. Lymphatic invasion is detected in 73 to 89 percent and vascular invasion in 78 percent of gastric NECs. Perineural invasion is less common (36.2 percent). The prevalence of lymphatic and venous invasion in NECs is higher than that reported for gastric adenocarcinomas (56.2 and 41.0 percent of cases, respectively) (fig. 10-18) (62,64,80).

Twenty seven to 35.3 percent of patients present with metastases at the time of diagnosis. Lymph node metastasis occurs in 59.5 to 88.0 percent of cases. The rate of liver metastasis ranges from 27 to 77 percent of cases. Other reported sites of metastases include peritoneum and lung/pleura (29,61,62,64,69,81).

Staging

NEC and MANEC are staged according to the classification used for gastric adenocarcinoma (see chapter 9) (82).

Treatment

Gastrectomy with lymphadenectomy is the first therapeutic approach when it can be tolerated by the patient. Platinum-based combination chemotherapy is also commonly used

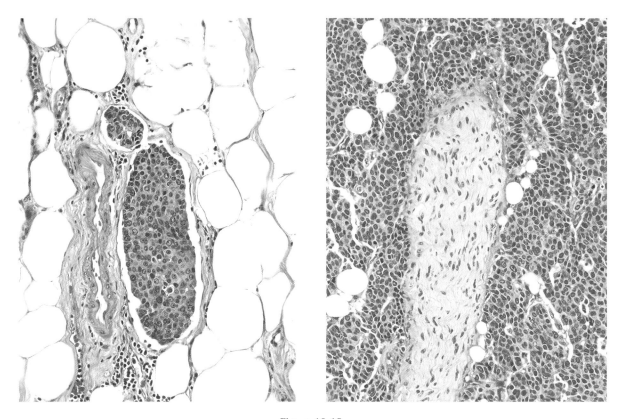

Figure 10-18

NEUROENDOCRINE CARCINOMA

Lymphovascular invasion is common in NEC (left), as is perineural invasion (right).

as a first-line treatment for gastric NEC. Combination irinotecan and cisplatin, and amrubicin monotherapy have also been used. As salvage therapy, second-line use of FOLFOX has been proposed. Thus far, the therapeutic efficacy has been poor (83–85).

Prognosis

NEC presents at an advanced stage and is associated with a poor prognosis. Stage I tumors represent only 25.5 percent of cases, while stage II, III and IV represent 32 to 40.5 percent, 12 to 34 percent, and 25 to 27 percent of all NECs, respectively (61,62,64).

The 3- and 5-year survival rates are 57.8 and 44.7 percent, respectively, after a median follow-up period of 30 months. A lower 5-year survival rate of 34.7 percent has been reported for a series of large cells NECs. Patients who have undergone curative surgery have a significantly better out-come than those without curative surgery (mean overall survival of 21 months) (61,62).

Due to the rarity of gastric NECs, few studies have examined the prognostic value of specific histologic subtypes. Ishida (62) showed no significant survival difference between patients with large cell NECs and small cell NECs, or between those with NECs and MANECs. Interestingly, Shia et al. (80) reported that the absence of an associated adenocarcinoma component was predictive of poorer disease-specific survival. Alternatively, the significance of immunohistochemical evidence of neuroendocrine differentiation below the 30 percent cutoff value to establish a diagnosis of MANEC is controversial. Several series have indicated that a threshold of 20 percent, or even as low as 10 percent, may be clinically significant since it is associated with a worse prognosis (61,62,64).

REFERENCES

1. Delle Fave G, O'Toole D, Sundin A, et al. ENETS Consensus Guidelines Update for Gastroduodenal Neuroendocrine Neoplasms. Neuroendocrinology 2016;103:119-24.
2. Modlin IM, Kidd M, Latich I, Zikusoka MN, Shapiro MD. Current status of gastrointestinal carcinoids. Gastroenterology 2005;128:1717-51.
3. Solcia E. Neuroendocrine neoplasms of the stomach. WHO classification of tumours of the digestive system. Lyon: IARC Press; 2010:64-8.
4. Modlin IM, Lye KD, Kidd M. A 5-decade analysis of 13,715 carcinoid tumors. Cancer 2003;97:934-59.
5. Yao JC, Hassan M, Phan A, et al. One hundred years after "carcinoid": epidemiology of and prognostic factors for neuroendocrine tumors in 35,825 cases in the United States. J Clin Oncol 2008;26:3063-72.
6. La Rosa S, Vanoli A. Gastric neuroendocrine neoplasms and related precursor lesions. J Clin Pathol 2014;67:938-48.
7. Modlin IM, Lye KD, Kidd M. Carcinoid tumors of the stomach. Surg Oncol 2003;12:153-72.
8. Godwin JD 2nd. Carcinoid tumors. An analysis of 2,837 cases. Cancer 1975;36:560-9.
9. Woltering EA, Bergsland EK, Beyer DT, et al. Neuroendocrine tumors of the stomach. In: Amin MB, Edge S, Greene F, et al., eds. AJCC cancer staging manual. 2017:351-9.
10. Modlin IM, Kidd M, Latich I, Zikusoka MN, Shapiro MD. Current status of gastrointestinal carcinoids. Gastroenterology 2005;128:1717-51.
11. Bordi C, D'Adda T, Azzoni C, Ferraro G. Classification of gastric endocrine cells at the light and electron microscopical levels. Microsc Res Tech 2000;48:258-71.
12. Rindi G, Necchi V, Savio A, et al. Characterisation of gastric ghrelin cells in man and other mammals: studies in adult and fetal tissues. Histochem Cell Biol 2002;117:511-9.
13. Tzaneva MA. Ultrastructural immunohistochemical localization of gastrin, somatostatin and serotonin in endocrine cells of human antral gastric mucosa. Acta Histochem 2003;105:191-201.
14. Tzaneva MA. Electron microscopic immunohistochemical investigation of chromogranin A in endocrine cells in human oxyntic gastric mucosa. Acta Histochem 2001;103:179-94.
15. Mitrovic O, Micic M, Radenkovic G, et al. Endocrine cells in human fetal corpus of stomach: appearance, distribution, and density. J Gastroenterol 2012;47:1212-20.
16. Klöppel G, Rindi G, Anlauf M, Perren A, Komminoth P. Site-specific biology and pathology of gastroenteropancreatic neuroendocrine tumors. Virchows Arch 2007;451(Suppl 1):S9-27.
17. Debelenko LV, Emmert-Buck MR, Zhuang Z, et al. The multiple endocrine neoplasia type I gene locus is involved in the pathogenesis of type II gastric carcinoids. Gastroenterology 1997;113:773-81.
18. Modlin IM, Kidd M, Malfertheiner MV, Gustafsson BI. Gastric neuroendocrine neoplasia. In: Wang TC, Fox JG, Girand AS, eds. The biology of gastric cancers. New York: Springer; 2009:185-216.
19. Royston CM, Brew DS, Garnham JR, Stagg BH, Polak J. The Zollinger-Ellison syndrome due to an infiltrating tumour of the stomach. Gut 1972;13:638-42.
20. Buyse S, Charachon A, Petit T, Marmuse JP, Mignon M, Soule JC. [The gastric antrum: a rare primitive location of a gastrinoma within a type I multiple endocrine neoplasia]. Gastroenterol Clin Biol 2006;30:625-8. [French]
21. Rindi G, Luinetti O, Cornaggia M, Capella C, Solcia E. Three subtypes of gastric argyrophil carcinoid and the gastric neuroendocrine carcinoma: a clinicopathologic study. Gastroenterology 1993;104:994-1006.
22. La Rosa S, Inzani F, Vanoli A, et al. Histologic characterization and improved prognostic evaluation of 209 gastric neuroendocrine neoplasms. Hum Pathol 2011;42:1373-84.
23. Gough DB, Thompson GB, Crotty TB, et al. Diverse clinical and pathologic features of gastric carcinoid and the relevance of hypergastrinemia. World J Surg 1994;18:473-9; discussion 479-80.
24. Gilligan CJ, Lawton GP, Tang LH, West AB, Modlin IM. Gastric carcinoid tumors: the biology and therapy of an enigmatic and controversial lesion. Am J Gastroenterol 1995;90:338-52.
25. Hirata Y, Sakamoto N, Yamamoto H, Matsukura S, Imura H, Okada S. Gastric carcinoid with ectopic production of ACTH and beta-MSH. Cancer 1976;37:377-85.
26. Tsuchiya K, Minami I, Tateno T, et al. Malignant gastric carcinoid causing ectopic ACTH syndrome: discrepancy of plasma ACTH levels measured by different immunoradiometric assays. Endocrine J 2005;52:743-50.
27. Ruszniewski P, Delle Fave G, Cadiot G, et al. Well-differentiated gastric tumors/carcinomas. Neuroendocrinology 2006;84:158-64.
28. Solcia E, Fiocca R, Rindi G, Villani L, Cornaggia M, Capella C. The pathology of the gastrointestinal endocrine system. Endocrinol Metab Clin North Am 1993;22:795-821.

29. Borch K, Ahrén B, Ahlman H, Falkmer S, Granérus G, Grimelius L. Gastric carcinoids: biologic behavior and prognosis after differentiated treatment in relation to type. Ann Surg 2005;242:64-73.

30. Sato Y, Iwafuchi M, Ueki J, et al. Gastric carcinoid tumors without autoimmune gastritis in Japan: a relationship with Helicobacter pylori infection. Dig Dis Sci 2002;47:579-85.

31. Rindi G, Bordi C, Rappel S, La Rosa S, Stolte M, Solcia E. Gastric carcinoids and neuroendocrine carcinomas: pathogenesis, pathology, and behavior. World J Surg 1996;20:168-72.

32. Berna MJ, Annibale B, Marignani M, et al. A prospective study of gastric carcinoids and enterochromaffin-like cell changes in multiple endocrine neoplasia type 1 and Zollinger-Ellison syndrome: identification of risk factors. J Clin Endocrinol Metab 2008;93:1582-91.

33. Hosoya Y, Fujii T, Nagai H, Shibusawa H, Tsukahara M, Kanazawa K. A case of multiple gastric carcinoids associated with multiple endocrine neoplasia type 1 without hypergastrinemia. Gastrointest Endosc 1999;50:692-5.

34. Bordi C, Corleto VD, Azzoni C, et al. The antral mucosa as a new site for endocrine tumors in multiple endocrine neoplasia type 1 and Zollinger-Ellison syndromes. J Clin Endocrinol Metab 2001;86:2236-42.

35. Solcia E, Capella C, Fiocca R, Rindi G, Rosai J. Gastric argyrophil carcinoidosis in patients with Zollinger-Ellison syndrome due to type 1 multiple endocrine neoplasia. A newly recognized association. Am J Surg Pathol 1990;14:503-13.

36. Bellorin O, Shuchleib A, Halevi AE, Aksenov S, Saldinger PF. Giant type III well-differentiated neuroendocrine tumor of the stomach: A case report. Int J Surg Case Rep 2016;25:62-5.

37. Abraham SC, Carney JA, Ooi A, Choti MA, Argani P. Achlorhydria, parietal cell hyperplasia, and multiple gastric carcinoids: a new disorder. Am J Surg Pathol 2005;29:969-75.

38. Ooi A, Ota M, Katsuda S, Nakanishi I, Sugawara H, Takahashi I. An unusual case of multiple gastric carcinoids associated with diffuse endocrine cell hyperplasia and parietal cell hypertrophy. Endocr Pathol 1995;6:229-37.

39. Moesta KT, Schlag P. Proposal for a new carcinoid tumour staging system based on tumour tissue infiltration and primary metastasis; a prospective multicentre carcinoid tumour evaluation study. West German Surgical Oncologists' Group. Eur J Surg Oncol 1990;16:280-8.

40. Kumashiro R, Naitoh H, Teshima K, Sakai T, Inutsuka S. Minute gastric carcinoid tumor with regional lymph node metastasis. Int Surg 1989;74:198-200.

41. Rindi G. Neuroendocrine tumors and non-neoplastic neudocrine cell changes. In: Tan D, Lauwers GY, eds. Gastric cancer. Philadelphia: Lippincott Williams & Wilkins; 2011:94-104.

42. Whitehead R, Cosgrove C. Mucins and carcinoid tumours. Pathology 1979;11:473-8.

43. Ordóñez NG, Mackay B, el-Naggar A, Bannayan GA, Duncan J. Clear cell carcinoid tumour of the stomach. Histopathology 1993;22:190-3.

44. Vanoli A, La Rosa S, Luinetti O, et al. Histologic changes in type A chronic atrophic gastritis indicating increased risk of neuroendocrine tumor development: the predictive role of dysplastic and severely hyperplastic enterochromaffin-like cell lesions. Hum Pathol 2013;44:1827-37.

45. Solcia E, Fiocca R, Villani L, Luinetti O, Capella C. Hyperplastic, dysplastic, and neoplastic enterochromaffin-like-cell proliferations of the gastric mucosa. Classification and histogenesis. Am J Surg Pathol 1995;19(Suppl 1):S1-7.

46. Solcia E, Bordi C, Creutzfeldt W, et al. Histopathological classification of nonantral gastric endocrine growths in man. Digestion 1988;41: 185-200.

47. Rindi G, Paolotti D, Fiocca R, Wiedenmann B, Henry JP, Solcia E. Vesicular monoamine transporter 2 as a marker of gastric enterochromaffin-like cell tumors. Virchows Arch 2000;436:217-23.

48. Thomas RM, Baybick JH, Elsayed AM, Sobin LH. Gastric carcinoids. An immunohistochemical and clinicopathologic study of 104 patients. Cancer 1994;73:2053-8.

49. Kölby L, Wängberg B, Ahlman H, et al. Gastric carcinoid with histamine production, histamine transporter and expression of somatostatin receptors. Digestion 1998;59:160-6.

50. D'Adda T, Keller G, Bordi C, Höfler H. Loss of heterozygosity in 11q13-14 regions in gastric neuroendocrine tumors not associated with multiple endocrine neoplasia type 1 syndrome. Lab Invest 1999;79:671-7.

51. Kidd M, Modlin IM, Mane SM, et al. Utility of molecular genetic signatures in the delineation of gastric neoplasia. Cancer 2006;106:1480-8.

52. Higham AD, Bishop LA, Dimaline R, et al. Mutations of RegIalpha are associated with enterochromaffin-like cell tumor development in patients with hypergastrinemia. Gastroenterology 1999;116:1310-8.

53. Dou D, Shi YF, Liu Q, et al. Hsa-miR-202-3p, up-regulated in type 1 gastric neuroendocrine neoplasms, may target *DUSP1*. World J Gastroenterol 2018;24:573-82.

54. Modlin IM, Lye KD, Kidd M. A 50-year analysis of 562 gastric carcinoids: small tumor or larger problem? Am J Gastroenterol 2004;99:23-32.

55. Rorstad O. Prognostic indicators for carcinoid neuroendocrine tumors of the gastrointestinal tract. J Surg Oncol 2005;89:151-60.
56. Saund MS, Al Natour RH, Sharma AM, Huang Q, Boosalis VA, Gold JS. Tumor size and depth predict rate of lymph node metastasis and utilization of lymph node sampling in surgically managed gastric carcinoids. Ann Surg Oncol 2011;18:2826-32.
57. Richards AT, Hinder RA, Harrison AC. Gastric carcinoid tumours associated with hypergastrinaemia and pernicious anaemia—regression of tumors by antrectomy. A case report. S Afr Med J 1987;72:51-3.
58. Cives M, Strosberg J. Treatment strategies for metastatic neuroendocrine tumors of the gastrointestinal tract. Curr Treat Options Oncol 2017;18:14.
59. Rindi G, Azzoni C, La Rosa S, et al. ECL cell tumor and poorly differentiated endocrine carcinoma of the stomach: prognostic evaluation by pathological analysis. Gastroenterology 1999;116:532-42.
60. Kang SH, Kim KH, Seo SH, et al. Neuroendocrine carcinoma of the stomach: A case report. World J Gastrointest Surg 2014;6:77-9.
61. Jiang SX, Mikami T, Umezawa A, Saegusa M, Kameya T, Okayasu I. Gastric large cell neuroendocrine carcinomas: a distinct clinicopathologic entity. Am J Surg Pathol 2006;30:945-53.
62. Ishida M, Sekine S, Fukagawa T, et al. Neuroendocrine carcinoma of the stomach: morphologic and immunohistochemical characteristics and prognosis. Am J Surg Pathol 2013;37:949-59.
63. Matsui K, Jin XM, Kitagawa M, Miwa A. Clinicopathologic features of neuroendocrine carcinomas of the stomach: appraisal of small cell and large cell variants. Arch Pathol Lab Med 1998;122:1010-7.
64. Park JY, Ryu MH, Park YS, et al. Prognostic significance of neuroendocrine components in gastric carcinomas. Eur J Cancer 2014;50:2802-9.
65. Xie JW, Sun YQ, Feng CY, et al. Evaluation of clinicopathological factors related to the prognosis of gastric neuroendocrine carcinoma. Eur J Surg Oncol 2016;42:1464-70.
66. Bordi C, Falchetti A, Azzoni C, et al. Aggressive forms of gastric neuroendocrine tumors in multiple endocrine neoplasia type I. Am J Surg Pathol 1997;21:1075-82.
67. Sweeney EC, McDonnell LM. Atypical gastric carcinoids. Histopathology 1980;4:215-24.
68. Domori K, Nishikura K, Ajioka Y, Aoyagi Y. Mucin phenotype expression of gastric neuroendocrine neoplasms: analysis of histopathology and carcinogenesis. Gastric Cancer 2014;17:263-72.
69. Boo YJ, Park SS, Kim JH, Mok YJ, Kim SJ, Kim CS. Gastric neuroendocrine carcinoma: clinicopathologic review and immunohistochemical study

70. of E-cadherin and Ki-67 as prognostic markers. J Surg Oncol 2007;95:110-7.
70. Campbell F, Lauwers GY. Tumors of the esophagus and stomach. In: Fletcher CD, ed. Diagnostic histopathology of tumors, 4th ed. Philadelphia: Elsevier/Saunders; 2013: 378-433.
71. al-Salman M, Taylor DC, Beauchamp CP, Duncan CP. Prevention of vascular injuries in revision total hip replacement. Can J Surg 1992;35:261-4.
72. Shida T, Furuya M, Kishimoto T, et al. The expression of NeuroD and mASH1 in the gastroenteropancreatic neuroendocrine tumors. Mod Pathol 2008;21:1363-70.
73. Ishida M, Sekine S, Fukagawa T, et al. Neuroendocrine carcinoma of the stomach: morphologic and immunohistochemical characteristics and prognosis. Am J Surg Pathol 2013;37:949-59.
74. Vijayvergia N, Boland PM, Handorf E, et al. Molecular profiling of neuroendocrine malignancies to identify prognostic and therapeutic markers: a Fox Chase Cancer Center Pilot Study. Br J Cancer 2016;115:564-70.
75. Furlan D, Cerutti R, Uccella S, et al. Different molecular profiles characterize well-differentiated endocrine tumors and poorly differentiated endocrine carcinomas of the gastroenteropancreatic tract. Clin Cancer Res 2004;10:947-57.
76. Pizzi S, Azzoni C, Bassi D, Bottarelli L, Milione M, Bordi C. Genetic alterations in poorly differentiated endocrine carcinomas of the gastrointestinal tract. Cancer 2003;98:1273-82.
77. Han HS, Kim HS, Woo DK, Kim WH, Kim YI. Loss of heterozygosity in gastric neuroendocrine tumor. Anticancer Res 2000;20:2849-54.
78. Ihler F, Vetter EV, Pan J, et al. Expression of a neuroendocrine gene signature in gastric tumor cells from CEA 424-SV40 large T antigen-transgenic mice depends on SV40 large T antigen. PLoS One 2012;7:e29846.
79. Sahnane N, Furlan D, Monti M, et al. Microsatellite unstable gastrointestinal neuroendocrine carcinomas: a new clinicopathologic entity. Endocr Relat Cancer 2015;22:35-45.
80. Shia J, Tang LH, Weiser MR, et al. Is nonsmall cell type high-grade neuroendocrine carcinoma of the tubular gastrointestinal tract a distinct disease entity? Am J Surg Pathol 2008;32:719-31.
81. Smith JD, Reidy DL, Goodman KA, Shia J, Nash GM. A retrospective review of 126 high-grade neuroendocrine carcinomas of the colon and rectum. Ann Surg Oncol 2014;21:2956-62.
82. Ajani JA, In H, Sano T, et al. Stomach. In: Amin MB, Edge, SB, eds. AJCC cancer staging manual /American Joint Committee on Cancer, 8th ed. Switzerland: Springer; 2017

83. Okita NT, Kato K, Takahari D, et al. Neuroendocrine tumors of the stomach: chemotherapy with cisplatin plus irinotecan is effective for gastric poorly-differentiated neuroendocrine carcinoma. Gastric Cancer 2011;14:161-5.

84. Ribeiro MJ, Alonso T, Gajate P, et al. Huge recurrent gastric neuroendocrine tumor: a second-line chemotherapeutic dilemma. Autops Case Rep 2018;8:e2018005.

85. Matsubara Y, Ando T, Hosakawa A, et al. Neuroendocrine carcinoma of the stomach: a response to combination chemotherapy consisting of ramucirumab plus paclitaxel. Intern Med 2018;57:671-5.

11 LYMPHOPROLIFERATIVE DISORDERS OF THE STOMACH

Despite the fact that the normal stomach contains little lymphoid tissue, it is, paradoxically, one of the most common sites for the development of extranodal lymphomas (1,2). Mucosa-associated lymphoid tissue (MALT) is thought to be induced as a response to persistent antigen stimulation prior to the development of lymphoma (3). Gastric lymphomas constitute 16 to 31 percent of all extranodal non-Hodgkin lymphomas and approximately 7 percent of all gastric malignancies (4,5). Any histologic subtype of lymphoma can arise in the stomach, but marginal zone B-cell lymphoma of mucosa-associated lymphoid tissue (MALT lymphoma) and diffuse large B-cell lymphoma constitute over 90 percent of gastric lymphomas.

Three common definitions are used to separate primary extranodal lymphomas from nodal lymphomas and these are outlined in Table 11-1 (1). All definitions accept involvement in organ systems other than lymph nodes, Waldeyer ring, spleen, or bone marrow as primary extranodal, but allow different degrees of nodal involvement. The first definition (#1) includes presen-

tation in a lymph node, Waldeyer ring, spleen, or bone marrow as primary nodal lymphoma. It also categorizes lesions with clinically dominant lymph node involvement and at most one extranodal organ involvement as primary nodal lymphoma. Presentation in other organs with no or minor lymph node involvement is considered primary extranodal. A separate category of "extensive involvement" is used for those patients with presentation involving both extranodal and nodal sites.

Definitions #2 and 3 eliminate the "extensive involvement" category, and such patients are included under primary nodal lymphoma. Definitions #1 and 2 share the same criteria for extranodal lymphoma, but definition #3 includes presentation in an extranodal site with regional lymph node involvement under extranodal lymphoma. Definitions #2 and 3 provide a more favorable outcome for patients with extranodal lymphomas since patients with more extensive disease are included in the primary nodal category. According to the most stringent definition (definition #1), patients

Table 11-1

THREE DEFINITIONS OF PRIMARY NODAL AND EXTRANODAL NON-HODGKIN LYMPHOMA[a]

Designation	Criteria
Definition 1	
Primary nodal	Presentation in lymph node, Waldeyer ring, spleen, or bone marrow; lymph node involvement clinically dominant; at most one extranodal organ involved (usually bone marrow)
Primary extranodal	Presentation in other organs; no or only minor lymph node involvement
Extensive involvement	Presentation in both extranodal and nodal sites (often other side of diaphragm)
Definition 2	
Primary nodal	As in definition 1, but also including patients with extensive involvement
Primary extranodal	As in definition 1
Definition 3	
Primary nodal	As in definition 1, but also including patients with extensive involvement and patients with disseminated disease presenting in an extranodal site
Primary extranodal	Presentation in an extranodal site with or without regional lymph node involvement

[a]Modified from a table in reference 1.

with primary nodal and extranodal lymphomas have comparable 5- and 10-year survival rates, but those with extranodal lymphomas have a more favorable event-free survival period (1).

Lymphoma classification has a relatively short (since 1934) but convoluted history (6,7). The most recent classification system is the product of collaborative efforts between the American Society and the European Society of Hematopathology, and is part of the World Health Organization (WHO) classification of tumors (8,9). In this classification, tumors that occur primarily in the stomach include extranodal MALT lymphoma and diffuse large B-cell lymphoma (8,9). Other lymphomas, such as Burkitt lymphoma, mantle cell lymphoma, and follicular lymphoma, rarely involve the stomach, either primarily or secondarily.

EXTRANODAL MARGINAL ZONE B-CELL LYMPHOMA OF MUCOSA-ASSOCIATED LYMPHOID TISSUE (MALT LYMPHOMA)

Definition. *Extranodal marginal zone B-cell lymphoma* is a discrete clinicopathologic entity that develops in MALT (10–12). Its distinction from nodal marginal zone B-cell lymphoma is based primarily on clinical criteria, although these two entities have different morphologies and genetic abnormalities (10–12).

Two types of MALT occur in the human body: primary "physiologic" lymphoid tissue, such as Peyer patches, and acquired MALT, which occurs in sites of inflammation such as with *Helicobacter pylori* gastritis or in Sjögren syndrome. Most MALT lymphomas arise from acquired MALT at anatomic sites that are normally devoid of lymphoid tissue, such as the stomach, salivary glands, lung, and thyroid gland (13).

MALT has strikingly similar histologic features to the normal Peyer patch. It consists of a reactive B-cell follicle surrounded by neoplastic cells that extend into the interfollicular regions and often infiltrate epithelium to form lymphoepithelial structures (14). MALT lymphomas, which are derived from marginal zone B cells, resemble normal MALT tissue, histologically, cytologically, phenotypically, and genotypically (14).

By definition, MALT lymphomas are small cell low-grade lymphomas. The existence of large cell high-grade MALT lymphomas is controversial. Some investigators believe that MALT

lymphomas undergo high-grade transformation (15–17). Most, however, agree to restrict the use of MALT lymphoma to "low-grade B-cell lymphomas" as originally described (18) in order to avoid mistaking "high-grade" MALT lymphoma as an entity that may respond to antibiotic therapy, as a low-grade MALT lymphoma sometimes does.

Incidence. Precise data regarding incidence rates of gastric MALT lymphomas are lacking. MALT lymphoma is the third most common type of non-Hodgkin lymphoma (7 to 8 percent of all non-Hodgkin lymphomas) (10,11). The stomach is the most common site of MALT lymphomas, comprising 70 percent of all cases (14). The incidence rate for all gastric non-Hodgkin lymphomas is 0.6 per 100,000 person-years according to the Surveillance, Epidemiology, and End Results (SEER) data in the United States (19). Depending on the type of study, MALT lymphomas constitute 30 to 60 percent of primary gastric lymphomas (10,20–23), an incidence rate of 0.18 to 0.36 per 100,000 person-years.

SEER data have shown a steady increase in the incidence of non-Hodgkin lymphomas between 1993 and 1998, including those not associated with human immunodeficiency virus (HIV) infection (19,24). Although recent data have shown an increase in the incidence of primary gastrointestinal non-Hodgkin lymphomas in a North American population (22), more specific data on gastric MALT lymphomas are sketchy. A population-based study in Italy showed a significant reduction in gastric MALT lymphomas, from 1.4 per 100,000 in 1997 to 0.2 per 100,000 in 2002, which then remained stable until 2007, the end of study period (25). In addition, the percentage of all gastric MALT lymphomas associated with *H. pylori* infection decreased from 61 to 17 percent between the period before and after 2002. Anti-*H. pylori* interventions likely contributed to this reduction.

Clinical Features. Gastric MALT lymphoma affects males slightly more than females, with a male to female ratio of 1.3 to 1.0 and a mean age of 57 years (23). Although there are no significant racial differences in the incidence of non-Hodgkin lymphomas (19), specific data related to MALT lymphomas are lacking.

The presenting symptoms of gastric MALT lymphomas are nonspecific epigastric/abdominal pain (28 percent), dyspepsia (69 percent), weight loss (49 percent), nausea and vomiting (17 percent), and gastric bleeding (27 percent) (23). Constitutional "B" symptoms (fever, night sweats, and weight loss) are uncommon (1 to 5 percent) (10,26,27). A small proportion of patients presents with elevated serum β_2-microglobulin (4 percent) or lactate dehydrogenase (1 percent) levels. In a small percentage of patients (3.2 percent), gastric MALT lymphoma was as incidental finding on endoscopy. Complications such as obstruction and perforation are rare (28).

Over 80 percent of patients present with disease localized to the stomach (stage IE, i.e., extranodal disease limited to the site of origin). Nevertheless, bone marrow involvement is seen in 5 to 10 percent of patients (10). The regional lymph nodes are involved (stage IIE) in 10 to 20 percent of patients (14). The high percentage of patients who present initially with low-stage disease may be a reflection of classification bias, since some authors consider only localized disease an indication of extranodal lymphoma (see Table 11-1).

Etiology. Of all MALT lymphomas, gastric tumors are the best understood with regard to etiology. *H. pylori* is a Gram-negative bacterium that colonizes the gastric mucosa and is associated with peptic ulcers and gastric adenocarcinomas. Gastric MALT lymphoma develops on a background of chronic inflammation and lymphoid infiltration displaying features of classic MALT architecture acquired from *H. pylori* infection. The combination of gastric MALT lymphoma and *H. pylori* infection is a model for infection-associated MALT lymphomas. *H. pylori* infection is a necessary component in the mechanism of gastric MALT lymphoma development, but is not sufficient alone for tumorigenesis.

Several lines of evidence support a link between *H. pylori*-induced chronic gastritis and the development of MALT lymphoma. First, *H. pylori* infection is present in the gastric mucosa in most, if not all, patients with gastric MALT lymphoma (29,30). An association between *H. pylori* infection and gastric MALT lymphoma has been established both in population-based studies (31) and on an individual level (32). An in vitro T-cell-dependent and *H. pylori* strain-specific stimulation of neoplastic cells from MALT lymphomas suggests that MALT lymphomas

mount an immunologic response to the *H. pylori* organism (33). Regression of MALT lymphoma after eradication of *H. pylori* infection occurs in 70 to 80 percent of patients (34–37). On progressive biopsy samples, MALT lymphomas have been shown to arise from B-cell clones at the site of chronic gastritis (38,39).

Interestingly, the prevalence rate of MALT lymphoma in patients with *H. pylori* infection is extremely low (1.8 percent) (29) and, thus, most patients with *H. pylori* infection do not develop MALT lymphoma. Virulence factors of the bacterium do not obviously determine this risk. Growing evidence suggests that genetic host factors play an important role in this context (40).

H. pylori infection in the stomach induces a vigorous systemic and mucosal humoral response (41). Antibody production does not lead to eradication of cellular infection, but instead contributes mainly to the induction of tissue damage and inflammation. The recognition of the *H. pylori* antigen by the immune system leads to T-cell activation, lymphoid follicle formation, and B-cell proliferation (42). *H. pylori*-specific gastric mucosal T cells show a phenotype that promotes gastritis. This biased T-cell response, combined with Fas-mediated apoptosis of *H. pylori*-specific T-cell clones, favors the persistence of *H. pylori* infection in the stomach. As a result of both direct and indirect immunologic stimulation (by auto-antigens and *H. pylori*-specific T cells, respectively), B cells infiltrate and proliferate within the stomach.

It has been proposed that the chronic active inflammation induced by *H. pylori* infection causes DNA damage, leading to various genetic abnormalities and the subsequent emergence of a neoplastic B-cell clone. For example, *H. pylori* infection attracts and activates neutrophils, which are stimulated to release reactive oxygen species (ROS). ROS has been shown to induce a wide range of genetic abnormalities, and has been proposed to play a role in the development of gastric MALT lymphoma (14). In in vitro experiments, growth and development of genetically altered lymphoid cells in the early phase of disease are not fully autonomous. Proliferation of malignant B cells, in the early stage of development, is partly dependent on *H. pylori*-related proteins and T cells (33,43). Intraclonal sequence variations, i.e., ongoing mutations, have been demonstrated in most cases. The finding of ongoing mutations strongly indicates that direct antigen stimulation has a direct role in the clonal expansion of MALT lymphoma. Preliminary data also indicate that the rate of ongoing mutations gradually declines during evolution from early- to late-stage MALT lymphomas. Therefore, the role of direct antigen stimulation in the pathogenesis of MALT lymphomas likely progressively decreases during tumor evolution (14).

Genetic Abnormalities. The most common nonrandom chromosomal aberration in gastric MALT lymphoma is the t(11;18)(q21;q21). In fact, in most translocation-positive cases, t(11;18) (q21;q21) is the only chromosomal aberration. This translocation causes reciprocal fusion of the *BIRC3* (*API2*) and *MALT1* genes (14). A functional *BIRC3-MALT1* fusion product develops the ability to activate the nuclear factor-kB (NF-kB) pathway (44). This translocation occurs specifically in MALT lymphomas, and not in other closely related nodal or splenic marginal zone B-cell lymphomas, non-Hodgkin lymphomas, or *H. pylori* gastritis, but it occurs at remarkably variable incidences in different anatomic sites. In gastric MALT lymphomas, it is present in up to 47 and 68 percent at stage IE and stage IIE or above lesions, respectively, in retrospective studies from several centers. This translocation is seen more frequently in tumors that disseminate to regional lymph nodes or distant sites compared to tumors confined to the stomach. The presence of this translocation is also associated with absence of *H. pylori* (45) and, thus, a lack of response to anti-*H. pylori* medication. Tumors with this translocation rarely transform to large cell lymphoma.

A second, less common, nonrandom translocation in MALT lymphoma is t(1;14)(p22;q32). This translocation occurs in approximately 5 percent of MALT lymphomas and is often associated with trisomy of chromosomes 3, 12, and 18 (14). It is also associated with a lack of response to *H. pylori* treatment and is typically seen in patients at an advanced stage of disease. This translocation brings the *BCL10* gene under the control of the Ig heavy-chain (*IGH*) gene enhancer, deregulating the expression of the *BCL10* gene, which is essential for both the development and function of mature B and T cells.

The t(14;18)(q32;q21) translocation, most often seen in nongastrointestinal MALT lymphomas, but occasionally (1.4 percent) occurring in gastric MALT lymphomas (14,46), brings the *MALT1* gene under the control of the enhancer region of *IGH* (47,48). This translocation is not to be confused with the t(14;18)(q32;q21) translocation seen in follicular lymphomas. Although bearing identical chromosomal band breakpoints, the translocation associated with follicular lymphoma brings the *BCL2* gene (49), which is located 5-Mb telomeric to the *MALT1* gene, under the influence of the *IGH* enhancer. Since the MALT t(14;18)(q32;q21) translocation involves the *MALT1* gene, its presence indicates that the tumor is not responsive to anti-*H. pylori* antibiotic therapy and will not likely undergo transformation to a large cell lymphoma type.

A fourth translocation, the t(3;14)(p14;q32), which is more common in extragastric MALT lymphoma, has also been observed in gastric MALT lymphoma. This translocation juxtaposes the *FOXP1* gene to the *IGH* enhancer, and interestingly has been associated with gastric MALT lymphomas with a large B-cell component (50).

Trisomy 3 was once reported as the most frequent (up to 60 percent) genetic abnormality in gastric MALT lymphomas (10), but its frequency in subsequent series ranged from 11 to 33 percent (46,51). It is also reported in several other subtypes of lymphoma (10). Trisomy 12 and trisomy 18 are detected in 15 percent and 6 to 18 percent of gastric MALT lymphomas, respectively (46,51,52).

Gross Findings. MALT lymphomas occur in any part of the stomach but are most common in the antrum or gastric body (75 percent combined) (23). Lymphomas are much more likely than gastric carcinomas to be multifocal (33 percent). Ulceration (39 to 48 percent) and nodule formation (30 to 52 percent) are the two most common patterns of presentation in gastric MALT lymphoma (53,54), although some grow as discrete polypoid lesions. Nodular lesions are often multiple and confluent (55). Some MALT lymphomas show a mixture of these patterns of growth or show normal or hyperemic mucosa. The most common presentation is a single or multiple, shallow or deep ulcer (53). These ulcers usually have vague margins and disorganized convergent rugae (56).

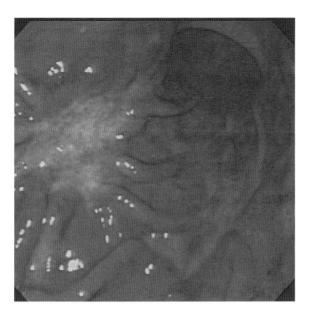

Figure 11-1

**GASTRIC MUCOSA-ASSOCIATED
LYMPHOID TISSUE (MALT) LYMPHOMA**

Endoscopically, a large superficial ulcer with long stellate branches is present.

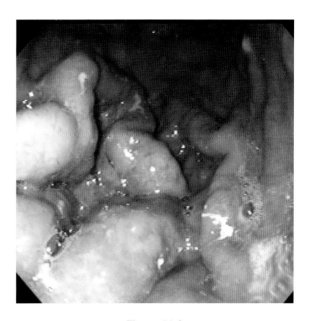

Figure 11-2

INFILTRATIVE MALT LYMPHOMA

Giant folds are evident in the stomach.

Surrounding or internal nodularity and focal masses, which mimic gastric carcinomas, are seen in a minority of cases.

By endoscopy, common findings include ulcers (47 percent), erythema (30 percent), and erosions (23 percent) (10). Diffuse infiltration and polypoid masses were noted in 18 percent and 25 percent of patients, respectively, in one series (57). Large superficial ulcers with long stellate branches are the most characteristic feature of lymphomas (fig. 11-1), but more penetrating ulcers are also present, although less commonly. On occasion, a diffuse infiltrative growth pattern with large nodular and occasional giant folds (fig. 11-2) may be difficult to distinguish from carcinoma of linitis plastica type, metastases, or Ménétrier disease. In up to 53 percent of the patients, the endoscopic findings are interpreted as benign, and in up to 15 percent the mucosa appears normal on endoscopy (27).

Microscopic Findings. Gastric MALT lymphoma has histologic features similar to those of the normal Peyer patch. Typical features include reactive appearing B-cell follicles surrounded by marginal zone cells interposed between the B-cell follicles and the overlying gastric mucosa.

Such an arrangement is typical of the "pseudolymphoma" described in the past in gastrectomy specimens, many of which contained bona fide MALT lymphoma (58). A characteristic feature of MALT lymphoma is the expansion of the marginal-like zone surrounding benign germinal centers (59) and infiltration by clusters of lymphocytes of the gastric-gland epithelium forming characteristic lymphoepithelial lesions (fig. 11-3) (14). The marginal zone B cells have small to medium-sized, slightly irregular nuclei with moderately dispersed chromatin and inconspicuous nucleoli, resembling those of centrocytes (fig. 11-4); they have abundant, pale cytoplasm (11).

In some cases, accumulation of pale-staining cytoplasm leads to a monocytoid appearance of the tumor cells (fig. 11-5). Marginal zone cells may also closely resemble small lymphocytes. Thus, the typical infiltrate of MALT lymphoma is characterized by sheets of centrocyte-like cells with a varying monocytoid appearance that often has a zonal distribution. Scattered large cells that resemble immunoblasts and centroblasts are often present (fig. 11-6). Any of these cellular patterns may predominate in any individual tumor, but usually these patterns are combined (10).

311

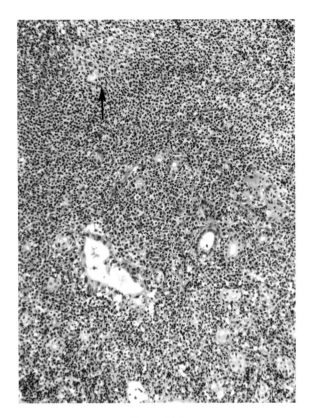

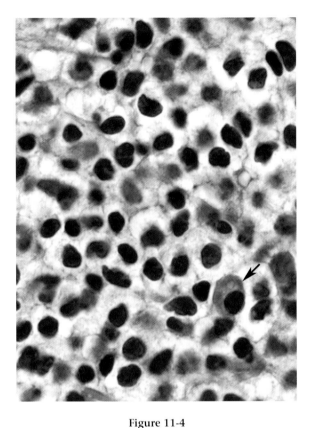

Figure 11-3

GASTRIC MALT LYMPHOMA WITH RESIDUAL REACTIVE FOLLICLE

At low magnification, a reactive follicle is present on the left (arrow). The rest of the field shows an intense infiltrate of monomorphic MALT lymphoma cells that destroy gastric glands to varying degrees (hematoxylin and eosin [H&E] stain).

Figure 11-4

GASTRIC MALT LYMPHOMA

High magnification of figure 11-1 shows an infiltrate consisting of small to medium-sized, slightly irregular nuclei with moderately dispersed chromatin and inconspicuous nucleoli. Many of the cells have abundant pale or vacuolated cytoplasm. A plasma cell is present in the right lower corner (arrow) (H&E stain).

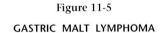

Figure 11-5

GASTRIC MALT LYMPHOMA

The abundant pale and vacuolated cytoplasm in this field gives the cells a monocytoid appearance. An immunoblast-like cell with a large central prominent nucleolus is in the center of the field (H&E stain).

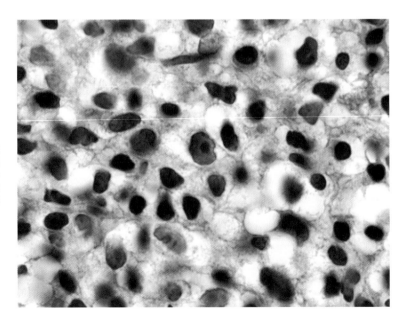

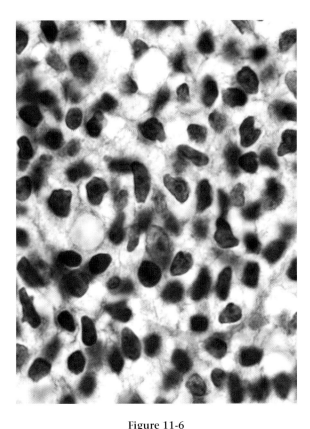

Figure 11-6

GASTRIC MALT LYMPHOMA

This field shows a heterogeneous mixture of small B cells, including marginal zone (centrocyte-like) cells, monocytoid cells, small lymphocytes, and scattered large cells that resemble immunoblasts and centroblasts (H&E stain).

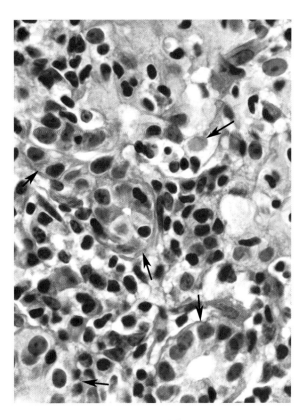

Figure 11-7

**GASTRIC MALT LYMPHOMA
WITH LYMPHOEPITHELIAL LESION**

Several lymphoepithelial lesions distort and destroy the epithelium to varying degrees (H&E stain).

Plasma cell differentiation is present in approximately 33 percent of cases. Plasma cells are occasionally so conspicuous that a diagnosis of extramedullary plasmacytoma may be considered in the differential diagnosis. Plasma cells present with varying degrees of atypia, Dutcher bodies, or other intracellular inclusions. The neoplastic plasma cells are often morphologically difficult to distinguish from benign lamina propria plasma cells. Neoplastic plasma cells are often detected beneath the luminal surface epithelium.

In later stages of progression, neoplastic cells may infiltrate into surrounding lamina propria and muscularis mucosae to form large confluent areas of tumor, which eventually may obliterate the preexisting reactive lymphoid follicles. Lymphoma cells may also colonize reactive germinal centers, and in rare cases, this can mimic the pattern seen in follicular lymphomas. Follicular colonization is usually accompanied by marked plasma cell differentiation.

Neoplastic cells commonly invade glandular epithelium and form lymphoepithelial lesions, which are defined as aggregates of three or more marginal zone cells in combination with distortion, or destruction, of the epithelium, often evident as eosinophilic degeneration of epithelial cells (fig. 11-7). Lymphoepithelial lesions are the pivotal diagnostic feature of gastric MALT lymphomas and are a particularly useful histologic feature in small mucosal biopsy specimens. The mere presence of a few scattered small lymphoid cells within the epithelial lining (fig. 11-8) is, however, insufficient for categorization as a lymphoepithelial lesion, and, in fact, such lymphoid cells are often T cells.

Histologic Grading. A variable number of "large cells" may be present in MALT lymphomas. When a solid or sheet-like

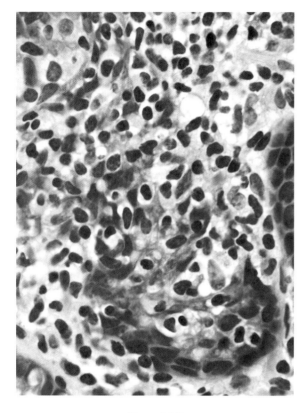

Figure 11-8

NON-NEOPLASTIC LYMPHOEPITHELIAL LESION

An isolated lymphoepithelial lesion seen in this gastric biopsy shows chronic gastritis with no evidence of MALT lymphoma (H&E stain).

proliferation of transformed centroblast- or immunoblast-like cells is present, the lymphoma is best categorized as a diffuse large B-cell lymphoma. In this case, the presence of accompanying MALT lymphoma should be noted in the pathology report (11). Unfortunately, there is controversy regarding the exact quantity of large cells needed to make this designation, although many advocate a "cutoff" of 30 percent large cells among the admixture of neoplastic cells (17).

Some data show clinical relevance for a grading system for gastric non-Hodgkin B-cell lymphomas. In a study by de Jong et al. (60), 106 such patients were divided into four groups according to both the percentage of diffusely intermingled large cells and the size of the clusters of large cells. Group A (n=30) included those without any diffuse large cell component, and the large cell clusters consisted of less than 5

cells. Group B (n=20) included cases with either 5 to 10 percent diffuse intermingled large cells, or with large cell clusters of more than 10 cells. Group C (n=23) included cases with a diffuse large cell component exceeding 10 percent of the overall quantity of tumor cells either with or without large cell clusters. Finally, group D (n=33) included cases that consisted of only large cells. The overall 5-year survival rates for the 4 groups were 95 percent, 64 percent, 46 percent, and 35 percent, respectively. The 10-year survival rates were 95 percent, 53 percent, 46 percent, and 29 percent, respectively. The differences between groups A and B were statistically significant, whereas the differences between groups C and D were not. Thus a designation such as "extranodal marginal zone B-cell lymphoma with increased large cells" seems justified for cases with more than 5 percent of large cells. As in other histologic classification/grading systems, this grading system may appear straightforward in theory; in practice, however, the interobserver reproducibility is fair at best ($\kappa \approx 0.3$) for simple gastritis, low-grade MALT lymphoma, and high-grade MALT lymphoma (61). Incorporation of clinical, immunophenotypic, and cytogenetic information improves diagnostic accuracy (59).

Immunohistochemical Findings. MALT lymphoma tumor cells typically express IgM and less often, IgA or IgG, and are always negative for IgD; they show light chain restriction (11). MALT lymphoma cells recapitulate the immunophenotype of marginal zone B cells: positive for CD20, CD21, CD35, and CD79a and negative for CD5, CD10, CD23, and cyclin D1. CD43 is expressed in approximately 50 percent of cases. Expression of CD11c is variable. Staining for CD21 and CD35 typically reveals an expanded meshwork of follicular dendritic cells, which corresponds to colonized lymphoid follicles.

Cytologic Findings. Cytologic specimens may be obtained by endoscopic brushing or by fine needle aspiration (FNA), either with or without ultrasound guidance. Brushing specimens often include normal or reactive gastric surface epithelium. FNA specimens may consist of abundant parietal and chief cells. Depending on the sampling technique, the lymphoid cell population shows a variable degree of cellularity, and is usually composed of a polymorphous

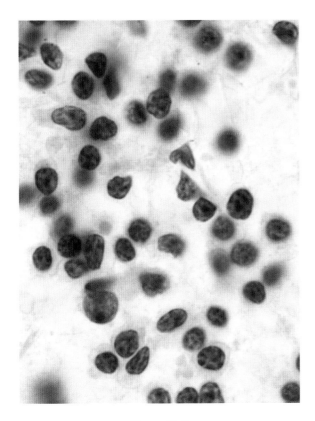

Figure 11-9

**GASTRIC FINE-NEEDLE ASPIRATION (FNA)
SPECIMEN OF MALT LYMPHOMA**

A polymorphous population of small, intermediate-sized, and large lymphoid cells is seen (Papanicolaou stain). (Courtesy of Dr. Martha Pitman, Boston, MA.)

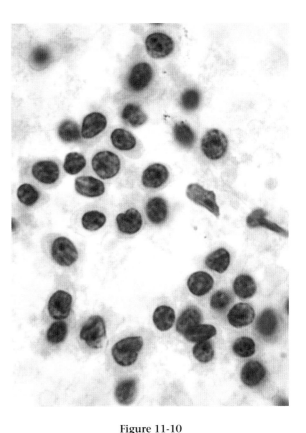

Figure 11-10

GASTRIC FNA OF MALT LYMPHOMA

There are predominantly intermediate-sized lymphoid cells with an indistinct cell border, a moderate amount of cytoplasm, when discernible, slight nuclear membrane irregularities, and inconspicuous or absent nucleoli (Papanicolaou stain). (Courtesy of Dr. Martha Pitman Boston, MA.)

population of small, intermediate- and large-sized cells (fig. 11-9) (62,63). The dominant cell population is usually intermediate-sized lymphoid cells that contain a moderate amount of cytoplasm, show slight nuclear membrane irregularities, and have inconspicuous or absent nucleoli (fig. 11-10). These cells often show a "plasmacytoid" morphology best appreciated on air-dried smears stained with either Diff-Quik® or Wright-Giemsa. Dendritic cells and lymphohistiocytic aggregates are also often present; monocytoid cells with pale cytoplasm, plasma cells, and tingible body macrophages are occasionally present as well. Large transformed cells have a fair amount of amphophilic to basophilic cytoplasm, slightly irregular nuclear membranes, vesicular chromatin, and usually multiple small nucleoli or a single centrally located large prominent nucleolus (fig. 11-11).

Diagnosing MALT lymphoma on cytologic specimens is challenging due to the polymorphous/heterogeneous nature of the lymphoid population and the predominance of small- to intermediate-sized lymphoid cells. A definitive diagnosis of lymphoma can be made in only 50 percent of cases (63,64), and reactive follicular hyperplasia is often erroneously diagnosed (62). When the cellularity of the specimen is sufficient, flow cytometric demonstration of light chain restriction in the B cells is diagnostic of lymphoma. A diagnosis of MALT lymphoma can be made on the basis of the morphologic appearance of the tumor cells in combination with an absence of immunophenotypic expression of CD5 and CD10 (63,65).

Differential Diagnosis. MALT lymphoma can be difficult to distinguish from reactive

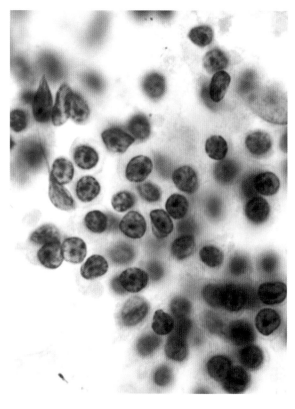

Figure 11-11

GASTRIC FNA OF MALT LYMPHOMA

Many of the lymphoid cells in this field are large transformed cells with slightly irregular nuclear membranes, vesicular chromatin pattern, and a single large prominent centrally located nucleolus or multiple small nucleoli (Papanicolaou stain). (Courtesy of Dr. Martha Pitman, Boston, MA.)

lymphoid hyperplasia, and from other small cell lymphomas. Its distinction from diffuse large B-cell lymphomas is discussed in the previous section on histologic grading.

For biopsies that show a prominent infiltrate of small lymphoid cells, the following features favor a diagnosis of lymphoma (61,66): an extensive confluent lymphoid infiltrate replacing and distorting mucosal glands and damaging the muscularis mucosae; the presence of convincing lymphoepithelial lesions; isolated or small groups of eosinophilic-appearing epithelial cells, which represent degenerated pit cells in lymphoepithelial lesions; a significant number of small cleaved cells which are larger than small lymphocytes, and show a more open chromatin pattern and irregular nuclear membranes; Dutcher

bodies or intranuclear inclusions in more than a few plasma cells; and monomorphism of the lymphoid infiltrate without admixed plasma cells. Unfortunately, some lymphomas are composed of lymphoid cells with only a minimal degree of cytologic atypia, and, conversely, lymphocytes within reactive lymphoid follicles may show an irregular nuclear contour. In a reactive lymphoid infiltrate, CD20-positive B cells are typically organized in nodules, while the interfollicular zone is rich in CD3-positive T cells. If immunostaining shows an extensive (at least half of a low power field using 4X objective), diffuse, densely packed infiltrate of CD20-positive B cells with a limited number of interspersed CD3-positive T cells, especially if the CD20-positive infiltrate percolates extensively between the residual gastric glands, this is supportive of a B-cell lymphoma. In contrast, a diffuse, dense infiltrate of CD3-positive T cells is inconclusive, because this may represent either a reactive lymphoid infiltrate or a T-cell lymphoma.

Demonstration of Ig light chain restriction is helpful in differentiating benign lymphoid infiltrates from MALT lymphoma. However, B-cell monoclonality as assessed by polymerase chain reaction (PCR) has been shown to be associated with reactive lymphoid follicles in chronic gastritis (67). Therefore, in order to firmly establish a diagnosis of MALT lymphoma, the above-mentioned histologic features should be present, i.e., centrocyte-like cells, lymphoepithelial lesions, and documented monoclonality of the lymphoid infiltrate by either immunohistochemistry or PCR (9). Although present only in a subset, demonstration by fluorescence in situ hybridization (FISH) of gene translocations such as t(11;18)(q21;q21) with *BIRC3-MALT1*, t(14;18)(q32;q21) with *MALT1-IGH*, or t(1;14)(p22;q32), strongly supports a diagnosis of MALT lymphoma.

MALT lymphoma also needs to be differentiated from other types of small B-cell lymphoma that rarely occur in the stomach, such as small lymphocytic lymphoma, mantle cell lymphoma, and diffuse follicular lymphoma, predominantly small cell type. These lymphomas are more likely to involve the intestine. Classification of diffuse small B-cell lymphomas can be difficult, particularly in small biopsies that contain crush artifact. Morphologic features suggestive of a MALT lymphoma include the presence of prominent lymphoepithelial

Table 11-2

SMALL B-CELL NEOPLASMS[a]

Neoplasm	Usual Immunolabeling Pattern
Mucosa-associated lymphoid tissue (MALT) lymphoma	CD20+, CD43+/–, CD5–, CD10–, cyclin D1–, IgM+, BCL2+, BCL6– (although may highlight follicular meshwork)
Small lymphocytic lymphoma/chronic lymphocytic leukemia	CD20+, CD43+, CD5+, cyclin D1-, CD10–, BCL2+, BCL6+/–, CD23+
Mantle cell lymphoma	CD20+, CD43+, CD5+, cyclin D1+, CD10–, BCL2+, BCL6–, CD23–, SOX11+
Follicular lymphoma	CD20+, CD43–, CD5–, cyclin D1–, CD10+, BCL2+, BCL6+, CD23 can be used to highlight follicular meshwork, SOX11–

[a]Data from reference 66.

lesions, abundant monocytoid cells, and reactive lymphoid follicles (66). In contrast, features suggestive of a mantle cell lymphoma include the presence of a monomorphic lymphoid population with interspersed cells with "naked" nuclei (follicular dendritic cells), a mantle zone growth pattern, solitary epithelioid histiocytes dispersed among the lymphoid infiltrate, and absence of lymphoepithelial lesions.

As shown in Table 11-2, immunohistochemical stains are helpful in differentiating MALT lymphoma from other small B-cell lymphomas (66,68). The BCL-2 immunostain is positive in all these types of lymphomas, but is negative in reactive lymphoid follicles, such as those that occur in MALT lymphomas. *BCL1* (cyclin D1; *CCND1*) gene rearrangement by molecular analysis strongly supports a diagnosis of mantle cell lymphoma (66). The presence of a *BCL2* gene rearrangement supports a diagnosis of follicular lymphoma. Demonstration of t(11;18)(q21;q21) (69), t(14;18)(q32;q21), or t(1;14)(p22;q32) supports a diagnosis of MALT lymphoma.

Spread. Despite a tendency for multifocality, more than 80 percent of gastric MALT lymphomas remain localized within the stomach, but can occasionally involve multiple mucosal sites simultaneously, such as the stomach and small bowel (10). MALT lymphomas often remain localized for prolonged periods of time; in some cases progression does not occur, even after several years, in patients without treatment. Tumors with t(11;18)(q21;q21) disseminate to regional lymph nodes or distant sites more frequently than tumors without this translocation (14).

Staging. The grade of malignancy (MALT lymphoma versus diffuse large B-cell lymphoma

with or without MALT components) and stage of the disease are the two major prognostic factors and therapeutic determinants. Accurate staging requires a thorough endoscopic biopsy protocol (gastric mapping) (28). A minimum of 10 biopsies should be obtained from macroscopic visible lesions: 4 biopsies each from normal mucosa in the corpus and the antrum, and 2 biopsies from fundus.

For accurate tumor staging the following tests should be performed: history (including duration and presence of local or systemic symptoms), physical examination (evaluation of all lymph node regions, inspection of the upper airway and tonsils, clinical evaluation of the size of liver and spleen, and detection of any palpable masses), laboratory tests (complete blood counts and peripheral blood smears, lactate dehydrogenase (LDH) and β_2-microglobulin levels, an evaluation of renal and liver function), bone marrow biopsy, standard posteroanterior and lateral chest radiographs, abdominal and pelvic computerized tomography scan, gastroduodenal endoscopy with multiple biopsies from each area of the stomach and from all the abnormal sites, and gastric endoscopic ultrasound to determine the depth of invasion and status of perigastric lymph nodes (2,10). The presence or absence of *H. pylori* infection must be determined by histology; serologic studies are mandatory when the results of histology are negative or equivocal.

Different staging systems are used for MALT lymphomas and there has been no agreement for use of a single system (Table 11-3). For centers that use endoscopic ultrasound, the TNM system (using the criteria initially proposed for gastric carcinoma by the American Joint Committee on Cancer and the International Union

Table 11-3

STAGING OF GASTRIC LYMPHOMA: COMPARISON OF DIFFERENT SYSTEMS[a]

Stage	Lugano Staging System for Gastrointestinal Lymphoma	TNM Staging System for Gastric Lymphoma	Ann Arbor Stage	Tumor Extension
I	Confined to GI tract (single primary or primary or multiple, noncontiguous)	T1N0M0	IE	Mucosa, submucosa
		T2N0M0	IE	Muscularis propria
		T3N0M0	IE	Serosa
II	Extending into abdomen			
	II1 = local nodal involvement	T1-3N1M0	IIE	Perigastric lymph nodes
	II2 = distant nodal involvement	T1-3N2M0	IIE	More distant regional lymph nodes
IIE	Penetration of serosa to involve adjacent organs or tissues	T4N0M0	IE	Invasion of adjacent structures
IV	Disseminated extranodal involvement or concomitant supradiaphragmatic nodal involvement	T1-4N3M0	IIIE	Lymph nodes on both sides of the diaphragm/
		T1-4N0-3M1	IVE	distant metastases (e.g., bone marrow or additional extranodal sites)

[a]Table 2 from Zucca E, Bertoni F, Roggero E, Cavalli F. The gastric marginal zone B-cell lymphoma of MALT type. Blood 2000;96:414.

Against Cancer) can be employed, based on the extent of gastric wall involvement (10).

Treatment. First-line treatment for gastric MALT lymphomas, particularly those with *H. pylori* infection, is antibiotics designed to eradicate the organism (28). According to a meta-analysis, 77.5 percent of patients with gastric MALT lymphoma achieve complete regression after successful eradication of *H. pylori* infection (37). Positivity for the *BIRC3-MALT1* fusion transcript, lack of demonstrable *H. pylori* infection, and high clinical stage are all features associated with a lack of response to eradication therapy (70,71), although some (16 to 29 percent) *H. pylori*-negative patients respond to antibiotic treatment (45,72). A watch-and-wait strategy with frequent endoscopic biopsies is recommended for those patients who show clinical/endoscopic response but with histologic residual disease (73).

Those patients who show local progression or transformation to high-grade disease and who do not show response to *H. pylori* eradication need to be referred for second-line treatment of radiotherapy and chemotherapy, either alone or in combination. In a study of pooled data analysis, radiotherapy achieved a higher remission rate than chemotherapy (97 versus 85 percent) (74).

Prognosis. In a large prospective study from Japan, an excellent 10-year overall survival rate of 95 percent and disease-free survival rate of

86 percent was achieved (71). The overall 3-year event-free survival rate for patients who received "second-line" treatment consisting of oral monochemotherapy was 89 percent (75). Those who received radiotherapy as the "second-line" treatment had a 10-year overall survival of 70 percent (76). Higher tumor stage and presence of a diffuse large B-cell lymphoma component are associated with a poorer prognosis.

In a long-term (average 122 months) follow-up study of 120 patients with localized gastric MALT lymphoma, 80 percent achieved complete remission (77); of those, 80 percent had histologic residual disease but without progression. A significantly higher incidence of gastric cancer with a hazard ratio of 8.6 (95 percent confidence interval of 3.6-21) and of non-Hodgkin lymphoma with a hazard ratio of 18 (95 percent confidence interval of 8.4-41) was found in those who achieved complete remission when compared to the general population.

DIFFUSE LARGE B-CELL LYMPHOMA

Definition. *Diffuse large B-cell lymphoma* (DLBCL) is a diffuse proliferation of large neoplastic B-lymphoid cells that contain nuclei of either equal or greater size than nuclei of normal macrophages, or are more than twice the size of normal lymphocytes (78). DLBCL represents a group of biologically and clinically heterogeneous lymphomas that derive from germinal center B cells or from B cells at a later stage of differentiation. The current WHO classification does not recommend the term "high-grade MALT lymphoma." Some authors, however, separate DLBCL with a MALT lymphoma component from those without, and demonstrate immunophenotypic and clinical differences between these two types of lesions (79–84).

Incidence. DLBCL is the most common (50 percent) primary extranodal lymphoma (1). Close to 40 percent of all DLBCLs are initially confined to extranodal sites (78). The gastrointestinal tract, and particularly the stomach, is the most common extranodal site for DLBCL (85). Although DLBCLs have not been as thoroughly investigated as MALT lymphomas, they are the most common type of non-Hodgkin lymphoma of the stomach after MALT lymphoma, constituting 55 to 65 percent of all gastric lymphomas (20,21,59,86). The SEER data in the United States have estimated the incidence rate of gastric DLBCL to be 0.4 per 100,000 person-years (19). The incidence rates of diffuse large B-cell lymphomas and primary gastric lymphomas, in general, have been increasing (22,24,87).

Clinical Features. The median age of affected patients is 65 years (range, 14 to 89 years), with a slight male predominance (male to female ratio, 1.0-1.4 to 1.0) (23,57,88). The presenting symptoms are similar to those of MALT lymphoma: nonspecific epigastric pain (76 to 84 percent), abdominal fullness (41 percent), nausea and vomiting (21 to 32 percent), and gastric bleeding (8 to 14 percent). More DLBCL patients present with weight loss and a palpable abdominal mass compared to patients with MALT lymphoma (26,27). Up to 10 percent of DLBCL patients have "B" type symptoms (88). A small percentage (2 percent) presents with perforation or ileus (0.6 percent). Elevated β_2-microglobulin and LDH levels have been reported in up to 39 percent and 30 percent of patients with gastrointestinal DLBCL, respectively (89). Seventeen to 27 percent of patients present with advanced stage disease (disseminated extranodal involvement or concomitant supradiaphragmatic nodal involvement). In fact, this value may be underestimated since some cases that present with disseminated disease are not considered extranodal in origin.

Etiology. Some (15 to 40 percent) patients with gastric DLBCL have a lesser component of low-grade (small cell) lymphoma (81,82,86, 88,90). This feature is considered strong evidence in favor of the development of DLBCL by progression/transformation from a less aggressive type of small cell lymphoma, such as chronic lymphocytic leukemia/small lymphocytic lymphoma, follicular lymphoma, nodular lymphocyte-predominant Hodgkin lymphoma, or MALT lymphoma. Nevertheless, most DLBCLs are believed to arise de novo (78).

Immunodeficiency disorders, such as primary immunodeficiency syndromes, human immunodeficiency virus (HIV) infection, and iatrogenic immunosuppression associated with organ transplantation or methotrexate therapy, are significant risk factors for the development of DLBCL. In immunodeficient patients, DLBCL is the most common type of non-Hodgkin lymphoma. In these patients, DLBCL is often associated with Epstein-Barr virus (EBV) infection.

Genetic Abnormalities. Most cases (over 80 percent) of gastric DLBCL show Ig heavy chain gene rearrangements and somatic mutations in the variable region of the rearranged Ig heavy chain genes (68,78,91). Translocation of the *BCL2* gene (t(14;18)(q32;q21)) occurs in 20 to 30 percent of gastric DLBCL (68,78,84). In up to 48 percent, abnormalities of the 3q27 regions, which involve the candidate proto-oncogene *BCL6,* are seen (9,84). Hypermutations of the *BCL6* gene, which are independent of the gene rearrangement, at the E1.11 segment have been reported in up to 73 percent of cases. Mutations at segment E1.12 occur in 14 percent of cases (92). Trisomy 12 and trisomy 18 are found in up to 20 percent and 13 percent of DLBCL cases, respectively (51,93).

Gross Findings. DLBCL develops in any portion of the stomach. More than 75 percent of the cases involve the corpus or antrum (23,27,88), and the remainder involve the stomach diffusely. The endoscopic findings are similar to those of advanced gastric cancer and include large ulcers (35 percent) (fig. 11-12), and intraluminal polypoid tumors (33 percent) (fig. 11-13) (57,88). Other cases show multiple small shallow ulcers or erosions, mucosal nodularity, enlarged gastric folds, or perforation (9,80,81). Diffuse infiltration (14 to 24 percent) and multiple small ulcers (11 percent) are also seen.

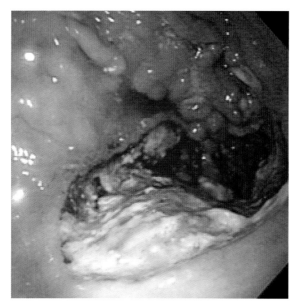

Figure 11-12

GASTRIC DIFFUSE LARGE B-CELL LYMPHOMA

A single large deep ulcer is partially surrounded by thickened folds.

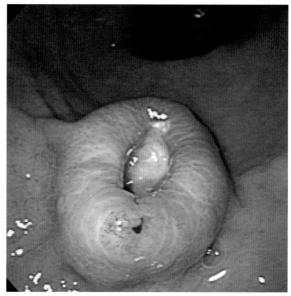

Figure 11-13

GASTRIC DIFFUSE LARGE B-CELL LYMPHOMA

A polyp with a deep central ulcer is seen endoscopically.

Microscopic Findings. DLBCLs are a heterogeneous group of lymphomas. They are typically composed of large cells (three times the size of normal lymphocytes) that resemble either proliferating germinal center cells (centroblasts/large noncleaved cells) or immunoblasts, but most tumors show a mixture of these two cell types (94). Several morphologic variants have been described, but their distinction shows poor intraobserver and interobserver reproducibility, and the clinical significance of the subclassification system is unclear (78,94). Unfortunately, immunophenotypic and genotypic parameters are generally not helpful in delineating distinctive morphologic subtypes.

The centroblastic type, which represents approximately 80 percent of the cases, is composed of medium-sized to large lymphoid cells that resemble centroblasts, and contain oval to round vesicular nuclei, fine chromatin, 1 to 4 peripherally located nucleoli, and a narrow rim of amphophilic to basophilic cytoplasm (fig. 11-14). Often a variable admixture of immunoblasts is present (fig. 11-15). This variant may have either a monomorphic or polymorphic appearance. Multilobated centroblasts with prominent immunoblasts are also present in

some cases, and contribute to the appearance of a polymorphous cellular infiltrate.

The immunoblastic type (10 percent of the cases) contains more than 90 percent immunoblasts. These cells show a single, prominent, centrally located nucleolus and an appreciable amount of basophilic cytoplasm, often with plasmacytoid differentiation (fig. 11-16). This type is more common in immunodeficient patients. Some studies suggest that this type has a worse prognosis in nonimmunodeficient patients (94), but this is controversial.

The anaplastic and T-cell/histiocyte-rich variants of DLBCL rarely occur in the stomach. In the T-cell/histiocyte-rich variant, the majority of cells represent non-neoplastic T cells, either with or without histiocytes; less than 10 percent of cells are neoplastic B cells. Histiocytes may be epithelioid in appearance. The large cells may resemble centroblasts, immunoblasts, Reed-Sternberg cells, or L&H cells of Hodgkin lymphoma. The anaplastic variant is characterized by large round, oval, or polygonal-shaped cells with bizarre pleomorphic nuclei that resemble Reed-Sternberg cells (fig. 11-17). In some cases, the cells grow in a cohesive pattern, mimicking carcinoma.

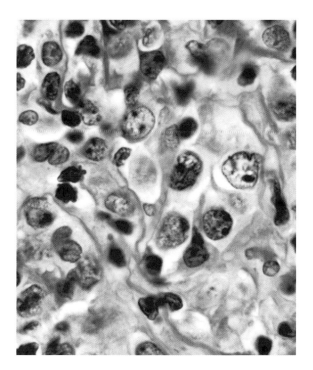

Figure 11-14

GASTRIC DIFFUSE LARGE B-CELL LYMPHOMA

Medium-sized to large lymphoid cells resemble centroblasts and contain oval to round vesicular nuclei, fine chromatin, 1-4 peripherally located nucleoli, and a narrow rim of amphophilic to basophilic cytoplasm (H&E stain).

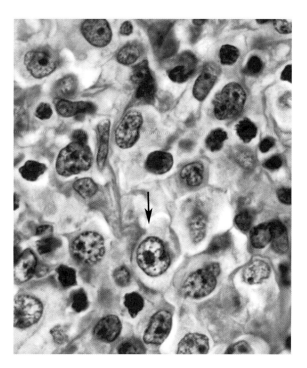

Figure 11-15

GASTRIC DIFFUSE LARGE B-CELL LYMPHOMA

In addition to centroblasts, an immunoblast (arrow) is seen with a large prominent central nucleus and amphophilic cytoplasm (H&E stain).

Immunohistochemical Findings. One or more B-cell markers, such as CD19, CD20, CD22, CD79a, and PAX5, are expressed in these tumors (78,94). Surface and/or cytoplasmic immunoglobulins (IgM>IgG>IgA) are expressed in 50 to 75 percent of cases. Some cases also express CD5 (10 percent) or CD10 (25 to 50 percent), and occasional tumors, especially those of the anaplastic type, stain for CD30. BCL-2 is positive in 30 to 50 percent of cases. Nuclear expression of BCL-6 is found in about 70 percent of cases, consistent with a germinal-center phenotype, independent of the *BCL6* gene rearrangement. The proliferation fraction, as detected by Ki-67 staining, is usually high (over 40 percent) and may even be greater than 90 percent in some cases.

Molecular Genetic Classification. Using gene expression profiling with complementary DNA microarrays, Alizadeh et al. (95) separated DLBCL, based on putative cells of origin, into two groups that resembled those of germinal center B cells (GC) and activated peripheral blood B cells

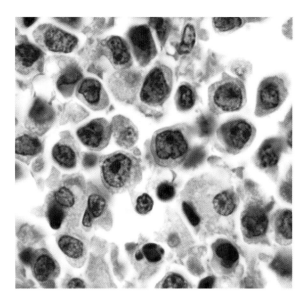

Figure 11-16

GASTRIC DIFFUSE LARGE B-CELL LYMPHOMA

Immunoblasts with a single prominent centrally located nucleolus and an appreciable amount of basophilic cytoplasm, often with a plasmacytoid appearance, are present (H&E stain).

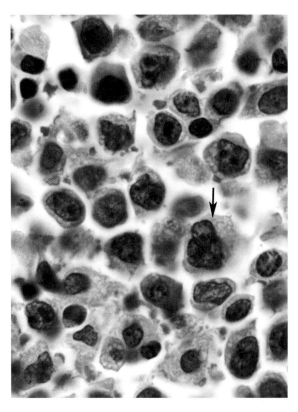

Figure 11-17

GASTRIC DIFFUSE LARGE B-CELL LYMPHOMA

Several anaplastic-appearing cells consisting of large round, oval, or polygonal-shaped cells with bizarre pleomorphic nuclei are present. One cell (arrow) resembles a Reed-Sternberg cell (H&E stain).

(ABC) (GC versus postgerminal center/peripheral blood). These two subgroups were distinguished by the differential expression of hundreds of genes that related each subgroup to a separate stage of B-cell differentiation and activation. DLBCL of the GC subtype was associated with a significantly better 5-year survival rate than the ABC subtype (76 percent versus 16 percent, P <0.01). In a subsequent study of 240 patients treated with anthracycline-based chemotherapy, those with the GC subtype had a 5-year survival rate of 60 percent, compared to 39 percent for patients with non-GC DLBCL (96). A third subtype demonstrated only minor expression of genes that are characteristic of the GC or ABC subtypes (97); the 5-year survival rate of this third subtype was similar that of the ABC subtype.

Immunohistochemical techniques can be used to classify DLBCL into GC or ABC sub-groups (98,99). GC subtype tumors are CD10 positive. Of the CD10-negative tumors, those that are BCL-6 positive, and MUM1 negative are also considered part of the GC subtype. In contrast, CD10-negative and BCL-6-negative tumors, and the CD10-negative, BCL-6-positive, and MUM1-positive tumors, are considered to represent the non-GC subtype. This approach demonstrated superior overall survival for the GC subgroup relative to the non-GC subgroup, similar to that reported using gene expression profiling. The sensitivity and positive predictive value for the GC and non-GC subtypes were 71/87 percent and 88/72 percent, respectively. Although other immunohistochemistry-based and nonimmunohistochemistry-based methods for molecular classification of DLBCL have been proposed (96), the Hans algorithm (99) described above is the most practical since it is based on readily available antibodies.

Cytologic Findings. If adequate material is present, a diagnosis of malignancy usually is established easily on cytology specimens (65). The presence of many isolated lymphoid cells favors a diagnosis of lymphoma. Nevertheless, immunocytochemical or flow cytometric studies may be needed to rule out carcinoma or malignant melanoma (see next section). Typical cytology specimens show a mixture of large centroblasts (fig. 11-18, left) and immunoblasts (fig. 11-18, right), with occasional smaller lymphoid cells, such as centrocytes and plasma cells. Depending on the type, centroblasts or immunoblasts may dominate the cellular profile.

Differential Diagnosis. Since some DLBCL tumor cells, such as immunoblasts, have a fair amount of cytoplasm, are polymorphic, and may even grow in a cohesive pattern, they may be difficult to distinguish from carcinoma or metastatic melanoma on H&E-stained sections. Immunohistochemical studies of epithelial, melanoma, lymphoid, and even B-cell markers, such as cytokeratins, S-100 protein/HMB-45/MART-1, CD45 (leukocyte common antigen), and CD20, are helpful in this differential. Carcinomas are positive for cytokeratins and negative for the other markers. Melanomas are negative for cytokeratins and lymphoid markers, but are usually positive for at least one of the above melanoma markers. DLBCL cells are positive for CD45 and usually one or more of the B-cell markers.

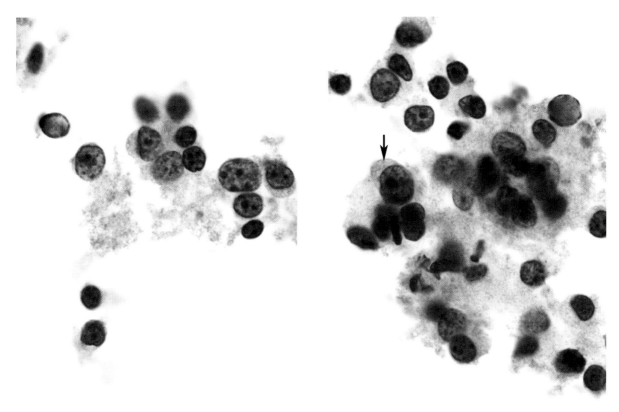

Figure 11-18

GASTRIC DIFFUSE LARGE B-CELL LYMPHOMA

Several centroblasts have oval to round, vesicular nuclei; fine chromatin; 1 to 4 peripherally located nucleoli; and a narrow rim of amphophilic to basophilic cytoplasm (Papanicolaou stain).

The current WHO classification acknowledges that a variable number of transformed centroblast- or immunoblast-like cells may be present in MALT lymphomas (9). Another difficult diagnostic issue occurs when most of the neoplastic cells appear medium-sized (with irregularly folded nuclei and fairly open chromatin) (8,9). In this situation it is difficult to determine whether they represent the small cells of MALT lymphoma or large cells of DLBCL. Immunohistochemical staining for Ki-67 is helpful in this regard. If the index is more than 40 percent, the lymphoma is best considered a large cell lymphoma.

On occasion, the immunoblastic variant of DLBCL may be difficult to distinguish from the plasmablastic variant of plasma cell myeloma. Clinical and immunophenotypic findings are critical in this distinction. The immunoblastic type of DLBCL is usually positive for CD20, whereas the plasmablastic variant of plasma cell myeloma is typically positive for CD138 and epithelial membrane antigen (EMA).

Since DLBCL is a heterogeneous group of lymphomas, there are often exceptions to typical immunophenotypic patterns (9). On occasion, immunoblastic DLBCL is negative for CD20 and CD79a, and may not express surface Ig. In addition, immunoblastic lymphomas with plasmablastic or plasmacytic differentiation may express EMA. A few tumors may lack CD45 expression but show intracytoplasmic positivity for cytokeratin. It is, thus, important to consider all available clinical, histologic, and immunophenotypic findings in order to establish a correct diagnosis. Based on histology, cells showing triangular-shaped cytoplasm with an eccentric nucleus, amphophilic cytoplasm on H&E-stained sections, and basophilic cytoplasm on Giemsa-stained sections, as well as demonstration of intracytoplasmic monotypic immunoglobulins, are consistent with DLBCL (9).

Spread. The muscularis propria is invaded in 77 to 85 percent of patients with gastric DLBCL (80). Regional lymph node involvement by lymphoma is significantly associated with depth of invasion. Lymph nodes are involved in 45 percent and 73 percent of cases with muscularis propria and subserosa/serosal involvement, respectively. In patients with tumor limited to submucosa and mucosa, less than 3 percent have lymph node involvement.

Advanced stages (Ann Arbor stages III and IV [disseminated extranodal involvement with lymph nodes on both sides of the diaphragm/ distant metastases]), have been reported in 18 to 27 percent of patients with primary gastric or gastrointestinal DLBCL (89,100). In one series of 312 patients with primary gastric DLBCL, however, 52 percent were confined to the gastrointestinal tract, 34 percent extended into the abdomen with local or distant nodal involvement, and 14 percent penetrated the serosa with involvement of adjacent organs or tissue, but none had disseminated involvement on both sides of the diaphragm (88).

Staging. See staging for MALT lymphoma.

Treatment. There are no recognized standard treatment strategies for patients with gastric DLBCL. Options include surgery, chemotherapy, and radiotherapy, either alone or in combination. The recent trend is toward stomach conservation, as the addition of surgery to conservative management (chemotherapy with or without radiotherapy) does not seem to change the outcome in a significant manner (101). Furthermore, DLBCL is a highly chemosensitive disease, and there is no evidence to suggest an advantage in the addition of radiotherapy (102). The addition of rituximab to standard chemotherapy has been shown to improve overall survival in patients with both subtypes (103). For patients with limited-stage DLBCL, *H. pylori* eradication resulted in a complete remission rate of 63 percent, a 5-year overall survival rate of 94 percent, and no deaths due to lymphoma in exploratory studies (104).

Prognosis. Patients with the localized form of gastric DLBCL have an overall 5-year survival rate of 90 percent (101,105–107). The survival rate is reduced to 50 percent, or less in some studies, for patients with advanced disease (88,100,105). The International Prognostic In-dex (IPI) (an index based on age, tumor stage, serum LDH concentration, performance status, and number of extranodal disease sites to stratify patients with aggressive non-Hodgkin lymphoma into various risk groups before treatment) (108) indices for DLBCL patients with low, intermediate, and high-risk categories are 45 percent, 38 percent, and 17 percent, respectively. The 5-year event-free survival rates for those in the low-, intermediate-, and high-risk categories are 70 percent, 50 percent, and 40 percent, respectively (108).

Factors associated with a favorable outcome include the centroblastic morphologic type, positive CD10 and BCL-6 expression, and the GC subtype (109). In contrast, the immuno-blastic type; positive CD5, BCL-2, and cyclin D2 expression; and the ABC subtype are associated with a poor prognosis. In fact, analysis of variables that include the molecular classification (GC versus non-GC subtypes), IPI risk group, cyclin D2, BCL-2, FOXP1 expression patterns, and the interactions between them, showed that a high IPI score and the non-GC subtype are independent adverse predictors of outcome for patients with DLBCL (99). Although most studies have shown a definite survival advantage in patients with DLBCL that presumably developed from MALT lymphoma or are *H. pylori* positive (79,82,84,110), one study showed that these patients have a significantly worse event-free survival rate compared to either those with MALT lymphoma or pure DLBCL (86).

BURKITT LYMPHOMA

Burkitt lymphoma comprises a heterogeneous group of highly aggressive B-cell malignancies (111). Burkitt lymphoma occurs primarily in three clinical settings: endemic, sporadic, and HIV associated. Burkitt originally described the endemic form that was often found in equatorial Africa and New Guinea.

This tumor typically arises at extranodal sites in adolescents and young adults. It is a tumor of B cells latently infected with EBV. A sporadic, morphologically identical form of Burkitt lymphoma that occurs in nonendemic regions also arises at extranodal sites in adolescents or young adults. Burkitt lymphoma accounts for 24 to 35 percent of HIV-associated non-Hodgkin lymphomas and often presents with extranodal and nodal involvement. Only a subset (25 to 40 percent) of sporadic and HIV-associated Burkitt lymphomas is EBV associated. The ileocecal region is the most common site for the sporadic form of Burkitt lymphoma. It only rarely occurs in the stomach and accounts for 1 to 3 percent of gastric lymphomas (20,86).

Burkitt lymphoma is a malignancy of intermediate-sized germinal center B cells that infiltrate in a diffuse pattern (111,112). The tumor cells usually express the B-cell–specific surface markers CD19, CD20, CD22, IgM, and Igκ or Igλ light chain restriction, as well as low to intermediate levels of CD10. Importantly, BCL-2 is not expressed in classic Burkitt lymphoma and this phenotypic trait is useful for differentiating classic Burkitt lymphoma from other high-grade lymphomas involving the stomach.

The histologic hallmark of Burkitt lymphoma is the "starry sky" microscopic appearance at low-power magnification that represents numerous apoptotic cells within scattered phagocytic macrophages. The rate of cell division in Burkitt lymphoma is among the highest of any human malignancy. It is reflected by the presence of numerous mitotic figures and a high fraction of actively growing cells. Stains for cell cycle-specific markers, such as Ki-67, typically show positivity in nearly 100 percent of the tumor cells.

All cases have a translocation of *MYC:* t(8;14) (q24;q32) in 80 percent, t(2;8)(p11/p12;q24) in 15 percent, and t(8;22)(q24;q11) in the remaining 5 percent (111,113). Therefore, *MYC* rearrangements are a sensitive marker for Burkitt lymphoma, but they are nonspecific since they are occasionally seen in large B-cell lymphomas, some aggressive transformed follicular lymphomas, and even a significant fraction of late-stage plasma cell myelomas. Certain aggressive B-cell lymphomas morphologically and immunophenotypically resembling Burkitt lymphoma (and thus are termed "Burkitt-like") usually lack *MYC* rearrangements. Therefore, the diagnosis of Burkitt lymphoma is based on a combination of clinical, histologic, immunophenotypic, and cytogenetic findings (114).

Recently, gene expression profiling has been found to be an accurate method for distinguishing Burkitt lymphoma from DLBCL (115,116). The genes identified may be useful for diagnosis with the use of fluorescence in situ hybridization (FISH), real-time polymerase chain reaction (PCR), or immunologic methods (114).

A correct diagnosis of Burkitt lymphoma is of clinical importance since this tumor shows a high response rate to intensive chemotherapy. Depending on tumor stage, a high event-free survival rate has been reported (80 to 90 percent) (112). Relapse, if it occurs, is usually detected within the first year after diagnosis. Patients without relapse for 2 consecutive years can be regarded as cured. Complications of gastric Burkitt lymphoma include perforation and infiltration into the esophagus (117).

MANTLE CELL LYMPHOMA

Mantle cell lymphoma is a B-cell neoplasm of the peripheral B cells located in the inner mantle zone of lymphoid follicles (118). Lymph nodes are the most common site of involvement, followed by spleen and bone marrow. Primary gastrointestinal mantle cell lymphomas are rare and constitute 4 to 9 percent of gastrointestinal B-cell lymphomas (119). The gastrointestinal tract, however, is the most frequently involved extranodal site, with up to 92 percent of patients with untreated mantle cell lymphoma showing upper or lower gastrointestinal tract involvement and 77 percent showing infiltration in the stomach with or without endoscopically abnormal mucosa (120).

Most cases of multiple lymphomatous polyposis of the small and large intestines used to be considered to represent mantle cell lymphoma. This phenomenon is now known to be present in follicular lymphomas and MALT lymphomas as well (119). The polyps range from 0.2 to 1.0 cm in size, but can occasionally produce a large tumor mass (9).

Histologically, mantle cell lymphoma demonstrates a vaguely nodular, diffuse, or mantle zone growth pattern composed of a monomorphic proliferation of small to medium-sized lymphoid cells with irregular nuclei. A true follicular pattern is only rarely seen. The tumor cells closely resemble centrocytes. The nuclei have moderately dispersed chromatin and inconspicuous nucleoli. Pseudofollicles are absent. In fact, blasts are only found as remnants of germinal centers. Sometimes lymphoepithelial lesions are observed.

The neoplastic cells are monomorphic B cells with intense surface IgM, with or without IgD.

They are positive for CD5, CD19, CD20, CD43, CD79A, BCL-2, and cyclin D1, and negative for CD10 and BCL-6. CD23 is often negative or only weakly positive. Ig heavy and light chain genes are usually rearranged. Igλ light chain is more commonly expressed than Igκ light chain.

The hallmark genomic abnormality is the presence of t(11;14)(q13;q32) translocation in virtually all mantle cell lymphomas (121), resulting in overexpression of cyclin D1. Overexpression of the transcription factor SOX11 is a newer diagnostic marker, identified in both cyclin D1-positive and cyclin D1-negative mantle cell lymphomas (119). Absence of SOX11 appears to be associated with an indolent mantle cell variant. Typically, mantle cell lymphomas do not transform to large cell lymphomas.

Patients with mantle cell lymphoma have a median survival period of 3 to 5 years, with an overall survival rate of 36 percent after 5 years. The most consistently reported adverse histologic prognostic factor is a high proliferation fraction as measured by mitotic rate or Ki-67 index. Due to poor prognosis, combined chemotherapy is the preferred upfront strategy, yet frequently yields low complete remission rates and short remissions.

FOLLICULAR LYMPHOMA

Follicular lymphoma is the second most common type of non-Hodgkin lymphoma after DLBCL, accounting for 20 percent of new lymphoma cases (119). Low- and intermediate-grade follicular lymphomas account for up to 12 percent of gastric lymphomas in older series (20,122), but they are virtually unseen in more recent series of gastric lymphomas (86). The median age of patients with gastrointestinal follicular lymphoma is 50 to 60 years with a 1 to 1 male to female ratio.

Follicular lymphoma is a neoplasm of follicle center B cells (centrocytes/cleaved follicle center cells and centroblasts/noncleaved follicle center cells) that show at least a partially follicular pattern (123). Some lymphomas are composed of follicle center cells, but do not form follicles and, therefore, do not fulfill the criteria for follicular lymphoma. The term "diffuse follicle center lymphoma" is used for these latter lymphomas, and they are considered a variant of follicular lymphoma.

Follicular lymphomas involve primarily lymph nodes, but also spleen, bone marrow, peripheral blood, and Waldeyer ring. Extranodal involvement occurs on occasion, but this is usually in the setting of widespread nodal disease. Primary gastrointestinal follicular lymphoma is rare and represents 1.0 to 3.6 percent of gastrointestinal non-Hodgkin lymphomas (124). They occur anywhere in the gastrointestinal tract but most frequently involve the small intestine, especially the duodenum and ileocecal region.

Gastrointestinal follicular lymphomas are most often multifocal, confined to the gastrointestinal tract, and present as multiple small polyps. Most are detected as an incidental finding on endoscopy, and over 90 percent are stage I to II disease (66 percent, stage I). Histologically, they demonstrate neoplastic follicles composed of small to medium-sized cells with angulated, elongated, twisted, or cleaved nuclei; inconspicuous nucleoli; and scant pale cytoplasm. The neoplastic cells are known as centrocytes or cleaved follicle center cells.

Follicular lymphomas are categorized into three grades according to the number of centroblasts (large nucleated cells) per high-power field. Less than five large transformed cells (cells with round or oval, but occasionally indented nuclei, vesicular chromatin, one to three peripheral nucleoli, and a narrow rim of cytoplasm, known as centroblasts or noncleaved follicle center cells) per high-power field are seen in grade 1 follicular lymphomas. The tumor cells do not usually infiltrate and destroy the glandular epithelium, i.e., there are no lymphoepithelial lesion (124).

The major differential diagnosis is with mantle cell lymphoma since both can present grossly as multiple polyps and microscopically with a nodular pattern of small to medium-sized lymphoid cells with irregular nuclei (9). The detection of lymphoepithelial lesions does not exclude a potential diagnosis of follicular lymphoma. Therefore, follicular lymphomas also may be difficult to distinguish from MALT lymphomas.

Immunohistochemistry is mandatory to establish a correct diagnosis (see Table 11-2). Tumor cells express surface Ig (IgM with or without IgD, IgG or rarely IgA), B-cell–associated antigens (CD19, CD20, CD22, and CD79a), as well as BCL-2 and CD10. They are negative for CD5, CD43, and cyclin D1. Ig heavy and light chains are typically rearranged. Most follicular lymphomas have cytogenetic abnormalities, such as t(14;18)(q32;q21)as described above (49,123).

Grade 1 follicular lymphoma has an indolent, but usually incurable, clinical course. Five-year survival rates of more than 70 percent are typically reported despite a nonaggressive (watch and wait) approach to initial management.

CHRONIC LYMPHOCYTIC LEUKEMIA/ SMALL LYMPHOCYTIC LYMPHOMA

Chronic lymphocytic leukemia/small lymphocytic lymphoma (SLL/CLL) is a neoplasm of monomorphic, small, round B lymphocytes in the peripheral blood, bone marrow, and lymph nodes, admixed with prolymphocytes and paraimmunoblasts (pseudofollicles) that express CD5 and CD23 (125). The liver and spleen are usually involved. Although it can involve virtually every type of tissue, gastrointestinal involvement is rare.

Histologically, SLL/CLL is characterized by a pseudofollicular pattern of regularly distributed large cells within a dark background of small cells (pseudofollicles, also known as proliferation centers, or growth centers). The predominant cells are small lymphocytes, which may be slightly larger than normal lymphocytes, that have clumped chromatin, round nuclei, and occasionally, a small nucleolus. Mitotic activity is usually very low. Pseudofollicles contain a continuum of small lymphocytes, medium-sized prolymphocytes (with dispersed chromatin and small nucleoli), and medium-sized to large paraimmunoblasts (with round to oval nuclei, dispersed chromatin, central eosinophilic nucleoli, and slightly basophilic cytoplasm).

The tumor cells express weak or dim surface IgM (with or without IgD), CD5, CD19, CD20 (weak), CD22 (weak), CD79a, CD23, CD43, and CD11c (weak), and are usually negative for CD10 and cyclin D1. Ig heavy and light chain genes are normally rearranged. Deletions at 13q14 are reported in up to 50 percent of cases, trisomy 12 in 20 percent, and deletions at 11q22-23 in 20 percent (125).

The clinical course of affected patients is indolent, but they are not usually cured. The overall 5-year survival rate is 51 percent, with a failure-free survival rate of 25 percent.

REFERENCES

1. Krol AD, le Cessie S, Snijder S, Kluin-Nelemans JC, Kluin PM, Noordijk EM. Primary extranodal non-Hodgkin's lymphoma (NHL): the impact of alternative definitions tested in the Comprehensive Cancer Centre West population-based NHL registry. Ann Oncol 2003;14:131-9.

2. Psyrri A, Papageorgiou S, Economopoulos T. Primary extranodal lymphomas of stomach: clinical presentation, diagnostic pitfalls and management. Ann Oncol 2008;19:1992-9.

3. Suarez F, Lortholary O, Hermine O, Lecuit M. Infection-associated lymphomas derived from marginal zone B cells: a model of antigen-driven lymphoproliferation. Blood 2006;107:3034-44.

4. Thomas RM, Sobin LH. Gastrointestinal cancer. Cancer 1995;75(1 Suppl):154-70.

5. Greiner TC, Medeiros LJ, Jaffe ES. Non-Hodgkin's lymphoma. Cancer 1995;75(1 Suppl):370-80.

6. Feller AC, Diebold J, Lennert K. History of lymphoma classification. In: Histopathology of nodal and extranodal non-Hodgkin's lymphomas: based on the WHO classification, 3rd ed. Berlin ; New York: Springer, 2004:1-5.

7. Trümper LH, Brittinger G, Diehl V, Harris NL. Non-Hodgkin's lymphoma: a history of classification and clinical observations. In: Mauch PM, Armitage JO, Coiffier B, Dalla-Favera R, Harris NL, editors. Non-Hodgkin's lymphomas. Philadelphia: Lippincott Williams & Wilkins; 2004:3-19.

8. Medeiros LJ, O'Mally DP, Caraway NP, Vega F, Elenitoba-Johnson KS, Lim MS. Tumors of the lymph nodes and spleen. AFIP Atlas of Tumor Pathology, 4th Series, Fascicle 25. Washington DC: American Registry of Pathology; 2017.

9. Swerdlow SH, Campo E, Harris NL, et al., eds. WHO classification of tumours of haematopoietic and lymphoid tissues, 4th ed. Lyon: IARC Press; 2017.

10. Zucca E, Bertoni F, Roggero E, Cavalli F. The gastric marginal zone B-cell lymphoma of MALT type. Blood 2000;96:410-9.

11. Isaacson PG, Müller-Hermelink HK, Piris MA, et al. Extranodal marginal zone B-cell lymphoma of mucosa-associated lymphoid tissue (MALT lymphoma). In: ology and genetics of tumours of haematopoietic and lymphoid tissues. Lyon: IARC Press, 2001:157-60.

12. Cook JR, Isaacson PG, Chott A, Nakamura S. Extranodal marginal zone lymphoma of mucosa-associated lymphoid tissue (MALT lymphoma). In: Swerdlow SH, Campo E, Harris NL, et al., eds. WHO classification of tumours of haematopoietic and lymphoid tissues, 4th ed. Lyon: IARC Press; 2017:259-62.

13. Yahalom J, Isaacson PG, Zucca E. Extranodal marginal zone B-cell lymphoma of mucosa-associated lymphoid tissue. In: Mauch PM, Armitage JO, Coiffier B, Dalla-Favera R, Harris NL, eds. Non-Hodgkin's lymphomas. Philadelphia: Lippincott Williams & Wilkins; 2004:345-60.

14. Isaacson PG, Du MQ. MALT lymphoma: from morphology to molecules. Nat Rev Cancer 2004; 4:644-53.

15. Chan JK, Ng CS, Isaacson PG. Relationship between high-grade lymphoma and low-grade B-cell mucosa-associated lymphoid tissue lymphoma (MALToma) of the stomach. Am J Pathol 1990;136:1153-64.

16. Du MQ, Diss TC, Dogan A, et al. Clone-specific PCR reveals wide dissemination of gastric MALT lymphoma to the gastric mucosa. J Pathol 2000; 192:488-93.

17. Maeshima AM, Taniguchi H, Toyoda K, et al. Clinicopathological features of histological transformation from extranodal marginal zone B-cell lymphoma of mucosa-associated lymphoid tissue to diffuse large B-cell lymphoma: an analysis of 467 patients. Br J Haematol 2016;174:923-31.

18. Harris NL, Jaffe ES, Diebold J, et al. The World Health Organization classification of neoplastic diseases of the hematopoietic and lymphoid tissues. Report of the Clinical Advisory Committee meeting, Airlie House, Virginia, November, 1997. Ann Oncol 1999;10:1419-32.

19. Groves FD, Linet MS, Travis LB, Devesa SS. Cancer surveillance series: non-Hodgkin's lymphoma incidence by histologic subtype in the United States from 1978 through 1995. J Natl Cancer Inst 2000;92:1240-51.

20. d'Amore F, Brincker H, Gronbaek K, et al. Non-Hodgkin's lymphoma of the gastrointestinal tract: a population-based analysis of incidence, geographic distribution, clinicopathologic presentation features, and prognosis. Danish Lymphoma Study Group. J Clin Oncol 1994;12:1673-84.

21. Nakamura S, Akazawa K, Yao T, Tsuneyoshi M. A clinicopathologic study of 233 cases with special reference to evaluation with the MIB-1 index. Cancer 1995;76:1313-24.

22. Howell JM, Auer-Grzesiak I, Zhang J, Andrews CN, Stewart D, Urbanski SJ. Increasing incidence rates, distribution and histological characteristics of primary gastrointestinal non-Hodgkin lymphoma in a North American population. Can J Gastroenterol 2012;26:452-6.

23. Zullo A, Hassan C, Andriani A, et al. Primary low-grade and high-grade gastric MALT-lymphoma presentation. J Clin Gastroenterol 2010;44:340-4.

24. Eltom MA, Jemal A, Mbulaiteye SM, Devesa SS, Biggar RJ. Trends in Kaposi's sarcoma and non-Hodgkin's lymphoma incidence in the United States from 1973 through 1998. J Natl Cancer Inst 2002;94:1204-10.

25. Luminari S, Cesaretti M, Marcheselli L, et al. Decreasing incidence of gastric MALT lymphomas in the era of anti-Helicobacter pylori interventions: results from a population-based study on extranodal marginal zone lymphomas. Ann Oncol 2010;21:855-9.

26. Morgner A, Bayerdorffer E, Neubauer A, Stolte M. Malignant tumors of the stomach. Gastric mucosa-associated lymphoid tissue lymphoma and Helicobacter pylori. Gastroenterol Clin North Am 2000;29:593-607.

27. Andriani A, Zullo A, Di Raimondo F, et al. Clinical and endoscopic presentation of primary gastric lymphoma: a multicentre study. Aliment Pharmacol Ther 2006;23:721-6.

28. Fischbach W. Gastric MALT lymphoma - update on diagnosis and treatment. Best Pract Res Clin Gastroenterol 2014;28:1069-77.

29. Wotherspoon AC, Ortiz-Hidalgo C, Falzon MR, Isaacson PG. Helicobacter pylori-associated gastritis and primary B-cell gastric lymphoma. Lancet 1991;338:1175-6.

30. Wotherspoon AC. Helicobacter pylori infection and gastric lymphoma. Br Med Bull 1998;54:79-85.

31. Doglioni C, Wotherspoon AC, Moschini A, de Boni M, Isaacson PG. High incidence of primary gastric lymphoma in northeastern Italy. Lancet 1992;339:834-5.

32. Parsonnet J, Hansen S, Rodriguez L, et al. Helicobacter pylori infection and gastric lymphoma. N Engl J Med 1994;330:1267-71.

33. Hussell T, Isaacson PG, Crabtree JE, Spencer J. The response of cells from low-grade B-cell gastric lymphomas of mucosa-associated lymphoid tissue to Helicobacter pylori. Lancet 1993;342:571-4.

34. Wotherspoon AC, Doglioni C, Diss TC, et al. Regression of primary low-grade B-cell gastric lymphoma of mucosa-associated lymphoid tissue type after eradication of Helicobacter pylori. Lancet 1993;342:575-7.

35. Roggero E, Zucca E, Pinotti G, et al. Eradication of Helicobacter pylori infection in primary low-grade gastric lymphoma of mucosa-associated lymphoid tissue. Ann Intern Med 1995;122:767-9.

36. Bayerdorffer E, Neubauer A, Rudolph B, et al. Regression of primary gastric lymphoma of mucosa-associated lymphoid tissue type after cure of Helicobacter pylori infection. MALT Lymphoma Study Group. Lancet 1995;345:1591-4.

37. Zullo A, Hassan C, Cristofari F, et al. Effects of Helicobacter pylori eradication on early stage gastric mucosa-associated lymphoid tissue lymphoma. Clin Gastroenterol Hepatol 2010;8:105-10.

38. Nakamura S, Aoyagi K, Furuse M, et al. B-cell monoclonality precedes the development of gastric MALT lymphoma in Helicobacter pylori-associated chronic gastritis. Am J Pathol 1998;152:1271-9.

39. Zucca E, Bertoni F, Roggero E, et al. Molecular analysis of the progression from Helicobacter pylori-associated chronic gastritis to mucosa-associated lymphoid-tissue lymphoma of the stomach. N Engl J Med 1998;338:804-10.

40. Fischbach W. Gastric mucosal-associated lymphoid tissue lymphoma. Gastroenterol Clin North Am 2013;42:371-80.

41. Suerbaum S, Michetti P. Helicobacter pylori infection. N Engl J Med 2002;347:1175-86.

42. Bhandari A, Crowe SE. Helicobacter pylori in gastric malignancies. Curr Gastroenterol Rep 2012;14:489-96.

43. Hussell T, Isaacson PG, Crabtree JE, Spencer J. Helicobacter pylori-specific tumour-infiltrating T cells provide contact dependent help for the growth of malignant B cells in low-grade gastric lymphoma of mucosa-associated lymphoid tissue. J Pathol 1996;178:122-7.

44. Ruskone-Fourmestraux A, Fischbach W, Aleman BM, et al. EGILS consensus report. Gastric extranodal marginal zone B-cell lymphoma of MALT. Gut 2011;60:747-58.

45. Nakamura S, Matsumoto T, Ye H, et al. Helicobacter pylori-negative gastric mucosa-associated lymphoid tissue lymphoma: a clinicopathologic and molecular study with reference to antibiotic treatment. Cancer 2006;107:2770-8.

46. Streubel B, Simonitsch-Klupp I, Mullauer L, et al. Variable frequencies of MALT lymphoma-associated genetic aberrations in MALT lymphomas of different sites. Leukemia 2004;18:1722-6.

47. Streubel B, Lamprecht A, Dierlamm J, et al. T(14;18)(q32;q21) involving IGH and MALT1 is a frequent chromosomal aberration in MALT lymphoma. Blood 2003;101:2335-9.

48. Sanchez-Izquierdo D, Buchonnet G, Siebert R, et al. MALT1 is deregulated by both chromosomal translocation and amplification in B-cell non-Hodgkin lymphoma. Blood 2003;101:4539-46.

49. Kridel R, Sehn LH, Gascoyne RD. Pathogenesis of follicular lymphoma. J Clin Invest 2012;122:3424-31.

50. Goatly A, Bacon CM, Nakamura S, et al. FOXP1 abnormalities in lymphoma: translocation breakpoint mapping reveals insights into deregulated transcriptional control. Mod Pathol 2008;21:902-11.

51. Hoeve MA, Gisbertz IA, Schouten HC, et al. Gastric low-grade MALT lymphoma, high-grade MALT lymphoma and diffuse large B cell lymphoma show different frequencies of trisomy. Leukemia 1999;13:799-807.

52. Remstein ED, Dogan A, Einerson RR, et al. The incidence and anatomic site specificity of chromosomal translocations in primary extranodal marginal zone B-cell lymphoma of mucosa-associated lymphoid tissue (MALT lymphoma) in North America. Am J Surg Pathol 2006;30:1546-53.

53. Kim YH, Lim HK, Han JK, et al. Low-grade gastric mucosa-associated lymphoid tissue lymphoma: correlation of radiographic and pathologic findings. Radiology 1999;212:241-8.

54. Park MS, Kim KW, Yu JS, et al. Radiographic findings of primary B-cell lymphoma of the stomach: low-grade versus high-grade malignancy in relation to the mucosa-associated lymphoid tissue concept. AJR Am J Roentgenol 2002;179:1297-304.

55. Yoo CC, Levine MS, Furth EE, et al. Gastric mucosa-associated lymphoid tissue lymphoma: radiographic findings in six patients. Radiology 1998;208:239-43.

56. Mendelson RM, Fermoyle S. Primary gastrointestinal lymphomas: a radiological-pathological review. Part 1: Stomach, oesophagus and colon. Australas Radiol 2005;49:353-64.

57. Taal BG, Boot H, van Heerde P, de Jong D, Hart AA, Burgers JM. Primary non-Hodgkin lymphoma of the stomach: endoscopic pattern and prognosis in low versus high grade malignancy in relation to the MALT concept. Gut 1996;39:556-61.

58. Abbondanzo SL, Sobin LH. Gastric "pseudolymphoma": a retrospective morphologic and immunophenotypic study of 97 cases. Cancer 1997;79:1656-63.

59. Burke JS. Lymphoproliferative disorders of the gastrointestinal tract: a review and pragmatic guide to diagnosis. Arch Pathol Lab Med 2011; 135:1283-97.

60. de Jong D, Boot H, van Heerde P, Hart GA, Taal BG. Histological grading in gastric lymphoma: pretreatment criteria and clinical relevance. Gastroenterology 1997;112:1466-74.

61. El-Zimaity HM, Wotherspoon A, de Jong D. Interobserver variation in the histopathological assessment of malt/malt lymphoma: towards a consensus. Blood Cells Mol Dis 2005;34:6-16.

62. Matsushima AY, Hamele-Bena D, Osborne BM. Fine-needle aspiration biopsy findings in marginal zone B cell lymphoma. Diagn Cytopathol 1999;20:190-8.

63. Crapanzano JP, Lin O. Cytologic findings of marginal zone lymphoma. Cancer 2003;99:301-9.

64. Chhieng DC, Cohen JM, Cangiarella JF. Cytology and immunophenotyping of low- and intermediate-grade B-cell non-Hodgkin's lymphomas with a predominant small-cell component: a study of 56 cases. Diagn Cytopathol 2001;24:90-7.

65. Zeppa P, Marino G, Troncone G, et al. Fine-needle cytology and flow cytometry immunophenotyping and subclassification of non-Hodgkin lymphoma: a critical review of 307 cases with technical suggestions. Cancer 2004;102:55-65.

66. O'Malley DP, Goldstein NS, Banks PM. The recognition and classification of lymphoproliferative disorders of the gut. Hum Pathol 2014;45:899-916.

67. Wündisch T, Neubauer A, Stolte M, Ritter M, Thiede C. B-cell monoclonality is associated with lymphoid follicles in gastritis. Am J Surg Pathol 2003;27:882-7.

68. Ansell SM, Armitage J. Non-Hodgkin lymphoma: diagnosis and treatment. Mayo Clin Proc 2005; 80:1087-97.

69. Wang G, Auerbach A, Wei M, et al. t(11;18)(q21;q21) in extranodal marginal zone B-cell lymphoma of mucosa-associated lymphoid tissue in stomach: a study of 48 cases. Mod Pathol 2009;22:79-86.

70. Inagaki H, Nakamura T, Li C, et al. Gastric MALT lymphomas are divided into three groups based on responsiveness to Helicobacter Pylori eradication and detection of API2-MALT1 fusion. Am J Surg Pathol 2004;28:1560-7.

71. Nakamura S, Sugiyama T, Matsumoto T, et al. Long-term clinical outcome of gastric MALT lymphoma after eradication of Helicobacter pylori: a multicentre cohort follow-up study of 420 patients in Japan. Gut 2012;61:507-13.

72. Zullo A, Hassan C, Ridola L, et al. Eradication therapy in Helicobacter pylori-negative, gastric low-grade mucosa-associated lymphoid tissue lymphoma patients: a systematic review. J Clin Gastroenterol 2013;47:824-7.

73. Fischbach W, Goebeler ME, Ruskone-Fourmestraux A, et al. Most patients with minimal histological residuals of gastric MALT lymphoma after successful eradication of Helicobacter pylori can be managed safely by a watch and wait strategy: experience from a large international series. Gut 2007;56:1685-7.

74. Zullo A, Hassan C, Andriani A, et al. Treatment of low-grade gastric MALT-lymphoma unresponsive to Helicobacter pylori therapy: a pooled-data analysis. Med Oncol 2010;27:291-5.

75. Nakamura S, Matsumoto T, Suekane H, et al. Long-term clinical outcome of Helicobacter pylori eradication for gastric mucosa-associated lymphoid tissue lymphoma with a reference to second-line treatment. Cancer 2005;104:532-40.

76. Wirth A, Gospodarowicz M, Aleman BM, et al. Long-term outcome for gastric marginal zone lymphoma treated with radiotherapy: a retrospective, multi-centre, International Extranodal Lymphoma Study Group study. Ann Oncol 2013;24:1344-51.

77. Wündisch T, Dieckhoff P, Greene B, et al. Second cancers and residual disease in patients treated for gastric mucosa-associated lymphoid tissue lymphoma by Helicobacter pylori eradication and followed for 10 years. Gastroenterology 2012;143:936-42.

78. Gatter KC, Warnke RA. Diffuse large B-cell lymphoma. In: Jaffe ES, Harris NL, Stein H, Vardiman JW, eds. Pathology and genetics of tumours of haematopoietic and lymphoid tissues. Lyon: IARC Press; 2001:171-4.

79. Ponzoni M, Ferreri AJ, Pruneri G, et al. Prognostic value of bcl-6, CD10 and CD38 immunoreactivity in stage I-II gastric lymphomas: identification of a subset of CD10+ large B-cell lymphomas with a favorable outcome. Int J Cancer 2003;106:288-91.

80. Yoshino T, Omonishi K, Kobayashi K, et al. Clinicopathological features of gastric mucosa associated lymphoid tissue (MALT) lymphomas: high grade transformation and comparison with diffuse large B cell lymphomas without MALT lymphoma features. J Clin Pathol 2000;53:187-90.

81. Hiyama T, Haruma K, Kitadai Y, Ito M, et al. Clinicopathological features of gastric mucosa-associated lymphoid tissue lymphoma: a comparison with diffuse large B-cell lymphoma without a mucosa-associated lymphoid tissue lymphoma component. J Gastroenterol Hepatol 2001;16:734-9.

82. Hsu C, Chen CL, Chen LT, et al. Comparison of MALT and non-MALT primary large cell lymphoma of the stomach: does histologic evidence of MALT affect chemotherapy response? Cancer 2001;91:49-56.

83. Kwon MS, Go JH, Choi JS, et al. Critical evaluation of Bcl-6 protein expression in diffuse large B-cell lymphoma of the stomach and small intestine. Am J Surg Pathol 2003;27:790-8.

84. Takeshita M, Iwashita A, Kurihara K, et al. Histologic and immunohistologic findings and prognosis of 40 cases of gastric large B-cell lymphoma. Am J Surg Pathol 2000;24:1641-9.

85. Møller MB, Pedersen NT, Christensen BE. Diffuse large B-cell lymphoma: clinical implications of extranodal versus nodal presentation—a population-based study of 1575 cases. Br J Haematol 2004;124:151-9.

86. Koch P, del Valle F, Berdel WE, et al. Primary gastrointestinal non-Hodgkin's lymphoma: I. Anatomic and histologic distribution, clinical features, and survival data of 371 patients registered in the German Multicenter Study GIT NHL 01/92. J Clin Oncol 2001;19:3861-73.

87. Severson RK, Davis S. Increasing incidence of primary gastric lymphoma. Cancer 1990;66:1283-7.

88. Cortelazzo S, Rossi A, Roggero F, et al. Stage-modified international prognostic index effectively predicts clinical outcome of localized primary gastric diffuse large B-cell lymphoma. International Extranodal Lymphoma Study Group (IELSG). Ann Oncol 1999;10:1433-40.

89. López-Guillermo A, Colomo L, Jiménez M, et al. Diffuse large B-cell lymphoma: clinical and biological characterization and outcome according to the nodal or extranodal primary origin. J Clin Oncol 2005;23:2797-804.

90. Cogliatti SB, Schmid U, Schumacher U, et al. Primary B-cell gastric lymphoma: a clinicopathological study of 145 patients. Gastroenterology 1991;101:1159-70.

91. Driessen A, Tierens A, Ectors N, et al. Primary diffuse large B cell lymphoma of the stomach: analysis of somatic mutations in the rearranged immunoglobulin heavy chain variable genes indicates antigen selection. Leukemia 1999;13: 1085-92.

92. Liang R, Chan WP, Kwong YL, et al. Bcl-6 gene hypermutations in diffuse large B-cell lymphoma of primary gastric origin. Br J Haematol 1997;99:668-70.

93. Skacel M, Paris PL, Pettay JD, et al. Diffuse large B-cell lymphoma of the stomach: assessment of microsatellite instability, allelic imbalance, and trisomy of chromosomes 3, 12, and 18. Diagn Mol Pathol 2002;11:75-82.

94. Armitage JO, Mauch PM, Harris NL, Dalla-Favera R, Bierman PJ. Diffuse large B-cell lymphoma. In: Mauch PM, Armitage JO, Coiffier B, Dalla-Favera R, Harris NL, eds. Non-Hodgkin's lymphomas. Philadelphia: Lippincott Williams & Wilkins; 2004:427-53.

95. Alizadeh AA, Eisen MB, Davis RE, et al. Distinct types of diffuse large B-cell lymphoma identified by gene expression profiling. Nature 2000;403:503-11.

96. Hill BT, Sweetenham J. Clinical implications of the molecular subtypes of diffuse large B-cell lymphoma. Leuk Lymphoma 2012;53:763-9.

97. Rosenwald A, Wright G, Chan WC, et al. The use of molecular profiling to predict survival after chemotherapy for diffuse large-B-cell lymphoma. N Engl J Med 2002;346:1937-47.

98. Colomo L, Lopez-Guillermo A, Perales M, et al. Clinical impact of the differentiation profile assessed by immunophenotyping in patients with diffuse large B-cell lymphoma. Blood 2003; 101:78-84.

99. Hans CP, Weisenburger DD, Greiner TC, et al. Confirmation of the molecular classification of diffuse large B-cell lymphoma by immunohistochemistry using a tissue microarray. Blood 2004;103:275-82.

100. Ibrahim EM, Ezzat AA, Raja MA, et al. Primary gastric non-Hodgkin's lymphoma: clinical features, management, and prognosis of 185 patients with diffuse large B-cell lymphoma. Ann Oncol 1999;10:1441-9.

101. Avilés A, Nambo MJ, Neri N, et al. The role of surgery in primary gastric lymphoma: results of a controlled clinical trial. Ann Surg 2004;240:44-50.

102. Raderer M, Paul de Boer J. Role of chemotherapy in gastric MALT lymphoma, diffuse large B-cell lymphoma and other lymphomas. Best Pract Res Clin Gastroenterol 2010;24:19-26.

103. Fang C, Xu W, Li JY. A systematic review and meta-analysis of rituximab-based immunochemotherapy for subtypes of diffuse large B cell lymphoma. Ann Hematol 2010;89:1107-13.

104. Ferreri AJ, Govi S, Ponzoni M. The role of Helicobacter pylori eradication in the treatment of diffuse large B-cell and marginal zone lymphomas of the stomach. Curr Opin Oncol 2013;25:470-9.

105. Popescu RA, Wotherspoon AC, Cunningham D, Norman A, Prendiville J, Hill ME. Surgery plus chemotherapy or chemotherapy alone for primary intermediate- and high-grade gastric non-Hodgkin's lymphoma: the Royal Marsden Hospital experience. Eur J Cancer 1999;35:928-34.

106. Koch P, del Valle F, Berdel WE, et al. Primary gastrointestinal non-Hodgkin's lymphoma: II. Combined surgical and conservative or conservative management only in localized gastric lymphoma--results of the prospective German Multicenter Study GIT NHL 01/92. J Clin Oncol 2001;19:3874-83.

107. Binn M, Ruskone-Fourmestraux A, Lepage E, et al. Surgical resection plus chemotherapy versus chemotherapy alone: comparison of two strategies to treat diffuse large B-cell gastric lymphoma. Ann Oncol 2003;14:1751-7.

108. International Non-Hodgkin's Lymphoma Prognostic Factors Project. A predictive model for aggressive non-Hodgkin's lymphoma. N Engl J Med 1993;329:987-94.

109. Wu G, Keating A. Biomarkers of potential prognostic significance in diffuse large B-cell lymphoma. Cancer 2006;106:247-57.

110. Huang WT, Kuo SH, Cheng AL, Lin CW. Inhibition of ZEB1 by miR-200 characterizes Helicobacter pylori-positive gastric diffuse large B-cell lymphoma with a less aggressive behavior. Mod Pathol 2014;27:1116-25.

111. Hecht JL, Aster JC. Molecular biology of Burkitt's lymphoma. J Clin Oncol 2000;18:3707-21.

112. Leoncini L, Campo E, Stein H, Harris NL, Jaffe ES, Kluin PM. Burkitt lymphoma. In: Swerdlow SH, Campo E, Harris NL, et al., eds. WHO classification of tumours of haematopoietic and lymphoid tissues, 4th ed. Lyon: IARC Press; 2017:330-3.

113. Gromminger S, Mautner J, Bornkamm GW. Burkitt lymphoma: the role of Epstein-Barr virus revisited. Br J Haematol 2012;156:719-29.

114. Harris NL, Horning SJ. Burkitt's lymphoma—the message from microarrays. N Engl J Med 2006; 354:2495-8.

115. Dave SS, Fu K, Wright GW, et al. Molecular diagnosis of Burkitt's lymphoma. N Engl J Med 2006;354:2431-42.

116. Hummel M, Bentink S, Berger H, et al. A biologic definition of Burkitt's lymphoma from transcriptional and genomic profiling. N Engl J Med 2006;354:2419-30.

117. Krugmann J, Tzankov A, Fiegl M, Dirnhofer S, Siebert R, Erdel M. Burkitt's lymphoma of the stomach: a case report with molecular cytogenetic analysis. Leuk Lymphoma 2004;45:1055-9.

118. Swerdlow SH, Campo E, Seto M, Müller-Hermelink HK. Mantle cell lymphoma. In: Swerdlow SH, Campo E, Harris NL, et al., eds. WHO classification of tumours of haematopoietic and lymphoid tissues, 4th ed. Lyon: IARC Press; 2017:285-9.

119. Hawkes EA, Wotherspoon A, Cunningham D. Diagnosis and management of rare gastrointestinal lymphomas. Leuk Lymphoma 2012; 53:2341-50.

120. Salar A, Juanpere N, Bellosillo B, et al. Gastrointestinal involvement in mantle cell lymphoma: a prospective clinic, endoscopic, and pathologic study. Am J Surg Pathol 2006;30:1274-80.

121. Bertoni F, Zucca E, Cotter FE. Molecular basis of mantle cell lymphoma. Br J Haematol 2004; 124:130-40.

122. Gurney KA, Cartwright RA. Increasing incidence and descriptive epidemiology of extranodal non-Hodgkin lymphoma in parts of England and Wales. Hematol J 2002;3:95-104.

123. Jaffe ES, Harris NL, Swerdlow SH, et al. Follicular lymphoma. In: Swerdlow SH, Campo E, Harris NL, et al., eds. WHO classification of tumours of haematopoietic and lymphoid tissues, 4th ed. Lyon: IARC Press; 2017:266-79.

124. Yamamoto S, Nakase H, Yamashita K, et al. Gastrointestinal follicular lymphoma: review of the literature. J Gastroenterol 2010;45:370-88.

125. Campo E, Ghia P, Montserrat E, et al. Chronic lymphocytic leukaemia/small lymphocytic lymphoma. In: In: Swerdlow SH, Campo E, Harris NL, et al., eds. WHO classification of tumours of haematopoietic and lymphoid tissues, 4th ed. Lyon: IARC Press; 2017:216-9.

12 MESENCHYMAL TUMORS OF THE ESOPHAGUS AND STOMACH

Similar to the gastrointestinal (GI) tract as a whole, by far the most common mesenchymal neoplasm of the stomach is GI stromal tumor (GIST): 60 percent of GISTs overall arise in the stomach (1). GIST should be the lead entity in the differential diagnosis (with rare exceptions), although awareness of the distinguishing histologic features of other mesenchymal and neural neoplasms should lead to consideration of alternative possibilities.

Gastric GISTs are among the most common human neoplasms: autopsy and surgical studies in which stomachs were entirely embedded or extensively sampled have revealed that small (under 1 cm) GISTs of the stomach are common, identified in up to 35 percent of older adults (and some adults harbor multiple minute, clinically inapparent gastric GISTs) (2–4). These minute GISTs, which have been referred to as "microGISTs" or GIST "tumorlets," arise in the muscularis propria (fig. 12-1), typically contain abundant sclerotic stroma with dystrophic calcifications, and show irregular infiltrative margins into the adjacent muscularis propria (fig. 12-2). Minute GISTs are positive for KIT (CD117) by immunohistochemistry (fig. 12-2) and harbor *KIT* mutations, similar to larger GISTs that present clinically (3,5). MicroGISTs are invariably benign.

The only other mesenchymal and neural tumors of the stomach that are common are leiomyomas and schwannomas; all others are rare. In contrast to the colon, where lipomas are frequently encountered during screening colonoscopy, gastric submucosal lipomas are uncommon. Such lesions are rarely biopsied or excised; lipomas are not discussed further in this chapter. Awareness of the incidence of these various tumor types is helpful when developing a differential diagnosis.

GISTs rarely arise in the esophagus. At that anatomic site, mural leiomyomas vastly outnumber GISTs; this is an important exception to keep in mind when encountering a spindle cell neoplasm in the wall of the esophagus. The only other common esophageal mesenchymal or neural tumors are granular cell tumors. Throughout this chapter, the key features that distinguish mesenchymal tumors of the esophagus and stomach from leiomyoma and GIST are emphasized.

Due to their submucosal/mural location, mesenchymal tumors are usually not accessible by endoscopic brush for cytologic sampling unless the overlying mucosa is ulcerated. Endoscopic fine-needle aspiration (FNA), with or without ultrasound guidance, is the preferred method of sampling (6–8). In some situations, diagnostic material is obtained by percutaneous computerized tomography (CT)- or ultrasound-guided FNA (9). Cytologic features of GIST, leiomyoma,

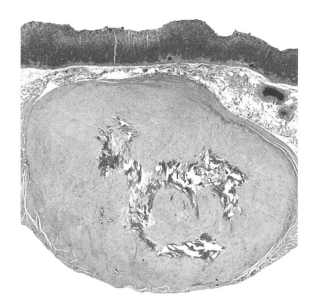

Figure 12-1

MICROGASTROINTESTINAL STROMAL TUMOR (GIST)

This tumor was discovered incidentally in a gastric sleeve resection specimen. This small tumor arose in the muscularis propria.

333

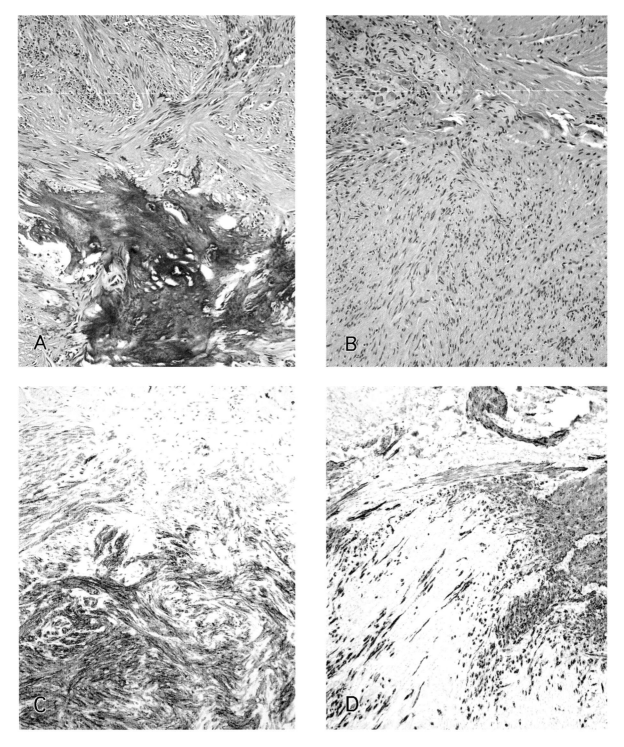

Figure 12-2

MICROGASTROINTESTINAL STROMAL TUMOR

A: Many minute GISTs contain sclerotic stroma and dystrophic calcifications.
B: The tumor entraps the adjacent muscularis propria.
C: Immunohistochemistry for KIT is positive in the tumor cells.
D: Desmin highlights the smooth muscle cells and the infiltrative margins of the tumor.

and leiomyosarcoma are discussed in the appropriate sections of the chapter.

GASTROINTESTINAL STROMAL TUMOR

Definition. Our understanding of *gastrointestinal stromal tumors* (GISTs) has evolved dramatically over the past several decades. Before 1998, when activating mutations in the tyrosine kinase receptor gene *KIT* and overexpression of the KIT protein were first identified in this tumor type (10), GISTs were often misclassified as smooth muscle or neural tumors; the terms "leiomyoblastoma" and "GI autonomic nerve tumor (GANT)" are obsolete. GISTs likely arise from a precursor to the interstitial cells of Cajal; they show phenotypic features of Cajal cell differentiation and most express both KIT and DOG1 (anoctamin 1, a calcium-activated chloride channel required for transmission of signals from the autonomic nervous system through Cajal cells to smooth muscle cells of the muscularis propria during peristalsis) (11,12).

General Features. As mentioned earlier, incidentally discovered microscopic GISTs of the stomach are very common (up to 35 percent of older adults have microGISTs) (2). In contrast, despite being the most common mesenchymal tumors of the GI tract, larger GISTs that present clinically are rare, with an annual incidence of approximately 15 per million (13). Approximately 60 percent of all GISTs arise in the stomach, whereas esophageal GISTs account for less than 1 percent of such tumors (1).

Clinical Features. GISTs most often affect middle-aged to elderly adults of a median age of 60 years (1,14). GISTs rarely arise during childhood (1 to 2 percent of all tumors), and nearly always in the stomach in this age group (15). GISTs range from incidentally discovered, small asymptomatic lesions to large tumors that present with anemia, GI bleeding, or an abdominal mass, although many patients only have vague abdominal complaints. Around 25 percent of gastric GISTs are clinically malignant (14). Patients with esophageal GISTs present with dysphagia (16,17).

Gastric GISTs are associated with two main tumor syndromes: Carney triad, the combination of gastric GIST, extra-adrenal paraganglioma, and pulmonary chondroma (18) and Carney-Stratakis syndrome, the dyad of gastric

GIST and paraganglioma (19). Carney triad is a nonfamilial syndrome that predominantly affects young women, whereas Carney-Stratakis syndrome is an inherited disorder caused by germline mutations in a succinate dehydrogenase (SDH) subunit gene (20). The tumors from patients with Carney triad usually show hypermethylation of the *SDHC* promoter (21). Tumors in both syndromes are clinically and pathologically similar, referred to as *SDH-deficient GISTs*; such tumors also arise in patients without these syndromes (22–24). SDH-deficient GISTs represent a large fraction of GISTs in children and young adults, 90 percent in the first two decades, 50 percent in the third decade, and 25 percent in the fourth decade; they rarely arise in patients over 50 years of age (22).

Gross Findings. Gastric GISTs may be limited to the wall of the stomach or protrude into the lumen; esophageal GISTs are usually confined to the wall. The cut surface ranges from fibrous to fleshy or gelatinous, often with cystic degeneration and hemorrhage (fig. 12-3). SDH-deficient GISTs show a multinodular appearance (fig. 12-3) (25).

Microscopic Findings. About 65 percent of gastric GISTs are composed exclusively of spindle cells; 25 percent show epithelioid cytomorphology and 10 percent contain an admixture of epithelioid and spindle cells (14). Most esophageal GISTs are of spindle cell type (16,17). Spindle cell GISTS are composed of fascicles or sheets of uniform cells with elongated nuclei, fine chromatin, indistinct or small nucleoli, and palely eosinophilic or basophilic fibrillary cytoplasm with a syncytial appearance (fig. 12-4). Nuclear palisading and paranuclear cytoplasmic vacuoles are typical (fig. 12-5), the latter nearly exclusive to gastric GISTs. A trabecular architecture is an uncommon feature (fig. 12-6). Some tumors contain dystrophic calcifications (fig. 12-2).

Epithelioid GISTs are usually composed of sheets of rounded or polygonal cells with central round nuclei, indistinct nucleoli, and eosinophilic cytoplasm (fig. 12-7). Some tumors show a nested, paraganglioma-like appearance (fig. 12-7). Rare epithelioid GISTs show rhabdoid features with eccentric nuclei and eosinophilic cytoplasmic inclusions (fig. 12-8) (26). A small amount of myxoid stroma is a common finding in epithelioid GISTs; in occasional examples, the myxoid stroma is abundant (fig. 12-9) (27).

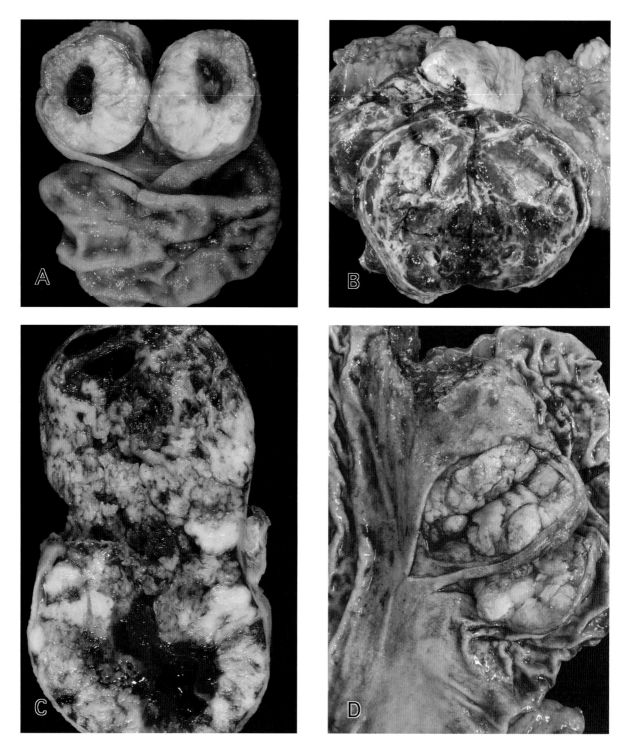

Figure 12-3

GASTROINTESTINAL STROMAL TUMORS OF THE STOMACH

A: Some GISTs show a fibrous cut surface, similar to leiomyomas.
B: Other tumors show a fleshy cut surface, similar to many sarcomas.
C: Central cystic degeneration and hemorrhage are common findings.
D: Succinate dehydrogenase (SDH)-deficient GISTs show a multinodular growth pattern.

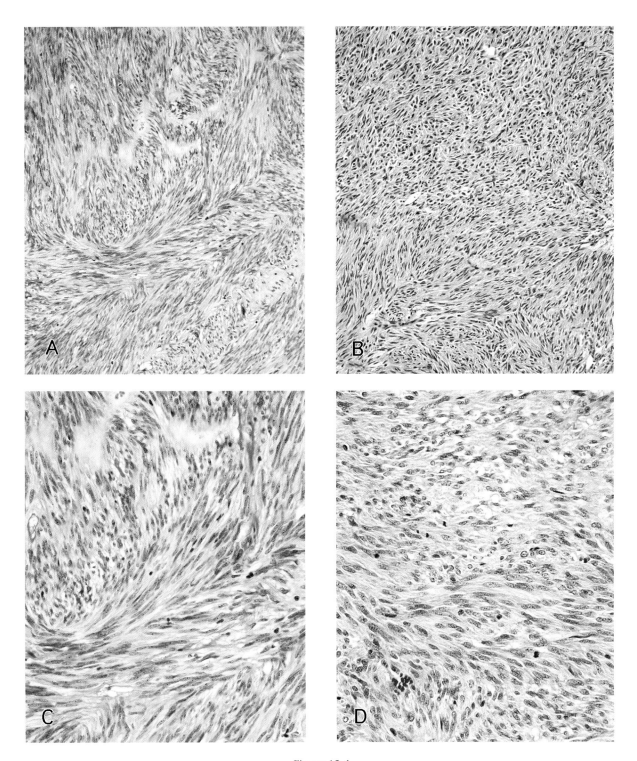

Figure 12-4

GASTROINTESTINAL STROMAL TUMOR, SPINDLE CELL TYPE

A,B: The tumors are composed of cellular fascicles of spindle cells with a palely basophilic (A) or eosinophilic (B) appearance.

C: The uniform spindle cells contain elongated nuclei with fine chromatin and eosinophilic cytoplasm.

D: This gastric GIST showed a high mitotic rate. Fibrillary, syncytial cytoplasm is seen.

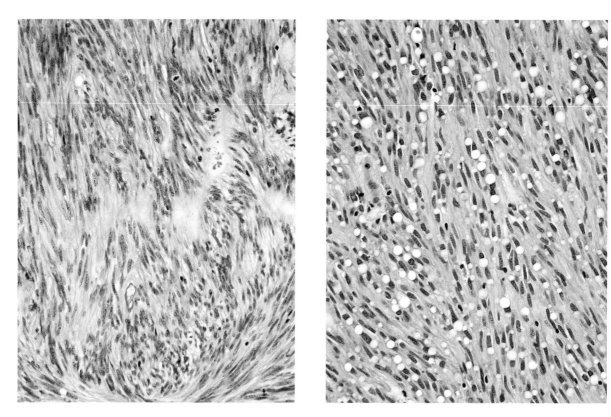

Figure 12-5

GASTROINTESTINAL STROMAL TUMOR, SPINDLE CELL TYPE

Left: Some spindle cell GISTs show nuclear palisading.
Right: Paranuclear vacuoles are a characteristic feature of gastric GISTs.

Figure 12-6

**GASTROINTESTINAL
STROMAL TUMOR,
SPINDLE CELL TYPE**

Rare GISTs show a trabecular architecture.

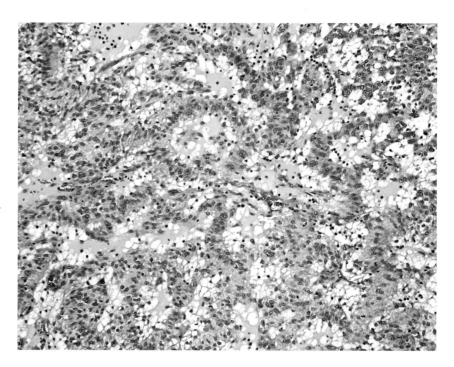

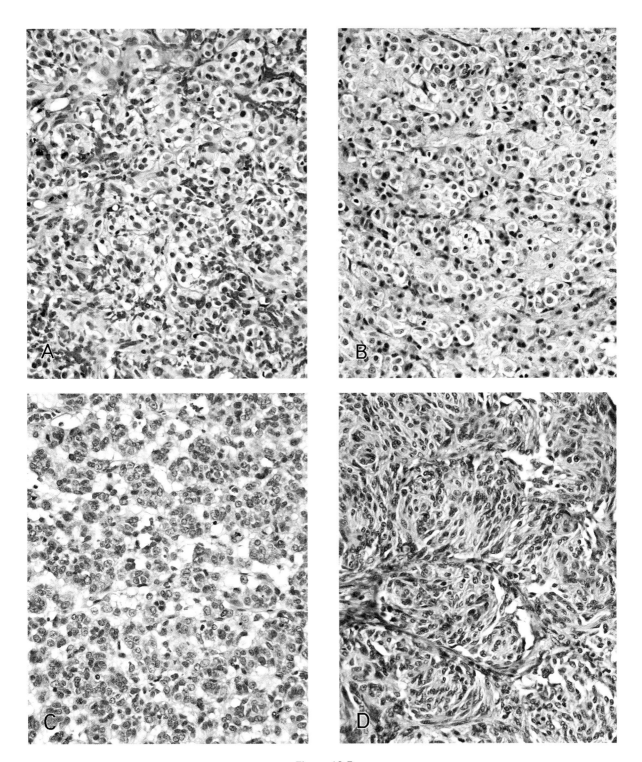

Figure 12-7

GASTROINTESTINAL STROMAL TUMOR, EPITHELIOID TYPE

A,B: The tumors are composed of sheets of epithelioid cells with round nucleoli, small nucleoli, and abundant palely basophilic (A) or eosinophilic (B) cytoplasm.

C: This example showed a somewhat nested appearance.

D: Occasional tumors show a striking resemblance to paragangliomas.

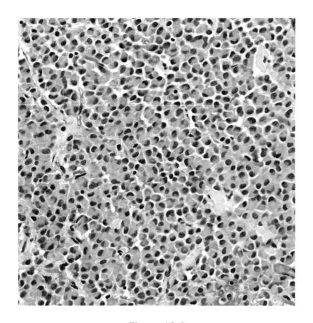

Figure 12-8

**GASTROINTESTINAL STROMAL
TUMOR, EPITHELIOID TYPE**

Rare epithelioid GISTs show rhabdoid features, with eccentric nuclei and eosinophilic cytoplasmic inclusions.

Epithelioid GISTs may show clear cell features or sclerotic stroma (fig. 12-10). Most GISTs show remarkable cytologic uniformity (even in aggressive tumors); pleomorphism is rare, most often seen in epithelioid tumors (fig. 12-10) (14). GISTs typically show a low mitotic rate (see below). Mucosal ulceration is common in gastric GISTs.

Rarely, GISTs undergo dedifferentiation (analogous to dedifferentiated chondrosarcoma or liposarcoma), either de novo or following prolonged tyrosine kinase inhibitor therapy (28). In such cases, a conventional, cytologically uniform, KIT-positive spindle cell or epithelioid GIST shows an abrupt transition to an anaplastic, often pleomorphic, KIT-negative component (fig. 12-11). The dedifferentiated component may express keratins or smooth muscle markers (28,29).

SDH-deficient GISTs show a distinctive multinodular or plexiform architecture that is recognized at scanning magnification (fig. 12-12) (25): nodules of tumor are separated by bands of smooth muscle of the muscularis propria

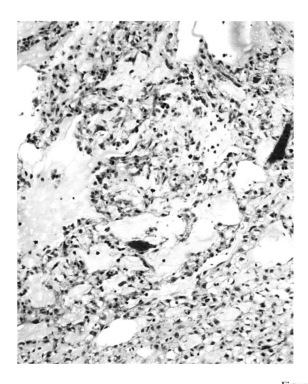
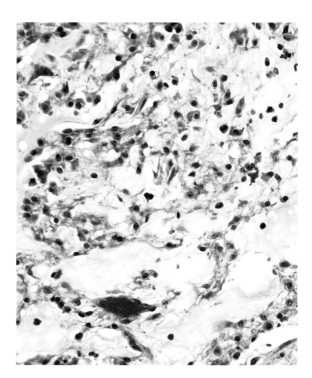

Figure 12-9

MYXOID GASTROINTESTINAL STROMAL TUMOR

Left: Occasional epithelioid GISTs contain abundant myxoid stroma.
Right: The round nuclei are uniform and the eosinophilic cytoplasm is wispy.

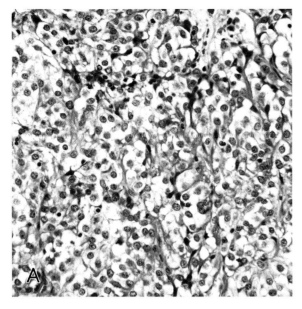

Figure 12-10

GASTROINTESTINAL STROMAL TUMOR, EPITHELIOID TYPE

A: Some epithelioid GISTs show clear cell features.
B: Sclerotic stroma is another variant feature.
C: Pleomorphism in GISTs is rare, mostly seen in epithelioid tumors. The tumor cells are multinucleated.

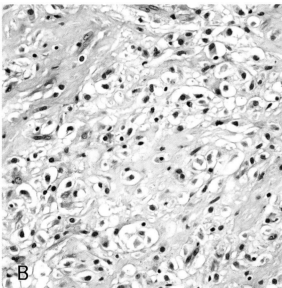

(fig. 12-12). Nearly all SDH-deficient GISTs are composed of sheets of epithelioid cells or, less often, an admixture of epithelioid and spindle cells (fig. 12-12) (22). The tumor cells in such cases may also contain cytoplasmic vacuoles (fig. 12-13). In contrast to conventional GISTs, vascular invasion is a common finding in SDH-deficient GISTs, as are lymph node metastases (fig. 12-14).

Cytologic Findings. The specimens are usually cellular, with a variable proportion of isolated cells and loose and crowded fragments of spindle or epithelioid cells. The individual cells often lose their wispy cytoplasm and become stripped nuclei (fig. 12-15) (30,31). The cytologic appearance depends upon the cell type.

Spindle Cell Type. Sheets of cells are often held together by small capillaries to sometimes form a complex branching pattern in which tumor cells are attached to capillaries and a prominent intercellular vascular network (fig. 12-16) (32,33). Eosinophilic or cyanophilic, delicate, fibrillary material separates the nuclei and represents either cytoplasmic processes or matrix (fig. 12-17) (32,34). Cytoplasmic borders are indistinct, if discernible (33,35). At the edges of groups and with single intact cells, numerous

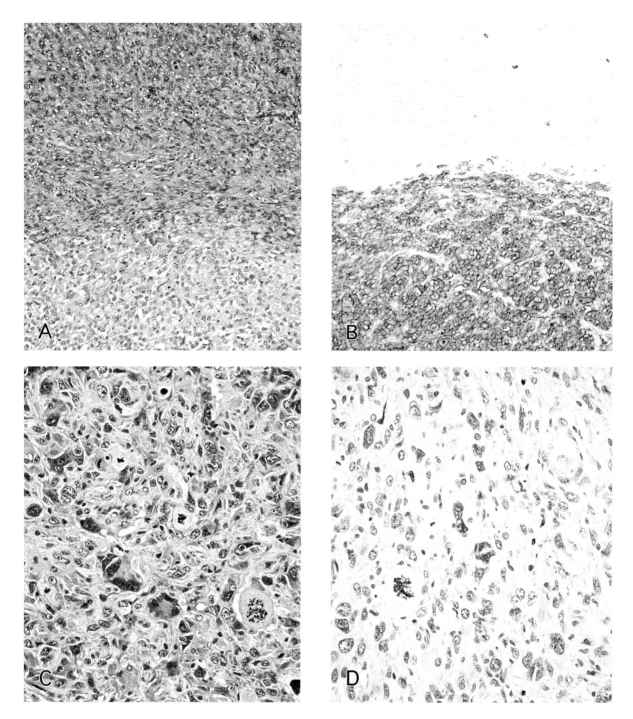

Figure 12-11

DEDIFFERENTIATED GASTROINTESTINAL STROMAL TUMOR

A: The tumor shows an abrupt transition from a typical GIST with epithelioid morphology and uniform, round nuclei (bottom) to a spindle cell component with marked nuclear atypia, pleomorphic forms, and brightly eosinophilic cytoplasm (top).

B: Immunohistochemistry for KIT is strongly positive in the conventional GIST but is completely negative in the anaplastic component.

C: The dedifferentiated component resembles an undifferentiated pleomorphic sarcoma with bizarre nuclei and striking mitotic activity.

D: KIT is negative in the tumor cells.

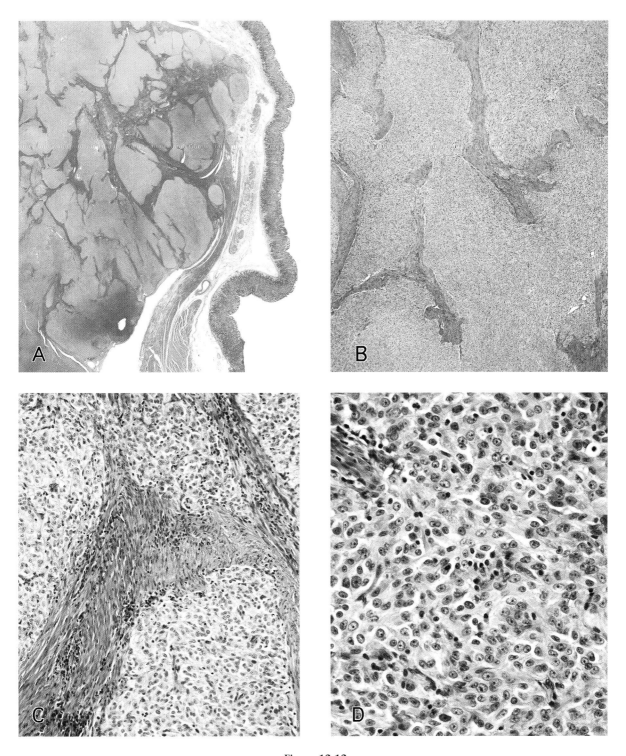

Figure 12-12

SUCCINATE DEHYDROGENASE (SDH)-DEFICIENT GASTROINTESTINAL STROMAL TUMOR

A: On scanning magnification, the tumor shows a multinodular architecture.
B: The muscularis propria is extensively infiltrated by tumor showing a plexiform growth pattern.
C: Bands of smooth muscle of the muscularis propria separate the nodules of tumor, which show epithelioid morphology.
D: The epithelioid tumor cells contain round nuclei, small nuclei, and abundant pale eosinophilic cytoplasm.

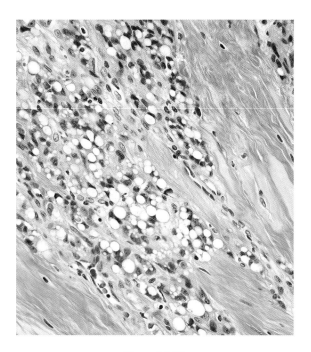

Figure 12-13

SUCCINATE DEHYDROGENASE-DEFICIENT GASTROINTESTINAL STROMAL TUMOR

In some cases, the epithelioid tumor cells contain prominent cytoplasmic vacuoles.

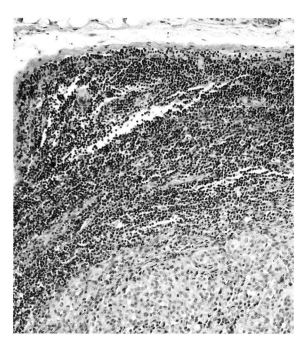

Figure 12-14

SUCCINATE DEHYDROGENASE-DEFICIENT GASTROINTESTINAL STROMAL TUMOR

Lymph node metastases are common with this variant, in contrast to conventional *KIT*-mutant GISTs, which almost never spread to lymph nodes.

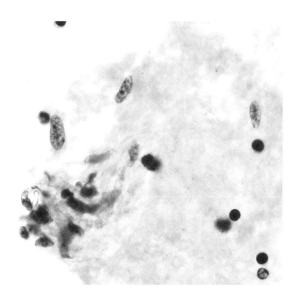

Figure 12-15

GASTROINTESTINAL STROMAL TUMOR, SPINDLE CELL TYPE

Scattered single stripped nuclei are embedded in a fibrillary matrix (Papanicolaou stain).

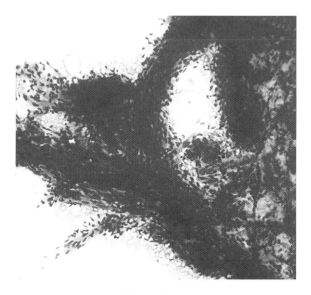

Figure 12-16

GASTROINTESTINAL STROMAL TUMOR, SPINDLE CELL TYPE

Sheets of cells are held together by small capillaries to form a complex branching pattern with tumor cells attached to capillaries. A prominent intercellular vascular network is apparent in the right half of the field (DiffQuik stain).

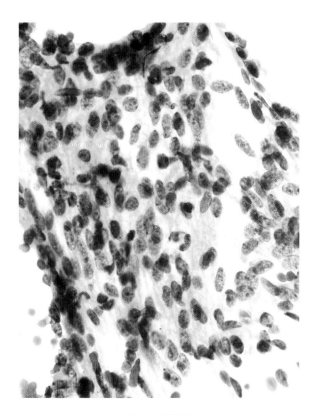

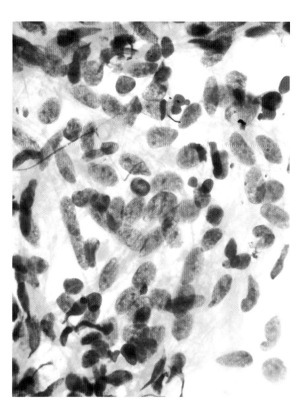

Figure 12-17

**GASTROINTESTINAL STROMAL
TUMOR, SPINDLE CELL TYPE**

Cyanophilic, delicate fibrillary material separates the nuclei and represents either cytoplasmic processes or matrix. Cytoplasmic borders are indistinct (Papanicolaou stain).

Figure 12-18

**GASTROINTESTINAL STROMAL
TUMOR, SPINDLE CELL TYPE**

The nuclei in this field are of uniform size and oval to spindle in shape. They have smooth nuclear membranes, a diffuse and homogeneous fine chromatin pattern, and inconspicuous nucleoli (Papanicolaou stain).

wispy cytoplasmic extensions/processes are noted. Cytoplasmic vacuoles may be present.

The nuclei are usually ovoid to spindled, and uniform in size and shape (fig. 12-18). They may appear wavy, as seen in tumors of nerve sheath origin, or with blunt or "squared off" ends as described in smooth muscle tumors (fig. 12-18) (33,36). Nuclei are occasionally arranged in a parallel, side-by-side (palisading) pattern (32,35). They characteristically have smooth nuclear membranes, a diffuse and homogeneous fine chromatin pattern, and inconspicuous nucleoli (fig. 12-18). Nuclear grooves are prominent in some cases (33), with occasional intranuclear inclusions (36). Mitoses are uncommon. Nuclear pleomorphism and other features of malignancy, such as evidence of dyshesion, hyperchromasia, irregular nuclear contours, increased nuclear/cytoplasmic (N/C) ratio, necrosis, and frequent mitoses are occasionally noted.

Epithelioid Type. This type of GIST shows more dyshesion on FNA, with tumor cells present singly or in small or loose clusters (fig. 12-19) (32,37). A variable number of spindle cells may be admixed with epithelioid cells. In some cases, vessels traverse aggregates of cells. Tumor cells are round, ovoid, or polygonal (fig. 12-20). The cytoplasm ranges from scant to abundant and may be eosinophilic, amphophilic, or cyanophilic. The cytoplasmic quality varies from granular to clear, with or without vacuoles.

The nuclei in epithelioid GISTs are more likely to show significant pleomorphism, such as hyperchromasia, coarsely granular or clumped chromatin, and irregular membranes (fig. 12-20). Nucleoli may be single and prominent or small and multiple. Intranuclear inclusions and binucleation have been reported to be prominent in some cases. The nuclear pleomorphism is

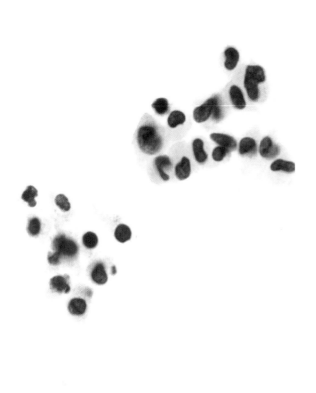

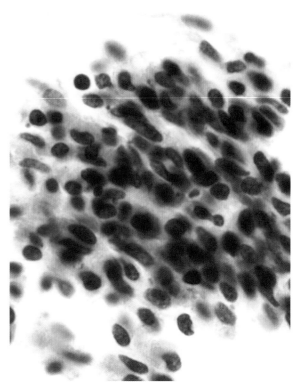

Figure 12-19

**GASTROINTESTINAL STROMAL
TUMOR, EPITHELIOID TYPE**

Epithelioid tumor cells are present singly and in loose clusters (Papanicolaou stain).

Figure 12-20

**GASTROINTESTINAL STROMAL
TUMOR, EPITHELIOID TYPE**

The nuclei in this type are more likely to show pleomorphism and are round, oval, or spindle in shape, as seen in this figure. Chromatin may be hyperchromatic, coarsely granular, or clumped. Cytoplasm ranges from scant to abundant in amount and may be granular to clear with or without vacuoles (Papanicolaou stain).

sometimes so pronounced that it mimics adenocarcinoma (fig. 12-21). Immunohistochemistry may be necessary to make the distinction (38). While adenocarcinomas are positive for keratins, GISTs are positive for KIT (fig. 12-22) and DOG1.

Immunohistochemical Findings. By immunohistochemistry, KIT is positive in 95 percent of GISTs, usually with strong and diffuse cytoplasmic staining (fig. 12-23) (12,14); some tumors show a dot-like staining pattern (fig. 12-24). Epithelioid GISTs (especially those with *PDGFRA* mutations) may be negative for KIT (15 percent of epithelioid tumors) (39,40) or show only limited (weak, patchy) staining. DOG1 shows similar sensitivity for GIST as KIT (fig. 12-23) (12). Around 50 percent of KIT-negative tumors express DOG1; DOG1 is most useful to confirm the diagnosis in cases with limited or no KIT expression (fig. 12-25). *PDGFRA*-mutant GISTs show strong and diffuse staining for PDGFRA (fig. 12-25), whereas *KIT*-mutant and

SDH-deficient GISTs generally show limited staining (41).

CD34 is usually positive in spindle cell GISTs of the stomach and esophagus, although epithelioid GISTs less often express CD34. Caldesmon is often positive in GISTs (about 70 percent of cases) (42). Expression of smooth muscle actin (SMA) may be seen (about 20 percent of cases, especially in spindle cell tumors), whereas desmin expression is uncommon (2 percent), except in gastric epithelioid GISTs, which show patchy staining for desmin in 10 percent of cases (1). Keratin expression (CK18) is limited and staining for S-100 protein is rare (around 1 percent).

Similar to conventional GISTs, SDH-deficient GISTs are usually positive for KIT, DOG1, and CD34 (fig. 12-26); loss of granular cytoplasmic staining for SDHB may be used to confirm the

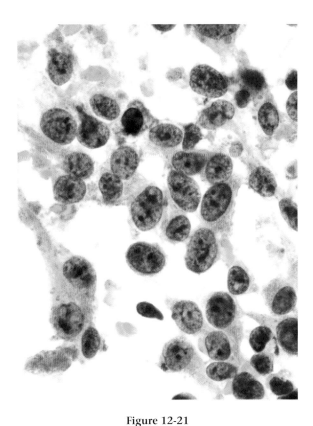

Figure 12-21

GASTROINTESTINAL STROMAL TUMOR, EPITHELIOID TYPE

The nuclear pleomorphism is so pronounced in this case that the tumor can be mistaken for an adenocarcinoma (Papanicolaou stain). (Courtesy of Dr. E. Cibas, Boston, MA.)

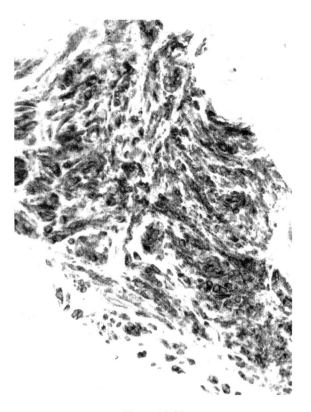

Figure 12-22

GASTROINTESTINAL STROMAL TUMOR

The tumor cells are strongly positive for KIT.

diagnosis (figs. 12-26, 12-27) (22,25,43,44). Loss of both SDHA and SDHB expression is only seen in SDH-deficient GISTs that harbor *SDHA* mutations (45,46). The correlation between immunophenotype and genotype in GISTs is summarized in Table 12-1.

Immunohistochemical studies have been successfully performed on cell blocks (31–34,37,47,48) and in some cases also on smears (33,37,48). If sufficient material is available, a panel of antibodies that includes KIT, DOG1, SMA, desmin, and S-100 protein on cell block preparations is recommended for spindle cell lesions. DOG1 has been shown to be 100 percent sensitive and specific for GIST, compared to 70 to 88 percent sensitivity and 76 percent specificity of KIT on FNA cell block preparations (49,50). The lower sensitivity of KIT in cell block preparations compared to surgical specimens is attributed to the alcohol-based fixative that is often used in endoscopic FNA samples, which decreases antigenicity for some markers (50).

Molecular Genetic Findings. Approximately 75 percent of gastric GISTs harbor *KIT* mutations, mostly in exon 11 (67 percent), and around 10 percent of gastric GISTs harbor mutations in *PDGFRA*, mostly in exon 18 (7 percent) (1,51,52). *KIT* mutations in exons 9, 13, or 17 and *PDGFRA* mutations in exons 12 or 14 are rarely identified in gastric GISTs. GISTs that lack mutations in *KIT* or *PDGFRA* have been referred to as "wild-type" GISTs; this is a heterogeneous group of tumors now known to include SDH-deficient GISTs (22), *BRAF* V600E-mutant GISTs (53), neurofibromatosis type 1 (NF1)-associated GISTs (54), GISTs with rare gene fusions (*NTRK3* and *FGFR1*) (55,56), and a small group of tumors with as yet unknown molecular pathogenesis.

SDH-deficient GISTs account for approximately 8 percent of gastric GISTs (1,22). The most commonly mutated SDH subunit is *SDHA* (35 percent) (45,46), whereas *SDHB*, *SDHC*, and

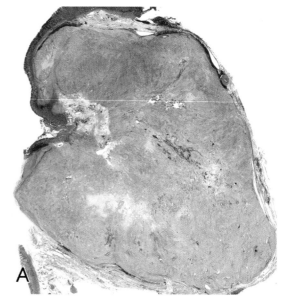

Figure 12-23

GASTROINTESTINAL STROMAL TUMOR

A: Scanning magnification of a spindle cell GIST of the stomach.

B,C: The tumor is strongly and diffusely positive for KIT (B) and DOG1 (C). More than 95 percent of spindle cell GISTs are positive for both of these markers.

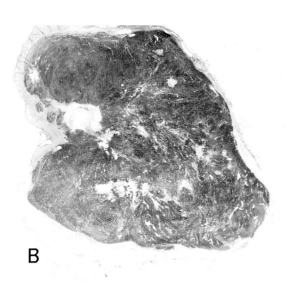

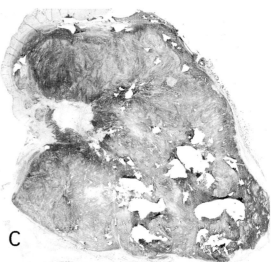

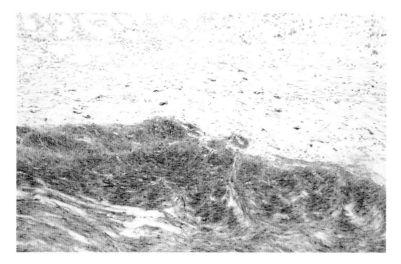

Figure 12-24

GASTROINTESTINAL STROMAL TUMOR

This gastric GIST shows both cytoplasmic and dot-like staining for KIT. KIT-positive mast cells are present in the adjacent mucosa and muscularis mucosae; these cells serve as a useful internal positive control.

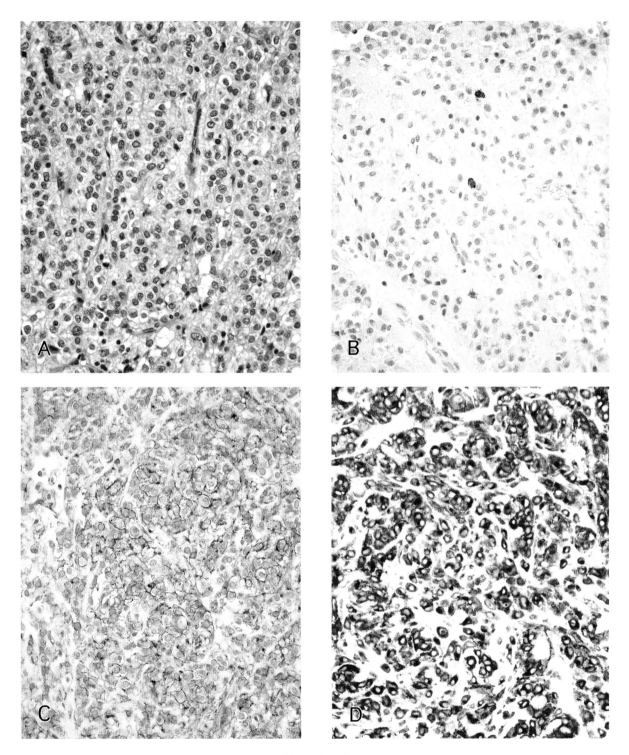

Figure 12-25

KIT-NEGATIVE GASTROINTESTINAL STROMAL TUMOR

A: This gastric epithelioid GIST harbored a *PDGFRA* D842V mutation.
B: Immunohistochemistry for KIT highlights rare mast cells but is negative in the tumor cells.
C: DOG1 is positive with a membranous staining pattern.
D: The tumor cells are strongly positive for PDGFRA, reflecting the underlying *PDGFRA* activating mutation.

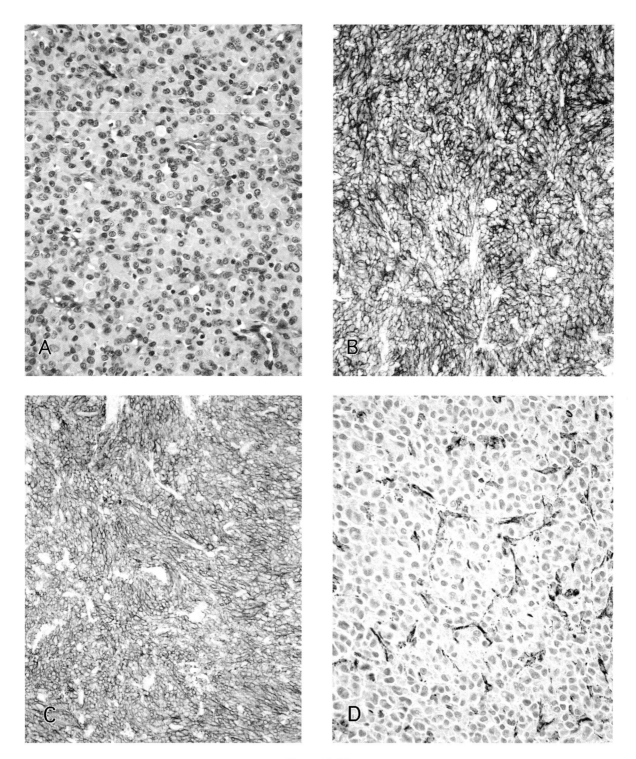

Figure 12-26

SUCCINATE DEHYDROGENASE-DEFICIENT GASTROINTESTINAL STROMAL TUMOR

A: The tumor is composed of sheets of epithelioid cells with uniform nuclei and eosinophilic cytoplasm.

B,C: SDH-deficient GISTs are positive for KIT (B) and DOG1 (C).

D: The tumor cells show loss of staining for SDHB. The endothelial cells lining delicate intratumoral blood vessels serve as a useful internal control.

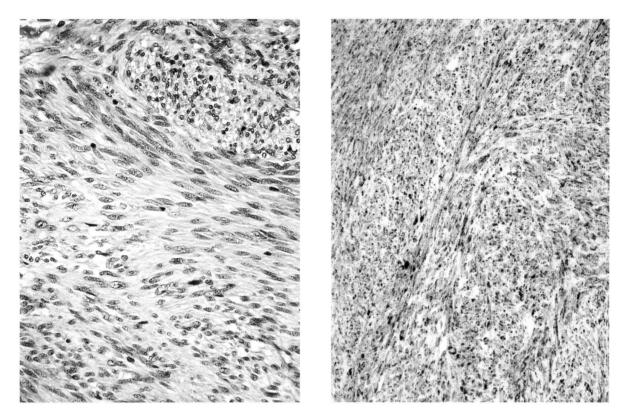

Figure 12-27

GASTROINTESTINAL STROMAL TUMOR, SPINDLE CELL TYPE

Left: This spindle cell GIST of the stomach harbored the common *KIT* exon 11 mutation.
Right: Expression of SDHB is retained (i.e., normal).

Table 12-1

**CORRELATION BETWEEN IMMUNOHISTOCHEMICAL FEATURES AND
GENOTYPE IN GASTROINTESTINAL STROMAL TUMORS OF THE STOMACH**

IHC[a] Marker	Genotype			
	KIT mutation	*PDGFRA* mutation	*SDHX*[b] mutation	*SDHA* mutation
KIT	+	– (or weak/focal)	+	+
DOG1	+	+	+	+
PDGFRA	– (or weak/focal)	+	– (or weak/focal)	– (or weak/focal)
SDHB	+	+	–	–
SDHA	+	+	+	–

[a]IHC = immunohistochemistry.
[b]SDHX refers to SDHA, SDHB, SDHC, or SDHD.

SDHD mutations together account for 25 percent of SDH-deficient GISTs (23,24); these mutations are nearly always germline. Most SDH-deficient GISTs without *SDHX* mutations instead show *SDHC* promoter hypermethylation (57). *BRAF* mutations in GIST are rare (less than 1 percent) (53). Although experience is limited owing to their rarity, esophageal GISTs appear to harbor *KIT* mutations with a similar distribution as gastric tumors, and rare *BRAF* mutations (17).

Table 12-2

DIFFERENTIAL DIAGNOSIS BETWEEN GASTROINTESTINAL STROMAL TUMOR,
SPINDLE CELL TYPE AND OTHER SPINDLE CELL TUMORS OF THE STOMACH

Tumor Type	Key Histologic Features	KIT	DOG1	SMA	Desmin	S-100 Protein
Gastrointestinal stromal tumor, spindle cell type	Uniform slender nuclei; fibrillary, syncytial palely eosinophilic or basophilic cytoplasm; +/- paranuclear vacuoles	98%	97%	20%	2%	<1%
Leiomyoma	Uniform, broad, blunt-ended nuclei; brightly eosinophilic cytoplasm; discernible cell borders; +/- cytoplasmic eosinophilic inclusions	0%	0%	100%	100%	0%
Leiomyosarcoma	Nuclear variability and atypia; broad, blunt-ended nuclei; pleomorphism; brightly eosinophilic cytoplasm	0%	0%	95%	70%	0%
Schwannoma	Peripheral lymphoid cuff; nuclear variability; tapering nuclei; collagenous stroma; +/- intratumoral lymphocytes	0%	0%	0%	0%	100%

Differential Diagnosis. The differential diagnosis for spindle cell GIST chiefly includes leiomyoma, leiomyosarcoma, and schwannoma (Table 12-2). Leiomyomas most often arise in the esophagus and less commonly in the stomach. In contrast to GIST, leiomyomas are composed of spindle cells with broad, blunt-ended ("cigar-shaped") nuclei, brightly eosinophilic cytoplasm, and discernible cell borders; strong and diffuse expression of desmin distinguishes leiomyoma from GIST, whereas KIT and DOG1 are negative. Esophageal mural leiomyomas often contain numerous KIT-positive mast cells and Cajal cells, which can lead to misinterpretation as positive staining in tumor cells (58).

Leiomyosarcomas rarely arise primarily in the stomach or esophagus. They show marked nuclear atypia and pleomorphism, as opposed to the cytologic uniformity of GIST; similar to leiomyomas, extensive desmin expression can help distinguish leiomyosarcoma from GIST.

Gastric schwannomas nearly always show a prominent peripheral lymphoid infiltrate, including follicles; this feature can help distinguish schwannoma from GIST. Gastric schwannomas also show more nuclear variability than GIST and prominent intercellular collagen, in contrast to the syncytial appearance of GIST. The presence of diffuse S-100 protein and SOX10 expression distinguishes schwannoma from GIST; KIT and DOG1 are negative.

The differential diagnosis for epithelioid GIST chiefly includes well-differentiated neuroendocrine tumors, paraganglioma, poorly differentiated adenocarcinoma, and glomus tumor. In contrast to GIST, well-differentiated neuroendocrine tumors are strongly positive for keratins and chromogranin. Paragangliomas are positive for chromogranin but negative for KIT and DOG1. Poorly differentiated adenocarcinomas of the stomach often contain a signet-ring cell component (with intracytoplasmic mucin-containing vacuoles); such cytology is rare in epithelioid GISTs. Diffuse expression of keratins and variable CDX2 expression distinguish adenocarcinoma from GIST, although a subset of gastric adenocarcinomas is positive for DOG1 (12), a potential diagnostic pitfall. Glomus tumors of the stomach are composed of rounded cells with well-defined cell borders, similar to a subset of gastric GISTs. Strong and diffuse SMA expression and negative KIT and DOG1 are typical of glomus tumors. Both GISTs and glomus tumors may be positive for caldesmon.

Treatment. Wedge resection or partial gastrectomy with narrow margins is adequate surgical therapy for most gastric GISTs; such tumors rarely recur locally at anastomotic sites. The one notable exception is SDH-deficient GIST, which often recurs locally (likely due to the infiltrative margins characteristic of this distinctive GIST variant) (22). In such cases (if the specific diagnostic category is known before surgery), more extensive resection may be indicated, in addition to lymph node dissection, since SDH-deficient GIST often spreads to lymph nodes (unlike GISTs with *KIT* or *PDGFRA* mutations, which almost never do).

Conventional chemotherapy is not effective for GIST. There are, however, three targeted systemic therapies for GIST approved by the US Food and Drug Administration (FDA): imatinib mesylate, sunitinib malate, and regorafenib (59–61). These agents target the tyrosine kinase receptors KIT and PDGFRA. Imatinib is first-line therapy for patients with metastatic or locally advanced disease; this drug is also used to treat patients in the adjuvant setting following resection of localized tumors with moderate or high-risk features (see below). Sunitinib is used for patients who fail (or are intolerant of) imatinib (60). Regorafenib is administered to patients who fail both other therapeutic agents (61).

The specific tumor genotype predicts the response to these targeted therapies (62,63). GISTs that harbor the most common *KIT* exon 11 mutations usually show an excellent response to imatinib (62). In contrast, tumors that harbor the most common *PDGFRA* exon 18 mutation (D842V) are completely imatinib resistant (62); such tumors are also resistant to sunitinib and regorafenib (affected patients should be enrolled in clinical trials). SDH-deficient GISTs also do not respond to imatinib, although limited data suggest that regorafenib has some benefit (64). Secondary resistance to imatinib, defined as initial response but tumor progression after 6 months of therapy, is a common finding: approximately 50 percent of treated patients show tumor progression within 2 years. In most cases, this form of progression is associated with secondary resistance mutations in *KIT*, particularly in regions that encode the kinase domains (65); these mutations block the binding of imatinib. Sunitinib and regorafenib are of benefit to patients whose tumors harbor secondary resistance *KIT* mutations. The rare GISTs with *BRAF* V600E mutations are treated effectively with BRAF inhibitors (66).

Patients with locally advanced GIST may undergo surgical resection following neoadjuvant imatinib therapy, which can "down-stage" the tumors in some cases. Stable, metastatic disease

Table 12-3

RISK STRATIFICATION IN GASTROINTESTINAL STROMAL TUMORS OF THE STOMACH ACCORDING TO MITOTIC INDEX AND TUMOR SIZE[a,b]

Mitotic Index (per 5 mm²)	Tumor Size (cm)	Risk of Progressive Disease
≤ 5	≤ 2	None
	> 2 and ≤ 5	Very low
	> 5 and ≤ 10	Low
	> 10	Moderate
> 5	≤ 2	None
	> 2 and ≤ 5	Moderate
	> 5 and ≤ 10	High
	> 10	High

[a]Adapted from Miettinen M, Lasota J. Gastrointestinal stromal tumors: pathology and prognosis at different sites. Semin Diagn Pathol 2006;23:70-83.
[b]Does not apply to succinate dehydrogenase-deficient gastrointestinal stromal tumors.

on targeted therapy may also be resected. In such cases, treated tumors rarely show frank necrosis (in contrast to other tumor types treated with cytotoxic chemotherapy); instead, a markedly hypocellular appearance with abundant hyalinized collagenous stroma is a characteristic finding (fig. 12-28) (29).

Assessment of treatment response does not play a role in patient management (and should be only descriptive), although highly cellular, mitotically active areas within an otherwise hypocellular, hyalinized tumor are usually associated with the acquisition of secondary resistance mutations. Resistance to therapy may sometimes be associated with loss of KIT expression (as described previously for "dedifferentiated" GIST) (28,29); even more rarely, heterologous rhabdomyosarcomatous differentiation (with tumors resembling embryonal or pleomorphic rhabdomyosarcoma) occurs as an unusual form of clonal evolution and tumor progression on targeted therapies (67).

Prognosis. GISTs are not categorized as benign or malignant; rather, a risk stratification system is applied, based on anatomic site, mitotic rate, and tumor size (Table 12-3) (68). This system is incorporated into the American Joint Committee on Cancer (AJCC) staging system, the National Comprehensive Cancer Network (NCCN) recommendations, and the College of American Pathologists (CAP) cancer synoptic

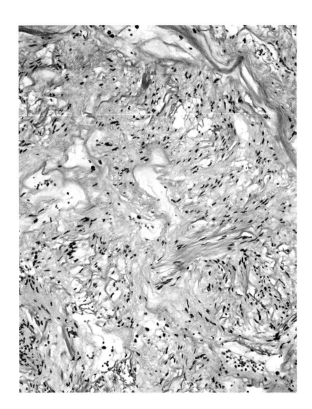 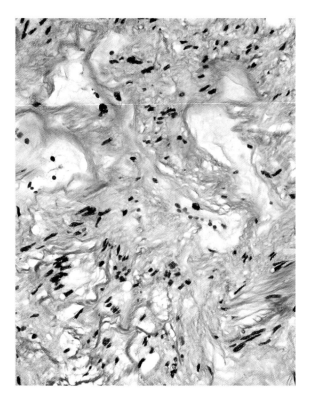

Figure 12-28

GASTROINTESTINAL STROMAL TUMOR, POST-IMATINIB THERAPY

This large spindle cell GIST of the proximal stomach was resected following neoadjuvant imatinib therapy, which caused the tumor to decrease in size, making the surgical approach more straightforward and allowing the resection to spare the gastroesophageal junction. The tumor has a hypocellular appearance with extensive stromal hyalinization (left), only scattered spindle cells, and occasional hemosiderin-laden macrophages (right). This appearance is characteristic of imatinib-sensitive GISTs that have responded well to therapy.

reporting, among other guidelines (69). The most important cut-offs are 5 cm and 5 mitotic figures per 5 mm². Initial guidelines included mitotic rate per 50 high-power fields until it was recognized that the studies establishing these criteria utilized a microscope with a field diameter markedly different from modern microscopes; 5 mm² on modern, wider field microscopes amounts to approximately 20 high-power fields.

Patients with gastric GISTs matched for size and mitotic rate have a better prognosis than those with intestinal tumors (68). This risk stratification system does not apply to SDH-deficient GIST; such tumors show a high rate of metastasis irrespective of mitotic rate and tumor size (70). Even with metastatic disease, however, many patients with SDH-deficient GISTs live for years or decades without therapy. The differences between SDH-deficient and conventional GISTs

are summarized in Table 12-4. Given the rarity of esophageal GISTs, there is no formal risk stratification system for such tumors.

LEIOMYOMA

General Features. Within the GI tract, mural *leiomyomas* are by far most common in the esophagus, where they outnumber GISTs by at least 50 to 1 (16,71). In contrast, although 10 percent of mural leiomyomas arise in the stomach (predominantly proximally), GISTs outnumber leiomyomas at this site by around 50 to 1. Microscopic leiomyomas of the esophagus may be found in nearly 50 percent of patients upon extensive sampling of GI resection specimens (4). Leiomyomas of the esophagus and stomach nearly always arise in the muscularis propria (in contrast to colorectal leiomyomas of the muscularis mucosae). They are somewhat more common in men,

Table 12-4

DIFFERENCES BETWEEN SUCCINATE DEHYDROGENASE-DEFICIENT GASTROINTESTINAL STROMAL TUMORS AND GASTROINTESTINAL STROMAL TUMORS WITH RETAINED SUCCINATE DEHYDROGENASE EXPRESSION

Feature	SDH[a]-Deficient Gastro-intestinal Stromal Tumors	Gastrointestinal Stromal Tumors with Retained SDH Expression
Age predilection	Children and young adults	Older adults
Anatomic site	Stomach	Entire gastrointestinal tract
Multifocality	Common	Rare
Multinodular architecture	Nearly always	Rare
Cytology	Epithelioid or mixed	Spindle cell >> epithelioid
Prognosis predicted by location, tumor size, and mitotic index	No	Yes
KIT or *PDGFRA* mutations	None	~85%
SDHX[b] mutations (germline)	~60%	None
Lymph node metastasis	Common	Exceptional
Clinical course of metastases	Indolent	Aggressive
Sensitive to imatinib	No	Most cases
Syndromic associations	Carney-Stratakis syndrome (germline *SDHX* mutations)	Neurofibromatosis type 1
	Carney triad (*SDHC* promoter hyper-methylation)	Familial GIST (germline *KIT* or *PDGFRA* mutation)

[a]SDH = succinate dehydrogenase.
[b]SDHX refers to SDHA, SDHB, SDHC, or SDHD.

with a wide size range (mean, 5 cm). Leiomyomas are benign and do not recur.

Microscopic Findings. Leiomyomas show a fibrous, trabeculated cut surface and are well circumscribed, and sometimes lobulated (fig. 12-29). Histologically, they are composed of intersecting fascicles of well-differentiated smooth muscle cells with blunt-ended or tapering nuclei and brightly eosinophilic cytoplasm (fig. 12-30); occasional cells contain eosinophilic cytoplasmic inclusions (fig. 12-30). Nuclear atypia is absent and mitotic figures are scarce, in contrast to the very rare leiomyosarcomas (see below).

Immunohistochemical Findings. By immunohistochemistry, leiomyomas are strongly positive for SMA, desmin (fig. 12-31), and caldesmon but negative for KIT and DOG1, although numerous intratumoral mast cells and Cajal cells may be identified by KIT stains (a potential diagnostic pitfall) (fig. 12-31) (58).

Cytologic Findings. FNA specimens of leiomyomas show scattered and small fragments of poorly cellular tissue composed of cohesive spindle cells arranged in parallel lines, with evenly spaced nuclei and abundant intercellular fibrillary matrix (fig. 12-32) (72). The cytoplasm appears fibrillary and is usually abundant and eosinophilic, with an ill-defined border (fig. 12-32). Groups of tumor cells thus often have a syncytial appearance and single tumor cells are rare. Elongated nuclei are separated from each other by a distance of two to three times their largest diameter (fig. 12-33). The nuclei have blunt ends (cigar-shaped) and finely granular and homogeneous chromatin (fig. 12-33).

Molecular Genetic Findings. *Esophageal leiomyomatosis* is a rare disorder characterized by extensive leiomyomas of varying size that replace large areas of the muscularis propria (figs. 12-34, 12-35) (73). This disorder may be sporadic or familial, the latter often associated with Alport syndrome (a hereditary glomerulonephritis), which is caused by germline deletions in one of the genes that encodes collagen type IV (*COL4A3*, *COL4A4*, or *COL4A5*) (73,74). Mutations of these genes may also be associated with some sporadic leiomyomas (75). An *FN1-ALK* gene fusion has recently been reported in an esophageal leiomyoma (76).

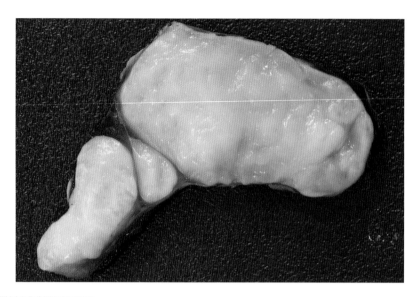

Figure 12-29

ESOPHAGEAL LEIOMYOMA

This lobulated tumor shows a fibrous cut surface. Leiomyomas of the esophagus are often marginally excised without esophagectomy.

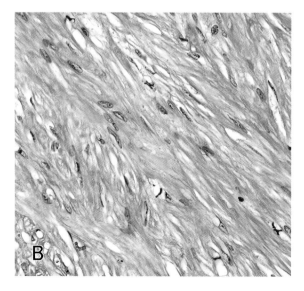

Figure 12-30

ESOPHAGEAL LEIOMYOMA

A: The tumor is composed of intersecting fascicles of spindle cells with brightly eosinophilic cytoplasm.

B: The tumor cells contain uniform, broad nuclei with fine chromatin, brightly eosinophilic cytoplasm, and discernible cell borders.

C: Occasional eosinophilic cytoplasmic inclusions are observed.

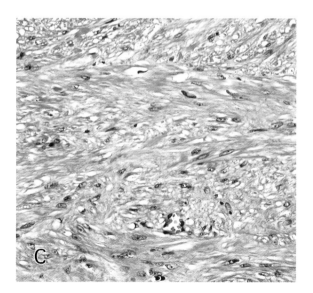

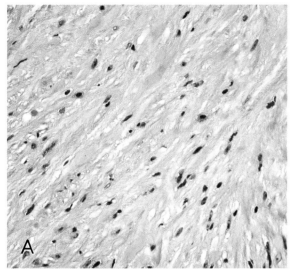

Figure 12-31

ESOPHAGEAL LEIOMYOMA

A: In this example, intratumoral mast cells can be appreciated with a hematoxylin and eosin (H&E) stain.

B: Immunohistochemistry for desmin is strongly and diffusely positive, a feature that distinguishes leiomyoma from GIST.

C: KIT highlights numerous intratumoral mast cells and Cajal cells, a potential diagnostic pitfall.

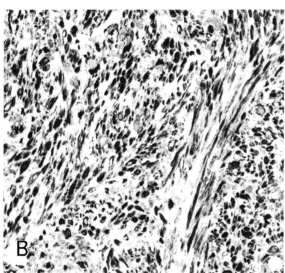

Figure 12-32

GASTRIC LEIOMYOMA

A fragment of tissue is composed of cohesive spindle cells arranged in parallel lines with evenly spaced nuclei and abundant intercellular fibrillary matrix. The cytoplasm is abundant and eosinophilic with an ill-defined border (DiffQuik Stain).

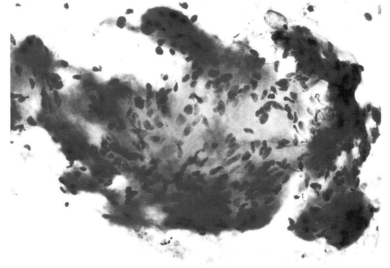

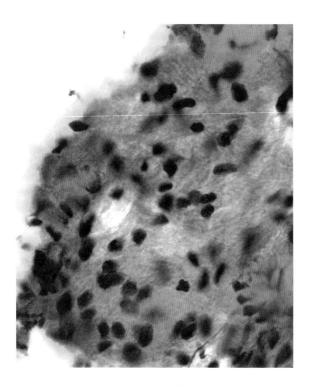

Figure 12-33

GASTRIC LEIOMYOMA

Elongated nuclei are separated from each other by a distance of two to three times their largest diameter. The nuclei have blunt ends (cigar-shaped) and finely granular and homogeneous chromatin (Papanicolaou stain).

LEIOMYOSARCOMA

General Features. As mentioned previously, GISTs were often classified as smooth muscle tumors (including leiomyosarcomas) before the modern era. It is now clear that bona fide primary *leiomyosarcomas* of the GI tract are rare, accounting for 1 percent of mesenchymal tumors at these locations (77,78). When a leiomyosarcoma is encountered in the GI tract, the possibility of a metastasis from the uterus or retroperitoneum (among other sites) should always be excluded. Primary GI leiomyosarcomas have a predilection for the small intestine and colon; esophageal and gastric primary tumors are rare (16,77,78).

Clinical Features. Patients with esophageal leiomyosarcomas may present with dysphagia, whereas those with gastric primary tumors typically present with anemia or hematemesis. Older adults are most often affected. The tumors are usually large when diagnosed, often with transmural involvement and mucosal ulceration. Leiomyosarcomas are aggressive tumors with significant metastatic potential to the peritoneal cavity, liver, lungs, and bone. Most affected patients die of disease despite systemic chemotherapy.

Microscopic Findings. GI leiomyosarcomas are histologically similar to those at other anatomic sites. Tumors show infiltrative margins

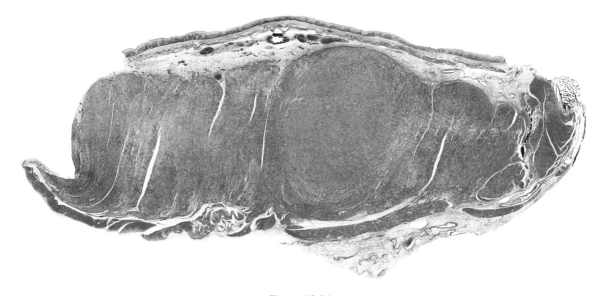

Figure 12-34

ESOPHAGEAL LEIOMYOMATOSIS

A scanning image of leiomyomatosis illustrates the extensive replacement of the muscularis propria by expansile nodules of smooth muscle.

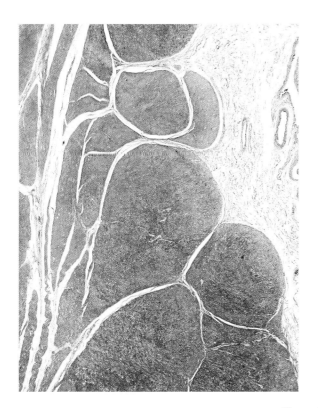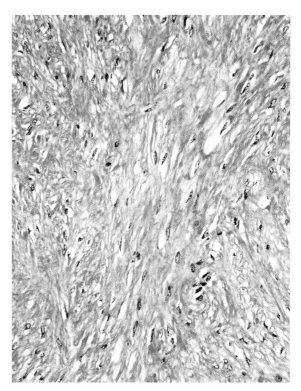

Figure 12-35

ESOPHAGEAL LEIOMYOMATOSIS

Left: In some areas, the tumor nodules are well-demarcated from the muscularis propria.
Right: The histologic features of the tumors are identical to sporadic esophageal leiomyomas.

and are composed of intersecting fascicles of spindle cells with broad, blunt-ended ("cigar-shaped") nuclei, coarse chromatin, and brightly eosinophilic cytoplasm (fig. 12-36).

Most GI leiomyosarcomas are high-grade tumors with marked nuclear atypia, pleomorphism, and a high mitotic rate (fig. 12-37); distinction from leiomyoma is usually straightforward. In occasional cases, leiomyosarcomas of the GI tract are well-differentiated and fairly uniform (fig. 12-37); in such examples, the presence of mitotic activity and nuclear atypia distinguishes leiomyosarcoma from leiomyoma. Rare gastric leiomyosarcomas show epithelioid morphology (fig. 12-38).

Nuclear atypia and variability also distinguish leiomyosarcomas from GISTs, which instead show uniform cytology. Since minimal criteria for malignancy have not been established, it is reasonable to use the designation "uncertain malignant potential" for mitotically active GI smooth muscle tumors without atypia.

Cytologic Findings. On FNA cytology, cells are predominantly arranged in large, three-dimensional, tightly cohesive cell clusters (fig. 12-39). Most cell groups have sharp, circumscribed borders (fig. 12-39), with an occasional coarse bundle of "pulled-out" stroma or cytoplasmic elements rather than the delicate strands of cytoplasm characteristic of GIST. Compared to GIST, leiomyosarcomas are more likely to show crush artifact, significant nuclear pleomorphism, and blunt-ended nuclei (fig. 12-40), and less likely to show delicate cytoplasmic processes, prominent vascular pattern, and wavy nuclei (33). Thus, most high-grade leiomyosarcomas have cytologic features that allow a diagnosis of sarcoma (79).

Within cell groups, cytoplasmic boundaries are indistinct. The cells appear embedded in an abundant wiry, refractile stroma or syncytial cytoplasm (fig. 12-41). This stroma/cytoplasmic material uncommonly appears wispy or in delicate thin strands as characteristic of GIST.

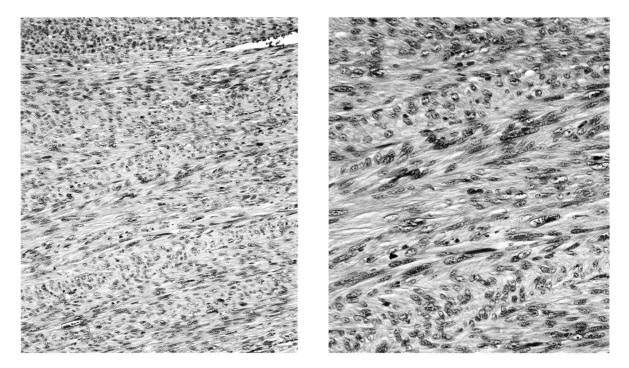

Figure 12-36

LEIOMYOSARCOMA

Left: This leiomyosarcoma of the stomach is composed of long fascicles of spindle cells with marked nuclear atypia and eosinophilic cytoplasm.

Right: The nuclei are broad and blunt-ended, and cell borders are appreciated.

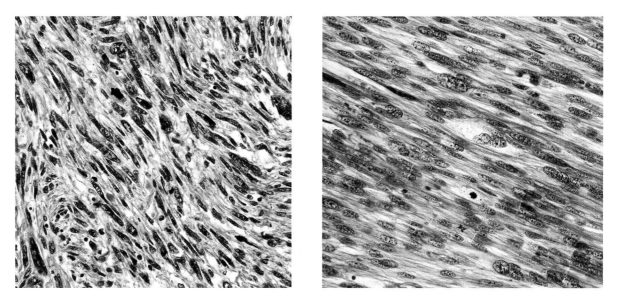

Figure 12-37

LEIOMYOSARCOMA

Left: This gastric leiomyosarcoma shows a more poorly differentiated appearance, with pleomorphic nuclei, a high mitotic rate, and less eosinophilic cytoplasm.

Right: This example is better differentiated, with classic cytologic features. The presence of nuclear atypia and mitotic activity distinguishes leiomyosarcoma from leiomyoma at this site.

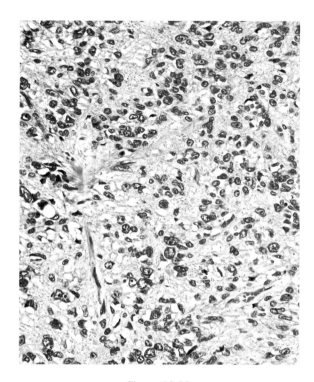

Figure 12-38

EPITHELIOID LEIOMYOSARCOMA

Rare gastric leiomyosarcomas show epithelioid cytomorphology. The nuclei are round to ovoid and the cytoplasm is eosinophilic.

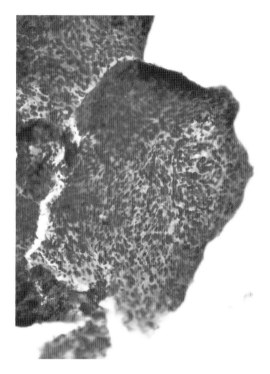

Figure 12-39

LEIOMYOSARCOMA

Large, three-dimensional, tightly cohesive cell clusters are present with sharp, circumscribed borders (Papanicolaou stain). (Courtesy of Dr. E. Cibas, Boston, MA.)

The most common cells are spindle cells with elongated, blunt-ended, segmented or fusiform nuclei, and round/polygonal cells with round or indented nuclei (78).

The nuclear features are more variable and pleomorphic and depend on the degree of differentiation. Most cases have a predominantly spindle cell morphology (fig. 12-41), but in a small number of cases, a substantial proportion (over 10 percent) of epithelioid cells is present. Well-differentiated tumors have ovoid, spindle-shaped, or elongated nuclei with blunt ends and finely or slightly coarsely granular chromatin. Their cytoplasm is scanty and ill defined, and is often stripped from the single cells. Perinuclear cytoplasmic vacuoles and multinucleation are infrequently seen. Poorly differentiated tumors show more dyshesion as demonstrated by many single tumor cells and loose cell groups. The nuclei are still ovoid to elongated but show more pleomorphism, with coarse clumping of chromatin. Multinucleation is present frequently and mitoses are frequent when present.

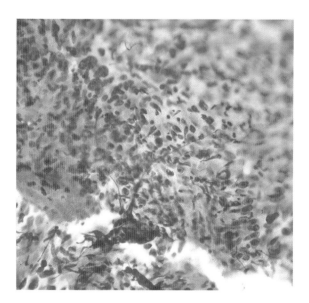

Figure 12-40

LEIOMYOSARCOMA

The nuclei show crush artifact and significant nuclear pleomorphism, and are blunt-ended (Papanicolaou stain). (Courtesy of Dr. E. Cibas, Boston, MA.)

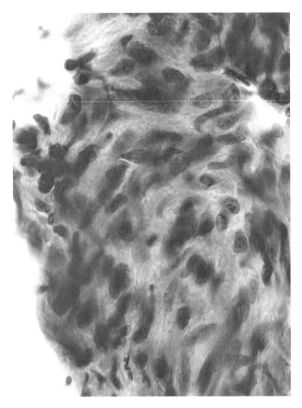

Figure 12-41

LEIOMYOSARCOMA

The cytoplasmic boundaries are indistinct, and the cells appear embedded in an abundant wiry, refractile stroma or syncytial cytoplasm (Papanicolaou stain). (Courtesy of Dr. E. Cibas, Boston, MA.)

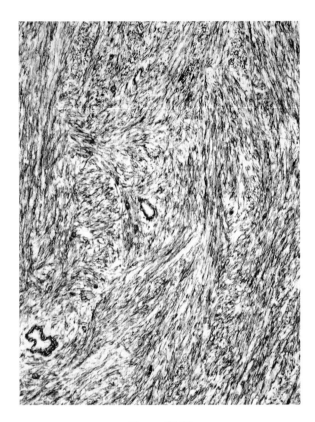

Figure 12-42

LEIOMYOSARCOMA

Immunohistochemistry for SMA shows strong and diffuse cytoplasmic staining. This is a consistent feature of leiomyosarcoma. Desmin and caldesmon are less consistently positive with more variable staining (not shown).

Immunohistochemical Findings. Leiomyosarcomas are nearly always uniformly and strongly positive for SMA (fig. 12-42); desmin and caldesmon are often also positive with more variable staining. KIT, DOG1, and S-100 protein are negative. Leiomyosarcomas often show focal expression of keratins.

SCHWANNOMA

GI schwannomas most often arise in the stomach (80-82), where they may present as mural or intraluminal masses, clinically invariably mistaken for GISTs. This is a critical distinction, since gastric schwannomas are benign and do not recur. GI schwannomas rarely arise in the esophagus (80,81). A yellow cut surface (similar to schwannomas of peripheral nerves) is typical (fig. 12-43).

Gastric schwannomas nearly always display a distinctive histologic feature that allows for their recognition under low magnification: a peripheral lymphoid cuff including germinal centers (figs. 12-44, 12-45) (80–82). Gastric schwannomas are well-circumscribed but unencapsulated. Although some show focal nuclear palisading, their histologic appearance differs from that of conventional schwannomas: they typically lack Antoni A and B zonation, Verocay bodies, and perivascular hyalinization. They are moderately cellular tumors composed of fascicles of elongated spindle cells with tapering nuclei, fine chromatin, and indistinct cytoplasm, often embedded in a dense collagenous stroma with scattered lymphocytes (fig. 12-45). Some tumors show a trabecular growth pattern. A degree of nuclear variability is common (fig. 12-46); this finding, along with the collagenous stroma, distinguish gastric schwannoma from GIST.

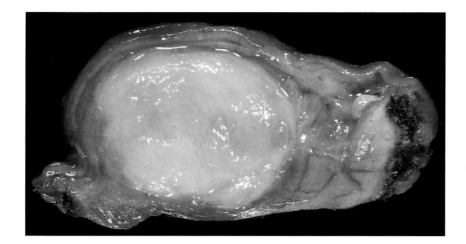

Figure 12-43

GASTRIC SCHWANNOMA

This tumor typically shows a yellow cut surface, similar to schwannomas of peripheral nerves.

Gastric schwannomas are strongly positive for S-100 protein (fig. 12-47), GFAP, and SOX10, but negative for KIT, DOG1, and desmin. In contrast to schwannomas of peripheral nerves (which show loss of the *NF2* gene locus), gastric schwannomas often show loss of *NF1* (83).

Rare gastric schwannomas show epithelioid morphology. *Epithelioid schwannomas* are composed of cords or sheets of epithelioid cells with round nuclei, small nucleoli, and eosinophilic cytoplasm (fig. 12-48). *Microcystic/reticular schwannoma* is another rare schwannoma variant that has a predilection for the stomach (84). This distinctive variant usually lacks the peripheral lymphoid cuff of other gastric schwannomas and is composed of a delicate meshwork of slender spindle cells embedded within an abundant myxoid or collagenous stroma (figs. 12-49, 12-50); such tumors may be mistaken for adenocarcinomas (and have also been reported as signet-ring cell schwannomas) (85).

GRANULAR CELL TUMOR

Within the GI tract, *granular cell tumors* are most common in the esophagus (86,87), where they are usually discovered incidentally at endoscopy; dysphagia is an uncommon presenting symptom. Esophageal granular cell tumors show a female predominance and are more common in African Americans (86,87). Most granular cell tumors arise in the distal esophagus (88). Most are less than 1 cm in size (fig. 12-51); multiple separate lesions are sometimes found (86,88).

Esophageal granular cell tumors often show overlying acanthosis of the squamous epithelium (fig. 12-52), and less often, pseudoepitheliomatous

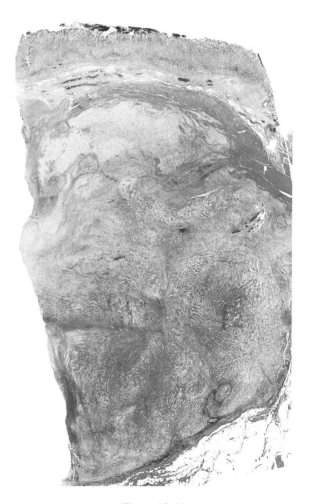

Figure 12-44

GASTRIC SCHWANNOMA

Schwannomas of the gastrointestinal tract display a distinctive peripheral lymphoid cuff, which can be appreciated on scanning magnification. This feature is a helpful diagnostic clue.

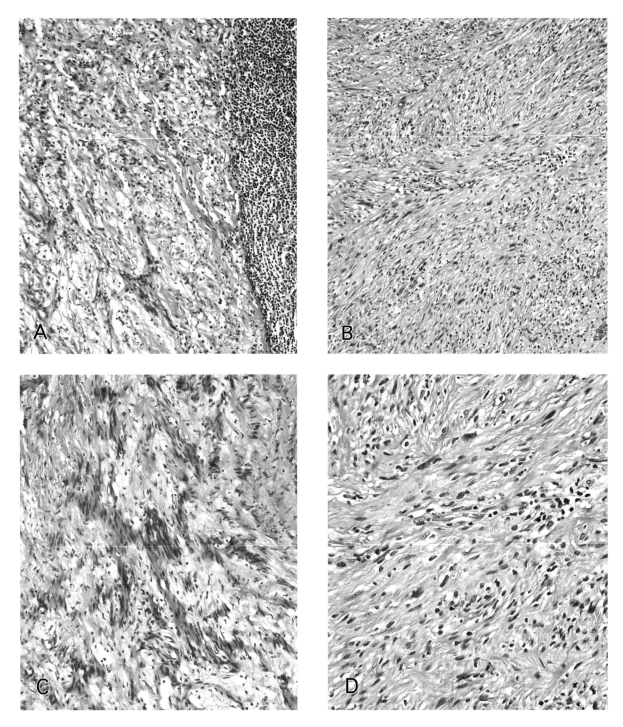

Figure 12-45

GASTRIC SCHWANNOMA

A: This well-circumscribed but unencapsulated tumor is composed of loose fascicles of eosinophilic spindle cells. There is an adjacent lymphoid cuff.

B: In this example, the fascicular architecture is better developed.

C: Focal areas of nuclear palisading are sometimes observed.

D: The spindled tumor cells contain elongated nuclei with fine chromatin. The nuclear size and shape vary and there is abundant collagenous stroma.

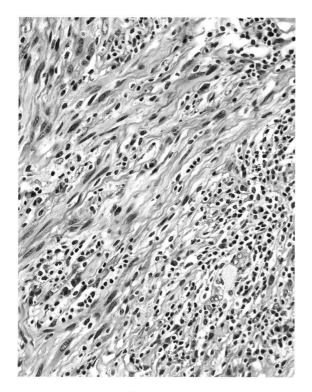

Figure 12-46

GASTRIC SCHWANNOMA

Gastric schwannomas often contain a prominent intratumoral lymphoid infiltrate. The cytologic features may resemble smooth muscle tumors.

Figure 12-47

GASTRIC SCHWANNOMA

Immunohistochemistry for S-100 protein is strongly positive. This feature distinguishes gastric schwannoma from GIST.

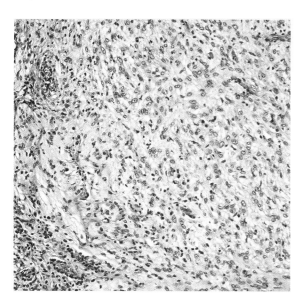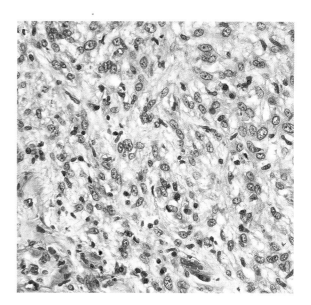

Figure 12-48

GASTRIC EPITHELIOID SCHWANNOMA

Left: Rare gastric schwannomas show epithelioid cytomorphology.
Right: The tumor cells contain rounded nuclei with fine chromatin and eosinophilic cytoplasm.

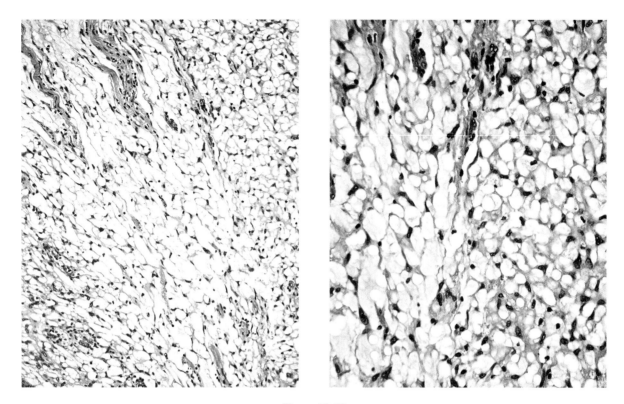

Figure 12-49

GASTRIC MICROCYSTIC/RETICULAR SCHWANNOMA

This rare schwannoma variant has a predilection for the stomach (left). The elongated spindle cells form a delicate net-like architecture with myxoid stroma (right). These tumors may be mistaken for adenocarcinomas.

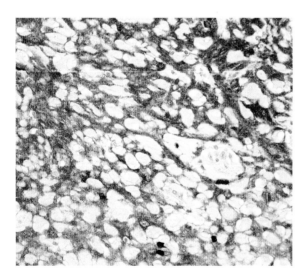

Figure 12-50

GASTRIC MICROCYSTIC/RETICULAR SCHWANNOMA

Similar to its staining pattern in other gastric schwannomas, S-100 protein is strongly positive with a nuclear and cytoplasmic pattern. The stain highlights the reticular growth pattern.

hyperplasia. They typically extend to the epithelium (fig. 12-53) and are composed of polygonal cells with small, round, hyperchromatic nuclei; indistinct nucleoli; and abundant granular eosinophilic cytoplasm (fig. 12-54) (89,90). Some tumors have a minor spindle cell component (fig. 12-55). Infiltrative margins are characteristic of this tumor type (fig. 12-56); this finding is of no clinical significance. The diagnosis is easily confirmed by immunohistochemistry: granular cell tumors are Schwann cell neoplasms positive for S-100 protein and SOX10.

Granular cell tumors of the esophagus are nearly always benign and rarely recur, even following incomplete excision. Very rare malignant esophageal granular cell tumors have been reported.

INFLAMMATORY FIBROID POLYP

Inflammatory fibroid polyps are distinctive neoplasms that occur throughout the GI tract; they most often arise in the gastric antrum,

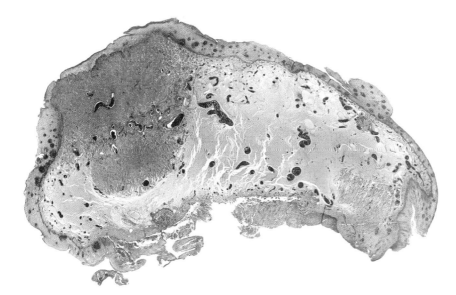

Figure 12-51

**ESOPHAGEAL GRANULAR
CELL TUMOR**

This large granular cell tumor was excised by endoscopic submucosal dissection. In this scanning image, the eosinophilic appearance is appreciated.

Figure 12-52

**ESOPHAGEAL GRANULAR
CELL TUMOR**

At this anatomic site, granular cell tumors are often associated with hyperplasia and acanthosis of the overlying squamous epithelium.

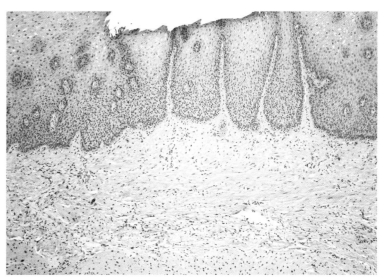

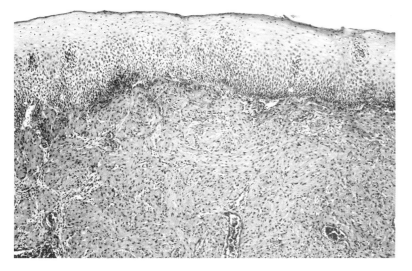

Figure 12-53

**ESOPHAGEAL GRANULAR
CELL TUMOR**

The tumor abuts the squamous epithelium, which shows basal cell hyperplasia. The tumor cells are large and polygonal with abundant eosinophilic cytoplasm.

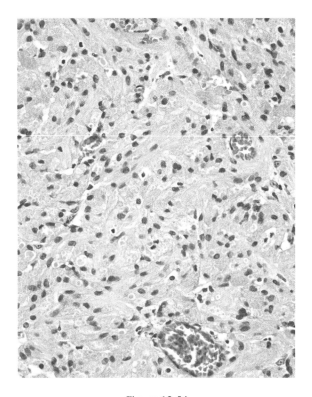

Figure 12-54

ESOPHAGEAL GRANULAR CELL TUMOR

The epithelioid tumor cells contain uniform round nuclei and abundant granular eosinophilic cytoplasm with a syncytial appearance

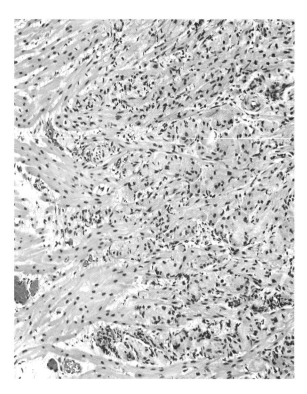

Figure 12-56

ESOPHAGEAL GRANULAR CELL TUMOR

Infiltrative margins are a typical finding of no clinical significance.

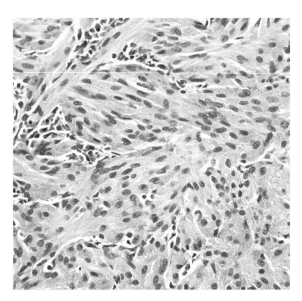

Figure 12-55

ESOPHAGEAL GRANULAR CELL TUMOR

Some cases contain a minor component of tumor cells with a spindle cell appearance. The nuclei are bland and uniform.

followed by the ileum (91). They may be discovered incidentally at endoscopy or occasional patients present with anemia or abdominal pain. Inflammatory fibroid polyps are benign and do not recur.

Most gastric examples are centered in the submucosa (fig. 12-57), and sometimes associated with mucosal ulceration. The size range is wide, with most gastric tumors between 1 and 3 cm.

Inflammatory fibroid polyps are usually hypocellular lesions (fig. 12-58), although occasional examples are more cellular (fig. 12-59). They are composed of haphazardly arranged, short spindled to stellate cells with fine chromatin, small nucleoli, and indistinct palely eosinophilic cytoplasm, embedded within a variably edematous, myxoid, or hyalinized stroma containing a mixed inflammatory cell infiltrate; eosinophils are often prominent (figs. 12-60, 12-61). Prominent intermediate-sized, rounded blood vessels, some with concentric perivascular ("onion-skin") fibrosis, are typically

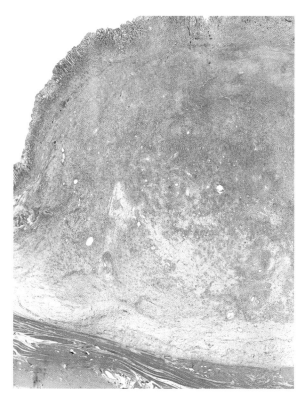

Figure 12-57

INFLAMMATORY FIBROID POLYP

This gastric inflammatory fibroid polyp involves the submucosa with ill-defined margins.

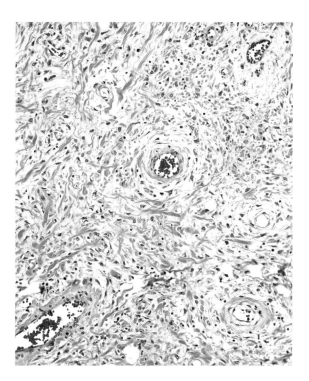

Figure 12-58

INFLAMMATORY FIBROID POLYP

This gastric inflammatory fibroid polyp has edematous stroma, haphazardly arranged tumor cells, and collagen fibers.

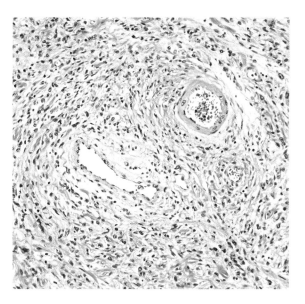

Figure 12-59

INFLAMMATORY FIBROID POLYP

This gastric tumor shows a more cellular appearance than the example in figure 12-58, and is composed of an admixture of spindle cells and more rounded cells. There are prominent, intermediate-sized blood vessels.

observed (fig. 12-62). Inflammatory fibroid polyps often show infiltrative margins into the mucosa and muscularis propria.

By immunohistochemistry, inflammatory fibroid polyps are positive for CD34 in about 95 percent of cases (fig. 12-63); focal expression of SMA is seen in about 10 percent (92,93). KIT, DOG1, S-100 protein, and desmin are negative.

Inflammatory fibroid polyps often harbor activating mutations in *PDGFRA*, most often in exon 18 (D842V) in gastric examples (94,95), similar to some gastric GISTs; immunohistochemistry for PDGFRA can be used to support the diagnosis (fig. 12-63). Rarely, inflammatory fibroid polyps may be familial and associated with germline *PDGFRA* mutations; carriers often develop multiple tumors (96,97).

PLEXIFORM FIBROMYXOMA

Plexiform fibromyxoma is a rare, distinctive mesenchymal neoplasm with a marked

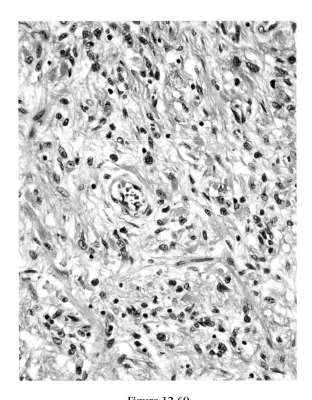

Figure 12-60

INFLAMMATORY FIBROID POLYP

The tumor cells contain ovoid nuclei with fine chromatin and indistinct cytoplasm. The stroma is collagenous, with scattered eosinophils.

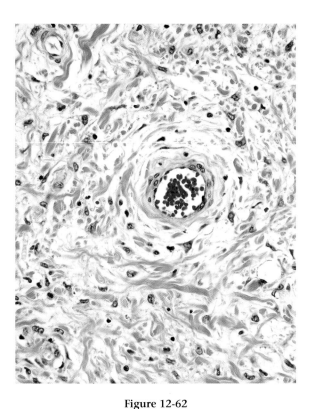

Figure 12-62

INFLAMMATORY FIBROID POLYP

Perivascular fibrosis is a characteristic finding but may be limited in extent or absent. The tumor cells are stellate.

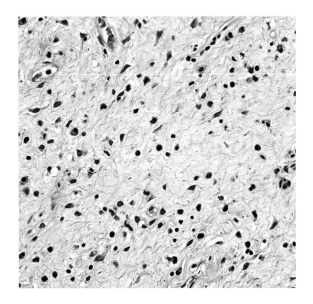

Figure 12-61

INFLAMMATORY FIBROID POLYP

In some cases, eosinophils are numerous. This gastric tumor contained fibrillary collagenous stroma.

predilection for the gastric antrum and pyloric region (98–100). This tumor type has also been referred to as *plexiform angiomyxoid myofibroblastic tumor* (99). Gastric outlet obstruction is common; hematemesis and anemia are typical presenting findings (98). This tumor type affects patients over a wide age range with no gender predilection. Plexiform fibromyxoma is benign and does not recur.

Plexiform fibromyxoma often manifests as a large transmural mass, which may protrude into the gastric lumen or bulge from the serosa; similar to other gastric mural mesenchymal tumors, the clinical diagnosis is usually GIST. There is a multinodular growth pattern through the muscularis propria (fig. 12-64), often extending to and ulcerating the mucosa. In most cases, the nodules contain abundant myxoid stroma (figs. 12-65, 12-66); a more fibrous stroma is sometimes observed (fig. 12-67). The tumor is composed of elongated spindle cells with slender nuclei, fine chromatin, and indistinct

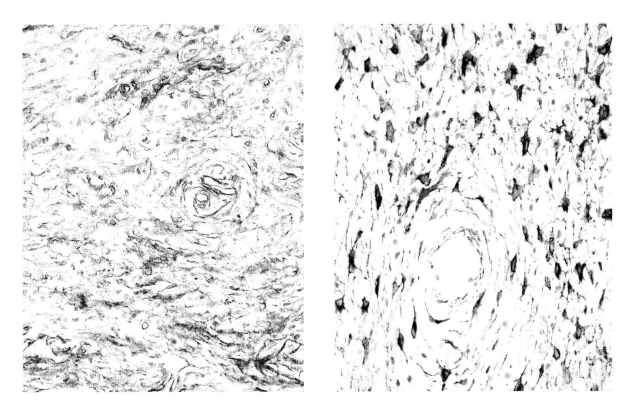

Figure 12-63

INFLAMMATORY FIBROID POLYP

Immunohistochemistry is usually positive for both CD34 (left) and PDGFRA (right), the latter reflecting the underlying *PDGFRA* activating mutation.

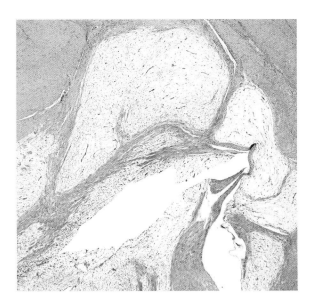

Figure 12-64

PLEXIFORM FIBROMYXOMA

This distinctive gastric tumor shows a plexiform architecture through the muscularis propria.

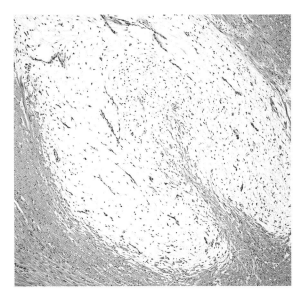

Figure 12-65

PLEXIFORM FIBROMYXOMA

The myxoid lobules are sharply demarcated from the adjacent muscularis propria.

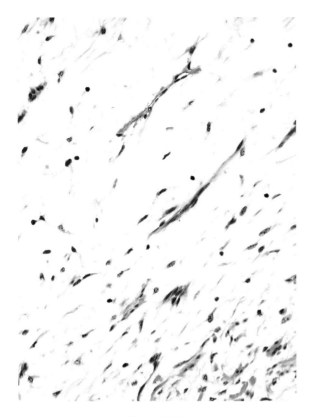

Figure 12-66

PLEXIFORM FIBROMYXOMA

The bland and uniform elongated spindle cells contain fine chromatin and indistinct cytoplasm. There are thin-walled blood vessels and abundant myxoid stroma.

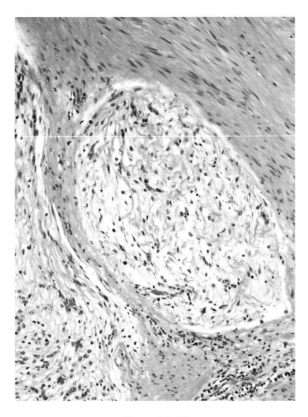

Figure 12-67

PLEXIFORM FIBROMYXOMA

In some cases, the tumor nodules contain more collagenous stroma.

cytoplasm; there is no nuclear atypia, and mitoses are scarce (fig. 12-66). Delicate, thin-walled blood vessels are characteristic (fig. 12-66).

By immunohistochemistry, plexiform fibromyxomas are usually positive for SMA and sometimes for desmin, whereas KIT, DOG1, and S-100 protein are negative (98). A *MALAT1-GLI1* gene fusion has been identified in a subset of plexiform fibromyxomas (101), the same fusion discovered in gastroblastoma (see below). The diagnosis is generally straightforward once plexiform fibromyxoma is considered.

GLOMUS TUMOR

When arising in the GI tract, *glomus tumors* have a marked predilection for the gastric antrum, although such tumors are rare at this site (102–104). Gastric glomus tumors usually affect adults, with a female predominance. They may either be discovered incidentally at endoscopy or patients present with abdominal pain, anemia, or melena. Gastric glomus tumors present as a mural mass, similar to GIST; most tumors are between 2 and 5 cm in size (102,103).

These tumors show a plexiform growth pattern through the muscularis propria (fig. 12-68) and are associated with prominent, slit-like and dilated blood vessels (figs. 12-69, 12-70). The histologic appearance is similar to that of glomus tumors of skin and subcutaneous tissue: the tumor cells show a sheet-like growth pattern and are rounded and uniform with round nuclei, fine chromatin, and moderate amounts of clear or eosinophilic cytoplasm with sharply defined cell borders (fig. 12-71). The tumor cells are arranged in close apposition to the blood vessels in a subendothelial location, a helpful diagnostic clue. Areas of hyalinized stroma are often observed (fig. 12-72). Vascular invasion is common but of no clinical significance.

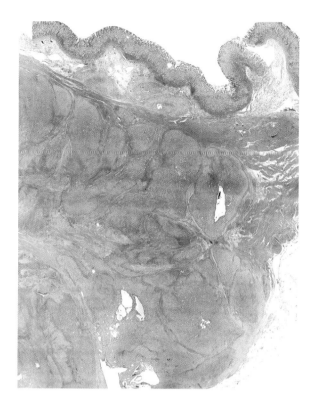

Figure 12-68

GLOMUS TUMOR

Gastric glomus tumors show a plexiform growth pattern through the muscular propria.

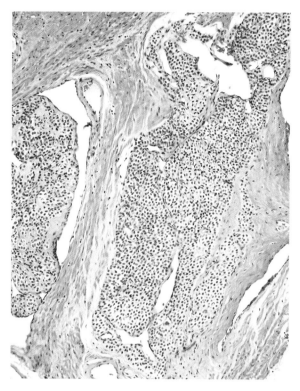

Figure 12-69

GLOMUS TUMOR

The tumor shows a multinodular architecture. Tumor nodules often protrude into thin-walled, dilated veins.

Glomus tumors are strongly positive for SMA (fig. 12-73) and often for caldesmon, whereas desmin, KIT, DOG1, CD34, keratins, and S-100 protein are negative. Weak staining for synaptophysin is common; this finding may lead to misdiagnosis as a well-differentiated neuroendocrine tumor (103). Glomus tumors harbor gene fusions involving *NOTCH* genes, most commonly *MIR143-NOTCH2* (105).

Gastric glomus tumors are usually benign, although some tumors metastasize to the liver (103). The histologic features do not correlate well with behavior, although a high mitotic rate is sometimes associated with an aggressive clinical course.

SYNOVIAL SARCOMA

Although exceedingly rare, GI *synovial sarcomas* nearly always arise in the stomach (106–108). They affect young to middle-aged adults. Gastric synovial tumors range from small mural tumors to large transmural masses.

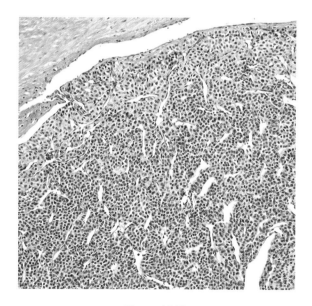

Figure 12-70

GLOMUS TUMOR

Gastric glomus tumors typically contain prominent slit-like blood vessels.

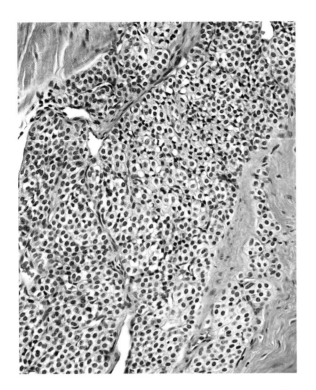
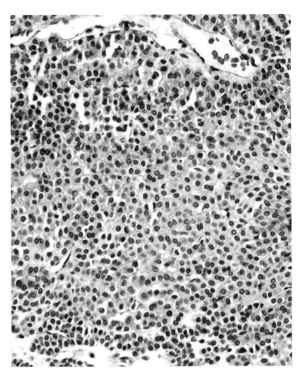

Figure 12-71

GLOMUS TUMOR

Left: The epithelioid tumor cells contain round and uniform central nuclei and clear cytoplasm with sharply defined cell borders.

Right: In some cases, the tumor cells contain eosinophilic cytoplasm.

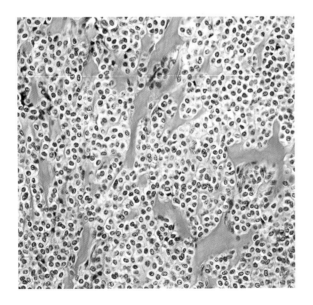
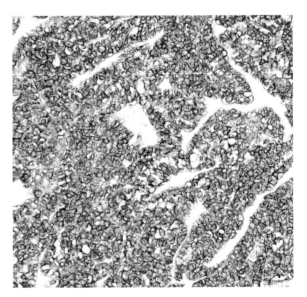

Figure 12-72

GLOMUS TUMOR

Hyalinized collagenous stroma is a characteristic finding. Uniform rounded cells with clear cytoplasm are seen.

Figure 12-73

GLOMUS TUMOR

Immunohistochemistry for smooth muscle actin (SMA) is strongly positive.

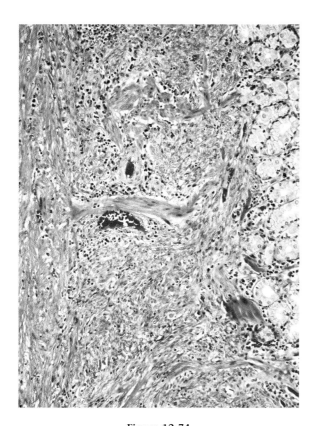

Figure 12-74

MONOPHASIC SYNOVIAL SARCOMA

Synovial sarcoma of the stomach infiltrates the muscularis mucosae.

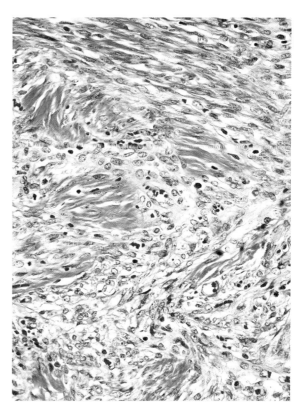

Figure 12-75

MONOPHASIC SYNOVIAL SARCOMA

This gastric tumor is composed of fascicles of uniform spindle cells with fine chromatin. The intercellular collagen bundles are prominent, some with a wiry appearance.

Most gastric synovial sarcomas are monophasic tumors, composed of highly cellular fascicles of uniform and bland, short spindle cells with fine chromatin and scant cytoplasm (figs. 12-74, 12-75). Wiry collagen fibers in the limited stroma between tumor cells is a characteristic finding (fig. 12-75). Some tumors contain thin-walled, dilated (hemangiopericytoma-like) blood vessels.

Synovial sarcomas are positive for EMA (fig. 12-76) and keratins, usually with limited staining in only a small subset of cells; strong and diffuse nuclear TLE1 is a highly sensitive but only moderately specific marker (fig. 12-76) (108). Synovial sarcomas may be positive for DOG1 but are negative for KIT (12). They harbor the pathognomonic t(X;18) translocation, resulting in *SS18-SSX1* or *SS18-SSX2* gene fusions; fluorescence in situ hybridization (FISH) for *SS18* rearrangement can be used to confirm the diagnosis.

Small gastric synovial sarcomas have a favorable outcome. Some affected patients, however, develop metastases to liver and lung and die of disease (107,108).

INFLAMMATORY MYOFIBROBLASTIC TUMOR

Inflammatory myofibroblastic tumors are rare mesenchymal neoplasms of intermediate biologic potential (rarely metastasizing) with a predilection for the GI tract and abdominal cavity; the stomach is commonly affected, whereas esophageal tumors are rare (109–111). This tumor type usually arises in children and young adults who typically present with abdominal pain, sometimes with fever. Abnormal laboratory tests include elevated leukocyte count, hypergammaglobulinemia, and elevated erythrocyte sedimentation rate (109,111).

Inflammatory myofibroblastic tumors show a wide size range and typically involve the

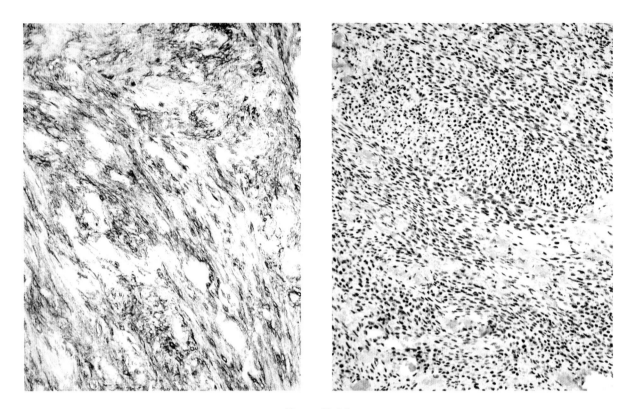

Figure 12-76

MONOPHASIC SYNOVIAL SARCOMA

Immunohistochemistry shows membranous staining for epithelial membrane antigen (EMA) (left) and nuclear staining for TLE1 (right).

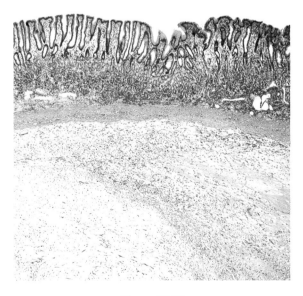

Figure 12-77

INFLAMMATORY MYOFIBROBLASTIC TUMOR

This gastric tumor arose in the submucosa. It has a hypocellular appearance and prominent myxoid stroma.

submucosa and muscularis propria (fig. 12-77). Tumors are composed of fascicles of plump spindle cells with vesicular chromatin, small nucleoli, and palely eosinophilic cytoplasm, admixed with a prominent chronic inflammatory infiltrate of plasma cells and lymphocytes; some examples contain myxoid stroma, whereas others are highly cellular (figs. 12-78, 12-79) (109).

By immunohistochemistry, inflammatory myofibroblastic tumors are consistently positive for SMA and often for desmin. ALK is expressed in around 60 percent of cases (fig. 12-80), correlating with the presence of *ALK* gene fusions; *ALK* fusions are common in tumors from young patients but are rare in older adults (111). Rarely, other tyrosine kinase receptor genes are involved, including *ROS1* and *NTRK3* (112–115).

Most GI inflammatory myofibroblastic tumors are benign; a small subset of patients develops metastases to the abdominal cavity and liver. Targeted systemic therapies benefit the rare patients with aggressive inflammatory

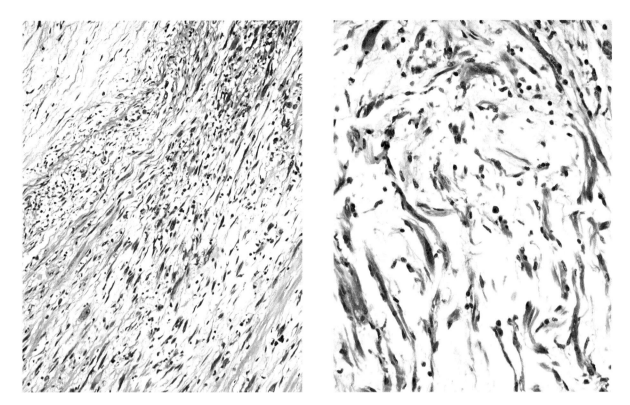

Figure 12-78

INFLAMMATORY MYOFIBROBLASTIC TUMOR

The tumor is composed of loose fascicles of elongated spindle cells (left) with plump nuclei, vesicular chromatin, and eosinophilic cytoplasm, embedded in a myxoid stroma (right). Scattered plasma cells and lymphocytes are present.

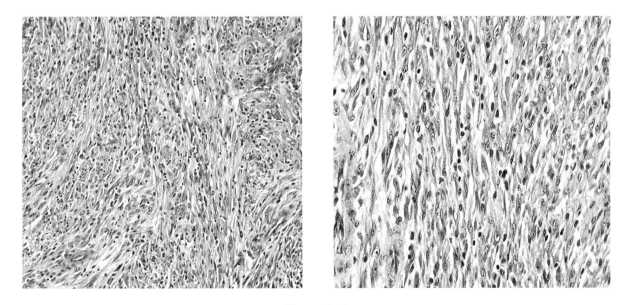

Figure 12-79

INFLAMMATORY MYOFIBROBLASTIC TUMOR

Left: This is a cellular, fascicular example mimicking GIST or a smooth muscle neoplasm.
Right: The tumor cells contain vesicular chromatin and eosinophilic cytoplasm with scattered lymphocytes.

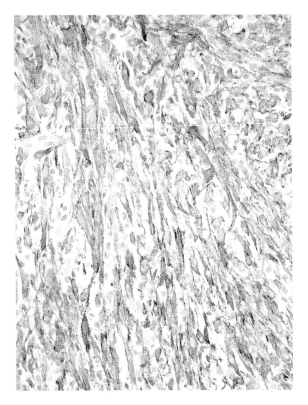

Figure 12-80

INFLAMMATORY MYOFIBROBLASTIC TUMOR

Immunohistochemistry for ALK is positive in about 60 percent of inflammatory myofibroblastic tumors, correlating with *ALK* gene rearrangements.

myofibroblastic tumors with *ALK* or *ROS1* rearrangements (112,116).

PERIVASCULAR EPITHELIOID CELL TUMORS

Perivascular epithelioid cell tumors (PEComas) are distinctive mesenchymal neoplasms that show an association with blood vessel walls and co-express smooth muscle and melanocytic markers (117,118). The most common member of this family of tumors is angiomyolipoma of the kidney; PEComas outside of the kidney are rare. The most common anatomic locations include retroperitoneum, abdominal cavity, GI tract, uterus, and pelvis (117,119). Unlike renal angiomyolipomas, PEComas of these other sites are rarely associated with the tuberous sclerosis complex (TSC) (119). Among GI tract PEComas, colon and small intestine are most often involved; gastric PEComas are rare (120). Patients typically present with a large mural mass, abdominal pain, and anemia.

PEComas are composed of epithelioid cells with round nuclei, small nucleoli, and clear to granular eosinophilic cytoplasm (fig. 12-81), arranged in nests and trabeculae with a delicate capillary vascular network (figs. 12-82, 12-83). The quality of the cytoplasm is a helpful clue to the diagnosis. Some GI PEComas contain a minor component of cells with spindle cell

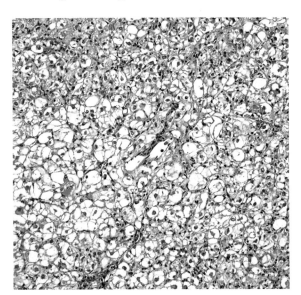
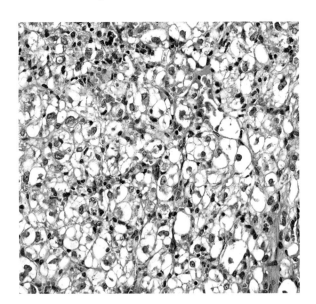

Figure 12-81

PECOMA

Most tumors are composed of large epithelioid cells (left) with abundant granular eosinophilic to clear cytoplasm (right).

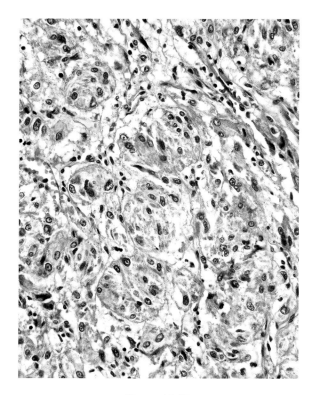

Figure 12-82

PECOMA

PEComas often show a nested appearance. The eosinophilic cytoplasm is granular.

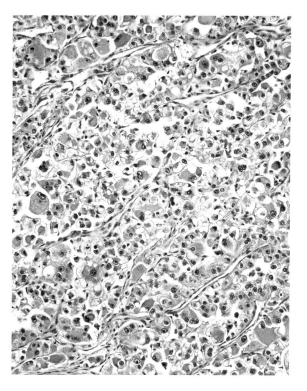

Figure 12-83

PECOMA

A malignant PEComa with a trabecular architecture. The tumor cells show marked nuclear atypia and contain macronucleoli, resembling metastatic melanoma.

morphology (120). Most PEComas show only mild atypia and contain rare mitotic figures.

By immunohistochemistry, GI PEComas often express SMA, desmin, HMB-45, and melan A (fig. 12-84); staining for each of these markers is variable, and all four may be required to demonstrate both smooth muscle and melanocytic differentiation (117). S-100 protein is weakly and focally positive in around 15 percent of cases, whereas KIT, DOG1, and keratins are negative. Most PEComas show biallelic inactivation of the *TSC2* gene, leading to mammalian target of rapamycin (mTOR) pathway activation (121–123).

Although many PEComas are benign, a small subset behaves as aggressive sarcomas. There are no firm minimal criteria for malignancy. Nevertheless, tumors showing the combination of marked nuclear atypia, pleomorphism, and mitotic activity (fig. 12-83) should be diagnosed as malignant PEComas; they pursue an aggressive clinical course with metastases to regional lymph nodes, liver, lungs, and bone (117,120). mTOR

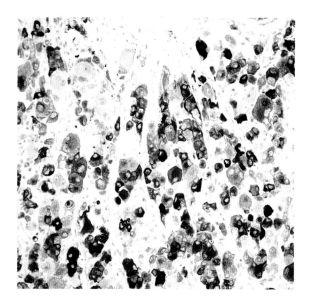

Figure 12-84

PECOMA

The most sensitive melanocytic marker for PEComa is HMB-45.

379

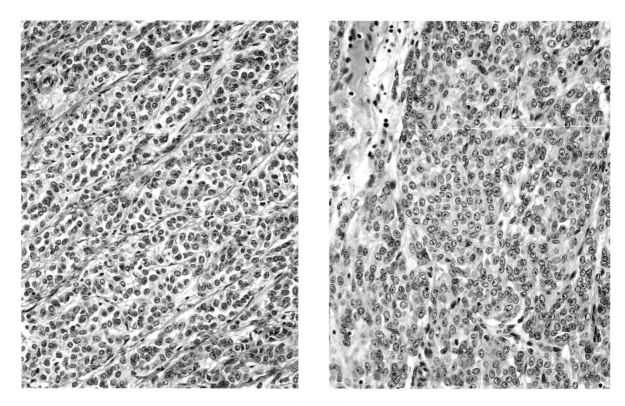

Figure 12-85

GASTROINTESTINAL NEUROECTODERMAL TUMOR (CLEAR CELL SARCOMA-LIKE TUMOR OF THE GI TRACT)

These tumors show a variably nested (left) or sheet-like (right) growth pattern. The nuclei are uniform, with small nucleoli.

inhibitors often prolong survival of patients with metastatic malignant PEComas (124,125).

GI NEUROECTODERMAL TUMOR

GI neuroectodermal tumor (GNET), also known as *clear cell sarcoma-like tumor of the GI tract*, is a distinctive GI sarcoma with a marked predilection for the small intestine; the stomach is more rarely affected (126–128). Despite some similar features, GNET shows significant histologic, immunophenotypic, and clinical differences from conventional clear cell sarcoma of tendons and aponeuroses, suggesting that this tumor type is not simply a GI variant of clear cell sarcoma (127,128). GNET predominantly affects young to middle-aged adults and presents as a large, transmural mass, often with mucosal ulceration (128).

GNETs show a multinodular, infiltrative growth pattern and are composed of sheets and nests of rounded or epithelioid cells with uniform nuclei, small nucleoli, and palely eosinophilic cytoplasm (figs. 12-85, 12-86), often with focally alveolar or pseudopapillary growth

patterns (fig. 12-87). Some tumors show clear cell features (fig. 12-88). Osteoclast-like giant cells are a characteristic feature (fig. 12-88) (128).

GNET is strongly and diffusely positive for S-100 protein (fig. 12-89) and SOX10, whereas HMB-45 and melan A are negative (unlike conventional clear cell sarcoma), as are KIT, DOG1, CD34, and keratins (128). GNET harbors *EWSR1* gene rearrangements, either *EWSR1-ATF1* or *EWSR1-CREB1*, with approximately equal distribution (126,128).

Once expression of S-100 protein or SOX10 is identified, the most important differential diagnostic consideration is metastatic melanoma, which has a predilection for the GI tract. Since metastatic melanoma is much more common that GNET (and metastatic melanomas often lack expression of HMB-45 and melan A), confirming the diagnosis by FISH for *EWSR1* is prudent (129).

GNET is an aggressive sarcoma that frequently presents with lymph node, liver, and peritoneal metastases (128). Most affected patients die of

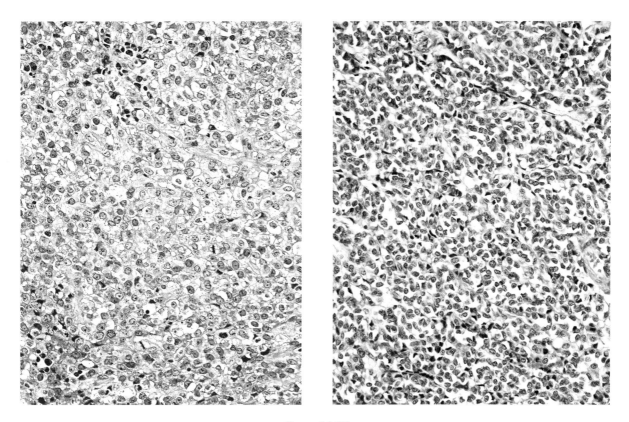

Figure 12-86

GASTROINTESTINAL NEUROECTODERMAL TUMOR (CLEAR CELL SARCOMA-LIKE TUMOR OF THE GI TRACT)

These tumors may be composed of small epithelioid cells (left) or round cells (right), with some cases resembling a small round blue cell tumor.

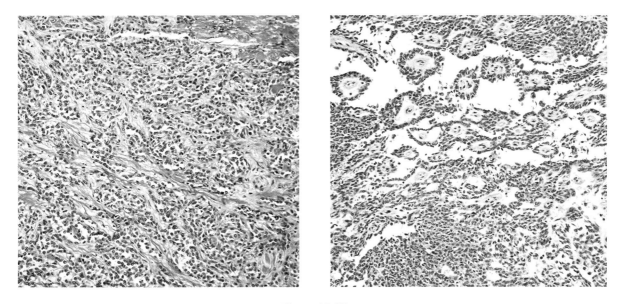

Figure 12-87

GASTROINTESTINAL NEUROECTODERMAL TUMOR (CLEAR CELL SARCOMA-LIKE TUMOR OF THE GI TRACT)

A focally alveolar (left) or pseudopapillary (right) growth pattern is a helpful diagnostic clue.

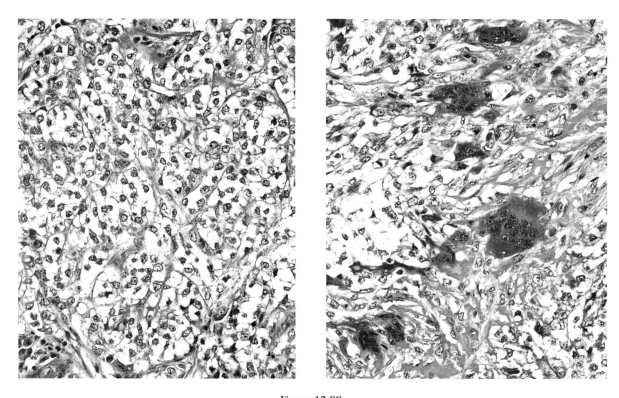

Figure 12-88

GASTROINTESTINAL NEUROECTODERMAL TUMOR (CLEAR CELL SARCOMA-LIKE TUMOR OF THE GI TRACT)

This tumor shows a focally nested, clear cell appearance (left) and contains prominent osteoclast-like giant cells (right).

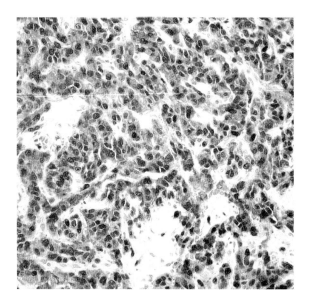

Figure 12-89

GASTROINTESTINAL NEUROECTODERMAL TUMOR (CLEAR CELL SARCOMA-LIKE TUMOR OF THE GI TRACT)

S-100 protein is strongly positive. Melanocytic markers such as HMB-45 and melan A are negative (not shown).

disease within several years. Effective systemic therapies for this sarcoma type have not yet been developed.

GASTROBLASTOMA

Gastroblastoma is a rare biphasic tumor of the stomach of uncertain lineage (130–132). Only small numbers of cases have been published. The biologic potential of this tumor type remains uncertain; reported cases have ranged from benign tumors to aggressive neoplasms with lymph node metastases and disseminated peritoneal disease (132).

Gastroblastoma usually presents as a large mass centered in the muscularis propria with infiltrative margins into the submucosa and mucosa, often with overlying ulceration (fig. 12-90). The tumor often shows a multinodular appearance (fig. 12-91).

Gastroblastoma contains both mesenchymal and epithelial components (fig. 12-92) (130). The relative proportions of epithelial cells and

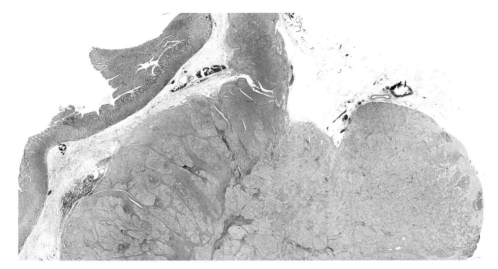

Figure 12-90

GASTROBLASTOMA

The infiltrative margins of this distinctive gastric tumor are appreciated at scanning magnification.

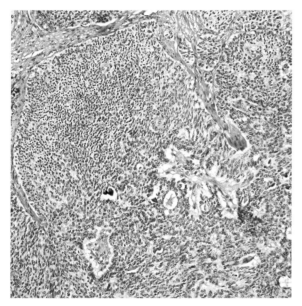

Figure 12-91

GASTROBLASTOMA

In this area, the tumor shows a predominantly spindle cell appearance.

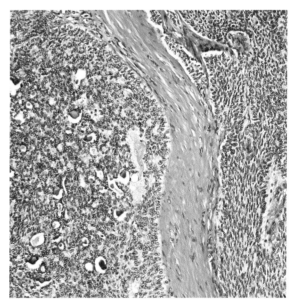

Figure 12-92

GASTROBLASTOMA

The biphasic nature of this tumor type is evident in this image, depicting both the spindle cell and epithelial components forming tubules with intraluminal secretions.

spindle cells are highly variable. The epithelial component is composed of tubules and nests of uniform cuboidal cells with small nuclei and eosinophilic or clear cytoplasm; the tubules often contain eosinophilic luminal secretions (fig. 12-93). The spindle cell component may show a fascicular or sheet-like growth pattern; in some cases, the spindle cells are embedded in myxoid stroma (fig. 12-94). The two components often appear to merge with one another.

By immunohistochemistry, the epithelial component is strongly positive for keratins; the spindle cell component is negative for keratins and markers of other lineages, although the nonspecific marker CD10 is often positive (130). Remarkably, gastroblastoma harbors the same *MALAT1-GLI1* fusion (133) as some cases of plexiform fibromyxoma. Given the histologic resemblance to biphasic synovial sarcoma, it is

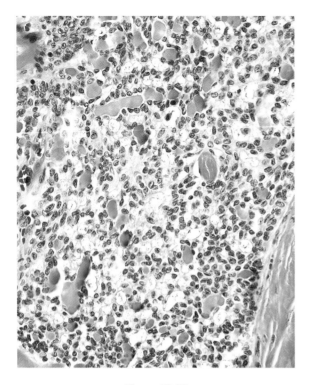

Figure 12-93

GASTROBLASTOMA

The tumor cells contain uniform nuclei and pale cytoplasm. Eosinophilic secretions are seen in the tubular structures.

important to exclude synovial sarcoma before rendering the diagnosis; *SS18* rearrangement by FISH is specific for synovial sarcoma.

WELL-DIFFERENTIATED LIPOSARCOMA (GIANT FIBROVASCULAR POLYP)

The term *giant fibrovascular polyp* has been applied to large, pedunculated esophageal polyps that contain adipose and fibrous tissue and blood vessels (134). It has recently become clear that the majority of (if not all) such polyps in fact represent *well-differentiated liposarcomas* presenting in a distinctive fashion in the esophagus (135–137).

Most polypoid well-differentiated liposarcomas at this site arise in the cervical esophagus and range in size from several to 20 cm (fig. 12-95) (137). They often contain prominent blood vessels, chronic inflammation (fig. 12-96), and an admixture of adipocytes and loose or sclerotic fibrous connective tissue (figs. 12-97, 12-98) (137); granulation tissue is commonly observed in superficial aspects of these polyps (areas of surface ulceration). Upon careful inspection, the adipocytes usually show some variation in cell size, and occasional hyperchromatic stromal cells are identified in the fibrous tissue

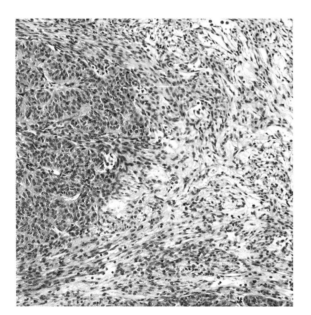
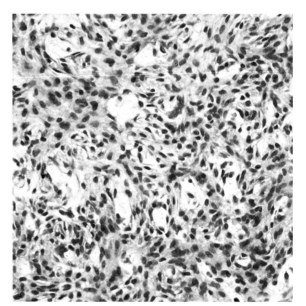

Figure 12-94

GASTROBLASTOMA

Left: The spindle cells are arranged in cellular bundles with areas of myxoid stroma.
Right: In the myxoid area, the uniform and bland nuclear morphology of the spindle cells is appreciated.

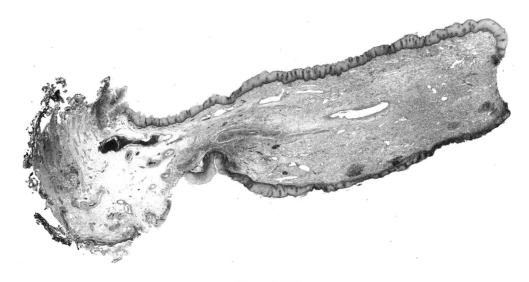

Figure 12-95

WELL-DIFFERENTIATED LIPOSARCOMA ("GIANT FIBROVASCULAR POLYP")

This is a scanning image of a well-differentiated liposarcoma presenting as a large pedunculated polyp arising from the cervical esophagus.

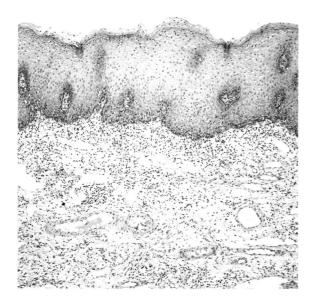

Figure 12-96

WELL-DIFFERENTIATED LIPOSARCOMA

When presenting as an esophageal polyp, well-differentiated liposarcomas often show areas of chronic inflammation and prominent blood vessels, which led to the original designation "giant fibrovascular polyp."

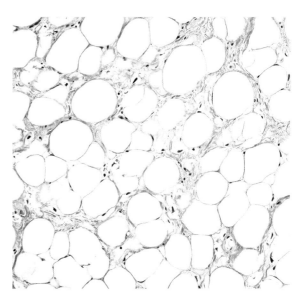

Figure 12-97

WELL-DIFFERENTIATED LIPOSARCOMA

In this esophageal polypoid example, the adipocytes are admixed with fine collagenous stroma containing occasional hyperchromatic nuclei.

component or in fibrous septa within the adipocytic component (fig. 12-97).

Scattered cells show nuclear staining for MDM2 (fig. 12-99) and CDK4, reflecting chromosome 12q13–15 amplification. *MDM2*

amplification as detected by FISH confirms the diagnosis (136,137).

Esophageal polypoid well-differentiated liposarcomas may recur locally; some cases are associated with well-differentiated or dedifferentiated

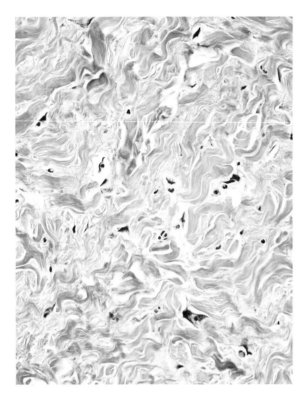

Figure 12-98

WELL-DIFFERENTIATED LIPOSARCOMA

Some cases in the esophagus show sclerosing features, similar to well-differentiated liposarcomas of the spermatic cord and retroperitoneum. The occasional hyperchromatic and multinucleated stromal cells are a helpful diagnostic clue.

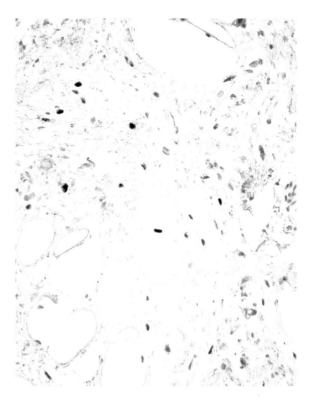

Figure 12-99

WELL-DIFFERENTIATED LIPOSARCOMA

MDM2 is positive in scattered nuclei, reflecting underlying *MDM2* gene amplification. Many laboratories use fluorescence in situ hybridization (FISH) for *MDM2* to confirm the diagnosis.

liposarcoma in the wall of the esophagus outside of the polyp or in the mediastinum (137). Dedifferentiated liposarcomas of the esophagus may result in metastases and patient death.

VASCULAR LESIONS

Various vascular tumors have been reported in the stomach and more rarely in the esophagus (138). *Hemangiomas* and *vascular malformations* may be discovered incidentally at endoscopy or present with upper GI bleeding (138). A clinically well-known form of malformation, known as *Dieulafoy lesion* (a tortuous arterial malformation in the gastric submucosa, most often found in the proximal stomach), is often associated with hemorrhage; hematemesis or melena are common presenting symptoms (139,140).

In the past, *Kaposi sarcoma* was frequently encountered in the GI tract of patients with acquired immunodeficiency syndrome (AIDS), including the stomach, often as multifocal lesions (141,142). With the development of effective therapies directed against human immunodeficiency virus (HIV), Kaposi sarcoma is now rare in the stomach. Gastric Kaposi sarcoma involves the mucosa and submucosa (fig. 12-100) and consists of fascicles of uniform and bland spindle cells with fine chromatin and eosinophilic cytoplasm, often accompanied by extravasated erythrocytes and scattered plasma cells (fig. 12-101). By immunohistochemistry, Kaposi sarcoma is positive for CD31, CD34, podoplanin (D2-40), and human herpesvirus-8 (HHV8); HHV8 is particularly useful to confirm the diagnosis (fig. 12-102).

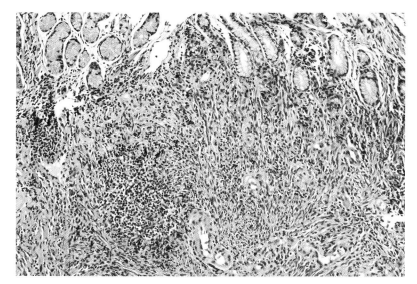

Figure 12-100

KAPOSI SARCOMA

Kaposi sarcoma in a patient with acquired immunodeficiency syndrome (AIDS). The tumor cells infiltrate between the gastric glands and are associated with chronic inflammation.

Figure 12-101

KAPOSI SARCOMA

This gastric example shows the characteristic histologic features, including fascicles of uniform spindle cells with fine chromatin, pale eosinophilic cytoplasm, and extravasated erythrocytes.

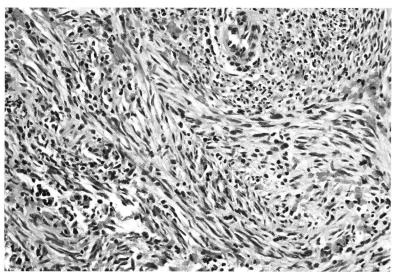

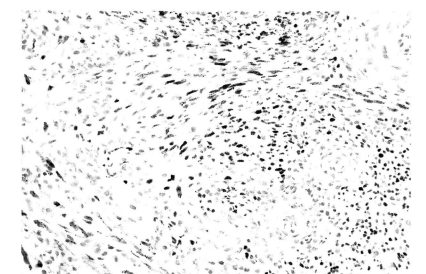

Figure 12-102

KAPOSI SARCOMA

Immunohistochemistry for human herpesvirus-8 (HHV8) shows granular nuclear staining in the tumor cells. This finding is a helpful confirmatory diagnostic feature.

REFERENCES

1. Doyle LA, Hornick JL. Gastrointestinal stromal tumours: from KIT to succinate dehydrogenase. Histopathology 2014;64:53-67.
2. Kawanowa K, Sakuma Y, Sakurai S, et al. High incidence of microscopic gastrointestinal stromal tumors in the stomach. Hum Pathol 2006;37:1527-35.
3. Agaimy A, Wunsch PH, Hofstaedter F, et al. Minute gastric sclerosing stromal tumors (GIST tumorlets) are common in adults and frequently show c-KIT mutations. Am J Surg Pathol 2007;31:113-20.
4. Abraham SC, Krasinskas AM, Hofstetter WL, Swisher SG, Wu TT. "Seedling" mesenchymal tumors (gastrointestinal stromal tumors and leiomyomas) are common incidental tumors of the esophagogastric junction. Am J Surg Pathol 2007;31:1629-35.
5. Corless CL, McGreevey L, Haley A, Town A, Heinrich MC. KIT mutations are common in incidental gastrointestinal stromal tumors one centimeter or less in size. Am J Pathol 2002;160:1567-wi72.
6. Wiersema MJ, Wiersema LM, Khusro Q, Cramer HM, Tao LC. Combined endosonography and fine-needle aspiration cytology in the evaluation of gastrointestinal lesions. Gastrointest Endosc 1994;40:199-206.
7. Turhan N, Aydog G, Ozin Y, Cicek B, Kurt M, Oguz D. Endoscopic ultrasonography-guided fine-needle aspiration for diagnosing upper gastrointestinal submucosal lesions: a prospective study of 50 cases. Diagn Cytopathol 2011;39:808-17.
8. Vander Noot MR 3rd, Eloubeidi MA, Chen VK, et al. Diagnosis of gastrointestinal tract lesions by endoscopic ultrasound-guided fine-needle aspiration biopsy. Cancer 2004;102:157-63.
9. Ballo MS, Guy CD. Percutaneous fine-needle aspiration of gastrointestinal wall lesions with image guidance. Diagn Cytopathol 2001;24:16-20.
10. Hirota S, Isozaki K, Moriyama Y, et al. Gain-of-function mutations of c-kit in human gastrointestinal stromal tumors. Science 1998;279:577-80.
11. Espinosa I, Lee CH, Kim MK, et al. A novel monoclonal antibody against DOG1 is a sensitive and specific marker for gastrointestinal stromal tumors. Am J Surg Pathol 2008;32:210-8.
12. Miettinen M, Wang ZF, Lasota J. DOG1 antibody in the differential diagnosis of gastrointestinal stromal tumors: a study of 1840 cases. Am J Surg Pathol 2009;33:1401-8.
13. Nilsson B, Bümming P, Meis-Kindblom JM, et al. Gastrointestinal stromal tumors: the incidence, prevalence, clinical course, and prognostication in the preimatinib mesylate era--a population-based study in western Sweden. Cancer 2005;103:821-9.
14. Miettinen M, Sobin LH, Lasota J. Gastrointestinal stromal tumors of the stomach: a clinicopathologic, immunohistochemical, and molecular genetic study of 1765 cases with long-term follow-up. Am J Surg Pathol 2005;29:52-68.
15. Miettinen M, Lasota J, Sobin LH. Gastrointestinal stromal tumors of the stomach in children and young adults: a clinicopathologic, immunohistochemical, and molecular genetic study of 44 cases with long-term follow-up and review of the literature. Am J Surg Pathol 2005;29:1373-81.
16. Miettinen M, Sarlomo-Rikala M, Sobin LH, Lasota J. Esophageal stromal tumors: a clinicopathologic, immunohistochemical, and molecular genetic study of 17 cases and comparison with esophageal leiomyomas and leiomyosarcomas. Am J Surg Pathol 2000;24:211-22.
17. Kang G, Kang Y, Kim KH, et al. Gastrointestinal stromal tumours of the oesophagus: a clinico-pathological and molecular analysis of 27 cases. Histopathology 2017;71:805-12.
18. Zhang L, Smyrk TC, Young WF Jr, Stratakis CA, Carney JA. Gastric stromal tumors in Carney triad are different clinically, pathologically, and behaviorly from sporadic gastric gastrointestinal stromal tumors: findings in 104 cases. Am J Surg Pathol 2010;34:53-64.
19. Carney JA, Stratakis CA. Familial paraganglioma and gastric stromal sarcoma: a new syndrome distinct from the Carney triad. Am J Med Genet 2002;108:132-9.
20. Pasini B, McWhinney SR, Bei T, et al. Clinical and molecular genetics of patients with the Carney-Stratakis syndrome and germline mutations of the genes coding for the succinate dehydrogenase subunits SDHB, SDHC, and SDHD. Eur J Hum Genet 2008;16:79-88.
21. Haller F, Moskalev EA, Faucz FR, et al. Aberrant DNA hypermethylation of SDHC: a novel mechanism of tumor development in Carney triad. Endocr Relat Cancer 2014;21:567-77.
22. Miettinen M, Wang ZF, Sarlomo-Rikala M, Osuch C, Rutkowski P, Lasota J. Succinate dehydrogenase-deficient GISTs: a clinicopathologic, immunohistochemical, and molecular genetic study of 66 gastric GISTs with predilection to young age. Am J Surg Pathol 2011;35:1712-21.

23. Janeway KA, Kim SY, Lodish M, et al. Defects in succinate dehydrogenase in gastrointestinal stromal tumors lacking KIT and PDGFRA mutations. Proc Natl Acad Sci U S A 2011;108:314-8.
24. Boikos SA, Pappo AS, Killian JK, et al. Molecular subtypes of KIT/PDGFRA wild-type gastrointestinal stromal tumors: A report from the National Institutes of Health gastrointestinal stromal tumor clinic. JAMA Oncol 2016;2:922-8.
25. Doyle LA, Nelson D, Heinrich MC, Corless CL, Hornick JL. Loss of succinate dehydrogenase subunit B (SDHB) expression is limited to a distinctive subset of gastric wild-type gastrointestinal stromal tumours: a comprehensive genotype-phenotype correlation study. Histopathology 2012;61:801-9.
26. Schaefer IM, Ströbel P, Cameron S, et al. Rhabdoid morphology in gastrointestinal stromal tumours (GISTs) is associated with PDGFRA mutations but does not imply aggressive behaviour. Histopathology 2014;64:421-30.
27. Sakurai S, Hasegawa T, Sakuma Y, et al. Myxoid epithelioid gastrointestinal stromal tumor (GIST) with mast cell infiltrations: a subtype of GIST with mutations of platelet-derived growth factor receptor alpha gene. Hum Pathol 2004;35:1223-30.
28. Antonescu CR, Romeo S, Zhang L, et al. Dedifferentiation in gastrointestinal stromal tumor to an anaplastic KIT negative phenotype: a diagnostic pitfall: morphologic and molecular characterization of 8 cases occurring either de novo or after imatinib therapy Am J Surg Pathol 2013;37:385-92.
29. Pauwels P, Debiec-Rychter M, Stul M, De Wever I, Van Oosterom AT, Sciot R. Changing phenotype of gastrointestinal stromal tumours under imatinib mesylate treatment: a potential diagnostic pitfall. Histopathology 2005;47:41-7.
30. Dodd LG, Nelson RC, Mooney EE, Gottfried M. Fine-needle aspiration of gastrointestinal stromal tumors. Am J Clin Pathol 1998;109:439-43.
31. Rader AE, Avery A, Wait CL, McGreevey LS, Faigel D, Heinrich MC. Fine-needle aspiration biopsy diagnosis of gastrointestinal stromal tumors using morphology, immunocytochemistry, and mutational analysis of c-kit. Cancer 2001;93:269-75.
32. Li SQ, O'Leary TJ, Buchner SB, et al. Fine needle aspiration of gastrointestinal stromal tumors. Acta Cytol 2001;45:9-17.
33. Wieczorek TJ, Faquin WC, Rubin BP, Cibas ES. Cytologic diagnosis of gastrointestinal stromal tumor with emphasis on the differential diagnosis with leiomyosarcoma. Cancer 2001;93:276-87.
34. Gu M, Ghafari S, Nguyen PT, Lin F. Cytologic diagnosis of gastrointestinal stromal tumors of the stomach by endoscopic ultrasound-guided fine-needle aspiration biopsy: cytomorphologic and immunohistochemical study of 12 cases. Diagn Cytopathol 2001;25:343-50.
35. Boggino HE, Fernandez MP, Logrono R. Cytomorphology of gastrointestinal stromal tumor: diagnostic role of aspiration cytology, core biopsy, and immunochemistry. Diagn Cytopathol 2000;23:156-60.
36. Elliott DD, Fanning CV, Caraway NP. The utility of fine-needle aspiration in the diagnosis of gastrointestinal stromal tumors: a cytomorphologic and immunohistochemical analysis with emphasis on malignant tumors. Cancer 2005;108:49-55.
37. Dong Q, McKee G, Pitman M, Geisinger K, Tambouret R. Epithelioid variant of gastrointestinal stromal tumor: diagnosis by fine-needle aspiration. Diagn Cytopathol 2003;29:55-60.
38. Laforga JB. Malignant epithelioid gastrointestinal stromal tumors: report of a case with cytologic and immunohistochemical studies. Acta Cytol 2005;49:435-40.
39. Medeiros F, Corless CL, Duensing A, et al. KIT-negative gastrointestinal stromal tumors: proof of concept and therapeutic implications. Am J Surg Pathol 2004;28:889894.
40. Debiec-Rychter M, Wasag B, Stul M, et al. Gastrointestinal stromal tumours (GISTs) negative for KIT (CD117 antigen) immunoreactivity. J Pathol 2004;202:430-8.
41. Agaimy A, Otto C, Braun A, Geddert H, Schaefer IM, Haller F. Value of epithelioid morphology and PDGFRA immunostaining pattern for prediction of PDGFRA mutated genotype in gastrointestinal stromal tumors (GISTs). Int J Clin Exp Pathol 2013;6:1839-46.
42. Miettinen MM, Sarlomo-Rikala M, Kovatich AJ, Lasota J. Calponin and h-caldesmon in soft tissue tumors: consistent h-caldesmon immunoreactivity in gastrointestinal stromal tumors indicates traits of smooth muscle differentiation. Mod Pathol 1999;12:756-62.
43. Gill AJ, Chou A, Vilain R, et al. Immunohistochemistry for SDHB divides gastrointestinal stromal tumors (GISTs) into 2 distinct types. Am J Surg Pathol 2010;34:636-44.
44. Gaal J, Stratakis CA, Carney JA, et al. SDHB immunohistochemistry: a useful tool in the diagnosis of Carney-Stratakis and Carney triad gastrointestinal stromal tumors. Mod Pathol 2011;24:147-51.
45. Wagner AJ, Remillard SP, Zhang YX, Doyle LA, George S, Hornick JL. Loss of expression of SDHA predicts SDHA mutations in gastrointestinal stromal tumors. Mod Pathol 2013;26:289-94.
46. Miettinen M, Killian JK, Wang ZF, et al. Immunohistochemical loss of succinate dehydrogenase subunit A (SDHA) in gastrointestinal stromal tumors (GISTs) signals SDHA germline mutation. Am J Surg Pathol 2013;37:234-40.

47. Li SQ, O'Leary TJ, Sobin LH, Erozan YS, Rosenthal DL, Przygodzki RM. Analysis of KIT mutation and protein expression in fine needle aspirates of gastrointestinal stromal/smooth muscle tumors. Acta Cytol 2000;44:981-6.

48. Lozano MD, Rodriguez J, Algarra SM, Panizo A, Sola JJ, Pardo J. Fine-needle aspiration cytology and immunocytochemistry in the diagnosis of 24 gastrointestinal stromal tumors: A quick, reliable diagnostic method. Diagn Cytopathol 2003;28:131-35.

49. Fatima N, Cohen C, Siddiqui MT. DOG1 utility in diagnosing gastrointestinal stromal tumors on fine-needle aspiration. Cancer Cytopathol 2011;119:202-8.

50. Hwang DG, Qian X, Hornick JL. DOG1 antibody is a highly sensitive and specific marker for gastrointestinal stromal tumors in cytology cell blocks. Am J Clin Pathol 2011;135:448-53.

51. Patil DT, Rubin BP. Genetics of gastrointestinal stromal tumors: a heterogeneous family of tumors? Surg Pathol Clin 2015;8:515-24.

52. Heinrich MC, Corless CL, Duensing A, et al. PDGFRA activating mutations in gastrointestinal stromal tumors. Science 2003;299:708-10.

53. Agaram NP, Wong GC, Guo T, et al. Novel V600E BRAF mutations in imatinib-naive and imatinib-resistant gastrointestinal stromal tumors. Genes Chromosomes Cancer 2008;47:853-9.

54. Miettinen M, Fetsch JF, Sobin LH, Lasota J. Gastrointestinal stromal tumors in patients with neurofibromatosis 1: a clinicopathologic and molecular genetic study of 45 cases. Am J Surg Pathol 2006;30:90-6.

55. Brenca M, Rossi S, Polano M, et al. Transcriptome sequencing identifies ETV6-NTRK3 as a gene fusion involved in GIST. J Pathol 2016;238:543-9.

56. Shi E, Chmielecki J, Tang CM, et al. FGFR1 and NTRK3 actionable alterations in "Wild-Type" gastrointestinal stromal tumors. J Transl Med 2016;14:339.

57. Killian JK, Miettinen M, Walker RL, et al. Recurrent epimutation of SDHC in gastrointestinal stromal tumors. Sci Transl Med 2014;6:268ra177.

58. Deshpande A, Nelson D, Corless CL, Deshpande V, O'Brien MJ. Leiomyoma of the gastrointestinal tract with interstitial cells of Cajal: a mimic of gastrointestinal stromal tumor. Am J Surg Pathol 2014;38:72-7.

59. Demetri GD, von Mehren M, Blanke CD, et al. Efficacy and safety of imatinib mesylate in advanced gastrointestinal stromal tumors. N Engl J Med 2002;347:472-80.

60. Demetri GD, van Oosterom AT, Garrett CR, et al. Efficacy and safety of sunitinib in patients with advanced gastrointestinal stromal tumour after failure of imatinib: a randomised controlled trial. Lancet 2006;368:1329-38.

61. Demetri GD, Reichardt P, Kang YK, et al. Efficacy and safety of regorafenib for advanced gastrointestinal stromal tumours after failure of imatinib and sunitinib (GRID): an international, multicentre, randomised, placebo-controlled, phase 3 trial. Lancet 2013;381:295-302.

62. Heinrich MC, Corless CL, Demetri GD, et al. Kinase mutations and imatinib response in patients with metastatic gastrointestinal stromal tumor. J Clin Oncol 2003;21:4342-9.

63. Heinrich MC, Owzar K, Corless CL, et al. Correlation of kinase genotype and clinical outcome in the North American Intergroup Phase III Trial of imatinib mesylate for treatment of advanced gastrointestinal stromal tumor: CALGB 150105 Study by Cancer and Leukemia Group B and Southwest Oncology Group. J Clin Oncol 2008;26:5360-7.

64. Ben-Ami E, Barysauskas CM, von Mehren M, et al. Long-term follow-up results of the multicenter phase II trial of regorafenib in patients with metastatic and/or unresectable GI stromal tumor after failure of standard tyrosine kinase inhibitor therapy. Ann Oncol 2016;27:1794-9.

65. Liegl B, Kepten I, Le C, et al. Heterogeneity of kinase inhibitor resistance mechanisms in GIST. J Pathol 2008;216:64-74.

66. Falchook GS, Trent JC, Heinrich MC, et al. BRAF mutant gastrointestinal stromal tumor: first report of regression with BRAF inhibitor dabrafenib (GSK2118436) and whole exomic sequencing for analysis of acquired resistance. Oncotarget 2013;4:310-5.

67. Liegl B, Hornick JL, Antonescu CR, Corless CL, Fletcher CD. Rhabdomyosarcomatous differentiation in gastrointestinal stromal tumors after tyrosine kinase inhibitor therapy: a novel form of tumor progression. Am J Surg Pathol 2009;33:218-26.

68. Miettinen M, Lasota J. Gastrointestinal stromal tumors: pathology and prognosis at different sites. Semin Diagn Pathol 2006;23:70-83.

69. von Mehren M, Randall RL, Benjamin RS, et al. Gastrointestinal stromal tumors, version 2.2014. J Natl Compr Canc Netw 2014;12:853-62.

70. Mason EF, Hornick JL. Conventional risk stratification fails to predict progression of succinate dehydrogenase-deficient gastrointestinal stromal tumors: a clinicopathologic study of 76 cases. Am J Surg Pathol 2016;40:1616-21.

71. Agaimy A, Wunsch PH. True smooth muscle neoplasms of the gastrointestinal tract: morphological spectrum and classification in a series of 85 cases from a single institute. Langenbecks Arch Surg 2007;392:75-81.

72. Stelow EB, Stanley MW, Mallery S, Lai R, Linzie BM, Bardales RH. Endoscopic ultrasound-guided fine-needle aspiration findings of gastrointestinal leiomyomas and gastrointestinal stromal tumors. Am J Clin Pathol 2003;119:703-8.

73. Antignac C, Zhou J, Sanak M, et al. Alport syndrome and diffuse leiomyomatosis: deletions in the 5' end of the COL4A5 collagen gene. Kidney Int 1992;42:1178-83.

74. Zhou J, Mochizuki T, Smeets H, et al. Deletion of the paired alpha 5(IV) and alpha 6(IV) collagen genes in inherited smooth muscle tumors. Science 1993;261:1167-9.

75. Heidet L, Boye E, Cai Y, et al. Somatic deletion of the 5' ends of both the COL4A5 and COL4A6 genes in a sporadic leiomyoma of the esophagus. Am J Pathol 1998;152:673-8.

76. Panagopoulos I, Gorunova L, Lund-Iversen M, Lobmaier I, Bjerkehagen B, Heim S. Recurrent fusion of the genes FN1 and ALK in gastrointestinal leiomyomas. Mod Pathol 2016;29:1415-23.

77. Aggarwal G, Sharma S, Zheng M, et al. Primary leiomyosarcomas of the gastrointestinal tract in the post-gastrointestinal stromal tumor era. Ann Diagn Pathol 2012;16:532-40.

78. Yamamoto H, Handa M, Tobo T, et al. Clinicopathological features of primary leiomyosarcoma of the gastrointestinal tract following recognition of gastrointestinal stromal tumours. Histopathology 2013;63:194-207.

79. Domanski HA, Akerman M, Rissler P, Gustafson P. Fine-needle aspiration of soft tissue leiomyosarcoma: an analysis of the most common cytologic findings and the value of ancillary techniques. Diagn Cytopathol 2006;34:597-604.

80. Daimaru Y, Kido H, Hashimoto H, Enjoji M. Benign schwannoma of the gastrointestinal tract: a clinicopathologic and immunohistochemical study. Hum Pathol 1988;19:257-64.

81. Prevot S, Bienvenu L, Vaillant JC, de Saint-Maur PP. Benign schwannoma of the digestive tract: a clinicopathologic and immunohistochemical study of five cases, including a case of esophageal tumor. Am J Surg Pathol 1999;23:431-6.

82. Hou YY, Tan YS, Xu JF, et al. Schwannoma of the gastrointestinal tract: a clinicopathological, immunohistochemical and ultrastructural study of 33 cases. Histopathology 2006;48:536-45.

83. Lasota J, Wasag B, Dansonka-Mieszkowska A, et al. Evaluation of NF2 and NF1 tumor suppressor genes in distinctive gastrointestinal nerve sheath tumors traditionally diagnosed as benign schwannomas: s study of 20 cases. Lab Invest 2003;83:1361-71.

84. Liegl B, Bennett MW, Fletcher CD. Microcystic/reticular schwannoma: a distinct variant with predilection for visceral locations. Am J Surg Pathol 2008;32:1080-7.

85. Tozbikian G, Shen R, Suster S. Signet ring cell gastric schwannoma: report of a new distinctive morphological variant. Ann Diagn Pathol 2008;12:146-52.

86. Johnston J, Helwig EB. Granular cell tumors of the gastrointestinal tract and perianal region: a study of 74 cases. Dig Dis Sci 1981;26:807-16.

87. Goldblum JR, Rice TW, Zuccaro G, Richter JE. Granular cell tumors of the esophagus: a clinical and pathologic study of 13 cases. Ann Thorac Surg 1996;62:860-5.

88. Voskuil JH, van Dijk MM, Wagenaar SS, van Vliet AC, Timmer R, van Hees PA. Occurrence of esophageal granular cell tumors in The Netherlands between 1988 and 1994. Dig Dis Sci 2001;46:1610-4.

89. Parfitt JR, McLean CA, Joseph MG, Streutker CJ, Al-Haddad S, Driman DK. Granular cell tumours of the gastrointestinal tract: expression of nestin and clinicopathological evaluation of 11 patients. Histopathology 2006;48:424-30.

90. An S, Jang J, Min K, et al. Granular cell tumor of the gastrointestinal tract: histologic and immunohistochemical analysis of 98 cases. Hum Pathol 2015;46:813-9.

91. Johnstone JM, Morson BC. Inflammatory fibroid polyp of the gastrointestinal tract. Histopathology 1978;2:349-61.

92. Kolodziejczyk P, Yao T, Tsuneyoshi M. Inflammatory fibroid polyp of the stomach. A special reference to an immunohistochemical profile of 42 cases. Am J Surg Pathol 1993;17:1159-68.

93. Hasegawa T, Yang P, Kagawa N, Hirose T, Sano T. CD34 expression by inflammatory fibroid polyps of the stomach. Mod Pathol 1997;10:451-6.

94. Schildhaus HU, Cavlar T, Binot E, Büttner R, Wardelmann E, Merkelbach-Bruse S. Inflammatory fibroid polyps harbour mutations in the platelet-derived growth factor receptor alpha (PDGFRA) gene. J Pathol 2008;216:176-82.

95. Huss S, Wardelmann E, Goltz D, et al. Activating PDGFRA mutations in inflammatory fibroid polyps occur in exons 12, 14 and 18 and are associated with tumour localization. Histopathology 2012;61:59-68.

96. Anthony PP, Morris DS, Vowles KD. Multiple and recurrent inflammatory fibroid polyps in three generations of a Devon family: a new syndrome. Gut 1984;25:854-62.

97. Ricci R, Martini M, Cenci T, et al. PDGFRA-mutant syndrome. Mod Pathol 2015;28:954-64.

98. Miettinen M, Makhlouf HR, Sobin LH, Lasota J. Plexiform fibromyxoma: a distinctive benign gastric antral neoplasm not to be confused with a myxoid GIST. Am J Surg Pathol 2009;33:1624-32.

99. Takahashi Y, Shimizu S, Ishida T, et al. Plexiform angiomyxoid myofibroblastic tumor of the stomach. Am J Surg Pathol 2007;31:724-8.

100. Yoshida A, Klimstra DS, Antonescu CR. Plexiform angiomyxoid tumor of the stomach. Am J Surg Pathol 2008;32:1910-2.

101. Spans L, Fletcher CD, Antonescu CR, et al. Recurrent MALAT1-GLI1 oncogenic fusion and GLI1 up-regulation define a subset of plexiform fibromyxoma. J Pathol 2016;239:335-43.

102. Appelman HD, Helwig EB. Glomus tumors of the stomach. Cancer 1969;23:203-213.

103. Miettinen M, Paal E, Lasota J, Sobin LH. Gastrointestinal glomus tumors: a clinicopathologic, immunohistochemical, and molecular genetic study of 32 cases. Am J Surg Pathol 2002;26:301-11.

104. Kang G, Park HJ, Kim JY, et al. Glomus tumor of the stomach: a clinicopathologic analysis of 10 cases and review of the literature. Gut Liver 2012;6:52-7.

105. Mosquera JM, Sboner A, Zhang L, et al. Novel MIR143-NOTCH fusions in benign and malignant glomus tumors. Genes Chromosomes Cancer 2013;52:1075-87.

106. Billings SD, Meisner LF, Cummings OW, Tejada E. Synovial sarcoma of the upper digestive tract: a report of two cases with demonstration of the X;18 translocation by fluorescence in situ hybridization. Mod Pathol 2000;13:68-76.

107. Makhlouf HR, Ahrens W, Agarwal B, et al. Synovial sarcoma of the stomach: a clinicopathologic, immunohistochemical, and molecular genetic study of 10 cases. Am J Surg Pathol 2008;32:275-81.

108. Romeo S, Rossi S, Acosta Marín M, et al. Primary Synovial Sarcoma (SS) of the digestive system: a molecular and clinicopathological study of fifteen cases. Clin Sarcoma Res 2015;5:7.

109. Coffin CM, Watterson J, Priest JR, Dehner LP. Extrapulmonary inflammatory myofibroblastic tumor (inflammatory pseudotumor). A clinicopathologic and immunohistochemical study of 84 cases. Am J Surg Pathol 1995;19:859-72.

110. Makhlouf HR, Sobin LH. Inflammatory myofibroblastic tumors (inflammatory pseudotumors) of the gastrointestinal tract: how closely are they related to inflammatory fibroid polyps? Hum Pathol 2002;33:307-15.

111. Gleason BC, Hornick JL. Inflammatory myofibroblastic tumours: where are we now? J Clin Pathol 2008;61:428-37.

112. Lovly CM, Gupta A, Lipson D, et al. Inflammatory myofibroblastic tumors harbor multiple potentially actionable kinase fusions. Cancer Discov 2014;4:889-95.

113. Antonescu CR, Suurmeijer AJ, Zhang L, et al. Molecular characterization of inflammatory myofibroblastic tumors with frequent ALK and ROS1 gene fusions and rare novel RET rearrangement. Am J Surg Pathol 2015;39:957-67.

114. Alassiri AH, Ali RH, Shen Y, et al. ETV6-NTRK3 is expressed in a subset of ALK-negative inflammatory myofibroblastic tumors. Am J Surg Pathol 2016;40:1051-61.

115. Yamamoto H, Yoshida A, Taguchi K, et al. ALK, ROS1 and NTRK3 gene rearrangements in inflammatory myofibroblastic tumours. Histopathology 2016;69:72-83.

116. Butrynski JE, D'Adamo DR, Hornick JL, et al. Crizotinib in ALK-rearranged inflammatory myofibroblastic tumor. N Engl J Med 2010;363:1727-33.

117. Hornick JL, Fletcher CD. PEComa: what do we know so far? Histopathology 2006;48:75-82.

118. Folpe AL, Kwiatkowski DJ. Perivascular epithelioid cell neoplasms: pathology and pathogenesis. Hum Pathol 2010;41:1-15.

119. Folpe AL, Mentzel T, Lehr HA, Fisher C, Balzer BL, Weiss SW. Perivascular epithelioid cell neoplasms of soft tissue and gynecologic origin: a clinicopathologic study of 26 cases and review of the literature. Am J Surg Pathol 2005;29:1558-75.

120. Doyle LA, Hornick JL, Fletcher CD. PEComa of the gastrointestinal tract: clinicopathologic study of 35 cases with evaluation of prognostic parameters. Am J Surg Pathol 2013;37:1769-82.

121. Kenerson H, Folpe AL, Takayama TK, Yeung RS. Activation of the mTOR pathway in sporadic angiomyolipomas and other perivascular epithelioid cell neoplasms. Hum Pathol 2007;38:1361-71.

122. Pan CC, Chung MY, Ng KF, et al. Constant allelic alteration on chromosome 16p (TSC2 gene) in perivascular epithelioid cell tumour (PEComa): genetic evidence for the relationship of PEComa with angiomyolipoma. J Pathol 2008;214:387-93.

123. Agaram NP, Sung YS, Zhang L, et al. Dichotomy of genetic abnormalities in PEComas with therapeutic implications. Am J Surg Pathol 2015;39:813-25.

124. Wagner AJ, Malinowska-Kolodziej I, Morgan JA, et al. Clinical activity of mTOR inhibition with sirolimus in malignant perivascular epithelioid cell tumors: targeting the pathogenic activation of mTORC1 in tumors. J Clin Oncol 2010;28:835-40.

125. Dickson MA, Schwartz GK, Antonescu CR, Kwiatkowski DJ, Malinowska IA. Extrarenal perivascular epithelioid cell tumors (PEComas) respond to mTOR inhibition: clinical and molecular correlates. Int J Cancer 2013;132:1711-7.

126. Antonescu CR, Nafa K, Segal NH, Dal Cin P, Ladanyi M. EWS-CREB1: a recurrent variant fusion in clear cell sarcoma—association with gastrointestinal location and absence of melanocytic differentiation. Clin Cancer Res 2006;12:5356-62.

127. Kosemehmetoglu K, Folpe AL. Clear cell sarcoma of tendons and aponeuroses, and osteoclast-rich tumour of the gastrointestinal tract with features resembling clear cell sarcoma of soft parts: a review and update. J Clin Pathol 2010;63:416-23.

128. Stockman DL, Miettinen M, Suster S, et al. Malignant gastrointestinal neuroectodermal tumor (GNET): clinicopathologic, immunohistochemical, ultrastructural and molecular analysis of 16 cases with a reappraisal of clear cell sarcoma-like tumors of the gastrointestinal tract. Am J Surg Pathol 2012;36:857-68.

129. Lyle PL, Amato CM, Fitzpatrick JE, Robinson WA. Gastrointestinal melanoma or clear cell sarcoma? Molecular evaluation of 7 cases previously diagnosed as malignant melanoma. Am J Surg Pathol 2008;32:858-66.

130. Miettinen M, Dow N, Lasota J, Sobin LH. A distinctive novel epitheliomesenchymal biphasic tumor of the stomach in young adults ("gastroblastoma"): a series of 3 cases. Am J Surg Pathol 2009;33:1370-7.

131. Shin DH, Lee JH, Kang HJ, et al. Novel epitheliomesenchymal biphasic stomach tumour (gastroblastoma) in a 9-year-old: morphological, ultrastructural and immunohistochemical findings. J Clin Pathol 2010;63:270-4.

132. Wey EA, Britton AJ, Sferra JJ, Kasunic T, Pepe LR, Appelman HD. Gastroblastoma in a 28-year-old man with nodal metastasis: proof of the malignant potential. Arch Pathol Lab Med 2012;136:961-4.

133. Graham RP, Nair AA, Davila JI, et al. Gastroblastoma harbors a recurrent somatic MALAT1-GLI1 fusion gene. Mod Pathol 2017;30:1443-52.

134. Ginai AZ, Halfhide BC, Dees J, Zondervan PE, Klooswijk AI, Knegt PP. Giant esophageal polyp: a clinical and radiological entity with variable histology. Eur Radiol 1998;8:264-9.

135. Jakowski JD, Wakely PE Jr. Rhabdomyomatous well-differentiated liposarcoma arising in giant fibrovascular polyp of the esophagus. Ann Diagn Pathol 2009;13:263-8.

136. Boni A, Lisovsky M, Dal Cin P, Rosenberg AE, Srivastava A. Atypical lipomatous tumor mimicking giant fibrovascular polyp of the esophagus: report of a case and a critical review of literature. Hum Pathol 2013;44:1165-70.

137. Graham RP, Yasir S, Fritchie KJ, Reid MD, Greipp PT, Folpe AL. Polypoid fibroadipose tumors of the esophagus: 'giant fibrovascular polyp' or liposarcoma? A clinicopathological and molecular cytogenetic study of 13 cases. Mod Pathol 2018;31:337-42.

138. Handra-Luca A, Montgomery E. Vascular malformations and hemangiolymphangiomas of the gastrointestinal tract: morphological features and clinical impact. Int J Clin Exp Pathol 2011;4:430-43.

139. Nojkov B, Cappell MS. Gastrointestinal bleeding from Dieulafoy's lesion: clinical presentation, endoscopic findings, and endoscopic therapy. World J Gastrointest Endosc 2015;7:295-307.

140. Chen X, Cao H, Wang S, et al. Endoscopic submucosal dissection for silent gastric Dieulafoy lesions mimicking gastrointestinal stromal tumors: report of 7 cases-a case report series. Medicine (Baltimore) 2016;95:e4829.

141. Saltz RK, Kurtz RC, Lightdale CJ, et al. Kaposi's sarcoma. Gastrointestinal involvement correlation with skin findings and immunologic function. Dig Dis Sci 1984;29:817-23.

142. Friedman SL, Wright TL, Altman DF. Gastrointestinal Kaposi's sarcoma in patients with acquired immunodeficiency syndrome. Endoscopic and autopsy findings. Gastroenterology 1985;89:102-8.

Index*

*In a series of numbers, those in boldface indicate the main discussion of the entity.